OXFORD MEDICAL PUBLICATIONS

Oxford Handbook of
Oncology

Published and forthcoming Oxford Handbooks

Oxford Handbook of
Oncology

THIRD EDITION

Edited by

Jim Cassidy

Professor of Oncology, Cancer Research UK
University of Glasgow, Glasgow

Donald Bissett

Consultant in Clinical Oncology,
Aberdeen Royal Infirmary, Aberdeen

Roy A.J. Spence OBE

Consultant Surgeon, Belfast Trust,
Honorary Professor, Queens University, Belfast,
Honorary Professor, University of Ulster

Miranda Payne

Specialist Registrar in Medical Oncology,
Oxford Radcliffe NHS Trust, Oxford

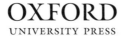

OXFORD
UNIVERSITY PRESS

OXFORD
UNIVERSITY PRESS

Great Clarendon Street, Oxford OX2 6DP

Oxford University Press is a department of the University of Oxford.
It furthers the University's objective of excellence in research, scholarship,
and education by publishing worldwide in

Oxford New York

Auckland Cape Town Dar es Salaam Hong Kong Karachi
Kuala Lumpur Madrid Melbourne Mexico City Nairobi
New Delhi Shanghai Taipei Toronto

With offices in

Argentina Austria Brazil Chile Czech Republic France Greece
Guatemala Hungary Italy Japan Poland Portugal Singapore
South Korea Switzerland Thailand Turkey Ukraine Vietnam

Oxford is a registered trade mark of Oxford University Press
in the UK and in certain other countries

Published in the United States
by Oxford University Press Inc., New York

British Library Cataloguing in Publication Data
Data available

Library of Congress Cataloging in Publication Data
Data available

Typeset by Glyph International, Bangalore, India
Printed in China
on acid-free paper through
Asia Pacific Offset

ISBN 978–0–19–956313–5

10 9 8 7 6 5 4 3 2 1

Preface

Welcome to the third edition of the handbook. Happily the last few years have seen significant progress in the treatment of a range of malignancies. The expansion in understanding of the molecular changes giving rise to cancer is now leading to the rational development of therapies specifically targeted against these changes. In addition technology facilitates a variety of new local treatments, both surgical and radiotherapeutic. The handbook has been extensively revised and updated by the co-editors to provide the reader with insights into these novel, often expensive therapies, the particular challenges of incorporating these alongside existing treatments, and of limiting their use to individuals most likely to benefit. Once again we have had valuable feedback from readers of the previous edition, and have endeavoured to address their varied suggestions for improvements. We have specifically enlisted the assistance of several new contributors to help produce a comprehensive and current introduction to oncology.

We hope that the breadth and style of the handbook will make it equally accessible for trainees embarking on their medical career and for more experienced non-oncological practitioners, few of whom do not come in contact with patients with cancer. As redesign of NHS services continues, increasing numbers of nurses, radiographers, pharmacists, and AHPs should find this a valuable source of information as their role in the care of cancer patients develops.

As always, apologies to our families for many hours spent with our laptops rather than them, hopefully time well spent.

Jim Cassidy
Donald Bissett
Roy A.J. Spence
Miranda Payne

Acknowledgements

This book would not have come into being without the support of our editorial team at Oxford University Press. In particular we would like to thank our assistant commissioning editor Anna Winstanley, who has very successfully achieved the challenging task of keeping the co-editors and other contributors to their promised schedule, providing encouragement and expert advice through the development of this edition of the *Oxford Handbook of Oncology*.

Roy A.J. Spence would especially like to acknowledge the enormous help from his academic secretary, Meg Alton, who helped with the references and who typed the surgical changes in this book. Meg sadly died of cancer as the book was completed.

We are indebted to the following contributors for their expert input to specific chapters:

Dr Dominic Culligan
Consultant in Haematooncology,
Aberdeen Royal Infirmary

Dr Rosemary Davidson
Consultant Clinical Geneticist,
Ferguson Smith Centre for Clinical
Genetics, Yorkhill, Glasgow

Professor Jeff Evans
Professor of Translational Cancer
Research, University of Glasgow

Dr Ann-Marie Kennedy
Specialist Registrar in
Clinical Oncology,
Aberdeen Royal Infirmary

Dr Tim Morgan
Consultant in Palliative Care,
Roxburghe House,
Aberdeen

Dr Nadeem Siddiqui
Consultant Gynaecological
Oncologist
Glasgow Royal Infirmary

We would also like to give special thanks to all those who have contributed either directly or indirectly to previous editions of the OH Oncology.

Contents

Detailed contents

Symbols and abbreviations

🔲	cross reference
↓	decreased
↑	increased
1°	primary
2°	secondary
AASLD	American Association for the Study of Liver Diseases
ABGs	arterial blood gases
ABVD	Adriamycin®–bleomycin–vinblastine–dacarbazine
AC	Adriamycin®–cyclophosphamide
ACh	acetylcholine
ACE	angiotensin-converting enzyme
ACTG	AIDS Clinical Trials Group
ACTH	adrenocorticotrophic hormone
ADA	adenosine deaminase
ADH	antidiuretic hormone
ADME	absorption, distribution, metabolism, excretion
AFP	alpha fetoprotein
AGC	absolute granulocyte count
AIDS	acquired immune deficiency syndrome
AIN	anal intra-epithelial neoplasia
AJCC	American Joint Committee on Cancer
ALG	anti-lymphocyte globulin
ALL	acute lymphoblastic leukaemia
ALMANAC	Axillary Lymphatic Mapping Against Nodal Axillary Clearance
ALT	alanine aminotransferase
AML	acute myeloid leukaemia
ANC	absolute neutrophil count
AP	area postrema
APC	adenomatous polyposis coli
APL	acute promyelocytic leukaemia
APUD	amine precursor uptake and decarboxylation (cell properties)
ara-C	cytosine arabinoside
ARDS	adult respiratory distress syndrome
ARF	acute renal failure
ASCO	American Society of Clinical Oncology
ASCT	autologous stem cell transplantation
ASPS	alveolar soft part sarcoma
AST	aspartate aminotransferase
ATLL	adult T-cell leukaemia/lymphoma
ATO	arsenic trioxide

ATRA	all-*trans* retinoic acid	CALGB	Cancer and Leukaemia Group B
AUC	area under the curve	CAP	cisplatin–doxorubicin–cyclophosphamide *or* cyclophosphamide–Adriamycin®–prednisolone
AV	arteriovenous		
AXR	abdominal X-ray		
B-ALL	Burkitt's leukaemia		
BCC	basal cell carcinoma		
BCG	bacillus Calmette–Guérin	CAR	cancer-associated retinopathy
B-CLL	B-cell chronic lymphocytic leukaemia	CAV	cyclophosphamide–doxorubicin–vincristine
BCNU	1,3-bis (2-chloroethyl)-1-nitrosourea	CCCR	Centre for Cancer Care and Research
BCPT	Breast Cancer Prevention Trial	CCNU	1-(2-chloroethyl)-3-cyclohexyl-1-nitrosourea
BCSH	British Committee for Standards in Haematology	CEA	carcinoembryonic antigen
bd	twice daily	CHART	continuous hyperfractionated accelerated radiotherapy
BEACOPP	bleomycin–etoposide–doxorubicin (Adriamycin®)–cyclophosphamide–vincristine (Oncovin®)–procarbazine–prednisolone		
		CHF	congestive heart failure
		$CH_2\text{-}FH_4$	5-10-methylene tetrahydrofolate
		ChlVPP	chlorambucil–vinblastine–procarbazine–prednisolone
BEP	bleomycin–etoposide–cisplatin		
bFGF	basic fibroblast growth factor	CHM	complete hydatidiform mole
BL	Burkitt's lymphoma	CHOP	cyclophosphamide–hydroxodoxorubicin–vincristine (Oncovin®)–prednisolone
BLL	Burkitt-like lymphoma		
BMP	bortezomib–melphalan–prednisolone		
		CIN	cervical intra-epithelial neoplasia
BMT	bone marrow transplantation	CIS	carcinoma *in situ*
BP	blood pressure	CK	creatine kinase
BSO	bilateral salpingo-oophorectomy	CLA	common leucocyte antigen

CLL	chronic lymphocytic leukaemia
CMF	cyclophosphamide–methotrexate–5-fluorouracil
CML	chroni myeloid leukaemia
CMML	chronic myelomonocytic leukaemia
CMV	cisplatin–methotrexate–vinblastine *or* cytogmegalovirus
CNS	central nervous systems *or* clinical nurse specialist
CO	cyclophosphamide–vincristine (Oncovin®)
CODOX-M	cyclophosphamide–vincristine (Oncovin®)–doxorubicin–methotrexate
COPD	chronic obstructive pulmonary disease
COX	cyclo-oxygenase
CPAP	continuous positive airways pressure
CPK	creatine phosphokinase
CPT	camptothecin
CR	complete response rate *or* complete remission
CRC	colorectal cancer
CRP	C-reactive protein
CRT	conformal radiotherapy
CSF	cerebrospinal fluid
CSI	craniospinal irradiation
CT	computerized tomography

CTC	common toxicity criteria *or* circulating tumour cell
CTD	cyclophosphamide–dexamethasone–thalidomide
cTn	cardiac troponin
CTV	clinical target volume
CUP	cancer of unknown primary *or* conventional chemotherapy, unpurged, purged (autograft)
CVA	cerebrovascular accident
C-VAD	cyclophosphamide–vincristine–Adriamycin®–dexamethasone
CVP	cyclophosphamide–vincristine–prednisolone *or* central venous pressure
CXR	chest X-ray
DAT	direct antiglobulin test
dATP	deoxyadenosine triphosphate
D&C	dilatation and curettage
DC	dendritic cell
DCIS	ductal carcinoma *in situ*
DFS	disease-free survival
DFSP	dermatofibrosarcoma protuberans
DHAP	cisplatin–ara-C–dexamethasone
DHFR	dihydrofolate reductase

DIC	disseminated intravascular coagulation	EGC	early gastric cancer
		EGF	epithelial growth factor
DLBL	diffuse large B-cell non-Hodgkin's lymphoma	EGFR	epidermal growth factor receptor
DL_{CO}	carbon monoxide diffusion capacity	EMA	etoposide–methotrexate–actinomycin D
DLT	dose-limited toxicity	EMG	electromyography
DMSA	dimercaptosuccinic acid	ENT	ear, nose, and throat
DPS	delayed primary surgery	EOC	epithelial ovarian cancer
DRE	digital rectal examination	EORTC	European Organisation for Research and Treatment of Cancer
DTIC	dacarbazine		
dTTP	2'-deoxythymidine 5'-triphosphate	EORTC-QLQ	EORTC Quality of Life Questionnaire
dUMP	2'-deoxyuridine 5'-monophosphate	EP	estramustine phosphate or etoposide–cisplatin
DVT	deep vein thrombosis		
EASL	European Association for the Study of the Liver	EPA	eicosapentanoic acid
		EPID	electronic portal imaging devices
EBMT	European Group for Blood and Marrow Transplantation	EPO	erythropoietin
		EPP	extrapleural pneumonectomy
		ER	(o)estrogen receptor
EBRT	external beam radiotherapy	ERCCI	excision repair cross-complementing rodent repair deficiency complementary group I
EBV	Epstein–Barr virus		
EC	etoposide–carboplatin (lung cancer) or epirubicin–cyclophosphamide (breast cancer)		
		ERCP	endoscopic retrograde cholangio-pancreatography
ECG	electrocardiograph	ESHAP	cisplatin–ara-C–etoposide–methyl-prednisolone
ECOG	Eastern Cooperative Oncology Group		
		ESPAC	European Randomized Adjuvant Study
EDTA	ethylendiaminetetra-acetic acid		

	Comparing Radiotherapy, 6 Months Chemotherapy and Combination Therapy versus Observation in Pancreatic Cancer	FIGO	International Federation for Gynaecology and Obstetrics
ESR	erythrocyte sedimentation rate	FISH	fluorescent *in situ* hybridization
EURAMOS	European and American Osteosarcoma Study Group	FL	follicular lymphoma
		FLIC	Functional Living Index – Cancer
EUS	endoscopic (or endo-oesophageal) ultrasound	FLIPI	follicular lymphoma prognostic index
EVA	etoposide–vincristine–doxorubicin	FNA	fine needle aspiration
		FOB	faecal occult blood
FAC	fluorouracil–doxorubicin (Adriamycin®)–cyclophosphamide	FOLFOX	folinic acid–fluorouracil–oxaliplatin
		FRS	fluid retention syndrome
FACT	Functional Assessment of Cancer Therapy	FSH	follicle-stimulating hormone
FAP	familial adenomatous polyposis	FSRT	fractionated stereotactic radiotherapy
FBC	full blood count	5-FU	5-fluorouracil
FC	fludarabine–cyclophosphamide	GABA	Gamma-aminobutyric acid
FCR	fludarabine–cyclophosphamide–rituximab	G-CSF	granulocyte colony-stimulating factor
FDG	fluorodeoxyglucose	GDEPT	gene-directed enzyme pro-drug system
FdUMP	5-fluoro-2-deoxyuridine 5-monophosphate	GDNF	glial-derived neurotrophic factor
FEC	fluorouracil–epirubicin–cyclophosphamide	GELA	Groupe d'Étude des Lymphomes des Adultes
FEV_1	forced expiratory volume in 1 s	GFR	glomerular filtration rate
		GGT	gamma-glutamyl transpeptidase
FFS	failure-free survival (rate)	GH	growth hormone

GI	gastrointestinal		HDR	high dose rate
GIST	gastrointestinal stromal tumours		HEDP	hydroxyethylidene diphosphonate
GnRH	gonadotrophin-releasing hormone		HER2	human epidermal growth factor receptor 2
GO	gemtuzumab ozogamicin		HGPRT	hypoxanthine guanine phosphori-bosyl transferase
G6PD	glucose-6-phosphate dehydrogenase		HHM	humoral hypercalcaemia of malignancy
GP	general practitioner		HHV	human herpes virus
GPAT	genetic pro-drug activation		5-HIAA	5-hydroxyin-doleacetic acid
GTAC	Gene Therapy Advisory Committee (UK)		HIF	hypoxia-inducible factor
GTD	gestational tropho-blastic disease		HIP	Health Insurance Plan
GTV	gross tumour volume		HIT	heparin-induced thrombocytopenia
GVHD	graft-versus-host disease		HIV	human immunode-ficiency virus
GVL	Graft versus leukaemia		HL	Hodgkin's lymphoma
Gy	gray		HLA	human leucocyte-associated antigen
HAART	highly active anti-retroviral therapy		HNPCC	hereditary non-polyposis colorectal cancer
HADS	Hospital Anxiety and Depression Scale		HPL	human placental lactogen
Hb	haemoglobin		HPV	human papilloma virus
HBV	hepatitis B virus		HRT	hormone replace-ment therapy
HCC	hepatocellular carcinoma		HSV	herpes simplex virus
HCG	human chorionic gonadotrophin		5-HT	5-hydroxytryptam-ine (serotonin)
HCV	hepatitis C virus		HTLV	human T-cell lymphocytotrophic virus
HD	Hodgkin's disease			
HDC	high-dose chemotherapy			
HDI	high-dose IV inter-feron-α		HUS	haemolytic–uraemic syndrome
HDP	hydroxymethylene diphosphonate			

ICE	ifosfamide–carbopl-atin–etoposide	IMID	immunomodulatory drug
ICH-GCP	International Conference for Harmonisation for Good Clinical Practice	IMRT	intensity-modulated radiotherapy
		INCH	Induction Chemotherapy and cHart
ICON	International Collaborative Ovarian Neoplasm	INR	international normalized ratio
ICP	intracranial pressure	IORT	intra-operative radiotherapy
ICRU	International Commission on Radiation Units	IPI	International Prognostic Index
		IPSS	International Prognostic Scoring System
ICSI	intracytoplasmic sperm injection	ITP	idiopathic thrombocytopenic purpura
ICT	intracavitary brachytherapy		
IESLG	International Extranodal Lymphoma Study Group	ITU	intensive therapy unit
		IV	intravenous
IFL	irinotecan–5-fluo-rouracil–leucovorin	IVAC	ifosfamide–etoposide–cytarabine
IFN	interferon (IFN-α, IFN-β, etc.)	IVC	inferior vena cava
IFR	involved field radiotherapy	IVE	ifosfamide–etoposide–epirubicin
IGCCC	International Germ Cell Consensus Classification	IVF	*in vitro* fertilization
		IVU	intravenous urography
IGF	insulin-like growth factor	JMML	juvenile myelomonocytic leukaemia
IGRT	image-guided radiotherapy		
IgM	Immunoglobulin M	KPS	Karnofsky Performance Status
IgVH	immunoglobulin heavy chain variable region	KS	Kaposi's sarcoma
		LAK	lymphokine-activated killer (cell)
IL	interleukin (IL-1, IL-4, etc.)		
IM	intramuscular	LCIS	lobular carcinoma *in situ*
^{131}I-MIBG	^{131}I-labelled meta-iodobenzyl-guanidine	LDH	lactate dehydrogenase

LDHL	lymphocyte-depleted classical Hodgkin's lymphoma		MDR	multidrug resistance
			MDS	myelodysplasia
LDR	low dose rate		MDS-U	myelodysplastic syndrome-unclassified
LEMS	Lambert–Eaton myasthenic syndrome		MDT	multidisciplinary team
LFT	liver function test		MEN	multiple endocrine neoplasia
LGL	large granular lymphocytic leukaemia		MFH	malignant fibrous histiocytoma
LH	luteinizing hormone		MGMT	O^6-methylguanine-DNA methyl transferase
LHRH	luteinizing hormone releasing hormone		MGUS	monoclonal gammopathy of uncertain significance
LLN	lower limit of normal			
LRHCL	lymphocyte-rich classical Hodgkin's lymphoma		MHC	major histocompatibility complex
			MIC	mitomycin–ifosfamide–cisplatin
LV	leucovorin		MIBG	meta-iodobenzyl-guanidine
mAb	monoclonal antibody			
MAGIC	MRC Adjuvant Gastric Infusional Chemotherapy		MLC	multi-leaf collimators
			MLL	mixed lineage leukaemia (protein)
MALT	mucosa-associated lymphoid tissue		MMC	mitomycin C
MAP	methotrexate–doxorubicin–cisplatin		MMMT	mixed mesodermal Müllerian tumours
			MMR	mismatch repair
MBC	metastatic breast cancer		MOPP	mechlorethamine–vincristine (Oncovin®)–procarbazine–prednisolone
MBL	monoclonal B-lymphocytosis			
MBP	methotrexate–bleomycin–cisplatin		MP	melphalan–prednisolone
MCL	mantle-cell lymphoma		6-MP	6-mercaptopurine
MCP	mitoxantrone–chlorambucil–prednisolone		MPM	malignant pleural mesothelioma
			MPNST	malignant peripheral nerve sheath tumour
MDP	methylene disphosphonate			

MPT	melphalan–prednisolone–thalidomide
MRC	Medical Research Council
MRD	minimum residual disease
MRI	magnetic resonance imaging
MRP	multidrug resistance-associated protein
MSI	microsatellite instability
MSM	men who have sex with men
MTD	maximal tolerated dose
MTX	methotrexate
MUGA	multigated acquisition (test)
MVAC	methotrexate–vinblastine–doxorubicin–cisplatin
MVP	mitomycin–vinblastine–cisplatin
MZL	marginal zone lymphoma
NACT	neoadjuvant chemotherapy
NCI	National Cancer Institute
NCIC	National Cancer Institute of Canada
NCIC–CTG	NCIC Clinical trials Group
NCRN	National Cancer Research Network
NF	neurofibromatosis
NG	nasogastric (tube)
NICE	National Institute for Health and Clinical Excellence (UK)
NHL	non-Hodgkin's lymphoma
NIH	National Institutes of Health
NK	natural killer (cell) or neurokinin
NLPHL	nodular lymphocyte predominant Hodgkin's lymphoma
NMDA	N-methyl-D-aspartate
NPI	Nottingham Prognostic Index
NSAID	Non-steroidal anti-inflammatory drug
NSCHL	nodular sclerosing classical Hodgkin's lymphoma
NSCLC	non-small-cell lung cancer
NSE	neurone-specific enolase
NSGCT	non-seminomatous germ cell tumour
NVB	vinorelbine
NWTSG	National Wilms' Tumour Study Group (US)
OAR	organ at risk
od	once daily
OGJ	oesophageal gastric junction
ONJ	osteonecrosis of the jaw
OPG	osteoprotegrin
OPSI	overwhelming post-splenectomy infection
ORR	overall response rate
OS	overall survival (rate)
PABLOE	prednisolone–doxorubicin–bleomycin–vincristine–etoposide

P_aCO_2	arterial carbon dioxide tension	PLL	prolymphocytic leukaemia
P_aO_2	arterial oxygen tension	PN	peripheral neuropathy
PBP	peripheral blood progenitors	PNET	primitive neuroec-todermal tumour
PCA	patient-controlled analgesia	PO	orally, by mouth
PCD	paraneoplastic cerebellar degeneration	POEMS	polyneuropathy–organomegaly–endocrinopathy–M protein–skin changes (syndrome)
PCI	prophylactic cranial irradiation		
PCL	primary CNS lymphoma	PPI	proton pump inhibitor
PCR	polymerase chain reaction	PR	progesterone receptor
PCV	procarbazine–CCNU–vincristine	pRBC	packed red blood cells
PDGF	platelet-derived growth factor	prn	as required
		PRPP	5-phosphoribo-sylpyrophosphate
PEG	percutaneous endoscopic gastrostomy	PS	paraneoplastic syndrome
PEI	percutaneous ethanol injection	PSA	prostate-specific antigen
PET	positron emission tomography	PSTT	placental site tro-phoblastic tumour
PFS	progression-free survival	PT	prothrombin time
PGDE	pharmacokineti-cally guided dose escalation	PTH	parathyroid hormone
		PTT	partial thrombo-plastin time
PgP	P glycoprotein	PTHrP	parathyroid hormone-related peptide
Ph	Philadelphia (chromosome)		
PHM	partial hydatidi-form mole	PTLD	post-transplant lymphoprolifera-tive disease
PLCO	Prostate Lung Colorectal and Ovarian Cancer (screening trial)	PTV	planning target volume
		PUO	pyrexia of unexplained origin
PIC	portable intensive care (system)	PVC	premature ventricular contraction
PICC	peripherally insert-ed central catheter		

QALY	quality-adjusted life years	RFA	radiofrequency ablation
qds	four times a day	RIC	reduced-intensity conditioning
QoL	quality of life	RMH	Royal Marsden Hospital (staging for testicular cancer)
RADICALS	Radiotherapy and Androgen Deprivation in Combination After Local Surgery		
		RMS	rhabdomyosarcoma
		RR	response rate
RAEB	refractory anaemia with excess blasts	RS	Reed–Sternberg (cell)
RANK	receptor activator of NF-κB	RTK	receptor tyrosine kinase
RARS	refractory anaemia with ringed sideroblasts	RTOG	Radiation Therapy Oncology Group
		RT-PCR	reverse transcription polymerase chain reaction
RATHL	RAndomized phase III Trial to assess response-adapted therapy using FDG-PET imaging in patients with newly diagnosed advanced Hodgkin's Lymphoma		
		s-AML	AML secondary to myelodysplasia
		SAS	subarachnoid space
		SBP	solitary bone plasmacytoma
		SC	subcutaneous
RCMD	refractory cytopenia with multilineage dysplasia	SCC	squamous cell carcinoma
		SCF	supraclavicular fossa
RCMD-RS	RCMD with ringed sideroblasts	SCLC	small-cell lung cancer
RCT	randomized controlled trial	SD	standard deviation
REACH	Randomized, Multicenter, Open-Label Study to Evaluate the Safety and Efficacy of Anti-TNF alpha Chimeric Monoclonal Antibody in Pediatric Subjects with Moderate to Severe Crohn's Disease	SEP	solitary extramedullary plasmacytoma
		SFLCR	Serum-free light chain ratio
		SGOT	serum glutamic oxaloacetic transaminase
		SGPT	serum glutamic pyruvic transaminase
RECIST	Response Evaluation Criteria in Solid Tumors	SIADH	secretion of inappropriate antidiuretic hormone (syndrome)

SIOP	International Society of Paediatric Oncology
SLL	small lymphocytic lymphoma
SLVL	splenic marginal zone lymphoma with circulating villous lymphocytes
SMC	Scottish Medicines Committee
SN-38	7-ethyl-10-hydroxycamptothecin
SOB	shortness of breath
SOCCAR	Sequential Or Concurrent Chemotherapy and Radiotherapy (study)
SPECT	single photon emission computerized tomography
SRS	stereotactic radiosurgery
SVC	superior vena cava
SVCO	superior vena cava obstruction
SVT	supraventricular tachycardia
T_3	triiodothyronine
T_4	thyroxine
TACE	trans-arterial chemo-embolization
t-AML	(chemo)therapy-related AML
TBI	total body irradiation
TCA	tricyclic antidepressant
TCC	transitional cell carcinoma
tds	three times a day
TENS	transcutaneous electrical nerve stimulation
TFT	thyroid function test
TG	thyroglobulin
6-TG	6-thioguanine
TK	tyrosine kinase
TKI	tyrosine kinase inhibitor
TI	thoracic irradiation
TIA	transient ischaemic attack
TIL	tumour-infiltrating lymphocyte
TME	total excision of the mesorectum
TNF	tumour necrosis factor (TNF-α)
TNM	tumour–node–metastasis (staging system for cancer)
TRAM	transverse rectus abdominis muscle
TRM	transplant-related mortality
TS	thymidylate synthase
TSH	thyroid-stimulating hormone
TTF	time to treatment failure
TTP	time to progression *or* thrombotic thrombocytic purpura
TURBT	transurethral resection of bladder tumour
TURP	transurethral resection of the prostate
U&E	urea and electrolytes

UICC	International Union Against Cancer
UKCCSG	UK Children's Cancer Study Group
UKLG	UK Lymphoma Group
ULN	upper limit of normal
USS	ultrasound scan
UV	ultraviolet
VAD	vincristine–Adriamycin®–dexamethasone
VATS	video-assisted thoracoscopy
VBL	vinblastine
VC	vomiting centre
VCR	vincristine
VDEPT	virus-directed enzyme pro-drug therapy
VEGF	vascular endothelial growth factor
VHL	von Hippel–Lindau (syndrome)
VIDE	vincristine–ifosfamide–doxorubicin–etoposide
VIP	etoposide–ifosfamide–cisplatin
VMA	vanillylmandelic acid
VOD	veno-occlusive disease
VTE	venous thromboembolism
WAGR	Wilms' tumour (associated with) aniridia–genitourinary abnormalities–mental retardation
WCC	white cell count
WHO	World Health Organization
WNL	within normal limits
WT	Wilms' tumour

List of plates

Part 1

Background

Multidisciplinary approach to cancer

Management of cancer involves a number of clinical disciplines. The majority require a variety of diagnostic tests including some form of pathological confirmation and imaging investigations to assess the extent of disease. Most patients have a primary surgical intervention. The development of more effective additional therapies for cancer such as chemotherapy, radiotherapy, hormones, etc. has made the overall management of cancer very complex.

No single clinician has all the skills needed to treat all cancers. This has led to the development of multidisciplinary teams that deal with certain types of cancer. Many professions allied to medicine have major roles to play in these teams (e.g. physiotherapists, stoma nurses, counsellors). The team may include individuals who are not directly involved in the treatment at presentation but have adjunctive roles at some stage in the course of the illness (e.g. palliative care). The composition of the team will vary considerably between institutions – and disease states. There must be a sufficient range of expertise to allow for informed discussion of the management policy for individual patients. The team's various roles include:

- planning diagnostic and staging procedures, primary treatment approach, and any adjuvant therapy to be delivered pre- or post-operatively
- preparing patients physically and psychologically for anti-cancer therapy and subsequent follow-up
- providing information on treatment, prognosis, side-effects, and any other pertinent matters (e.g. stoma care)
- efficiently planning and delivering surgery, radiotherapy, and chemotherapy as appropriate
- aiding rehabilitation from the illness
- providing appropriate follow-up care
- ensuring that the transition from curative to palliative care is appropriately managed
- promoting recruitment to appropriate clinical trials.

Management within such a team structure results in better outcomes for patients. Studies demonstrate survival advantages but, equally importantly, patients also have functional, psychological, cosmetic, and quality of life benefits.

The team should also formally audit its procedures and performance to ensure continued development of the team and to allow for comparisons with other teams.

Aetiology and epidemiology

Genetic factors

- Approximately 7 million deaths worldwide can be attributed to malignancy each year.
- The interplay between the hereditary and environmental risk factors underlying the development of malignancy is becoming clearer.
- It is thought that at least 50% of cases are preventable.
- Primary prevention strategies focus on modifiable lifestyle and environmental risk factors.
- Most cancers are monoclonal, i.e. a single cell accumulates sufficient mutations in key genes to cause uncontrolled cell proliferation.
- Genes involved in the development of cancers fall into three categories:

Tumour suppressor genes

- Genes whose function is lost during carcinogenesis.
- Both allele copies must be inactivated before the tumour suppressor function is completely lost (absence of normal protein product), i.e. can be classified as recessive.
- Functional mutations result in loss of growth inhibitory mechanisms.
- Mutations can be hereditary (germline mutations) or acquired.
- An example of a tumour suppressor gene – the *p53* gene:
  - produces a transcriptional regulator involved in cell cycle control and maintaining genomic integrity
  - ~50% of human cancers possess *p53* mutations including breast, lung, pancreas, colon, and brain tumours and malignancies seen in the inherited Li–Fraumeni syndrome.

Proto-oncogenes

- Genes whose function becomes enhanced in carcinogenesis.
- Usually play an essential role in controlling cell proliferation, encoding growth factors, growth factor receptors, transcription factors, etc.
- Mutations of oncogenes may impede normal cell cycle regulation causing uncontrolled cellular replication.
- Mutation in only one of the proto-oncogene alleles is needed for the mutant gene product to influence downstream events, i.e. mutations are dominant at the cellular level.
- An example of a proto-oncogene – the *Ras* gene:
  - encodes a membrane-associated G protein responsible for cellular signal transduction
  - mutated *Ras* products remain activated even in the absence of the appropriate growth factor receptor signal
  - mutations in *Ras* are implicated in 30% of all cancers including melanoma, lung, and pancreas.

DNA repair genes

- Genes whose usual function is to carry out DNA repair.
- Functional mutations of DNA repair genes accelerate accumulation of mutated tumour suppressor genes and proto-oncogenes.
- An example of a DNA repair gene – the *ATM* gene:
  - encodes a protein involved in the detection of DNA damage with an important role in cell cycle progression

- multiple double-stranded DNA breaks lead to high rates of chromosomal rearrangements
- produces the syndrome of ataxia–telangiectasia, associated with:
  - progressive cerebellar ataxia
  - ↑ incidence of malignancies (usually lymphomas/leukaemias)
  - hypersensitive response to treatment with ionizing radiation.

The relative contribution of the genetic mutation to the cancer varies:

Specific genes that confer a high probability of susceptibility to specific cancer

- Comprise 5% of total incidence of fatal cancers.
- Usually:
  - highly penetrant
  - dominantly inherited.
- Examples include:
  - *BRCA1/2* genes – mutations account for the majority of hereditary breast carcinomas. Female carriers have 55–85% lifetime risk of breast carcinoma and 40% (*BRCA1*) or 18% (*BRCA2*) lifetime risk of ovarian cancer. ↑ incidence of pancreatic and male breast and prostate cancers also reported
  - *RB1* gene – on chromosome 13. Encodes a nuclear protein, which acts as a tumour suppressor. Mutations may be hereditary or acquired. Inactivation of both alleles causes retinoblastoma
  - *APC* gene – on chromosome 5. Mutations result in familial adenomatous polyposis, which classically causes the development of numerous colonic adenomas with subsequent malignant transformation.

Genes with modest effects that may interact with environmental factors

- For example, tumour viruses expressing genes that disrupt activity of tumour suppressor genes.

Genetic (somatic) mutations caused by recognizable carcinogens causing sporadic cancers

- Many exogenous carcinogens cause somatic mutations.
- Examples include:
  - aromatic hydrocarbons
  - UV radiation.

Gender

- Many cancers occur more frequently in one or other sex, e.g. stomach cancer – twice as frequent in men.
- It is difficult to distinguish innate differences in susceptibility from differences caused by other risk factors, e.g. the greater incidence of carcinoma of the bladder in men was thought to represent an innate difference in susceptibility – but, when exposed to the same occupational carcinogens and tobacco smoke, women are at least as susceptible to the disease.

External factors

Smoking

- Tobacco smoking is:
  - the most important known carcinogen
  - the largest single avoidable cause of premature death in the developed world.
- 15% of all cancer cases worldwide and >30% of cases in men from developed countries are attributed to smoking.
- Associated particularly with lung cancer, which is the commonest cause of cancer death. Smoking is responsible for ~90% of cases of lung cancer. The relative risk in a lifelong smoker compared to a lifelong non-smoker is between 10- and 30-fold dependent on intensity and duration of exposure. It has been estimated that smoking was responsible for 0.85 million avoidable deaths from lung cancer in 2000 worldwide.
- Also has a definite causative role in many other cancers including:
  - mesothelioma
  - myeloid leukaemia
  - gastrointestinal (GI) tract including oral cavity, oesophageal, gastric, and pancreatic
  - ear, nose, and throat (ENT) including pharyngeal, laryngeal, nasopharyngeal, cancers of the nasal cavity and paranasal sinuses
  - urinary tract including bladder and renal
  - liver
  - cervical.
- An association has been suggested, but not proven, between smoking and an increased incidence of breast and colonic carcinomas.
- Cigarette smoking has a synergistic (multiplicative) effect on the risk of development of neoplasms caused by other carcinogens, e.g. alcohol, asbestos.
- A substantial increase in the cancer burden may be expected unless measures to control consumption are strengthened – a consequence of the ongoing increase in global cigarette consumption, especially amongst women and in developing countries.
- Smoking cessation reduces the risk of cancer, but programmes promoting cessation have had only limited success.
- Passive exposure to tobacco smoke also contributes. Estimates are that 15–30% of lung cancer in patients who have never smoked can be attributed to environmental tobacco smoke exposure.

Alcohol

- Alcohol is implicated as causative in several malignancies including:
  - **head and neck cancer, and cancer of the oropharynx** – the risk increases linearly with alcohol intake
  - **oesophageal cancer**, particularly squamous – the risk is strongly related to alcohol intake and again appears to be increased even at low levels of consumption.
  - **breast cancer** – studies suggest that moderate to heavy alcohol intake (>2 units/day) is associated with an increased incidence of

carcinoma of the breast; 2–10% of all breast cancers may be related to alcohol intake. The mechanism of carcinogenesis is unclear but it is thought it could be related to an increase in circulating oestrogens and androgens
  • **hepatocellular carcinoma** – moderate to heavy drinking is a risk factor for alcoholic cirrhosis and this is a risk factor for hepatocellular cancer. Excessive alcohol intake in the absence of cirrhosis has a less clear role.
• A confounding factor in many studies is that excess alcohol intake has a positive association with tobacco consumption. These two factors can have a synergistic rather than additive effect on cancer incidence but the association between the two can make assessment of the relative contribution of each difficult to elucidate.

Diet

Obesity

• Adult obesity is a risk factor for many solid tumours including:
  • endometrial cancer
  • post-menopausal breast cancer
  • cancer of the kidney
  • oesophageal carcinoma
  • colorectal carcinoma.
• Has also been suggested to contribute to the development of prostate, liver, ovarian, gastric, and pancreatic malignancies.
• May have a role in up to 20% of cancer deaths in the developed world.
• The mechanisms underlying the association between obesity and malignancy are poorly understood.

General dietary risk factors

• High levels of vegetable consumption appear to be associated with a reduced risk of colon cancer, particularly distal tumours, although the prospective evidence is not strong.
• Consistent evidence that a high intake of vegetables and fruit reduces the risk of other tumours is lacking.
• High levels of red meat consumption appear to increase the risk of colonic and rectal cancer.
• A high-fibre diet has previously been reported as being associated with a lower risk of carcinoma of the colon. However, these results may have been influenced by confounding dietary factors, such as folate intake, and the association has not been confirmed.
• Fat consumption – there is ongoing interest in whether the various types of dietary fats influence cancer risk differently, with most concern over the saturated and trans fats found in meats and some dairy produce.

Specific dietary risk factors

• Appropriate dietary modifications may significantly influence the incidence of certain cancers.
• Examples include:
  • **salt fish** – reducing the intake of salt fish could reduce the incidence of nasopharyngeal cancer in developing countries by 33–50%

- **aflatoxins** – a mycotoxin produced by *Aspergillus* species of mould which frequently contaminates corn, peanuts, and soybeans. Halving the median daily intake of aflatoxins may reduce the incidence of hepatocellular carcinoma (HCC) in Africa and Asia by up to 40%.

Exercise
- Physical inactivity appears to be associated with an increased risk of many adult tumours.
- Current evidence is greatest for breast and colonic cancers.
- The benefit appears to be independent of associated obesity.

Infections

Sixteen per cent of the worldwide incidence of cancer is due to infection. For developed countries, the proportion is 9% and for developing countries >20%.

Viral infections

- Most tumour viruses are ubiquitous; the prevalence of infection is much higher than the incidence of the respective form of tumour.
- Development of associated tumours requires many years of infection.
- Viral infection plays a significant role in the initial step towards carcinogenesis. However, other co-factors are necessary for development of virally linked tumours including genetic, immunological, and environmental factors.
- Some viruses increase the risk of multiple malignancies (see 📖 Chapter 29, AIDS-related malignancies, pp. 625–640).
- Other viruses are directly linked to human tumours. Examples include:

Human papillomavirus (HPV)

- The most frequent sexually acquired infection in the developed world.
- Genital infection is via unprotected sexual intercourse or close contact with an infected area.
- Small, double-stranded DNA viruses (*Papoviridae* family).
- Specifically infect squamous epithelial cells.
- >100 different genotypes identified.
- HPV infection accounts for >80% of cervical cancers worldwide.
- Also associated with vaginal, vulval, penile, and anal carcinoma.
- Strongest evidence for carcinogenicity is for HPV types 16 and 18 (cervical cancer).
- A quadrivalent vaccine is now available for girls/unvaccinated women, a national (UK) programme for immunization has been introduced. Cervical screening programmes in developed countries have reduced the incidence of cervical carcinoma.

Hepatitis B and C virus (HBV, HCV)

- 81% of cases of hepatocellular carcinoma (HCC) are attributable to chronic infection.
- 75% with 1° HBV infection develop lifelong hepatic infection → hepatocellular injury → chronic hepatitis.
- Chronic HBV infection is associated with ↑ 100-fold risk of HCC.
- Prevalence of HBV carriers in SE Asia, China, and sub-Saharan Africa may be >20%.

Epstein–Barr virus (EBV)

- An endemic *Herpes* virus.
- Hodgkin's lymphoma – EBV may account for:
  - up to 60% of Hodgkin's disease in developed countries
  - ≥80% in developing countries.
- Burkitt's lymphoma:
  - EBV is thought to be causative in >90% of Burkitt's lymphoma in equatorial Africa (>90% of children are infected with EBV by the age of 3 years and Burkitt's is the most common childhood malignancy)

- has a lesser role elsewhere (<25% of cases outside Africa, the Middle East, and South America)
- malaria infection is considered a co-factor in the genesis of Burkitt's lymphoma. Putative mechanisms for this include chronic stimulus for B-cell proliferation or depression of cytotoxic T-cell function such that EBV infection may escape T-cell surveillance
- Greater uncertainty about the role of EBV in other types of non-Hodgkin's lymphoma.
- Highly consistent association with nasopharyngeal carcinoma. EBV can be found in every anaplastic nasopharyngeal carcinoma cell.

Bacterial infections

Helicobacter pylori

- Clear association between *H. pylori* infection and gastric adenocarcinoma.
- One-third of gastric adneocarcinomas in developed countries can be attributed solely to *H. pylori* and this figure is likely to be closer to 50% in developing countries.
- The mechanism of carcinogenesis is not fully understood.
- *H. pylori* is also likely to a role in the development of gastric lymphoma.
- Different strains may have different carcinogenic potential.

Parasitic infections

Schistosomiasis haematobium (bilharzial bladder disease)

- Linked to hyperplasia, metaplasia, dysplasia, and invasive carcinoma of the bladder.
- 8% of cases of bladder cancer in the developing world may be attributable to infection – the majority of which are squamous cell.
- It is not relevant in bladder cancer seen in the developed world.

Exposures

Solar exposure
- >1 million cases of skin cancer are diagnosed worldwide each year.
- Epidemiological evidence suggests >90% of malignant melanoma is attributable to solar radiation.
- The most frequent 1° sites are areas exposed intermittently but intensely, e.g. skin of back.
- Australians (mostly white and intensely exposed to ultraviolet (UV) radiation) have the highest incidence of melanoma in the world.
- Sun exposure in childhood is a particular risk factor.
- Exposure to solar radiation is also likely to account for the great majority of non-melanoma skin cancer.
- Basal cell and squamous cell carcinomas are associated with cumulative sun exposure, typically in maximally sun-exposed areas, e.g. face and ears.

Other radiation exposure
- Initiating factor in carcinogenesis is probably a mutation in a tumour suppressor/proto-oncogene → aberrant loss/gain of function.
- High-dose exposure:
  - doses of 500–2000 mSv are known to be carcinogenic, potentially causing several malignancies, e.g. acute leukaemias, thyroid cancer
  - exposures of this magnitude are unusual – much of the data come from complex epidemiological studies performed in the wake of Nagasaki, Hiroshima, and Chernobyl, or in studies of second malignancies in patients previously treated for cancer.
- Low-dose exposure:
  - the average per capita dose from all sources of ionizing radiation is ~3.4 mSv per year (~88% from natural sources and the remainder primarily from medical exposures)
  - most data have been collated from studies on secondary malignancies in survivors previously treated with radiotherapy, and epidemiological studies of miners
  - extrapolation from data on exposure to ≥500 mSv suggests that 1–3% of all cancers may be attributable to radiation arising largely from natural sources.
- Radiation sensitivity:
  - ~3% of the population show undue sensitivity to conventional doses of ionizing radiation without any obvious pre-treatment phenotype apart from the presence of cancer. This group is at risk of excess toxicity from standard radiation therapy regimens. Greater understanding of underlying defects in DNA repair, cell cycling, and DNA damage signal transduction would allow appropriate tailoring of therapy
  - rare radiosensitivity syndromes also exist, predisposing to early development of cancer, e.g. ataxia–telangiectasia, Bloom's syndrome. Susceptibility to DNA damage is enhanced and both radiotherapy and chemotherapy regimens need adjustment accordingly.

Other exposures
Other exposures account for <5% of the cancer burden. Many chemical carcinogens have been identified.

Industrial exposure
- Dye/textile workers (naphythylamines) – bladder cancers.
- Chemical, rubber workers (benzene) – haematological malignancies.
- Asbestos exposure – lung cancer, mesothelioma (notifiable).

Pharmacological exposure
- Many chemotherapeutic agents used in the treatment of cancer are carcinogenic, e.g. alkylating agents.
- High-dose diethylstilbesterol during pregnancy (used in the 1960s to reduce the risk of miscarriage) → small percentage of female offspring developed clear cell carcinoma of the vagina as they reached menarche.

Environmental exposure
- Few causal links with environmental pollutants have been firmly established.
- Estimates suggest ~1% of lung cancer deaths (US figures) are attributable to air pollution.
- Incidence of many cancers varies greatly between geographical areas – this includes variation between countries and between different regions within countries.
- Variations reflect complex interactions between genetic, environmental, economic, and behavioural factors.
- Migration between areas of contrasting incidence → migrant population usually acquires the cancer pattern of their adopted country, i.e. environmental rather than genetic factors dominate, except in rare familial cases.
- Cancer incidence can vary between socio-economic groups.
- Epidemiological studies help further understanding of the aetiology of different cancers and allow development of strategies for disease prevention.

Further reading

Jemal A, Siegel R, Ward E, et al. (2008) Cancer statistics 2008. *CA Cancer J Clin* **58**, 71.

Schottenfeld D, Fraumeni JF (eds) (2006) *Cancer Epidemiology and Prevention*, 3rd edn. Oxford: Oxford University Press.

Dumitrescu RG (2009) Epigenetic targets in cancer epidemiology. *Methods Mol Biol* **471**, 457–67.

Danaei G, Vander Hoorn S, Lopez AD, et al. (2005) Causes of cancer in the world: comparative assessment of nine behavioural and environmental risk factors. *Lancet* **366**, 1784.

Coyle YM (2009) Lifestyle, genes and cancer. *Methods Mol Biol* **472**, 25–56.

Genetics of cancer

The cancer phenotype

Cancer is a genetic disease, arising as a result of a number of genetic alterations accumulating in stepwise manner within the cell, leading to uncontrolled proliferation and selection of those clones that acquire a growth advantage over their neighbouring cells. In the majority of cancers, these changes are acquired as somatic events, and are then passed on to daughter cells. In a small number of cancers, there are inherited changes in the genes of all cells which make the development of cancer more likely. The same genes may be involved in both acquired and inherited mutations, and hence better understanding of the molecular and cellular processes involved may apply to all cancers. In addition, susceptibility to the effects of environmental carcinogens which may lead to these acquired mutations can itself be genetically determined.

Characteristics of cancer cells include:
- proliferation in the absence of exogenous factors (such as growth factors)
- failure to respond to normal 'brakes' on proliferation, e.g. growth inhibitors, cell cycle control check points
- resistance to apoptosis and senescence
- ability to recruit blood vessels
- ability to invade surrounding tissues and metastasize

Many of the corresponding genes in which alterations can occur and which may facilitate these features have now been characterized.

Which genes are involved?

Genes in which mutations are known to occur in cancers include:
- oncogenes
- tumour suppressor genes:
  - cell cycle control genes
  - 'mutator' genes (DNA repair)
  - apoptosis genes
  - telomerase associated genes.

Oncogenes

Oncogenes are mutated proto-oncogenes, and in normal cells promote cellular proliferation. They encode growth factors, growth factor receptors, signal transducers, or transcription factors. In the normal situation they are activated in response to cellular signals, but when mutated may become inappropriately active in the absence of the relevant signal, or resistant to inactivation (i.e. they show a 'gain of function'). An example would be RET, which acts as a cell surface receptor for ligands such as glial-derived neurotrophic factor (GDNF), and activation leads to intracellular signal transduction via RAS/ERK, P13 kinase or JNK pathways. Mutations are activating, so that the receptor and pathway are activated in the absence of GDNF, usually because of permanent dimerization and autophosphorylation. These mutations may be inherited in the case of multiple endocrine neoplasia (MEN)2a (see 🕮 p.357), or may be acquired as somatic mutations in a variety of tumours. Their importance is the insight they provide to pathogenesis, which may lead to novel treatments. Due to the activating nature of the mutations, only one copy of the gene needs to be affected in order to confer a growth advantage to the cell, and hence mutations in these genes behave in a dominant manner. Oncogenes may become activated by:

- point mutation (e.g. in *RET* in MEN2, in *RAS* in 30% of all tumours, V600E in *BRAF* in sporadic microsatellite instability (MSI)-positive bowel cancers)
- gene amplification, with multiple copies appearing within the tumour (e.g. N-Myc in neuroblastoma)
- chromosome rearrangement to create a novel fusion gene, or for the gene to become associated with the promotor region of a different gene, making it active in a different situation (e.g. *ELKS-RET* in papillary thyroid cancer).

Inherited mutations in oncogenes are in fact rather uncommon in inherited cancer predispositions, but are seen much more commonly as somatic mutations in sporadic tumours, or during the progression to malignancy of tumours in individuals carrying a predisposition gene (see Table 3.1).

Table 3.1 Examples of tumour suppressor genes and oncogenes

Gene	Normal function	Associated cancers
Tumour suppressor genes		
p53	Regulates transcription, G1–S checkpoint control and apoptosis trigger	Breast, lung, colon, glioma, sarcoma
Rb	Cell cycle control	Retinoblastoma, small-cell lung cancer, osteosarcoma
MTS1	Cell cycle control	Glioma, melanoma, lung, bladder, mesothelioma
BRCA1 & 2	Involved in DNA repair by homologous recombination	Familial breast and ovarian cancer
Oncogenes		
Ras	Signal transduction	Colon, lung, melanoma
Myc	Transcription factor	Lung, breast, cervix
erb-B	Growth factor receptor	Breast, lung, stomach
Src	Signal transduction	Colon

Tumour suppressor genes

Tumour suppressor genes are genes that act as inhibitors of cellular growth, and mutations in these genes results in 'loss of function'. Consequently, in most cases, both copies of the gene need to be lost before the cellular effects are evident. This would usually mean both copies are lost in the same cell as a somatic event, but in the case of an inherited tumour predisposition, the first 'hit' is inherited (and so is present in all the cells), and the second occurs somatically, often by deletion detected by 'loss of heterozygosity' when tumour is compared to blood. This is the 'two-hit hypothesis' described by Knudson, typically exemplified by retinoblastoma. This explains why the same genes can be involved in both inherited and sporadic tumours, and why inherited tumours typically occur at a younger age and more than once (e.g. a high proportion of retinoblastomas are bilateral and occur at an earlier age than sporadic, unilateral retinoblastomas). It also explains why the cancer predisposition itself is inherited in an autosomal dominant manner (only one copy of the gene mutated) and yet acts in an autosomal recessive manner within the cancer cell (where both copies are inactive). Tumour suppressor genes include:

- cell cycle control genes e.g. *RB1* (G1/S checkpoint), *p53* (transcription of genes for G1/S cell cycle arrest)
- apoptosis genes e.g. *p53* (promotes Bcl2 path to apoptosis)
- telomerase-associated genes
- 'mutator' genes involved in DNA repair (e.g. xeroderma pigmentosum, ataxia telangiectasia and *BRCA1*/*BRCA2*).

Loss of function mutations in *p53* are the most common genetic changes in human cancers, with both alleles inactivated in over 50% of all tumours. Mutation of *p53* can also be inherited, causing Li–Fraumeni syndrome. This is a relatively rare cancer predisposition, characteristically leading to very early-onset breast cancer (under 30 years), childhood tumours (sarcoma, brain tumour, leukaemia, adrenocortical carcinoma) and other adult-onset cancers.

'Mutator' genes leading to genetic instability

This is exemplified by inherited bowel cancer (hereditary non-polyposis colorectal cancer, HNPCC) which is caused by mutations in a group of genes called mismatch repair genes – loss of this crucial function leads to genomic instability, with mutation rates in other genes 2–3-fold increased, so mutations in other crucial genes accumulate more quickly. In the case of HNPCC, the genetic instability can be identified by the finding of microsatellite instability within tumour tissue, which is due either to a germline mutation in one of these genes, or inactivation of one of the same genes within the tumour, most commonly by promoter methylation (an **epimutation**).

Multistep carcinogenesis

The multistep process, whereby a number of these genetic alterations accumulate over time, has been particularly well characterized for colorectal cancer (see Fig. 3.1). Loss of function of an important gatekeeper gene such as *APC* can lead to benign cellular proliferation (polyps or adenomas) that predisposes to the development of malignancy, as further mutations accumulate in the cells. Mutations in mismatch repair genes speed up this process, so that the transition from polyp to cancer is more likely to happen and to happen more quickly.

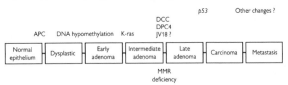

Fig. 3.1 Genetic alterations associated with colorectal carcinogenesis. Mutation frequencies in mismatch repair (MMR)-deficient cells are 2–3 times higher than in normal cells – such mismatch repair mutations are found in >70% of hereditary non-polyposis colorectal cancer (HNPCC) cases and >65% of sporadic colorectal cancers exhibiting microsatellite instability (by sporadic promoter silencing). These cases account for 15–17% of colorectal cancers. (Adapted from Kinzler KW, Vogelstein B (1996) The lessons from hereditary colorectal cancer. *Cell* **87**, 159–70, with permission from Elsevier.)

What is the relevance of genetic changes in sporadic cancers?

Knowledge of the genetic alterations found within individual tumours may provide insights into the molecular processes involved in the aetiology of the tumour, may be useful in classifying tumour subtypes, and has potential to target therapies more effectively (see 📖 pp.196–205). Examples include *HER2* amplification in breast cancers and resistance to taxols/response to herceptin; *BCR-ABL* fusion gene in chronic myeloid leukaemia (CML), or *KIT* mutation in gastrointestinal stromal tumours and response to the tyrosine kinase inhibitor, imatinib. The presence of the abnormal copies of the genes, or the level of amplification, can be used to monitor the response to treatment and has the potential to identify which patients have a high risk of relapse and need further treatment, or to identify relapse at an early stage.

Genetic predisposition to cancer

Epidemiological studies of most cancers have demonstrated a moderate (2–3 times) increase in risk among first-degree relatives of affected individuals. In a minority, this may represent families where an inherited gene alteration confers a high risk of developing a specific cancer; in others, relatives may have an increased susceptibility to developing cancer in response to environmental carcinogens, or may simply share environmental risk factors.

Familial cancers may be recognized by:
• occurrence of rare tumours known to be genetic, e.g. bilateral retinoblastoma
• associated phenotypic features, e.g. multiple polyps in familial adenomatous polyposis, mucosal pigmentation in Peutz–Jegher syndrome, or chromosome breakage in a DNA repair disorder.

In other situations, clues must be sought from the family history:
• unusually early age of onset of the tumour
• multiple or bilateral tumours
• familial clustering of the same tumour type, or of related types (such as breast and ovary, or colon and uterus)

In general, the following may raise suspicion of a familial predisposition:
• three or more close relatives (on the same side of the family) with the same common cancer (or related cancers)
• two or more close relatives (on the same side of the family) with the same common cancer (or related cancers), where one is affected under 50 years
• one close relative with early-onset cancer, e.g. breast cancer under 40 years, bowel cancer under 45 years
• one close relative with multiple primary cancers
• two or more relatives with the same uncommon cancer, e.g. sarcoma, glioma, pancreatic cancer, etc.

Such families should be referred to clinical genetics services, so that the family histories can be verified and risk assessments performed. Sometimes, clinical examination may be needed to seek features of a specific genetic syndrome such as Cowden syndrome (mucosal 'cobblestone' papules, facial trichilemmomas, acral keratoses, craniomegaly), Gorlin syndrome (hypertelorism, frontal bossing, palmar and plantar pits), or neurofibromatosis (café-au-lait patches, cutaneous neurofibromas, axillary freckling). More commonly, there are no specific signs and assessment is based on the family history itself but, if appropriate, cancer surveillance can be arranged for at-risk relatives, although evidence of effectiveness is often lacking and recruitment to trials is important where available.

In a small number of families, molecular genetic testing may be possible, but only where the causative germline mutation can be identified in a blood sample from an affected relative. Thus for many families, no genetic test is possible, either because the family is not thought likely to harbour a mutation in a known predisposition gene, because a sample is not available from an affected relative, or because analysis of the relevant predisposition genes has not identified the causative mutation in the family.

Predictive genetic testing

Where a mutation has been identified in a family, and consent to share the results is available, relatives can be offered a genetic test to find out whether they have inherited the familial predisposition. This would normally be offered via a clinical genetics service, after consultation with a genetic counsellor and with sufficient time to consider all the implications. It is important for the individual to appreciate that a positive result does not make cancer inevitable, and a negative result is not a guarantee against cancer developing. However, it may help guide who needs surveillance, allow decisions to be made about potential risk-reducing surgery, and clarify risks to the next generation. The potential for psychological distress, and for the effect of the findings on other family members as well on the individual being tested, should all be considered. There have been concerns that there may be implications for insurance premiums, which has led to guidelines being drawn up to address these issues in the UK and elsewhere.

Implications of genetic testing for the affected individual

Much of the discussion around predictive genetic testing is often focused on the healthy 'at-risk' individual in the family, rather than on the affected relative whose blood is needed to start the testing process. There may be implications for the affected individual as well that need to be considered:

- many genetic analyses result in a negative result, as no mutation has been identified, but this should NOT be taken to mean that there is no genetic predisposition in the family, merely that it has not been identified
- sometimes no clear result is obtained, i.e. a 'sequence change' is found in the individual's blood, but it is unclear whether this is a benign variant or pathogenic, and further testing may be needed to try to understand its significance
- a positive result may cause some distress to the affected individual, and feelings of guilt if this has been passed on to other family members, especially children
- there may be implications for the individual themselves, such as an increased risk of metachronous cancers, or of cancers at associated sites which may not have been foreseen from the family history (e.g. ovarian cancer risk where a *BRCA1* mutation is found in a breast cancer family).

Common cancer predispositions

Breast cancer family history (see □ Genetics of breast cancer, p.280)
Concern about a family history of breast cancer is a common referral to both clinical genetics and breast clinics. Many women can be reassured, if there is a single relative affected over the age of 40 years, or two relatives but on different sides of the family.

Where it appears that there may be a 'moderate' increase in risk, mammographic surveillance under the age of 50 years may be offered, but in most families genetic testing is unlikely to be useful. This is because the majority of families, if they do harbour breast cancer predisposition genes, will have genes conferring low or moderate increased risk, which are not yet identified or amenable to testing. It may be appropriate to store samples from affected relatives if they wish to do so, or submit such families to research studies with the aim of identifying these genes. An exception may be for families in whom there is Ashkenazi Jewish ancestry, in whom specific mutations in BRCA1 and BRCA2 genes are more likely, and testing for these could be offered after counselling.

For families where there is a higher likelihood of a predisposition gene, and where an affected relative is willing to give a blood sample, genetic analysis for the two major high-risk genes, BRCA1 and BRCA2, can be offered. At present, this is suggested where the chance of identifying a mutation is estimated to be at least 20%, which would include most families with ovarian as well as breast cancers, families with two breast cancers under 30 years, three breast cancers under 40 years, or four breast cancers under 50 years. Occasionally, testing for other genes such as PTEN (Cowden syndrome), or p53 (Li–Fraumeni syndrome) may be considered, depending on the spectrum of cancers that have occurred in the family.

Where a woman is found to carry a BRCA1 or BRCA2 gene mutation, options include mammographic and magnetic resonance imaging (MRI) surveillance, or risk-reducing surgery, and the risk to the ovaries must also be considered.

Bowel cancer family history

An increased risk of bowel cancer may occasionally be due to a recognizable syndrome, identified by the presence of polyps such as familial adenomatous polyposis (FAP) or one of the hamartomatous polyp syndromes (Cowden's syndrome, Peutz–Jegher, juvenile polyposis), and genetic testing can find the causative mutation in the majority of these conditions.

Where adenomatous polyps are present in significant numbers the conditions to consider are:
- FAP – classically over 100 polyps are present in the bowel
- attenuated FAP – presents with fewer than 100 polyps, with an older onset but still has a high risk of progressing to bowel cancer, and the risk for upper gastrointestinal (GI) malignancy. Both these conditions are autosomal dominant and due to mutations in the same gene, but the site of the mutation determines the phenotype

- *MYH*-associated polyposis – this is an autosomal recessive predisposition to adenomatous bowel polyps, so usually presents with a history of bowel cancer in siblings within the family. The majority of affected individuals have one or both of two common mutations within the *MYH* gene, so testing is relatively straightforward.

More commonly, a bowel cancer predisposition is marked only by the familial aggregation of bowel cancer cases, with fewer polyps, and hence is known as hereditary non-polyposis colon cancer (HNPCC), also referred to as Lynch syndrome. In most cases where a genetic predisposition is proven, this is due to mutation in one of the mismatch repair genes (see above), *MLH1*, *MSH2*, *MSH6*, or *PMS2*. The genetic defect leads to defective mismatch repair of DNA, which leads to an increase in mutation rate and faster progression of bowel polyps to cancers. Another consequence is microsatellite instability, which can be observed in the laboratory in tumour tissue, and can be used to identify patients in whom a mismatch repair mutation is more likely.

Thus for individuals concerned about their family history of bowel cancer, the family history can be assessed. Those with only one affected relative over the age of 45 years, or two relatives who are over 55 years, or on different sides of the family may be reassured. Where the family appears to be at 'moderate' risk (one relative under 45 years, two relatives where one is under 55 years at diagnosis, or three affected relatives at any age), permission is sought to access tumour tissue from one of the affected relatives. If this shows microsatellite instability, it may indicate a mismatch repair mutation is present. In this situation, the tumour tissue is also tested to see if there is loss of expression of the mismatch repair proteins, which may help guide which gene to analyse first, and if blood is available from the affected individual, the commonly involved mismatch repair genes are analysed (*MLH1* and *MSH2*). The tumour may also be tested for the common *BRAF* mutation (V600E) found in sporadic bowel cancers with MLH1 promoter hypermethylation and MSI, as finding this mutation would make it unlikely a germline mutation would be found.

Where the family fits the 'Amsterdam criteria' for a high risk of harbouring a mutation, the mismatch repair genes can be analysed irrespective of the tumour analysis. (These families have at least three individuals with bowel cancer in two generations of the family, where at least one is affected under the age of 50 years, and familial polyposis excluded).

If a mutation is found, then relatives can be offered genetic testing to guide surveillance. In the absence of a genetic test, those families thought to be at 'moderately' increased risk are offered colonoscopic surveillance, which may involve a single examination at presentation and repeat at age 55 years, whereas those who are thought to be at 'high risk' of harbouring a predisposition gene (or known gene carriers) are offered two-yearly colonoscopy from age 25 or 35 years, depending on the family history. For families with known mismatch repair genes, the risk of endometrial cancer (40%+) in the women must be remembered, and surveillance for other cancers may also be appropriate (e.g. for gastric cancer in over 50s).

Part 2

Principles of treatment

Surgical oncology

General principles

Surgery is the mainstay of treatment – and principal hope of cure – for most patients with solid tumours. Surgery is most effective when cancer is localized, but substantial numbers of long-term survivors can be achieved with some tumour types that show metastatic disease at presentation. This applies in particular to thyroid and testicular cancer.

Surgery has an advantage over radiotherapy as long-term morbidity of treating tissues without the primary tumour is significantly less; this must be balanced against disruption of normal anatomy inherent in radical resection of cancer, with potential loss of cosmesis and function.

Surgery has three main roles in the management of cancer patients:
- diagnosis and staging
- curative
- palliative.

In addition, there is now growing evidence that surgery in patients with metastases should be considered in selected patients, particularly if the primary tumour has been removed.

There is also a role, in certain tumours, for prophylactic surgery. For example, in familial polyposis coli colon cancer, in the patient who is known to be a *BRCA1* gene carrier (breast cancer), and in some of the multiple endocrine neoplasia (MEN) syndromes (thyroid cancer).

Tumour behaviour

An understanding of tumour biology is essential in the planning of surgical treatment for cancer.

The behaviour of solid tumours is diverse and the implications for surgery are often paradoxical. The three principal methods of spread are:
- direct infiltration
- lymphatic
- blood-borne.

Most cancers disseminate by all three methods, although one method of spread may be predominant. Breast and colorectal cancer exhibit both blood and lymphatic spread, whereas cancers arising in the upper gastrointestinal (GI) tract and the upper airways metastasize via the lymphatics. Even cancers arising from the same cell type behave differently – papillary and follicular tumours of the thyroid give rise to lymphatic and haematogenous metastases, respectively. Different surgical approaches will be required depending on tumour type.

Surgical techniques

The en-bloc technique is most often used in cancers with a pre-dominantly lymphatic spread and is best developed in surgery of head and neck cancer. It is increasingly being used for stomach and oesophageal cancers. No advantage has been reported for aggressive en-bloc resection of loco-regional lymphatics in surgery of large bowel cancer. However, in other areas of cancer surgery there are developments to minimize morbidity.

Sentinel node biopsy has been used for some years in melanoma surgery where the most likely lymph node, which contains metastatic cells, is identified by a radioisotope and/or blue dye. Thereafter, if the gland is positive (on frozen section), the surgeon will proceed to a block resection of the regional nodes. This has now led to the avoidance of block resection of regional nodes in patients who are node negative (with the avoidance of morbidity). The ALMANAC trial of sentinel node biopsy in the UK has provided strong evidence that this will be the management of choice for the axilla in breast cancer patients. However, interesting new controversies have arisen with detailed pathological studies of sentinel nodes. The management of patients with isolated tumour cells and micrometastases (over 0.2 mm and less than 2 mm) is currently debated, with the latter being considered node positive in most centres and the former being node negative (see Rutgers 2008). Sentinel node biopsy is now also used in anal cancer.

One of the major changes in the past two decades is the avoidance of unnecessary surgery in cancer patients. Twenty years ago, the procedure of exploratory laparotomy was not uncommon. Patients were opened and closed with all the associated morbidity and occasional mortality. This is rare, nowadays, with the advances in modern pre-operative imaging, such as ultrasound, computerized tomography (CT), magnetic resonance imaging (MRI), and positron emission tomography (PET) scanning, and also pre-operative image-directed fine needle biopsy. The advances in laparoscopy, as a staging procedure, have also decreased the need for unnecessary surgery.

Minimally invasive cancer surgery

There has been an exponential growth in minimally invasive cancer surgery during the past decade. There are theoretical advantages of decreased hospital stay, rapid return to work, and decreased wound problems. With modern instrumentation and training, there is now a role for laparoscopic cancer surgery in certain areas. Initially, early reports of port site recurrences after laparoscopic surgery for colorectal carcinoma were discouraging. But this is now known to be uncommon (in the region of 1%). Laparoscopic resection is becoming the gold standard in colorectal cancer, renal cancer surgery, and radical prostatectomy. The place of thoracoscopic surgery in oesophageal cancer is less clear but thoracoscopic lung tumour resection is now established. Laparoscopy is used widely in the staging of malignancy and is now part of the work-up protocol in oesophageal, gastric, pancreatic, hepatobilary, and urological tumours.

Conservative and radical surgery

There are increasing data to support conservative resections for selected tumours. For example, minimally invasive follicular carcinoma of the thyroid gland can be dealt with by thyroid lobectomy, as opposed to total thyroidectomy; wide local excision (when followed by radiotherapy) is adequate treatment for selected breast cancer patients provided the resection margin is at least 0.5 cm. Limb-conserving surgery, often with endoprosthetic bone and joint replacement, is suitable for young patients with bone tumours around the knee in highly specialized centres to avoid amputation.

Similarly, multiple liver resections can now be performed, provided the resection margins are clear, without performing formal lobectomy.

Radical surgery still has its place in the patient with large hepatomas, and total mastectomy is still required for large breast cancers. Occasionally, liver transplantation is performed for primary liver cancer or secondary endocrine tumours of the liver but the benefits of such a transplant are debatable.

Reconstructive surgery

To return patients to an adequate and reasonable quality of life after cancer surgery, reconstruction should be offered, where possible (if the patient wishes). For example, after mastectomy the breast can be reconstructed using either an implant, tissue expander, transverse rectus abdominis muscle (TRAM), or latissimus dorsi flaps. This topic has been well reviewed by Cordeiro in 2008. After major head and neck resections, oncological plastic surgeons use free vascularized flaps to replace skin, muscle, and bone. Examples include radial and fibular free flaps. Although the hand transplant is technically feasible, fewer than ten have been performed worldwide because of poor functional results and considerable psychological morbidity.

Prophylactic cancer surgery

Surgery has a very definite role in the prevention of cancer in selected patients. There are a number of conditions, either acquired or inherited, in which preventative surgery has a major role after careful counselling of the patient. These include:

- orchidopexy or occasionally orchidectomy in the patient with a maldescended testis
- total colectomy with pouch procedure, in patients with polyposis coli
- the occasional patient with ulcerative colitis involving the entire colon (over 10 years) and who has changes of dysplasia on mucosal biopsies may require a total colectomy
- patients at risk of medullary cell carcinoma of the thyroid gland, who have the MEN syndrome (type 2) require total thyroidectomy at an early age
- patients carrying the *BRCA1* gene may require prophylactic bilateral mastectomy (and reconstruction); similarly patients with familial ovarian cancer may require a laparoscopic oophorectomy.

Further reading

Colon Cancer Laparoscopic Group (2009) Survival after laparoscopic surgery versus open surgery for colon cancer: long term outcome of a randomised clinical trial. *Lancet Oncol* **10**, 44–52.

Cordeiro P (2008) Breast reconstruction after surgery for breast cancer. *N Engl J Med* **359**, 1590–601.

Damber JE, Aus G (2008) Prostate cancer. *Lancet* **371**, 1710–21.

Depue RH, Pike MC, Henderson BE (1986) Cryptorchidism and testicular cancer. *J Natl Cancer Inst* **77**, 830–3.

Galmiche JP, Pallone F (2005) Barrett's oesophagus and oesophageal adenocarcinoma. *Gut* **54**, 11–142.

Goyal A, Mansell RE (2004) Sentinel lymph node biopsy in breast cancer. *Adv Breast Cancer* **1**, 11–14.

Gretschel S, Warnick P, Bembenek A, *et al.* (2008) Lymphatic mapping and sentinel node biopsy in epidermoid carcinoma of the anal canal. *Eur J Surg* **34**, 890–4.

Killeen SD, O'Sullivan MJ, Coffey JC, *et al.* (2005) Provider volume and outcomes for oncological procedures. *Br J Surg* **92**, 389–402.

Lynch, HT (1996) Is there a role for prophylactic subtotal colectomy among hereditary non-polyposis colorectal cancer germ line mutation carriers? *Dis Colon Rectum* **39**, 109–10.

Lynch HT, De la Chapelle A (2003) Hereditary colorectal cancer. *N Engl J Med* **348**, 919–32.

Machens A, Niccoli-Sire P, Hoeel J, *et al.* (2003) Early malignant progression of hereditary medullary thyroid cancer. *N Engl J Med* **349**, 517–25.

Patel NA, Bergamaschi R (2005) Laparoscopic surgery – beyond mere feasibility. *Surg Clin North Am* **85**, 49–74.

Rutgers EJT (2008) Sentinel node biopsy: interpretation and management of patients with immunohistochemistry-positive sentinel nodes and those with micrometastases. *J Clin Oncol* **26**, 698–702.

Diagnosis and staging

The development of cross-sectional radiology, ultrasound, CT, and MRI – together with the radiologist's ability to perform core biopsies or fine-needle aspiration cytology combined with use of endoscopy and biopsies or cytological brushing – allows pre-operative diagnosis to be made in most cases.

- While fine needle aspiration and core biopsy often give the cancer diagnosis, it is important that the physician, pathologist, or radiologist performing these investigations directs their needle bearing in mind the possibility of tumour seeding. Tumour seeding is not a problem with a fine needle aspiration generally, but may be more of a problem with core biopsy, especially with soft tissue sarcomas. Here, the needle track should be placed after discussion with the surgeon so that the needle track will be excised in the definitive surgery. Fine needle biopsy interpretation requires an experienced and specialized cytopathologist. Core biopsy is especially useful in breast cancer, giving architecture and receptor status.

- The surgeon may still be required to perform either an incisional or an excisional biopsy. In the former, compromise to the future definitive operation must not occur. The excisional biopsy should in many cases be carried out by the appropriate specialist who will be carrying out the definitive surgery. This applies particularly in melanoma where there is controversy over the excision margins (depending upon the depth of the melanoma). A suspicious lesion should be excised for histology with a 2 mm margin.

- When taking biopsies for diagnostic purposes, the surgeon needs to be in close consultation with his pathologist as some tissue samples will need to be sent 'fresh' if electron microscopy or other specialized stains or cytogenetics are required. This applies especially to lymph node excision for lymphoma, where tissue should always be sent fresh to the haematology laboratory.

- Laparoscopy is now accepted as being an excellent tool in the diagnosis and staging of malignancy. While image-directed biopsy can give a diagnosis in a large proportion of patients, some areas are not easily amenable to image-directed biopsy and instead laparoscopic biopsy will often provide the answer. This can include tumours in the mesentery and the retroperitoneal space.

- A further benefit of laparoscopic diagnosis in staging is the use of intra-operative ultrasonography via the laparoscope. This allows detection and biopsy of masses (and staging) in solid organs such as the liver. Lesions smaller than 1 cm can be identified and biopsied and even treated by laparoscopic ablation techniques. The addition of Doppler ultrasound allows the identification of vascular structures and their avoidance (intra-operatively). The oncologist must be aware of the possibility of port site recurrences in the patient with ascites and widespread carcinomatosis.

- Laparoscopy is used for staging the following malignancies prior to definitive surgery:
  - oesophageal cancer
  - gastric cancer
  - pancreatic cancer
  - liver cancer
  - prostatic cancer
  - ovarian cancer.

Laparosopic staging is useful in selected patients with lymphoma.

- Surgery will provide the pathologist with specimens, including the adjacent lymph nodes to help stage the tumours. The advent of sentinel node biopsy in melanoma and breast cancer allows staging of these tumours with much less morbidity. Sentinel node biopsy is also being investigated for other tumours, including gastric, colon, head, and neck.

Curative surgery

The long-term outcome after cancer surgery depends on tumour type and the stage of presentation. Survival rates for some cancers have improved due to earlier presentation following public awareness and screening programmes, e.g. breast cancer, cervical cancer, and the current colon cancer screening programme. Improving techniques mean larger resections can be carried out with low risk, often with excellent functional results, e.g. limb-preserving surgery for osteosarcoma; many liver resections today require little (or no) blood transfusion. In the central nervous system (CNS), vital structures continue to inhibit the extent of resection.

For some cancers, results are good – 5-year survival rate in breast cancer is over 80% and for large bowel cancer in the USA it approaches 70%. Unfortunately, the cure rate for pancreatic and gastric cancer remains low with 5-year survival figures less than 10% in Europe. Lung cancer patients still have an overall survival of only 15% at 5 years. Ideally, long-term tumour control can be obtained if all the cancer is removed at surgery.

- The limits of cancer clearance are extremely important, and close co-operation between the surgeon and the pathologist is essential. For example, wide local excision for breast cancer needs to have a clearance of between 0.5 and 1 cm and most patients require radiotherapy following partial mastectomy to prevent local recurrence.
- Similarly it is now recognized that in colorectal cancer surgery a 5 cm limit proximally and a 2 cm limit distally are required for adequate clearance. It is important that limits of excision are not compromised in the learning curve of laparoscopic colonic resection.
- Total mesorectal excision is essential to prevent local recurrence in the pelvis after rectal cancer. There is now clear evidence of the benefit of specialization in rectal cancer surgery.
- Cancers that are prone to multiple foci require consideration of wider resection to excise all the tumour. This occurs, for example, in papillary carcinoma of the thyroid gland where total thyroidectomy in some cases is appropriate.
- There is now increasing evidence that in major oncological surgery the procedure should be carried out by a specialist in a unit doing a high volume of that particular procedure. The evidence is now growing that this applies to rectal, oesophageal, gastric, and pancreatic cancer.

The use of laparoscopy in the definitive treatment of malignancy is evolving. Concerns in evolution have included a satisfactory oncological resection, i.e. clear margins and lymph node removal, and whether there is proven benefit over conventional surgery, with decreased morbidity, more rapid return to work, and finally, and most important, to ensure that there is no negative impact on survival. Multiple trials are ongoing in a number of cancer areas.

The following cancers are currently being evaluated as being suitable for laparoscopic resection:
- oesophageal
- gastric
- pancreatic (difficult, specialized surgery, data unclear)

- liver – resection (increasing evidence of safe laparoscopic approach with as good survival as open)
- colon (a standard resection including that of the colon and rectum and especially including mesorectal resection can now be performed safely laparoscopically). Several trials show as good results as open surgery. Long-term survival is equal to conventional surgery
- the kidney and prostate – over 1000 patients in Germany have been reported. In the hands of an experienced laparoscopic surgeon, these resections appear to be safe. Long-term data are just coming through (equal survival to open surgery)
- gynaecological – laparoscopic resection in specialized centres, is safe, with equally good long-term survival as open surgery.

Further reading

Alexakis N, Halloran C, Raraty M, et al. (2004) Current standards of surgery for pancreatic cancer. Br J Surg **91**, 1410–27.

Carpelan-Holmstrom M, Nordling S, Pukkala E, et al. (2005) Does anyone survive pancreatic ductal adenocarcinoma? Gut **54**, 385–7.

Hogan AM, Kennelly R, Winter DC (2009) Volume–outcome analysis in rectal cancer. A plea for enquiring, evidence and evolution. Eur J Surgl Oncol **35**, 111–12.

Lo CM, Fan ST (2004) Liver transplantation for hepatocellular carcinoma. Br J Surg **91**, 131–3.

Ryder S (2005) Predicting survival in early hepatocellular carcinoma. Gut **54**, 328–9.

Thirlwell C, Nathan P (2008) Melanoma management. BMJ **337**, 1345–8.

Thompson JF, Scolyer RA, Kefford RF (2005) Cutaneous melanoma. Lancet **365**, 687–701.

Tsang WWC, Chung CC, Kwok SY, Li MKW (2005) Minimally invasive surgery for rectal cancer. Surg Clin North Am **85**, 61–73.

Tsao H, Atkins MB, Sober AJ (2004) Medical progress – management of cutaneous melanoma. N Engl J Med **351**, 998–1012.

Wu CC, Cheng SB, Ho WM, et al. (2005) Liver resection for hepatocellular carcinoma in patients with cirrhosis, Br J Surg **92**, 348–55.

Palliative surgery

Surgical palliation falls into several different categories, requiring a broad range of expertise and knowledge. A patient's life expectancy may vary from weeks to years depending on their condition, and the surgeon must know when not to operate and to utilize palliative care teams and interventional radiology, as well as being able to decide when and what operation is required. Discussion at a multidisciplinary meeting is essential.

Bowel obstruction

Patients with colon or ovarian cancer make up the bulk of those developing small or large bowel obstruction. In a colon cancer patient, confirmation of incurability will usually be made at laparotomy, following a decision to treat a large bowel obstruction. Where possible, these patients should have the primary cancer excised and intestinal continuity restored by primary anastomosis. In selected patients endoscopic stent placement is appropriate but there is a 4% perforation risk and 12% incidence of stent migration. Management of the obstructed ovarian cancer patient is usually more difficult, as the key decision is often whether or not the patient should have the operation. A multidisciplinary team discussion of these difficult patients, in consultation with the patients and their families, is essential. Generally, a combined approach involving a colorectal surgeon and a cancer gynaecologist is best.

Many patients will have multiple obstruction sites, with small and large bowel studded with tumours on the serosal surface. Such patients are not suitable for surgical palliation. Others will have one or two site obstructions, e.g. a segment of terminal ileum embedded in pelvic tumour. They can benefit from debulking, resection, and anastomosis or bypass surgery.

Differentiating these categories of patient can usually be done by a history of crampy abdominal pain, clinical examination revealing a distended tympanitic abdomen (as opposed to an abdomen with multiple sites of palpable tumour and ascites), plain X-rays revealing many loops of distended bowel with air-fluid levels, and CT evidence of pelvic or other single-site tumour deposit.

Laparoscopy will sometimes be helpful in the obstructed patient who has not had previous abdominal surgery. With modern techniques, laparoscopic bypass can be carried out by suitably trained surgeons in selected patients. This requires great care in the obstructed patient.

Fistulas

Fistulas caused by pelvic tumours or post-radiotherapy include:
- rectovaginal
- enterovaginal
- colovesical
- vesicovaginal
- a combination of the above.

Pre-operative assessment to determine the exact type of fistula is important. A proximal end sigmoid colostomy, which can usually be performed without a formal laparotomy, is the treatment of choice for most rectovaginal fistulas if definitive surgery is not possible. Patients with combined rectovaginal and vesicovaginal fistulas may need an end colostomy and ileal conduit. A covered stent, delivered endoscopically or radiologically, should be considered for patients with a colovesical fistula. Patients with an enterovesical fistula will require laparotomy, resection of small bowel segment, and anastomosis. For low vaginal fistulas colo-anal sleeve procedures may be helpful. This should be done by an appropriate colorectal specialist.

Jaundice

Obstructive jaundice can be palliated surgically by choledochoenterostomy or cholecystenterostomy, although these procedures have been largely superseded by endoscopic and radiological placement of stents. Stents can become blocked, resulting in repeated cholangitis. A trial has demonstrated a shorter overall hospital stay and decreased morbidity for surgical palliation of jaundice compared to endoscopic stenting and this should be considered in medically fit patients. Selected patients with inoperable hilar tumours will be best treated by segment III biliary enteric bypass. In those patients who require surgical bypass of obstructive jaundice, laparoscopic techniques by appropriately trained surgeons have a role in selected patients.

Ascites

Peritoneal-venous (LeVeen) shunts can be inserted to relieve ascites in selected cases. Patients with ascites due to ovarian cancer have the longest survival and occasionally such patients, where the ascites has not responded to chemotherapy, may be suitable for a shunt. Careful preoperative assessment should be undertaken to ensure that the ascites is not loculated and that the tumour is not mucinous; otherwise the shunt will become blocked. These are usually inserted using local anaesthetic and sedation, with >50% of patients achieving good, long-term palliation. Post-operative coagulopathy may be a problem.

Pain

There are a number of options open to oncological surgeons to help patients with pain:

- surgical debulking of large, slow-growing tumours (e.g. intra-abdominal, soft-tissue sarcomas in otherwise fit patients where the expected morbidity of the procedure is low)
- stabilization of pathological fractures and prophylactic pinning of bone metastases involving >50% of cortex
- neurosurgical approaches for pain control including cordotomy (rare nowadays with modern pain teams)
- thoracoscopic splanchnectomy for intractable pain secondary to pancreatic cancer (again rare with the advent of the coeliac plexus block).

Generally, with modern pain management and specialist pain clinics, the requirement for a surgical approach to the spinal cord or to peripheral nerves is now rare.

Gastrointestinal bleeding

A wide array of endoscopic and radiological techniques is available to stop bleeding from benign and malignant causes in incurable cancer patients, including injection sclerotherapy (benign ulceration), laser coagulation (neoplastic ulcers), and radiological embolization (should other methods fail). Surgery should be reserved for those with a life expectancy of 3 months or more, for whom other methods fail. Usually the interventional radiologist can deal with most bleeding sources in the cancer patient.

Cytoreductive surgery

In some patients, extensive local disease may prevent removal of all disease by surgery but partial resection is still appropriate. This applies particularly to ovarian cancer where subsequent chemotherapy can lead to good results, even in advanced disease. Indeed several debulking procedures following chemotherapy are appropriate in specialized centres.

Palliative resection of the primary tumour

Up to 10% of patients with breast cancer will present with metastatic disease; patients with visceral metastases have a poor prognosis but patients with bone metastases have a median survival of over 2 years. Resection of the primary tumour to achieve loco-regional control will often improve patients' quality of life, preventing fungation or uncontrolled axillary metastases.

Patients with colorectal cancer are staged prior to surgery to determine the most appropriate therapy. In those in whom unresectable liver metastases are identified, primary tumour resection, especially laparoscopic, should still be considered to minimize the risk of bleeding, perforation, or obstruction, which may subsequently occur.

Laparoscopic surgery has a definite role in the palliation of malignancy. For example, gastric outlet obstruction, intestinal obstruction, biliary bypass for obstructive jaundice (pancreatic cancer); feeding tubes for nutrition can also be placed laparoscopically, the colon and small bowel can be decompressed, and stomata can be created using minimally invasive techniques.

Further reading

Avantumde AA, Parsons SL (2007) Pattern and prognostic factors in patients with malignant ascites: a retrospective study. *Ann Oncol* **18**, 945–9.

Baron TH (2001) Expandable metal stents for the treatment of cancerous obstruction of the gastrointestinal tract. *N Engl J Med*. **344**, 1681–7.

Chao TC, Wang CS, Chen MF (1999) Gastroduodenal perforation in cancer patients. *Hepatogastroenterology* **46**, 2878–81.

Helyer LK, Law CH, Butler M *et al.* (2007) Surgery as a bridge to palliative chemotherapy in patients with malignant bowel obstruction from colorectal cancer. *Ann Surg Oncol* **14**, 1264–71.

Hill J (2008) Stenting and colorectal cancer. *Br J Surg* **95**, 1195–6.

Mittal A, Windsor J, Woodfield J, *et al.* (2004) Matched study of three methods for palliation of malignant pyloroduodenal obstruction. *Br J Surg* **91**, 205–9.

Randall TC, Rubin SC (2000) Management of intestinal obstruction in the patient with ovarian cancer. *Oncology* **14**, 1159–63.

Rose PG, Nerenstone S, Brady MF (2004) Secondary surgical cytoreduction for advanced ovarian carcinoma. *N Engl J Med* **351**, 2489–97.

Zanon C, Grosso M, Apra F, *et al.* (2002) Palliative treatment of malignant refractory ascites by positioning of Denver peritoneovenous shunt. *Tumori* **88**, 123–7.

Surgery for metastatic disease

In principle, patients with a single site of metastatic disease, and the occasional patient with multiple metastases, should be considered for resection. Some patients with limited secondary deposits in the lung, liver, or brain may have prolonged survival, but the patients should be carefully assessed at a multi-disciplinary team meeting to consider fitness for major surgery, likely benefit, potential complications, and patient and family wishes.

Lymphatic clearance
- May be curative.
- May avoid need for adjuvant chemotherapy or radiotherapy (avoids the need for axillary radiotherapy in breast cancer).
- Useful in:
  - breast cancer
  - colorectal cancer and gastric cancer – limited role
  - head and neck cancer
  - penile cancer
- No role for prophylactic nodal block surgery in melanoma.
- There is a role for sentinel node dissection in breast and melanoma. In the UK the ALMANAC (2004) trial showed benefit in breast cancer. Once UK breast surgeons have been trained, routine axillary clearance will be uncommon.

Liver metastases
- Some secondaries are unsuitable for resection.
- The natural history of liver metastases must be considered – mean survival of 16 months without treatment. Benefit of surgery to selected patients with colorectal secondaries:
  - 40% 5-year survival
  - 1% operative mortality in specialized centres
  - 20% post-operative morbidity.
- Better survival if:
  - one lobe (compared to two)
  - size of secondary <5 cm
  - margin >1 cm – now debate that lesser margin is safe
  - metachronous resection as opposed to synchronous.
- Repeated liver resection is possible.
- Benefit of liver resection for non-colorectal cancer is controversial and uncertain because of the frequency of recurrent tumour at other sites.
- Liver resection for endocrine liver metastases gives a 5-year survival up to 50%.
- Up to 60% 5-year survival has been reported for resection of liver secondaries from the genitourinary tract (including testis, ovary, kidney, uterus).
- Resection of liver secondaries from other primary sites is of unproven benefit. No benefit for breast secondaries.
- Laparoscopic liver resection is now used widely.

Other treatment options
- Cryotherapy
- Laser (may have a role but unproven currently)

- Radiofrequency ablation – good early results in USA for small tumours
- Injection of alcohol (used in Japan) (percutaneous under image guidance)

Lung metastases

- Spread to lung is via lymphatics or blood-borne.
- The lung is the second commonest site for metastases. In one-fifth of patients, the lung is the sole site of metastases.
- Diagnosis: combination of chest X-ray, CT, MRI, and PET.
- Criteria for lung resection include metastatic disease limited to the lung, primary tumour controlled, and medically fit patient.
- Metastasectomy can be formed with low morbidity and mortality and can be performed repeatedly (thoracoscopic techniques now commonplace).
- 10–60% 5-year survival after resection of solitary lung secondary has been reported.
- Long-term survival in patients with primary tumours of:
  - kidney
  - testis
  - colon
  - sarcoma.
- Median survival of over 36 months for completely resected patients is now possible in patients with sarcoma
- Very rarely, lung transplantation has been carried out with preliminary data of 50% survival in 5 years – this is still a controversial area.
- Survival data after resection of lung metastases (usually performed thoracoscopically):
  - osteosarcoma, 40% 5-year survival
  - soft tissue sarcoma, 25–40% 5-year survival
  - cancer of the colon, 35% 5-year survival
  - renal cell carcinoma, 40% 5-year survival
  - breast carcinoma, 38% 5-year survival (rarely done)
  - head and neck cancer, 50% 5-year survival
  - gynaecological cancer, 35% 5-year survival
  - melanoma, 20% 5-year survival (in selected cases)
  - germ cell tumours, 86% 5-year survival, 74% 10-year survival (some germ cell secondaries contain only necrotic cells following chemotherapy).

Bone metastases

- Presentation is usually that of a pathological fracture.
- Breast and prostate are the most common primary sites followed by lung, thyroid, and renal cancer.
- Mean survival is 3 months with lung cancer to over 4 years with breast cancer.
- Investigations: MRI and PET scanning are the most accurate investigations, followed by bone scanning.
- Internal fixation is useful if:
  - weight-bearing bone, especially if lesion is >2.5 cm or involves circumference
  - painful secondary after radiotherapy
  - will improve mobilization and nursing care

- patient is fit
- bone quality will support fixation.
- Considerations in spinal secondary:
  - stability of spine
  - spinal cord compression.

Treatment options
- Radiotherapy.
- Hormone manipulation.
- Surgery – stabilization preceded by bone tumour biopsy (occasionally it is possible to excise the secondary deposit).
- Internal fixation techniques include plates, intramedullary nails, prosthetic replacement of metaphyseal lesions.
- Occasionally cast or brace immobilization or external fixation is used for patients with extensive localized disease that cannot be immobilized by internal methods. Rarely is amputation appropriate, except for fungating tumours, recurrent infections, and intractable pain.
- Minimally invasive treatment of metastatic bone lesions with radiographically guided percutaneous injection of bone cement is currently used in selected cases, e.g. in the spine.

Brain metastases
- Common: up to 10% of cancer patients have brain secondaries.
- The 5-year cumulative incidence of brain metastases is 16%, 10%, 7%, 5%, and 1% for patients with lung cancer, renal cell cancer, melanoma, breast cancer, and colorectal cancer, respectively. The lung and breast are the commonest primary sites.
- Blood-borne: the distribution of brain metastases reflects blood flow – 80% of lesions are found in the cerebrum, 15% in the cerebellum, and 5% in the brainstem.
- Presentations include headache, focal weakness, altered mental status, and epilepsy.
- Haemorrhage within brain metastases may cause an acute neurological state.
- Diagnosis is by MRI (this picks up smaller secondaries).
- Mean survival without therapy is 2 months, 3 months with steroid therapy, 6 months with radiotherapy.
- Surgery is useful to confirm diagnosis, relieve pressure effects, improve local control and survival (in selected cases).
- Survival is poor in patients with systemic uncontrolled disease, poor general medical condition, tumours lying infratentorially, poor neurological status, and a short interval from the diagnosis of the primary tumour to the diagnosis of the brain metastases.
- Tumour deposits in the thalamus, brainstem, and basal ganglia are usually irresectable.
- Resection of a single secondary can lead to prolonged survival (melanoma 7 months, lung cancer 12 months, renal cell cancer 10 months, breast cancer 1 year, and colon cancer 9 months). Occasionally resection of multiple metastases is worthwhile:
  - good palliation
  - underused

- occasionally curative
- post-operative radiotherapy helps
- anatomical site important.

Malignant pleural effusion

- Surgery is rarely indicated as these can usually be managed medically.
- Occasional role for thoracoscopy to drain fluid, break down adhesions, biopsy the pleura, and instill sclerosing agents such as talc or bleomycin.
- Rarely, pleurectomy is performed in malignant mesothelioma but there is significant morbidity and the mortality is 10%. The procedure can only be performed in very selected patients.
- Occasionally the insertion of a pleuroperitoneal shunt has been used with limited benefit.

Malignant pericardial effusion

In selected patients the creation of a pericardial window compares favourably with pericardial percutaneous drainage.

Malignant ascites

While most patients with malignant ascites can be treated medically, peritoneal venous shunting (Denver shunt) is useful in those with a reasonable life expectancy. Shunt occlusion and coagulopathy are limiting factors.

Further reading

Abu Hilal M, McPhail MJW, Zeidan B, et al. (2008) Laparoscopic versus open left lateral hepatic sectionectomy. Eur J Surg Oncol **34**, 1285–8.

Assal M, Zanone X, Peter A (2000) Osteosynthesis of metastatic lesions of the proximal femur with a solid femoral nail and interlocking spinal plate inserted without reaming. J Orthop Trauma **14**, 394–7.

Cheung G, Chow E, Holden L (2006) Percutaneous vertebroplasty in patients with intractable pain from osteoporotic or metastatic fratures. Can Assoc Rad J **57**, 13–21.

Fuchs B, Ossendorf D, Leerapun T, Sim FH (2008) Intercalary segmental reconstruction after bone tumour resection. Eur J Surg Oncol **34**, 1271–6.

Inoue M, Kotake Y, Nakagawa K, et al. (2000) Surgery for pulmonary metastases from colorectal carcinoma. Ann Thorac Surg **70**, 380–3.

Kaibara N, Sumi K, Yonakawa M, et al. (1990) Does extensive dissection of lymph nodes improve the result of surgical treatment of gastric cancer? Am J Surg **159**, 218–21.

Ko AS, Lefor AT (2005) Laparoscopic surgery in cancer. In: Devita VT, Hellman S, Rosenberg SA, eds. Principles and practice of oncology, 7th edn. Philadelphia: Lippincott, pp. 253–66.

Lodge JPA, Menon KV, Fenwick SW, et al. (2005) In-contiguity and non-anatomical extension of right trisegmentectomy for liver metastases. Br J Surg **92**, 340–7.

Prasad D, Schiff D (2005) Malignant spinal cord compression. Lancet Oncol **6**, 15–24.

Sciubba DM, Gokaslan ZL, Suk I, et al. (2007) Positive and negative prognostic variables for patients undergoing open surgery for metastatic breast disease. Eur Spine J **16**, 1659–67.

Thompson JF, Scolyer RA, Kefford RF (2005) Cutaneous melanoma. Lancet **365**, 687–701.

Vogelsang H, Haas S, Hierholzer C, et al. (2005) Factors influencing survival after resection of pulmonary metastases from colorectal cancer. Br J Surg **91**, 1066–71.

Wilkinson AN, Viola R, Brandege MD (2008) Managing skeletal related events resulting from bone metastases. BMJ **337**, 1101–105.

Yim AP, Ho JK (1995) Video assisted subxiphoid pericardiectomy. J Laparoendosc Surg **5**, 193–8.

Principles of radiation oncology

Introduction

Radiation oncology or radiotherapy is the treatment of malignant disease with ionizing radiation, most commonly using high-energy X-ray beams, external beam radiotherapy (EBRT). This treatment modality has been developed over the last 100 years, with considerable technical and clinical advances. It is now arguably the most important non-surgical cancer therapy, used in more than 50% of all patients with malignant disease.

Historical perspective

1896   Discovery of X-rays
1898   Discovery of radium
1899   Successful treatment of skin cancer with X-rays
1915   Treatment of cervical cancer with radium implant
1922   Cure of laryngeal cancer with a course of X-ray therapy
1928   Roentgen defined as unit of radiation exposure
1934   Dose fractionation principles proposed
1950s   Radioactive cobalt teletherapy (1 MV energy)
1960s   Production of megavoltage X-rays by linear accelerators
1990s   3-dimensional radiotherapy planning
2000s   Intensity-modulated (IMRT), image-guided (IGRT), and stereotactic radiotherapy

When X-rays pass through living tissue, energy is absorbed, resulting in ionization of a number of molecules, with generation of fast-moving electrons and free radicals. Biologically, the most important effects involve DNA, where radiation may cause damage including breaks in the DNA double helix.

SI unit for dose of radiation is the gray (Gy), energy absorbed per unit mass (joules/kilogramme).

Biological effects of radiotherapy relate to both the dose of radiation and the timing of delivery of this treatment. Early clinical experience with radiotherapy demonstrated that delivery of small daily doses or fractions of radiotherapy allowed the administration of a larger total dose of radiation than could be safely given as a single fraction, with preferential reduction in normal tissue damage while maintaining cell kill in malignant tissue. This provides the basis of fractionated radiotherapy in modern radiation oncology, in which the majority of treatments are delivered using small daily doses over consecutive days/weeks.

Fractionation is the division of a total dose of EBRT into small, often once-daily doses. It results in preferential sparing of normal tissue damage, allowing safe delivery of higher total doses of radiation with increased cancer cell kill.

Radiobiology of normal tissues

Effects of radiation on tissues are generally mediated by one of two mechanisms:
- loss of mature functional cells by apoptosis (programmed cell death, usually within 24 h of irradiation)
- loss of cellular reproductive capacity.

In general, these effects are dose dependent; increasing doses of radiation produce greater cell loss. However, different cell types show large differences in radiosensitivity to either of these processes. A limited number of cell types predominantly respond by apoptosis. These include some cells of haemopoietic lineage, and salivary glands. As most tissues or organs have redundant functional cells, they may lose a significant fraction of this cell population by apoptosis without clinical impairment of tissue function. Usually lost cells are replaced by proliferation of surviving stem cells or progenitor cells. These may be cells surviving in irradiated tissue or cells migrating from unirradiated margins.

Radiosensitivity of normal tissues

Highly sensitive	Lymphocytes, germ cells
Moderately sensitive	Epithelial cells
Resistant	Central nervous system (CNS), connective tissue

When cell loss occurs predominantly through loss of proliferative capacity, the rate of cell renewal of a particular organ determines the time of appearance of tissue damage, varying from days to even years after irradiation. This has led to the arbitrary distinction of acute and late effects of radiation, with acute effects being restricted to changes developing during a course of radiotherapy of up to 8 weeks.

Acute effects of radiation

Acute effects involve mainly the skin, mucosa, and haemopoietic system. Although initial cell loss may be partly through apoptosis, the predominant effect is loss of reproductive capacity, interfering with the replacement of lost cells. Thus, tissues with fast normal cellular turnover (epithelia of skin and gut, bone marrow) display effects of irradiation earliest.

The timing of radiation effects also depends on the rate of dose administration or fractionation. After a single dose of 10 Gy to the abdomen, the mucosal lining of the intestinal tract is depleted in a few days, while it may take several weeks during a fractionated course of radiotherapy with daily doses of 2 Gy.

The speed of recovery of acute reaction depends on the level of stem cell depletion, and varies from a few days to several months. If the number of surviving stem cells is too low, severe epithelial damage may persist as a chronic ulcer.

Acute effects of radiotherapy

- Occur within 8 weeks of treatment
- Skin, gastrointestinal (GI) tract, bone marrow
- Severity depends on total dose of radiation and length of time over which radiotherapy delivered
- Treatment doses selected so that complete recovery is usual

Late effects of radiotherapy

Late effects occur predominantly in slowly proliferating tissues (such as the lung, kidney, heart, liver, and CNS) but are not restricted to these slowly renewing cell systems. For example, in the skin, in addition to the acute epidermal reactions, late changes can develop several years later.

By definition, late radiation reactions are not apparent until a considerable time after irradiation and these are not always predicted by the severity of the acute reaction. Although the total dose of radiation is most important, another major determinant of late radiation effect is the dose of radiation per fraction of treatment.

Late effects of radiotherapy

- Lung, kidney, CNS, heart, connective tissue
- Severity depends on total dose of radiation and dose per fraction (small dose per fraction protects)
- Recovery may be incomplete

The distinction between acute and late effects has important clinical implications. Since acute reactions are observed during the course of a conventionally fractionated radiotherapy schedule (~2 Gy per fraction, 5 times a week), it is possible to reduce the total dose in the event of unexpectedly severe reactions, allowing a sufficient number of stem cells to survive. Surviving stem cells will repopulate and restore the integrity of the rapidly proliferating tissue, preventing irreparable damage.

If the overall treatment time is reduced, for example by the use of dose fractions >2 Gy, the acute reactions may not reach maximal intensity until after completion of treatment. This precludes adjustment of the dose regimen to the severity of reactions. If intensive fractionation schedules reduce the number of surviving stem cells to below the level needed for effective tissue restoration, acute reactions may persist as chronic injury.

Radiation effects in specific tissues

Skin: acute effects

- Erythema 'sunburn' reaction:
  - starting week 2–3
  - skin feels hot, itchy, sore
- Desquamation:
  - initially dry peeling of epidermis
  - later moist and painful with exposure of dermis
  - usually heals within 6 weeks of treatment completion; residual pigmentation fades over months
- Ulceration only if above reaction fails to heal.

Skin: late effects (months/years)
- Atrophy
- Fibrosis
- Telangiectasia.

Oral mucosa
- Erythema starting week 2–3
- Painful ulceration week 4–6
- Usually healed 4 weeks post-radiotherapy
- Dry mouth may persist as late effect depending on volume of salivary glands irradiated and dose.

Gastrointestinal tract
- Acute mucositis causes site-specific effects starting weeks 1–4
- Oesophagitis
- Gastric/small bowel – 5-hydroxytryptamine ($5\text{-}HT_3$)-mediated nausea and vomiting
- Distal small bowel/colon – diarrhoea
- Rectum – tenesmus, mucous discharge, bleeding
- Late effects – mucosal ulceration, fibrosis/obstruction, necrosis.

CNS
- No acute reaction
- 2–6 months – demyelination effects:
  - brain – somnolence
  - spinal cord – Lhermitte's syndrome (shooting pains radiating down limbs below the level of injury, sometimes provoked by spinal flexion)
- 1–2 years, radiation necrosis (irreversible neurological deficit).

Lung
- Acute deterioration airways obstruction after large (e.g. 8 Gy) single fractions
- 2–6 months – radiation pneumonitis:
  - cough, dyspnoea, reversible X-ray changes
  - may improve with steroid therapy
- 6–12 months – irreversible lung fibrosis.

Kidney
- No acute response
- Large reserve capacity, effects occur up to 10 years post-radiotherapy
- Radiation nephropathy:
  - proteinuria
  - hypertension
  - renal failure.

Heart
- 6–24 months: pericarditis (self-limiting)
- >2 years: cardiomyopathy and conduction blocks.

Normal tissue tolerance to re-treatment

Previously it was believed that the late effects of radiotherapy were irreversible, and treatment of an area of the body that had previously been irradiated to high dose carried risk of serious morbidity. Recent studies have shown that some tissues and organs have a substantial ability to recover from subclinical radiation injury, allowing the retreatment of previously irradiated sites. The large capacity of the CNS for long-term regeneration allows the safe retreatment of parts of the brain or the spinal cord and offers new clinical possibilities for tumours recurring in or near these critical structures.

Carcinogenesis

DNA damage caused by radiotherapy may cause the development of a new cancer. Secondary malignancy may occur 5–30 years after radiation exposure. Leukaemias occur most frequently at 6–8 years after radiotherapy. Solid cancers may occur after 10–30 years, and certain organs such as the thyroid and breast are particularly susceptible to developing secondary cancer, especially when exposure to radiation occurs in childhood/young adulthood.

- Induction of a second cancer is a rare but serious consequence of exposure to ionizing radiation, often with a long latent period.
- For oncology patients such risks must always be weighed against the risk of recurrence of cancer.

Repair of radiation-induced DNA damage

Some of the DNA lesions caused by radiation can be repaired. When more than one fraction of radiotherapy is delivered daily, a minimum gap of 6–8 h between fractions is required to allow repair, without which excessive normal tissue damage occurs. A number of rare hereditary defects in DNA repair exist, and some of these predispose to cancer (e.g. ataxia telangiectasia). The use of conventional doses of radiotherapy to treat these cancers may result in severe normal tissue reactions.

Hypoxia

Hypoxic cells are 2–3 times less sensitive to radiotherapy than oxygenated cells, and in many cancers there are areas of hypoxia relating to the abnormal blood supply of the cancer. Anaemia may aggravate this. During a fractionated course of radiotherapy, response of the cancer to treatment may result in reoxygenation of areas of initial hypoxia, further enhancing tumour cell kill.

Radiotherapy fractionation

Objective

To choose for a course of EBRT the most appropriate combination of:
- total dose of radiotherapy (Gy) to achieve the required effect on the cancer
- number of doses or fractions
- overall treatment time (determined by number of fractions per week).

Linear quadratic model

At clinically relevant doses, cancers and early-reacting tissues respond to ionizing radiation with a linear relationship between dose and cell kill – the linear or α component. In the late-reacting tissues, a large part of the effect of radiation is related to the square of the individual dose given – the quadratic element or β component.

The important implication of the linear quadratic model is that, by giving radiotherapy in many small doses, damage in the late-reacting tissues should be minimized, with little or no alteration in the response of the early-reacting normal tissues and, most importantly, the cancer.

Number of treatments

Traditionally radiotherapy has been delivered once daily, Monday to Friday, and two different fractionation schedules are widely used.

Few large daily fractions

- Advantages:
  - fewer attendances
  - sparing of resources
  - fast tumour response
  - reduces risk of tumour repopulation during treatment course
- Disadvantages:
  - limits total dose that can be safely delivered
  - increases risk of late normal tissue damage
  - reduced potential for reoxygenation
  - total dose is usually inadequate to eradicate all cancer cells in target

Many small daily fractions

- Advantages:
  - less severe acute reactions (longer treatment time)
  - reduced late normal tissue damage
  - maximizes total dose that can be delivered
  - maximizes reoxygenation
  - total dose may be sufficient to eradicate all cancer cells
  - total dose may be reduced if unexpectedly severe acute reaction
- Disadvantages:
  - demand on resources and patient
  - potential for repopulation of fast-growing tumours during radiotherapy
  - prolonged acute reaction may need supportive treatment, e.g. dietary support for sore mouth/oesophagitis

Radiosensitivity of tumours

Some tumours, such as lymphoma and seminoma, may be controlled by doses (30–40 Gy) approximately half that required for many carcinomas (60–70 Gy); others including gliomas and sarcomas may be resistant to the highest doses that can be safely delivered.

Tolerance doses of normal tissues

Some tissues are particularly radiosensitive and doses to them must be limited in order to minimize the risk of late damage. If 2 Gy/fraction is given, then tolerance doses are:

- testis   2 Gy
- lens of the eye   10 Gy
- whole kidney   20 Gy
- whole lung   20 Gy
- spinal cord   50 Gy
- brain   60 Gy

The risk of significant late and irreparable damage rises acutely above these levels.

The inter-fraction interval

After a radiation treatment, some of the damage induced is irreversible but some can be repaired. With once-daily fractionation, nearly all of the repair process is complete before the next treatment is given. If more than one treatment is given during a day, the duration of time between fractions should be at least 6 h to allow as much repair as possible in normal tissues.

Hyperfractionation

By giving many fractions of <2 Gy, a higher total radiation dose may be delivered without an increase in late normal tissue damage. In order to avoid increasing the total time for the treatment course, treatment may be given at weekends, or more than once daily.

Overall treatment time and accelerated radiotherapy

There is now evidence that some cancers (e.g. lung cancer) have the capacity for rapid proliferation, with significant potential for growth during a conventional 6-week course of radiotherapy. By shortening the overall duration of a treatment course, the opportunity for this to occur is reduced. This approach may be combined with hyperfractionation by treating 2–3 times daily to minimize late normal tissue damage.

In a randomized controlled trial, the CHART regimen (Continuous Hyperfractionated Accelerated RadioTherapy), in which 54 Gy is given in 1.5 Gy fractions 3 times on each of 12 consecutive days, proved superior to conventional radiotherapy (60 Gy in 30 fractions in 6 weeks) in non-small-cell lung cancer without any increase in late normal tissue damage.

The optimum fractionation regimen

The clinical circumstances dominate the choice of regimen for each individual patient. Treatment is broadly divided by intention, either curative or palliative.

Radical radiotherapy
- The highest tolerable dose is usually given to maximize probability of eradication of cancer.
- Lower doses for highly radiosensitive malignancies and to eradicate microscopic residual disease of moderate radiosensitivity e.g. adjuvant therapy post surgery.
- Multiple daily fractions of around 2 Gy employed to minimize the risk of late radiation damage.
- Considerable acute toxicity acceptable because of anticipated survival benefit.
- Patients must be fit enough for daily attendance over several weeks.

Palliative radiotherapy
- Aim is to achieve quick symptom relief.
- May have little or no impact on survival time.
- Prefer lowest dose and number of fractions that will achieve the desired response.
- Avoid prolonged acute normal tissue damage.
- Late normal tissue effects may be irrelevant.
- High-dose palliative radiotherapy may be appropriate in patients with disease too advanced for radical treatment, where durable local disease control is the aim, in tumours which have not disseminated widely, and where life expectancy is at least many months.

External beam radiotherapy

Basic principles

Treatment with beams of ionizing radiation produced from a source external to the patient is known as external beam radiotherapy (EBRT).

Superficial X-ray therapy

Superficial tumours (e.g. skin, ribs) may be treated with X-rays of low energy, in the range 80–300 kV. Electrons, emitted from a heated cathode, are accelerated across an X-ray tube, strike a tungsten anode, and undergo bremsstrahlung interactions to produce X-rays. The beam size is selected by using metal applicators of different sizes.

Cobalt teletherapy

Deeper-seated tumours are usually treated using megavoltage photons. One option is to use a source of cobalt, Co-60, emitting gamma rays of average energy 1.25 MeV. Source strengths of about 350 TBq are required to achieve a sufficiently high dose rate.

Megavoltage radiotherapy

However, much more commonly, megavoltage X-rays are produced by linear accelerators, in which electrons are accelerated to near the speed of light in a waveguide, before striking a thin transmission target. The resultant X-rays can have energies in the range 4–20 MV. Such beams offer advantages of higher penetration, higher dose rate, and better collimation (restriction of the radiation to the treatment field) than beams of Co-60.

Electron therapy

Some linear accelerators are also configured to produce beams of electrons of various energies, usually in the range 4–20 MeV. Such beams can uniformly treat from the skin surface down to a specified depth (related to the energy), with a fairly rapid fall-off in dose beyond that. For example, 6 MeV electrons will treat to about 1.5 cm deep and 20 MeV to about 5.5 cm. Electrons offer a good alternative to kilovoltage X-rays for treating superficial tumours.

The main limitations of low energy X-ray beams are:
- unsuitability for the treatment of deep-seated malignancies, e.g. thorax, abdomen, pelvis
- inherent delivery of high dose to the skin
- relatively rapid 'fall-off' of dose with depth
- higher absorbed dose in bone compared with soft tissue.

Features of megavoltage X-rays

- High dose delivered at depth through tissue
- Maximum dose below skin surface
- Skin sparing
- Absorbed dose falls off exponentially with depth in tissue
- Sharp 'fall-off' of dose at beam edge (penumbra)
- Beam shape can be modified by metal blocks or multileaf collimators, now an integral part of modern linear accelerators
- Metal filters or wedges can be used to create a gradient in the dose across the beam
- Treatment from any direction is feasible
- Crossfire technique with 2–4 beams gives higher target dose and relative sparing of adjacent normal tissues.

The planning process

There are six major steps in designing and delivering EBRT treatment.

1. Beam dosimetry

The pattern of dose distribution from each linear accelerator has to be measured prior to clinical use (Fig. 5.1). Due to absorption properties at such high energies, these measurements can be made using a small ionization chamber dosimeter in a tank of water. It is also essential to measure calibration factors (known as output factors) that define the irradiation time required for a specified absorbed dose for each treatment machine.

2. Planning computer

Simple planning can be carried out using tables or plots of measured beam data. However, most planning is performed using computers with specialized application software. Calculations are based on measured beam data but also depend on algorithms that allow for varying attenuation and scatter of X-rays in tissues of different densities. This density information is often based on computerized tomography (CT) scans performed with the patient in the treatment position.

3. Target drawing

The most important step in planning radiotherapy is defining the target, i.e. volume of tissue to be irradiated. This includes the gross tumour volume (GTV – e.g. as visualized clinically or on CT scan) together with surrounding tissues that might have microscopic invasion of tumour cells (CTV – clinical target volume). A further margin has to be allowed for uncertainties in treatment set-up; these include variations in patient positioning, internal organ movement, and tolerances of machine calibration (PTV – planning target volume). It is also essential to define the position of critical organs, i.e. those with a lower tolerance to radiation such as the spinal cord, eyes, and kidneys. All can be drawn directly into the planning computer on a set of CT images covering the full extent of the involved area. For less sophisticated treatments, the target and critical organs are defined clinically, e.g. by palpation of soft tissue tumour or using surface anatomy, and by plain radiographs, often obtained on a fluoroscopic simulator.

4. Dose planning

The objective of dose planning is to design a treatment plan such that the target is uniformly irradiated to an appropriate dose, while ensuring that critical organs do not exceed tolerance doses. Parameters that can be varied include:

- patient position
- beam size
- beam shape
- beam direction
- number of beams
- relative dose per beam (beam weight)
- wedging
- use of compensators.

5. Treatment verification

It is essential that beams are correctly positioned and critical organs not over-irradiated. Beams for CT planned radiotherapy are commonly verified by taking radiographs on a radiotherapy simulator prior to treatment; alternatively this can also be done during any treatment with megavoltage radiographs or electronic portal imaging devices (EPIDs).

Increasingly, *in vivo* dosimetry, direct measurement of the dose delivered to the target and to adjacent critical normal structures, is being used as the gold standard of treatment verification for radical treatments. For this, thermoluminescence dosimeters are attached to relevant sites on the patient during one fraction of radiotherapy.

6. Treatment prescription and delivery

The clinical oncologist prescribes the appropriate dose and fractionation schedule. Together with beam configuration information, these form a dataset completely describing the intended treatment. They are entered into a computer verification system on the linear accelerator and control set up and delivery of each treatment.

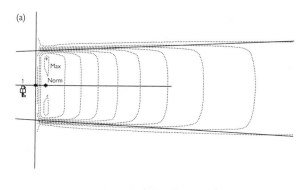

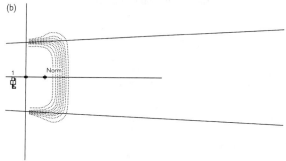

Fig. 5.1 (a) Isodose curves for open beams of 6 MV X-rays. (b) Isodose curves for 12 Mev electrons.

Progress in external beam radiotherapy

3D planning

Perhaps the most significant change in radiotherapy practice in the past 15 years has been the direct use of cross-sectional imaging (most commonly using CT scanning) for radiotherapy planning (Fig. 5.2). The advantages of CT planning are significant:

- tumour and critical structures are more accurately defined
- dose calculation is more precise
- the planning process can be truly 3D, offering potential for reduction in normal tissue damage, escalation of total dose to tumour, and improvement in the therapeutic index.

Conformal treatment/multileaf collimators

It has always been the aim of radiotherapy to conform high dose volume to the target. Normal practice until the 1990s was to use rectangular beams with limited use of blocking. Inevitably, some normal tissue was unnecessarily irradiated to high doses. Improved levels of conformation can be achieved by positioning shaped alloy blocks in the beam and, automatically, with a feature on the modern linear accelerator known as multileaf collimators (MLCs). Here, the beam can be shaped under computer control by sliding a series of 0.5 cm-wide leaves into the beam.

By minimizing the amount of normal tissue irradiated to high dose, it may be possible to deliver higher doses to the target, thereby improving tumour control without increasing morbidity.

Further reading

Royal College of Radiologists. *Radiotherapy Dose–Fractionation*. Guidance BFCO(061). London: Royal College of Radiologists. http://www.rcr.ac.uk/publications.aspx?PageID=149&Publication ID=229 (accessed 30 June 2009).

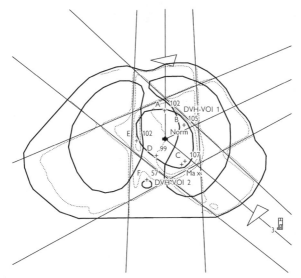

Fig. 5.2 Three radiotherapy beams converging on CT-defined volume of lung cancer.

Recent advances in external beam radiotherapy

In recent years, major technological advances have contributed to important changes in the practice of EBRT. Together they have improved:
- the accuracy and precision of treatment
- the minimization of radiation exposure to organs at risk
- the ability to deliver higher doses of radiation to the tumour, with improved local tumour control.

Volume definition

Most centres now have their own high-resolution CT simulator, while previously planning scans were performed on diagnostic scanners. The tumour volume for even palliative treatments can now be accurately defined in 3D. For radical treatments it is now possible to fuse CT images with other diagnostic modalities including magnetic resonance imaging (MRI) and positron emission tomography (PET), further improving the accuracy of definition of the tumour volume.

Image-guided radiotherapy

Radiotherapists have always recognized the need to allow for discrepancies between the planned treatment volume and the volume of tissue that actually receives irradiation. Traditionally, a margin of ~1 cm was added to the clinical target volume to allow for errors in patient positioning and set-up, and movement of the patient, the tumour, and organs at risk both between and during fractions of radiotherapy.

Previously, confirmation of the accuracy of treatment required the taking of a megavoltage X-ray of the exit beam during a small part of the treatment exposure. These images are of limited value because of their poor quality.

Port films have now been replaced by electronic portal imaging devices (EPIDs). So-called online imaging can be performed at the start of a treatment fraction in order to correct any misalignment, while offline images can be reviewed by radiographers or clinicians after the treatment fraction has been delivered (e.g. to compare a series of fractions to look for repeated errors in set-up).

While previously confirmation of correct set-up relied simply on comparison of bony landmarks between the the treatment plan and the portal images, the tumour itself can now be imaged during radiotherapy:
- fiducial markers, e.g. gold seeds, can be implanted into the prostate
- ultrasound imaging can confirm the position of e.g. the prostate gland
- cone beam CT, mounted on the linear accelerator, allows online 3D imaging of the tumour target.

Inverse planned intensity-modulated radiotherapy

While conventional radiotherapy uses treatment beams that deliver a uniform dose across the beam, this dose can be varied in a computerized optimization process based on a set of dose constraints for the relevant normal organs at risk, and prescribed doses to the tumour targets (CTV and GTV). To achieve these dose constraints, the distribution of radiation beam intensity is modulated across each beam:

- step and shoot technique – the beam intensity is modulated by superimposing a number of static uniform intensity segments
- dynamic multileaf collimator delivery – a shaped sliding window passes across the field during treatment
- tomotherapy – treatment delivered with multiple arcs, with the intensity of each modulated by special dynamic MLCs.

Stereotactic radiotherapy

Since the 1990s, this treatment modality has become established for the treatment of a number of intracranial conditions including benign tumours and arteriovenous (AV) malformations. Using an external 3D co-ordinate system, along with a stereotactic fixation system, it is possible to treat small lesions (<1 cm^3) with high precision (1–2 mm).

Typically treatment comprises 1–3 large fractions (12–20 Gy).

Recently this approach has been used successfully in the treatment of small malignancies in the brain, lung, and liver. The accuracy of these treatments at sites unsuitable for localization frames is facilitated by IGRT techniques as above.

Electron beam therapy

Although electron radiation is radiobiologically equivalent to photon radiation in terms of its effects on normal and malignant cells, the physical characteristics of electron beams have advantages over photon beams in the treatment of some anatomical sites. Unlike photons, electrons possess charge and so interact frequently as they penetrate tissue; the resulting energy loss leads to a well-defined range in tissue. Radiation dose deposited beyond a certain depth in tissue is negligible (Fig. 5.3). This allows treatment of target volumes lying within a few centimetres of the skin's surface while sparing any underlying critical structures.

Electron versus photon radiotherapy

Electrons
• Limited tissue penetration
• Negligible exit dose from beam
• Particularly useful for superficial tumours, e.g. skin cancer, head and neck cancer, breast cancer
• Reduced dose to normal tissues beneath target, e.g. spinal cord, lung

Photons
• Suitable tissue penetration characteristics for the treatment of deep-seated cancers
• Skin sparing
• Beam characteristics facilitate beam matching and crossfire treatment plans

Production of electron beams

Most radiation therapy facilities have high-energy linear accelerators capable of producing both X-ray and electron beams.

Since electrons scatter significantly in air, beam-defining cones or 'trimmer' bars are fitted to the head of the treatment machine in order to collimate the beam near the skin's surface. The beam may be shaped further either by fitting a lead or 'cerrobend' aperture at the end of the cone (an electron cut-out), or by using lead sheet laid directly on skin to restrict exposure of electrons to the target area.

Dosimetric characteristics of electron beams

The various dosimetric aspects of electron beams in **homogeneous** tissue are as follows.

Depth dose characteristics
Dose builds up slowly to a maximum value and then falls off rapidly, reaching nearly zero at a depth equal to the practical electron range.

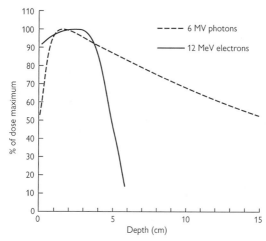

Fig. 5.3 Tissue penetration of different types of radiotherapy beams.

Effect of incident energy

The depth of penetration of an electron beam is determined by its incident energy. The practical range (in centimetres) of an electron beam in water is approximately

$$R_p \approx \frac{E_0}{2}$$

where E_0 is incident beam energy expressed in mega-electron volts (MeV).

Similarly, the clinically useful range – the depth at which the dose falls to 80% of its maximum value – is estimated as

$$d_{80} \approx \frac{E_0}{3}.$$

The surface dose (commonly defined as dose at 0.5 mm depth) is significantly higher for an electron beam than for a megavoltage photon beam and ranges from about 85% of dose maximum at low energies (less than 10 MeV) to about 95% at higher energies.

Accelerators that offer an electron beam mode generally allow selection of one of several available electron beam energies, most commonly in the range 6–15 MeV.

Beam profile and penumbra

Beam penumbra tend to be larger for electron beams than for photon beams. For electron beams, the dose falls to 90% of central axis value approximately 1 cm inside the geometric field edge for depths near the dose maximum; a 10 × 10 cm^2 beam, for instance, produces an 'effective' field size of only 8 × 8 cm^2. The corresponding distance for a photon beam is only about 0.5 cm. Thus, a larger electron beam is required to cover a given target to a clinically useful dose. This property of electron beams makes abutting of photon and electron beams problematical, since a uniform dose across a field junction cannot be achieved at all depths.

Brachytherapy

A form of radiation treatment where the radiation sources are placed within, or close to, the tumour, or target volume.

Indications

- The extent of the neoplasm must be known precisely, as treatment is often given to a relatively small volume, and 'geographic miss' of tumour is a significant risk, resulting in recurrence of the tumour at the edge of the target volume.
- The site should be accessible for both inserting and removing sources and allowing satisfactory geometric positioning of those sources.

Advantages

- The probability of local tumour control increases with increasing radiation dose, but so does the probability of normal tissue damage. Brachytherapy allows the delivery of a localized high radiation dose to a small tumour volume, increasing the chance of local control. There is a sharp fall-off of radiation dose in the surrounding normal tissue; therefore the risks of complication are reduced.
- The overall duration of brachytherapy is short, generally 2–7 days. The constant low-dose irradiation takes advantage of the different rates of repair and repopulation of normal and malignant tissue to produce differential cell killing, enhancing the therapeutic ratio.
- Hypoxic cells are relatively resistant to radiation treatment. Reoxygenation may occur during low-dose-rate radiotherapy, with initially resistant hypoxic cells becoming oxygenated and more radiosensitive during the course of brachytherapy.
- The dose distribution within the tumour volume is often not homogeneous. Treatment is often prescribed to the minimum dose received around the periphery of the treated volume. Areas close to the radiation sources in the centre of the tumour volume often receive up to twice this dose. Hypoxic cells are situated in avascular, sometimes necrotic areas in the centre of tumours, and the higher doses received in the centre may help to compensate for the relative radioresistance of these hypoxic cells.
- Irregular-shaped tumours can be treated by judicious positioning of radiation sources, and critical surrounding normal tissues can be avoided.

Disadvantages

- Many sources emit gamma rays, and nursing and medical staff may be exposed to low but significant doses of radiation from the patient. Staff exposure can be minimized by after-loading techniques or the use of low-energy radionuclides.
- Large tumours are usually unsuitable, although brachytherapy may be employed as a boost treatment following reduction in size by EBRT and/or chemotherapy.
- Radiation dose falls off rapidly from the sources according to the inverse square law. In order to treat the required tissue volume adequately, accurate geometric positioning of the sources is critical.

The spatial arrangement of sources used varies, depending on the type of source applicator, the anatomical position of the tumour, and the surrounding dose-limiting normal tissue. Accurate positioning of sources or applicators requires special skill and training and this is not universally available.

- Surrounding structures such as lymph nodes that may contain overt or microscopic cancer will not be irradiated by the implant or intracavity treatment.

Types

- Intracavity – radioactive material inserted into body cavities:
  - cervix/uterine cancer
  - bronchial cancer
  - oesophageal cancer
  - bile duct cancer
- Interstitial – radioactive material inserted into tissues:
  - prostate cancer
  - breast cancer
  - head and neck cancer
  - anal cancer
- Surface – radioactive material placed over tumour:
  - skin
  - eye

Implants can be classified as manually inserted, after-loading, or remote after-loading. Manual insertion of radiation sources should be avoided if possible, owing to the radiation hazards to operating staff and nurses. After-loading is when radioactive material is loaded into hollow needles, catheters, or applicators that have been inserted into the tumour area previously. Manipulation of these 'cold' applicators carries no radiation hazard to medical and nursing staff, so that time can safely be taken to ensure optimal source geometry.

After-loading with radioactive material can be manual or remote (using machines such as the Selectron, commonly used to treat gynaecological cancer). For remote after-loading, stainless steel pellets containing, e.g., caesium in glass, are moved pneumatically from a computer-controlled lead-lined safe into intrauterine and vaginal applicators. This completely eliminates irradiation of theatre and nursing staff.

Some remote after-loading devices work at a very high dose rate, e.g. the Microselectron (high-intensity iridium sources) or the Cathetron (high-intensity cobalt sources) and treatment is delivered in a matter of minutes. Low-dose-rate brachytherapy may require the sources to remain in place for many hours.

Most implants are of the removable type – the radiation sources are removed after delivery of the prescribed treatment dose. However, permanent implantations can be performed using relatively short half-life isotopes such as ^{125}I or ^{198}Au, which are implanted into the tumours in the form of seeds that remain in place after the radiation has decayed.

Radionuclides

Gamma emitters

Radium was used for many years as the source of gamma rays for brachytherapy. This is now obsolete. The major source of gamma rays is not radium but the gaseous daughter product, radon. Radium tubes and needles must be gas-tight and frequently checked for leaks. The gamma rays produced are relatively high energy (average 830 keV), and thick lead shields are required to provide adequate radiation protection. Caesium-137 has no gaseous daughter products, a useful half-life of 30 years, and a less penetrating 660 keV gamma ray, and it has largely replaced radium, especially for gynaecological work.

Iridium-192 is manufactured in the form of flexible wire and has many advantages over traditional radium or caesium needles for interstitial brachytherapy. Thin wires (0.3 mm in diameter) can be inserted into flexible nylon tubes or after-loading needles previously implanted into the tumour. Thicker wires (0.6 mm diameter), in the form of hairpins, can be inserted directly into a tumour through suitable introducers. In the USA, iridium is also available in the form of seeds sealed in thin plastic coating. Iridium produces a gamma ray of 330 keV, and lead shields 2 cm in thickness provide good protection for medical and nursing staff. The major disadvantage of iridium is the relatively short half-life (74 days), so that fresh material should be used for each implant.

Iodine-125 has a half-life of 59.6 days and is used for permanent implants of the prostate. As well as having a relatively short half-life, the gamma rays produced by this radionuclide are of low energy (27–35 keV) and little radiation is emitted from a patient following the implant, allowing early discharge from hospital.

Beta emitters

The major use of plaques emitting beta radiation is in the treatment of eye tumours. Plaques can be made of strontium-90 or ruthenium-106/rhodium-106.

Dosimetry

Radioactive material is implanted into tissues according to distribution rules that vary according to the system used. In Europe the classical Parker–Paterson and Quimby systems have largely been superseded by the Paris system, which is particularly suitable for iridium wire implants. Wire of the same linear intensity is used and sources are arranged in parallel, straight, equidistant lines, 8–20 mm apart. To compensate for 'uncrossed' ends, the wires are 20–30% longer than the length required to treat the tumour. In a volume implant, sources in cross-section should be arranged in either equilateral triangles or squares.

The dose to the tumour can be calculated manually, using graphs such as Oxford cross line curves, or by computer. The basal dose rate (the mean of minimum values between sources) is first calculated. The treatment dose (e.g. 65 Gy in 7 days) is prescribed to the reference dose line (85% of the basal dose).

The prescription point for surface applicators such as moulds and some intracavity treatment is usually 0.5–1 cm from the applicator. A special case is intracavitary gynaecological treatment. The most frequently used prescribing point is the Manchester A point, defined as a point 2 cm lateral to the uterine canal and 2 cm above the cervical os. The dose calculated at this point is a good predictor of late radiation damage to the ureter, bladder, rectum, and other pelvic organs. The International Commission of Radiation Units (ICRU) Report 38 has proposed that the volume (defined in height, thickness, and width enclosed by a 60 Gy isodose line) should be used for reporting absorbed dose following gynaecological treatments.

Future developments

There is increasing use of sophisticated 3D planning techniques incorporating CT or MRI scans to determine the dosage to the whole tumour and to critical normal tissues. As well as defining the dose in purely physical terms, the biological effects in different tissues may be expressed as biological effective doses.

Radiation exposure to staff has been reduced by the increased use of high-dose-rate remote after-loading machines. The complication rate following fractionated high-dose gynaecological insertions is less than that following manually inserted low-dose sources. Continuous low-dose-rate implants may be replaced by high-dose 'pulsed' insertions with optimization of the dose distribution and more homogeneous irradiation of the target volume.

Further reading

International Commission on Radiation Units (ICRU) (1985) *Report 38: Dose and volume specification for reporting intra-cavity therapy in gynecology.* Bethesda: International Commission on Radiation Units.

Nag S, ed. (1997) *Principles and practice of brachytherapy.* New York: Futura.

Intra-operative radiotherapy

A fundamental problem with radiotherapy is targeting diseased tissues while avoiding unaffected normal structures. Various approaches are possible including intra-operative radiotherapy (IORT). Involved tissues can be surgically exposed and selectively treated with a single fraction of EBRT (either orthovoltage X-rays or electrons) with reduced morbidity to non-affected tissues. The principal drawbacks are:

- need for specialist additional equipment in the operating theatre
- need for radiation protection for staff in the presence of therapeutic (as opposed to diagnostic) radiation exposure
- need for the radiation oncologist to be present in theatre
- radiobiological effects of a single large exposure on adjacent normal tissues.

Long-term follow-up data are limited but animal studies suggest that IORT exposures up to 30 Gy carry little risk of long-term sequelae as long as radiosensitive normal structures such as major nerves, blood vessels, the spinal cord, or the small bowel are kept out of the radiation field. The threshold for nerve damage is 20–25 Gy with a latent period of 6–9 months.

A further risk to be considered is the induction of malignancy. A number of studies in dogs have reported a high incidence of sarcomas induced by IORT compared to other treatment modalities. Issues such as treatment planning are clearly complex, as only limited treatment volume data can be available pre-operatively.

Specific tumours

- **Rectal cancer**: may be helpful in both primary and recurrent tumours.
- **Stomach and oesophagus**: doses of up to 20 Gy appear safe.
- **Bile duct**: may have role in minimal residual disease rather than for unresectable disease.
- **Pancreas**: although feasible, no proven benefits as yet.
- **Head and neck cancer**: safe, well tolerated, and encouraging results from limited number of centres; may be helpful if minimal residual disease or recurrent disease.
- **Brain**: poor results.
- **Other tumours**: may be of value in some paediatric cancers, breast cancer, and soft-tissue sarcomas.

Conclusions

IORT is a promising technique but limited by the technical and logistic problems already outlined. The continued development of conformal planning and delivery techniques for EBRT may reduce the therapeutic gain that can be obtained from intra-operative treatment. In addition, conformal radiotherapy (CRT) is more reproducible in set-up and poses no special problems in dosimetry and fractionation. The development of IORT continues to be restricted to clinical trials within a few specialist centres.

The role of unsealed radionuclides

Nuclear medicine in oncology may be used to:
• localize the primary tumour
• detect metastases
• monitor the response to therapy and detect recurrences
• deliver targeted radiotherapy.

Radiolabelled tracers

A radiopharmaceutical consists of a ligand attached to a radionuclide that emits gamma rays. The distribution of the radiopharmaceutical may vary from the normal because of a pathological process, e.g. a malignant tumour. Such biochemical or functional changes in tumours cannot be detected by cross-sectional imaging such as CT or MRI. However imaging by detection of radiopharmaceutical – scintigraphy – lacks the anatomical detail of CT or MRI, and information from different imaging modalities is often complementary.

Several radiopharmaceuticals are used for both diagnosis and treatment. Examples are iodine-123 and -131, which localize avidly in functioning thyroid tissue. Other simple radiopharmaceuticals are thallium-201 (^{201}Tl) and gallium-67 (^{67}Ga). The ideal radionuclide for scintigraphic imaging does not exist, but technetium-99m (^{99m}Tc) has many favourable characteristics.

Scintigraphic methods

Traditionally, gamma cameras are used for scintigraphic imaging. Planar images and whole-body images are acquired during a period of several minutes by a stationary gamma camera. With single photon emission computerized tomography (SPECT), cross-sectional images can be obtained using computer techniques similar to those in CT. The main advantages of SPECT are greater sensitivity and accurate 3D localization of lesions.

Positron emission tomography (PET)

PET employs radionuclides that emit positrons and provides quantitative tomographic images. Glucose utilization is measured with ^{18}F-labelled fluorodeoxyglucose and cerebral blood flow has been studied with ^{15}O-labelled water. PET scanning may be useful to identify primary tumours and metastases, and to study tumour vitality, cell turnover rates, and metabolic response to therapy.

Applications in diagnosis and follow-up

Bone scintigraphy

Bone scintigraphy is normally performed 2–4 h after the injection of 550 MBq of ^{99m}Tc-labelled methylene disphosphonate (^{99m}Tc-medronate, MDP) or hydroxymethylene disphosphonate (^{99m}Tc-oxidronate, HDP). Multiple planar images or a whole-body survey of the skeleton are obtained. Skeletal scintigraphy has high sensitivity for the detection of primary and metastatic bone lesions. In the absence of reactive osteoblastic activity, the lesion itself may appear on the bone scan as a 'cold' defect.

High sensitivity (80–100%) has been reported in patients with bone metastases from breast carcinoma, prostatic carcinoma, bronchogenic carcinoma, gastric carcinoma, osteogenic sarcoma, cervical carcinoma, Ewing's sarcoma, head and neck carcinoma, neuroblastoma, and ovarian carcinoma. Lower sensitivity, around 75%, has been found in melanoma, small-cell lung tumours, Hodgkin's disease, renal cell carcinoma, rhabdomyosarcoma, multiple myeloma, and bladder carcinoma.

Thyroid scintigraphy

^{131}I as radioiodine, ^{123}I as sodium iodide, and ^{99m}Tc as sodium pertechnetate are the radionuclides used for scintigraphic visualization of the thyroid gland. Although ^{131}I is cheap and readily available, its major disadvantages are its long physical half-life and α-emissions, resulting in a considerable radiation dose to the thyroid and the GI tract. ^{123}I has excellent physical properties for imaging and a physical half-life of 13 h, but its use is limited due to its cost. ^{99m}Tc is trapped in the thyroid, but is not organified, and washes out from the gland over time.

The indications for thyroid scintigraphy in oncology are:

- evaluation of a solitary or dominant nodule
- follow-up after surgery for differentiated thyroid cancer.

Therapy with unsealed radioactive sources

Targeted radiotherapy using tumour-seeking radiopharmaceuticals has been employed for almost half a century. The radiopharmaceutical should have specific affinity for tumour tissue with a high target-to-background ratio and long retention time; the radiation emitted by the radioisotope should be sufficiently energetic for a therapeutic effect, but be absorbed over a short distance to irradiate the tumour target only. Some of the clinically useful radiopharmaceuticals for therapy are ^{131}I, ^{89}Sr, ^{32}P, ^{186}Re, ^{153}Sm, and ^{90}Y.

Iodine-131 therapy in differentiated thyroid cancer

^{131}I has been used extensively in the treatment of thyrotoxicosis and in differentiated thyroid carcinoma after thyroidectomy. ^{131}I is used for ablation of the remaining thyroid tissue following total thyroidectomy and for treatment of recurrent and metastatic thyroid cancer.

^{131}I-meta-iodobenzylguanidine (MIBG) therapy in neural crest tumours

^{131}I-MIBG has been used successfully for radionuclide therapy of neural crest tumours. Post-therapy scintigrams, 1 week after administration, can be obtained for further documentation. In patients with malignant phaeochromocytoma, response is achieved in >50% of patients; with neuroblastoma the response rate is 35%. Some success is reported with ^{131}I-MIBG therapy for paraganglioma and medullary thyroid carcinoma.

Bone-seeking radiopharmaceuticals for metastatic bone disease

Bone metastases occur in up to 85% of patients who have breast, lung, or prostate cancer. Bone-seeking radiopharmaceuticals have pharmacokinetic properties similar to those of either calcium or phosphate. Strontium-89 (^{89}Sr) is a calcium analogue. ^{32}P, ^{86}Re, hydroxyethylidine diphosphonate (HEDP), and ^{153}Sm are all phosphate analogues.

Historically, intravenous injection of ^{32}P-orthophosphate for the treatment of bone pain was effective, but bone marrow toxicity limited its widespread use. ^{89}Sr was the first radioisotope licensed as a systemic treatment for bone metastases in prostate cancer. After intravenous (IV) administration of 150 MBq of ^{89}Sr, the radiopharmaceutical is avidly accumulated in areas of high bone turnover, such as reactive bone surrounding a metastasis. Myelosuppression can be expected after 6 weeks. After a single administration of ^{89}Sr, in 75–80% of patients pain is promptly relieved and progression of further bone disease is delayed, with the response lasting 1–6 months.

Intracavitary therapy

Injection of radiopharmaceuticals directly into the pleural cavity, pericardium, peritoneum, urinary bladder, cerebrospinal fluid, or cystic tumours offers the potential advantage of direct access of radiopharmaceuticals to tumour tissue without a systemic burden. Colloids and monoclonal antibodies labelled with ^{32}P, ^{90}Y, or ^{131}I can be used for this purpose.

Monoclonal antibodies

Monoclonal antibodies were considered the ultimate 'magic bullets' for cancer therapy when introduced 20 years ago. The goal has been to develop antibodies that target active tumour cells specifically and act as carriers of radiation to treat the disease. At present radio-immunotherapy has met with more problems than successes and its future is uncertain.

Total body irradiation (TBI)

Treatment intensification with high doses of chemotherapy and/or radiotherapy is used to try to improve cure rates for sensitive tumours and to eradicate remaining bone marrow stem cells prior to transplantation, most commonly with donor stem cells.

Aims of TBI

- To eliminate any residual malignant disease
- To ablate residual marrow to permit engraftment of donor peripheral stem cells or bone marrow
- To produce immune suppression (especially for non-haplotype identical grafts)

Indications for high-dose therapy

Haematological malignancies

- Prior to bone marrow or stem cell transplantation for relapsed disease, e.g. acute leukaemia, high-grade non-Hodgkin's lymphoma (NHL), myeloma

Other malignancies

These include neuroblastoma.

Types of haemopoietic reconstitution

- Autologous: transplant may be peripheral stem cells or cryopreserved marrow obtained before high-dose therapy
- Allogeneic: matched or mismatched (1 haplotype identical) bone marrow is usually used, and may be obtained from a family member or from a donor panel

Pre-treatment screening

- The patient's disease should be in remission.
- There should be adequate renal, cardiac, hepatic, and pulmonary function to cope with the toxicity of chemotherapy and TBI.
- Exposure to medication with the same side-effects as TBI, or likely to potentiate its side-effects, should be assessed:
  - neurotoxicity with asparaginase
  - renal toxicity with platinum or ifosfamide
  - pulmonary toxicity with methotrexate or bleomycin
  - cardiac toxicity with cyclophosphamide or anthracyclines
- Consider the need for additional therapy to sites such as the central nervous system, testes, mediastinum, i.e. areas of sanctuary or bulk disease.

Preparation

Anti-emetics, including a 5-HT antagonist, are given with dexamethasone, intravenously, 1 h before treatment starts. If additional sedation is required, phenobarbitone or diazepam may be used. For very young children, anaesthesia with ketamine may be necessary.

Technique

- Linear accelerator – optimum energy around 6 MV.
- Fractionated TBI is preferred for reasons of convenience.
- Patient lies on couch behind a Perspex sheet (to provide full dose to skin) either on their side or back and side alternately.
- Treatment is given by opposed fields for half of each treatment time.
- The couch is placed at an extended distance from the machine to obtain the field size required to cover the whole body.
- The dose distribution will be inhomogeneous because of variation in AP/PA separation along the body and because of density differences (especially the lung). This can be compensated for by using bolus or lung shielding but is unnecessary using schedules described here, where doses do not exceed tolerance for any normal tissues.
- The organ most at risk is the lung.

Calculation of dose

Paired lithium fluoride dose meters or diodes are used to measure dose distribution throughout the body. These are placed on the skin at defined sites in the upper and lower lung, mediastinum, abdomen, and pelvis. Midline doses are taken as the average of AP and PA dose meter readings, or CT scanning of the whole body can be used with a planning computer to calculate doses throughout the body.

Dose schedules

Adults

The optimum fractionated doses are determined as 13.2–14.4 Gy depending on the point of dose prescription. The maximum lung dose is preferred, as this is the dose-limiting organ, and should not exceed 14.4 Gy.

Children

May tolerate slightly higher doses than adults. In the Medical Research Council (MRC) protocol, treatment is given in 8 fractions of 1.8 Gy over 4 days. Many other dose schedules are in common use and have been found by experience to be satisfactory.

Toxicity of treatment

Acute effects

- Nausea and vomiting commonly start about 6 h after the first fraction
- Parotid swelling – occurs in the first 24 h and then resolves spontaneously, although often leaving a dry mouth
- Hypotension
- Fever – abolished by steroids
- Diarrhoea – occurs at day 5 as a result of GI mucositis
- Delayed toxicity
- Pneumonitis presenting with dyspnoea and characteristic X-ray appearances
- Somnolence due to transient demyelination occurs at 6–8 weeks and is characterized by sleepiness, anorexia, and in some cases nausea which settles spontaneously within 7–10 days.

Late toxicity

- Cataracts occur in <20% of patients; incidence increases at 2–6 years, but then appears to plateau.
- Hormonal changes – azoospermia and amenorrhoea with consequent sterility are the norm; very occasionally fertility has been maintained, leading to normal pregnancies with no increased incidence of abnormalities in the offspring.
- Hypothyroidism may result from damage to the thyroid alone or in combination with pituitary damage.
- In children, there may be impaired production of growth hormone which, added to the effect of early epiphyseal fusion from TBI, results in stunting of growth.
- Induction of second malignancy – there is a 5-fold increase in the risk of second malignancies. Brain tumours may be attributed to the TBI, and oral and rectal carcinomas have been reported.
- Malignancy of the lymphoid system may result from the prolonged immune suppression.

Principles of chemotherapy

Rationale for combination therapy

Cytotoxic chemotherapy destroys cancer cells. Currently available drugs target:
- chemistry of nucleic acids
- DNA or RNA production
- mechanics of cell division (e.g. spindle poisons).

The discovery and development of cytotoxic agents has paralleled the understanding of the chemical processes involved. The lack of selectivity inherent in this approach has limited the ability to kill cancer cells while leaving normal dividing cells unscathed.

Cytotoxic agents can be classified by:
- chemical properties or mechanisms of action
- source (e.g. natural products)
- propensity to be cell cycle or phase specific.

The following principles underlie the design of a potential combination chemotherapy regimen:
- each drug should have single-agent activity in that tumour type
- each drug should have a different mechanism of activity
- drugs with non-overlapping toxicity patterns are preferable
- drugs that work in different parts of the cell cycle should be selected
- drugs should not all share the same resistance mechanisms.

Combination therapy aims to increase 'fractional cell kill', leading to improved overall response of the tumour. Higher doses of cytotoxic drugs tend to produce increased cell kill (at least within certain limits); thus it is important not to compromise on the dose of each agent (hence the need to select drugs with non-overlapping toxicity).
- Tumour mass is usually composed of cells that are asynchronously dividing – thus combinations of drugs that act at different points in the cell cycle will theoretically kill more cells.
- 'Multidrug resistance' is displayed by some tumour types, resulting from e.g. expression of an efflux pump on the cell surface that drives the drug out of the cell.

More recently, so-called targeted therapies have been developed which aim to specifically inhibit some process of fundamental importance to the cancer cell – good examples are angiogenesis inhibition and blockade of the epithelial growth factor receptor. These drugs often target some aspect of oncogene function. These drugs already have an established place in the therapy of some cancers. However, there is still a lot of clinical research that needs to be done to determine the optimal way of integrating these agents with existing therapies to maximize benefits to the patient. See 📖 Chapter 10 and appropriate site-specific chapters in 📖 Part 4.

Alkylating agents

The oldest anti-cancer cytotoxics – alkylating agents – are antiproliferative drugs because they bind covalently via alkyl groups to DNA. Following cross-linking there is thought to be arrest in G1–S transition followed either by DNA repair or apoptosis.

Clinical use

Extensively used to treat leukaemia and lymphoma and they are also active in a wide range of solid cancers.

Resistance

Resistance to alkylating agents is multifactorial and may differ between classes of alkylating agents, e.g. resistance to nitrosoureas is probably mediated by increased expression of the enzyme O^6-alkyl transferase. In addition to enhanced DNA repair, resistant cells may exhibit an increased ability to detoxify alkylating agents. Such mechanisms include increased:

- glutathione
- metallothionein
- glutathione-S-transferase.

Examples of alkylating agents

- *Melphalan* is a derivative of nitrogen mustard and the amino acid phenylalanine. The rationale behind this is that dividing cells might take up amino acids more rapidly (and hence melphalan), thus providing some tumour selectivity.
- *Chlorambucil* is the phenylbutyric acid derivative of nitrogen mustard, a well-absorbed alkylating agent that can be orally administered – with activity in both solid and haematological malignancies.
- *Cyclophosphamide* is extensively used in cytotoxic chemotherapy. Its major toxicities are marrow suppression, alopecia, nausea, and vomiting. As a result of its relative lack of non-haematological toxicities, it is used in high-dose chemotherapy regimens.
- *Ifosfamide* is an isomer of cyclophosphamide. Extensive metabolism of this agent occurs, liberating chloroacetaldehyde, which is thought to be responsible for some of the toxicity profile. It nearly always causes alopecia and haemorrhagic cystitis, but this can be circumvented by co-administration of thiol mesna which is thought to chemically combine with acrolein, the metabolite thought to be responsible for this toxicity.
- *Both cyclophosphamide and ifosfamide* are prodrugs activated by hepatic cytoshrome P450 metabolism to produce nitrogen mustards.
- *Busulphan* has a special place in the treatment of chronic myeloid leukaemia. It is well absorbed from the GI tract. The dose-limiting toxicities are myelosuppression and hepatic veno-occlusive disease. It can also cause hyperpigmentation and, rarely, pulmonary interstitial fibrosis.
- *BCNU* (1,3-bis (2-chloroethyl)-1-nitrosourea, carmustine) is a small lipophilic molecule and is used to treat CNS tumours and as a conditioning agent in high-dose therapy.
- *Temozolomide* is a more recently developed agent that is active in glioma and melanoma.

Anti-tumour antibiotics

Anthracyclines

Anthracyclines (doxorubicin, daunorubicin, epirubicin, and idarubicin) are closely related structurally and have similar mechanisms of action and resistance, but have different patterns of clinical activity and toxicity.

Pharmacology

The anthracyclines have several effects, and their specific mode of action is unclear.

- There are direct effects at the cell surface and also on signal transduction, specifically activation of protein kinase C-mediated cell signalling pathways. The role of these actions in mediating anthracycline cytotoxicity is undefined.
- Their ability to undergo reduction to highly reactive compounds and to generate free radicals has clinically important implications. Characteristic cardiotoxicity of anthracyclines appears due to the generation of free radicals in the heart where defence systems are less active.
- The major target of anthracyclines is the enzyme topoisomerase II. During cell division, topoisomerase II binds to DNA forming a 'cleavable complex' that makes transient 'nicks' in DNA, allowing torsional strain in DNA to be released, after which strands rejoin. Anthracyclines bind to the cleavable complex, disrupting this process, leading to DNA strand breaks and cell death.

Drug resistance

Some tumours are inherently resistant to anthracyclines, whereas others initially respond but later become resistant.

The *MDR1* gene codes for a P-170 glycoprotein (Pgp) that is a naturally occurring cell-surface pump. Its physiological function appears to be a protective mechanism, expelling toxic substances from the cell. Though expression is increased in some human cancers before treatment or at relapse, attempts to manipulate Pgp have had limited success.

A second efflux pump associated with expression of multidrug resistance-associated protein (*MRP*) gene has been implicated in anthracycline resistance in the lab.

Pharmacokinetics and metabolism

After intravenous (IV) administration, anthracycline levels fall rapidly as it is distributed and binds to tissue DNA. Subsequent metabolism and elimination lead to a slow fall in plasma concentrations over several days. Dose reductions are recommended for patients with abnormal liver biochemistry, as they are at risk of increased toxicity.

Clinical use

The anthracyclines are among the most active cytotoxic agents.

- Doxorubicin and epirubicin are commonly used in IV regimens against breast cancer, sarcoma, and haematological cancers.
- Daunorubicin and idarubicin (oral) have a major role in treatment of acute leukaemia.

Toxicity

The dose-limiting acute toxicities are:

- myelosuppression and mucositis, both occurring 5–10 days after treatment
- alopecia – occurs but is reversible
- extravasation injury – can be severe and there is no proven, effective treatment.

Cumulative cardiotoxicity is specific to anthracyclines and appears to be caused by accumulation of free radicals in the heart. It typically presents with heart failure, the risk of which is dose related. At doxorubicin doses below 450 mg/m^2, the risk is less than 5%, but increases substantially at higher doses. In most cases this threshold allows a full course of anthracycline to be given without risk. Irradiation of the heart increases risk of cardiotoxicity, as does pre-existing cardiac disease.

- Liposomal encapsulation of doxorubicin reduces cardiotoxicity.
- Epirubicin, daunorubicin, and idarubicin have less effect on the myocardium than doxorubicin.

Mitoxantrone

This agent binds to DNA and interacts with topoisomerase II but appears less potent in generating free radicals. It is also a substrate for Pgp. The main clinical use of mitoxantrone has been as an alternative to doxorubicin in advanced breast cancer, as it is substantially less cardiotoxic, less vesicant, and causes less alopecia. However, mitoxantrone is less effective than doxorubicin. It has some activity against other solid tumours, including non-Hodgkin's lymphoma and non-lymphocytic leukaemia.

Actinomycin D (dactinomycin)

Actinomycin D binds strongly to DNA by intercalation, and inhibits synthesis of RNA and proteins. It also appears to be a substrate for the Pgp pump. It is especially active against childhood tumours.

Mitomycin C (MMC)

MMC is active against a range of solid tumours but is also used as a radiosensitizer in chemo-irradiation. MMC is used in combination with other cytotoxics to treat breast cancer, non-small-cell lung cancer, and GI cancer. It is used as a radiosensitizer in the treatment of anal cancer.

The most important toxicity of MMC is myelosuppression, especially thrombocytopenia, which is delayed and can be cumulative. Accordingly, MMC is given systemically every 6 weeks in contrast to the 3-weekly schedules usually used for other anti-tumour antibiotics. Haemolytic–uraemic syndrome, pulmonary fibrosis, and cardiac complications are all uncommon side-effects.

Anti-metabolites

Anti-metabolites interfere with normal cellular metabolism of nucleic acids; they act with S-phase specificity (Fig. 6.1). They include some of the most widely prescribed cytotoxic agents, whose indications are not confined to treating malignancies.

Anti-folates

Understanding anti-metabolite action necessitates knowledge of folate biochemistry. The enzyme thymidylate synthase (TS) acts as rate-limiting step in the synthesis of thymidylate, converting dUMP (2'-deoxyuridine 5'-triphosphate) into dTTP (2'-deoxythymidine 5'-triphosphate) by transferring a methyl group from CH_2-FH_4. The supply of reduced folate is maintained by the enzyme dihydrofolate reductase (DHFR).

Methotrexate (MTX)

Widely used in many cancers, MTX is frequently used in breast cancer, osteogenic sarcoma, GI cancers, and choriocarcinoma.

Pharmacology

MTX is well absorbed orally below 25 mg/m^2, but is usually administered IV, except in maintenance regimens and treatment of benign connective tissue diseases. There is some hepatic metabolism to the active drug 7-OH-MTX and approximately 10% of the drug is cleared by biliary excretion. Dose adjustments are not usually necessary with hepatic dysfunction. Significant third-space effects occur in the presence of fluid collections (e.g. ascites, pleural effusions) and can increase toxicity through reduced clearance. MTX excretion can also be inhibited by probenecid, penicillins (and cephalosporins), and non-steroidal anti-inflammatory agents.

Common toxicities include mucositis, myelosuppression, and nephrotoxicity.

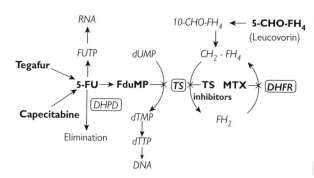

Fig. 6.1 Main sites of action of anti-metabolites.

MTX — Cytotoxics (MTX—methotrexate; 5-FU –5–fluorouracil; TS inhibitors include ralitrexed)

dTTP — Normal metabolites

—✕ Indicates enzyme inhibition

⟨DHPD⟩ Enzyme (TS—thymidylate synthase; DHPD—dihydropyrimidine dehydrogenase; DHFR—dihydrofolate reductase)

Thymidylate synthase (TS) inhibitors

New agents have been developed that directly inhibit TS (in contrast to indirect inhibitors, e.g. 5-fluorouracil (5-FU) and MTX) and interact with the folate-binding site of TS.

Raltitrexed (Tomudex®) causes prolonged inhibition of TS by enhanced retention in cells due to polyglutamation of the parent molecule. After IV administration it has triphasic elimination, with a rapid initial fall in concentration but very prolonged final phase; 50% of the drug is renally excreted unchanged. It is active in breast and colorectal cancer with toxicities including myelosuppression, diarrhoea and transaminitis. It has not been licensed in many situations because of unpredictable severe toxicities.

Fluoropyrimidines

These pro-drugs are intracellularly activated and their products inhibit pyrimidine synthesis.

5-fluorouracil (5-FU)

This is a widely prescribed agent with particular activity in breast cancer, GI cancers, and head and neck tumours.

It is metabolized to FdUMP (5-fluoro-2-deoxyuridine 5′-monophosphate), which, in the presence of CH_2-FH_4, forms a stable complex inhibiting TS. It also inhibits RNA synthesis and pre-ribosomal RNA processing.

Pharmacology

5-FU is given IV both as a bolus and a prolonged infusion. It has a short initial half-life, with significant hepatic, renal, and lung clearance. Active metabolites (e.g. 5dUMP and FUTP) have variable pharmacokinetics.

Toxicities of 5-FU include myelosuppression and, particularly with longer administration schedules, stomatitis and diarrhoea. Prolonged infusion overcomes the initial rapid clearance, resulting in differing toxicities with minimal bone marrow effects. Instead, cutaneous toxicity known as hand–foot syndrome occurs. Neurotoxicity and cardiotoxicity may also occur.

5-FU pro-drugs

Uftoral® (tegafur with uracil)

Orally active this is a mixture of tegafur given in combination with uracil in a molar ratio of 1:4. This agent is licensed and used in many countries but not in the USA. It has shown activity mainly in colorectal and other GI cancers.

Capecitabine

This is an orally active pro-drug of 5-FU. It is preferentially activated in tumour and liver tissue and has the potential to replace prolonged or continuous infusion 5-FU. It has been shown to be active in a wide range of cancers and is licensed for breast and GI cancers. Further development and clinical trial work is ongoing to try to substitute this drug for 5-FU in other clinical scenarios.

2-fluoro-2'-deoxyuridine (floxuridine)

Given IV, this agent can be metabolized both into 5-FU and also directly into FdUMP, theoretically giving increased efficacy. Its clinical use has largely been confined to hepatic artery infusion because it is less toxic than single-agent 5-FU used by this route for treating colon cancer. It is not licensed for use in the UK.

Modulation of 5-FU

A number of agents have been combined with 5-FU in order to increase either its efficacy or therapeutic index.

5-FU and folinic acid combinations are the mainstay of treatment of colon cancer. Folinic acid is given by infusion, before or concomitant with 5-FU. By increasing supply of CH_2-FH_4, folinic acid potentiates interaction between 5-FU and TS. Although more toxic, it has a higher response rate in advanced colorectal cancer with combined treatment than single-agent 5-FU.

Anti-purines

Purine analogues are widely used to treat leukaemias and as immunosuppressives (azathioprine) and antivirals (aciclovir, ganciclovir).

Pemetrexed is a novel TS inhibitor which also inhibits DHFR and GARFT. It is licensed for the treatment of mesothelioma and non-small cell lung cancer. Its toxicity is reduced by the concomitant administration of B12 and folate supplements. 6-Mercaptopurine (6-MP) and 6-thioguanine (6-TG) both inhibit *de novo* purine synthesis, and their nucleotide products are incorporated into DNA. Hypoxanthine guanine phosphoribosyl transferase (HGPRT) produces monophosphates, that inhibit early stages of purine synthesis, and then convert into triphosphates that are incorporated into DNA, causing strand breaks. There are synergistic effects with MTX, due to 5- phosphoribosylpyrophosphate (PRPP) build-up, facilitating phosphorylation by HGPRT. Resistance develops due to HGPRT deficiency and reduced substrate affinity. Variable oral bioavailability may contribute to some treatment failures in childhood acute lymphoblastic leukaemia (ALL).

Both drugs have a short half-life and are primarily metabolized – the important difference is that 6-MP is a substrate for xanthine oxidase, and dose alterations are necessary when co-administered with allopurinol. There is poor CSF penetration, but otherwise these agents are widely distributed.

The main toxicity is myelosuppression, but 6-MP can also cause hepatotoxicity. Nausea, vomiting, and mucositis can also occur, more commonly with 6-MP. The commonest indication is haematological malignancy: 6-MP is used for maintenance therapy of ALL, and 6-TG is used for both remission induction and maintenance in acute myeloid leukaemia (AML).

Cytosine analogues

Cytarabine (cytosine arabinoside, ara-C)

Cytarabine is actively transported, and its metabolite ara-CTP is incorporated into DNA, inhibiting DNA polymerases and possibly phospholipid synthesis. Unlike gemcitabine, no further normal nucleotides are added, so that damaged DNA is susceptible to DNA repair.

Cytarabine is active in non-Hodgkin's leukaemia (NHL) and AML, but not in solid tumours. There is renal excretion of deaminated compound and because of rapid clearance better activity is observed when cytarabine is given by continuous infusion. Side-effects are emesis, alopecia, and myelosuppression.

It can also cause 'ara-C syndrome' with fevers, myalgias, rash, keratoconjunctivitis, and arthralgias. Rarely, lung and pancreatic damage occur.

2,2-Difluorodeoxycytidine (gemcitabine)

This fluorinated analogue has better membrane permeation and affinity for deoxycytidine kinase than cytarabine. Intracellular retention is prolonged, partly due to a unique self-potentiation in which the bi- and triphosphates facilitate the phosphorylation of the parent compound, as well as inhibiting its catabolism.

The active metabolite dF-CTP is incorporated into DNA, followed only by one more normal nucleotide, resulting in protection of the DNA from repair enzymes ('masked termination'). It is probably the saturable formation of dF-CTP that contributes to the clinical schedule dependency of gemcitabine, usually given IV, weekly for 3 weeks out of 4.

Toxicities include flu-like symptoms, transaminitis, peripheral oedema, myelosuppression, and possible nephrotoxicity.

There is some evidence for synergy with cisplatin, the extent of which appears to be schedule dependent. Gemcitabine is active in a wide range of cancers – most notably in pancreatic carcinoma where it is one of a very few drugs that have modest survival advantage.

Adenosine analogues

Three adenosine analogues have come into clinical practice, active in low-grade NHL, Waldenström's macroglobulinaemia, and chronic lymphocytic leukaemia (CLL). All have similar effects and interact with the enzyme adenosine deaminase (ADA), a deficiency of which causes severe combined immunodeficiency. Toxicity includes myelosuppression with particular effects on lymphocytes, including depression of CD3 and CD4 levels, and reduced natural killer cell (NK) activity.

Fludarabine

Resistant to ADA, it is particularly useful in treating CLL. It is actively transported into the cells and its mode of action is a consequence of phosphorylation, following which it is incorporated into DNA, and probably RNA, and may even cause topoisomerase II inhibition. Can cause haemolytic anaemia.

2'-Deoxycoformycin (pentostatin)

Has a very high affinity for ADA, and the resultant complex is stable for over 24 hours, resulting in enzyme inhibition. Its major indication is treatment of hairy-cell leukaemia. Actively transported into cells, it is phosphorylated and incorporated into DNA and also produces inhibitory dATP. It inhibits both DNA synthesis and DNA repair.

2-Chlorodeoxyadenosine (cladribine)

Resistant to ADA, phosphorylated and incorporated into DNA, and is used for hairy-cell leukaemia.

Hydroxyurea

This oral agent inhibits ribonucleotide reductase, which reduces the availability of all deoxynucleotides. It crosses the blood–brain barrier, and is used in myeloproliferative disorders. Toxicities are myelosuppression, GI toxicities, and sometimes hyperpigmentation of the skin.

Cisplatin and derivatives

Cisplatin is one of the most active anti-cancer drugs in clinical use, with a very wide spectrum of anti-tumour activity. In view of its considerable toxicity profile, many attempts have been made to develop analogues with less toxicity, increased efficacy, or both.

Carboplatin

A large number of analogues have been subject to clinical trials but only carboplatin has emerged as a viable clinical candidate.

There is still a degree of controversy regarding the clinical equivalence of cisplatin and carboplatin; there are limited situations such as germ cell tumours where cisplatin still appears to be the agent of choice. However, carboplatin in most other circumstances has supplanted the use of cisplatin.

Side-effects of carboplatin
Significant
- Thrombocytopenia, worse at day 14
- Leucopenia, worse at day 14

Less significant toxicities
- Renal
- Neurological
- Otological
- Nausea and vomiting – occasionally
- Alopecia – absent/mild
- Visual disturbances – rarely
- Allergy – in 2%

Dosage of carboplatin
Initially, a dosage of carboplatin based on body-surface area resulted in a variable degree of thrombocytopenia with a number of patients requiring platelet transfusion. Pharmacokinetically based dosing is now the adopted standard.

The simple pharmacokinetics of carboplatin with clearance being dependent almost exclusively on renal mechanisms allow a dosing formula to be derived. The dose required to achieve a specific AUC (area under the curve) can be calculated for an individual patient. The most widely used formula is:

$$\text{Dose} = H(\text{GFR} + 25)$$

where:
- dose is the total dose in mg to be given to the patient
- H is the desired area under the curve (AUC) in mg/ml.mm. Typical AUCs are between 4 and 7, depending on frequency of administration, previous treatment, and the drugs being used in combination
- GFR is the glomerular filtration rate of the patient (ml/min), unadjusted for surface area (should ideally be measured by an isotope method such as ^{51}CrEDTA clearance, but a carefully performed 24-h urinary creatinine clearance is also acceptable).

Activity of carboplatin

Carboplatin can be regarded as a less toxic substitute for cisplatin and is used for similar indications. Patients resistant to cisplatin will also be resistant to carboplatin and vice versa. However, the increased thrombocytopenia seen with carboplatin may be a disadvantage in some combinations, while reduced non-haematological toxicities may be an advantage in others. Further, a low level of non-haematological toxicity makes carboplatin suitable for inclusion in high-dose regimens with bone marrow or stem cell rescue.

Pharmacokinetic interactions with carboplatin

Unlike cisplatin, carboplatin does not affect hepatic cytochrome P450 enzyme, and pharmacokinetic interactions with other drugs seem to be rare.

Summary

Carboplatin has major advantages over cisplatin in terms of ease of administration and non-haematological toxicities, although the higher incidence of thrombocytopenia may be a problem in some circumstances. In the main, it can be regarded as an alternative to cisplatin, but current data suggest cisplatin should still be used for treating testicular teratoma. Unlike cisplatin, carboplatin can be used in high-dose regimens. Carboplatin should generally be dosed on a pharmacokinetic basis.

Cisplatin mechanism of action

Cisplatin binds directly to DNA, inhibiting synthesis by altering the DNA template via formation of intra-strand and inter-strand cross-links.

These cross-links are generated by an aquated complex that acts as a bifunctional alkylating agent. Cytotoxic effects of cisplatin are cell-cycle independent, and synergy between cisplatin and anti-metabolites has been demonstrated both *in vitro* and in clinical trials. The mechanism behind this synergy has not been fully explained; the most commonly held hypothesis is that this is due to a malfunction in DNA repair processing.

Side-effects of cisplatin

Cisplatin is highly emetogenic, it produces a dose-dependent nephrotoxicity, it can also cause peripheral neuropathy, and due to ototoxicity it can produce tinnitus and high tone deafness. Cisplatin is not very toxic to white cells or platelets but has the propensity to cause anaemia.

Dosage of cisplatin

Cisplatin is used in a variety of dosage schedules. The standard dose limit is 100 mg/m^2 as a single daily dose; higher doses have been explored in clinical trials, particularly in conjunction with neuroprotective agents. Alternate schedules such as five daily injections of 20 mg/m^2 are favoured in the treatment of teratoma.

The initial clearance of cisplatin is rapid, followed by a much slower decline due to binding to plasma proteins. Clearance is prolonged in patients with renal insufficiency. Unlike carboplatin, there is no clear evidence of a pharmacodynamic/pharmacokinetic relationship with cisplatin; therefore dosage is usually based on empirical body-surface calculations.

Clinical indications for cisplatin

Cisplatin has been a major step forward in the treatment of testicular cancer. In patients with metastatic disease, cisplatin-based combination therapy results in a complete clinical response in over 80% of patients, with the majority of these achieving long-term cure. Cisplatin is also a major component of treatment of ovarian cancer, genitourinary tumours, and other squamous carcinomas, particularly those in the head and neck and non-small-cell bronchogenic carcinoma.

Combinations of cisplatin with other cytotoxic agents are common and are used in a variety of human solid cancers and paediatric tumours.

Oxaliplatin

Oxaliplatin is a platinum analogue that differs from carboplatin and cisplatin, in both chemical behaviour and possibly its mechanism of action. *In vitro* oxaliplatin has a broad spectrum of activity with marked differences from the spectrum seen with cisplatin or carboplatin. In clinical practice it is used extensively in colorectal cancer both in the adjuvant and advanced disease settings. It has broad-spectrum activity and is also used in many other cancer types – such as upper GI. Unfortunately, its cumulative dosage is limited by the development of a characteristic peripheral neuropathy, which in most cases is reversible on withdrawal of the drug.

Dosage of oxaliplatin

Two commonly used regimens exist:
- 85 mg/m^2 every 2 weeks as a 2–6 h infusion
- 130 mg/m^2 over a similar length of time repeated every 3 weeks.

However, a multitude of studies exist using a variety of different dosing regimens, including chronomodulated infusion together with 5-FU.

Topoisomerase inhibitors

Topoisomerase enzymes are a family of nuclear proteins with essential functions in regulating the topology of the DNA helix. Eukaryotics have two forms of topoisomerase enzyme.

- Topoisomerase I (topo I) binds to double-stranded DNA and cleaves and relegates one strand of duplex DNA. Relaxation of supercoiled DNA is then used during processes of replication, transcription, and recombination.
- Topoisomerase II (topo II) creates transient double-stranded breakage of DNA, allowing subsequent passage of a second intact DNA duplex through the break.

Topoisomerase I inhibitors

Camptothecin (CPT) has been identified as the active constituent of an extract isolated from the Chinese tree, *Camptotheca acuminata*. Mechanism of action studies demonstrated that CPT stabilized covalent adducts between genomic DNA and topoI. Early clinical studies with CPT observed anti-tumour activity in a variety of common solid tumours. However, a high rate of severe and unpredictable toxicities led to discontinuation of CPT's development.

To date, two main derivatives have been licensed, irinotecan and topotecan.

Both agents can be administered in a variety of IV schedules with claimed differences in response and/or toxicity profile.

Side-effects

- Neutropenia – common
- Diarrhoea – common (early or late)
- Thrombocytopenia
- Anaemia
- Alopecia
- Nausea, vomiting.

Clinical pharmacology

Both CPT-11 and topotecan can be absorbed orally, with topotecan bioavailability of 30–50%; both are widely distributed throughout the body, with cerebrospinal fluid topotecan concentrations 30–50% of simultaneous plasma concentrations.

Topotecan undergoes negligible metabolism and is primarily eliminated by the kidneys, with evidence for renal tubular secretion. A linear relationship between creatinine clearance and clearance of both total topotecan and lactone form has been demonstrated.

CPT-11 is in itself relatively inactive and must be converted by carboxylesterases to 7-ethyl10-hydroxycampothecin (SN-38), which has potent topoI inhibitory activity. Glucuronidation and biliary excretion are the principal mechanisms of elimination for SN-38. Particular caution and dose reduction are recommended for patients with liver dysfunction or Gilbert's syndrome.

Topoisomerase II inhibitors

Etoposide and teniposide exert their action on topo II by:
- inhibiting the ability of the enzyme to relegate the cleaved DNA complex
- generating high levels of DNA with potentially toxic double-stranded breaks
- promoting mutation
- permanent double-stranded breaks
- illegitimate recombination
- apoptosis.

Etoposide and teniposide are poorly water soluble and are formulated with a number of excipients including polysorbate (etoposide) or teniposide (Cremophor® EL). Etoposide can be administered by either oral or intravenous routes, teniposide only by IV injection.

Teniposide and etoposide are widely used in treatment of adult and paediatric malignancies. Etoposide has been more broadly used in front-line therapy, particularly for small-cell lung cancer and germ-cell tumours. The pattern of toxicity is very similar between both agents and includes neutropenia, alopecia, mucositis, infusion-related blood pressure changes, and hypersensitivity reactions. Teniposide is not licensed for use in the UK.

Clinical pharmacology

Etoposide absorption appears to be non-linear with decreased bioavailability at doses above 200 mg. Both etoposide and teniposide are heavily protein bound; use in patients with low albumin concentrations will result in greater than expected systemic toxicity due to the larger free (unbound) drug concentrations.

Both etoposide and teniposide are extensively metabolized. Etoposide is more rapidly eliminated than teniposide. Linear relationships between etoposide systemic clearance and creatinine clearance have been described for both adult and paediatric patients.

Anti-microtubule agents

Tubulin-interactive agents, commonly known as 'spindle poisons', have a long history of use in cancer treatment. They act by binding to specific sites on tubulin, a protein that polymerizes to form cellular microtubules.

Table 6.1 focuses on important anti-microtubule agents in clinical use. Tubulin is an important target for anti-cancer drug development; several anti-tubulin agents have significant anti-cancer activity in the clinic. The taxanes (Taxol® and Taxotere®) were the most encouraging development in anti-cancer chemotherapy of the 1990s.

Recent progress observed with taxanes has led to renewed interest in anti-microtubule analogues or drugs interacting with different sites on tubulin. In particular, agents with an improved pharmacological profile and/or activity in vinca/taxane-resistant cell lines are of interest. Several new anti-tubulin agents are in preclinical development, and methods of enhancing cellular delivery of taxanes whilst avoiding the toxic side-effects are the focus of many drug-development efforts.

Table 6.1 Anti-microtubule agents

Class of spindle poison (mechanism of action)	Useful indications	Drug administration (IV doses in mg/m²)	Main toxicities	Pharmacokinetics and metabolism	Comments of clinical interest
Vincristine (VCR) (destabilization of polymerized tubulin (β-tubulin))	Leukaemias, lymphomas, paediatric tumours, small-cell lung cancer, multiple myeloma	0.5–1.4 q 1–4 weeks (maximum total individual dose: 2 mg)	Neuropathy	Metabolized in the liver	VCR induces multidrug resistance (MDR) by P-glycoprotein (Pgp). Mutations in α– and β-tubulin proteins enhance stability against depolymerization
Vinblastine (VBL) (same as VCR)	Lymphomas, germ cell tumours, Kaposi's sarcoma, breast cancer	6–10 q 2–4 weeks	Neutropenia, neuropathy	Metabolized in the liver	Neuropathy occurs less frequently than with VCR
Vindesine (VDS) (same as VCR)	Non-small-cell lung cancer (NSCLC), breast cancer, prostate, lymphomas	2–4 q 1–3 weeks	Neutropenia, neuropathy	Metabolized in the liver	Randomized trials (breast, NSCLC, sarcomas, and melanoma) with VDS showed no advantage over treatments without VDS
Vinorelbine (NVB) (same as VCR)	NSCLC, breast cancer	25–30 weeks combinations: cisplatin (NSCLC) and doxorubicin or 5-FU (breast); Oral form in clinical development	Neutropenia, constipation, neuropathy	Metabolized in the liver	Selective binding to the tau family of microtubule- associated proteins → tubulin aggregation into spirals and paracrystals

(continued)

Table 6.1 (Cont'd)

Class of spindle poison (mechanism of action)	Useful indications	Drug administration (IV doses in mg/m²)	Main toxicities	Pharmacokinetics and metabolism	Comments of clinical interest
					NVB not active and associated with severe neurotoxicity in paclitaxed pre-treated breast cancer patients.
Paclitaxel (P) (microtubule stabilizer) (also anti-angiogenesis effect, disruption of Ki-Ras function, apoptosis induction by phosphorylation of bcl-2)	Ovarian, breast, and lung cancers (other tumours). Reproducible anti-tumour activity (response rate 15–25%) in platinum-resistant ovarian cancer stimulated further clinical development	135 (24 h)–175 (3 h) q 3 weeks. Weekly schedule is under investigation. Combinations: mainly with cisplatin or carboplatin (ovary) and doxorubicin (breast)	Neutropenia, neurotoxicity	Metabolized in the liver. Cisplatin → P: severe neutropenia; P → doxorubicin: more mucositis than the reverse sequence	Toxicities are sequence- and schedule-dependent. Steroid pre-medication is used to reduce hypersensitivity reactions. Water-soluble analogues and derivatives active in resistant cells of P are under development.Mutations in P53 cell lines confer sensitization to P. Resistance to P due to Pgp and/or alterations in the expression or structure of β-tubulin

| Docetaxel (D) (microtubule stabilizer) | Breast cancer, lung cancer (other tumours). Reproducible anti-tumour activity (response rate 35–50%) in anthracycline-resistant breast cancer stimulated further clinical development | 100 (1 h) q 3 weeks, 75 q 3 weeks (if elevated liver function tests). Weekly schedule is under investigation | Neutropenia, fluid retention syndrome (FRS) | Metabolized in the liver | Steroid pre-medication reduces and delays FRS. Tau and β4-tubulin expression correlate with D sensitivity in adenocarcinoma models |
| Estramustine phosphate (EP) (binds to the microtubule-associated proteins to promote microtubule disassembly) | Prostate cancer | 560 mg × 2/day orally (with meal) | Gastrointestinal | 75% of oral EP is absorbed. Terminal half-life: 20–40 h | Most responses observed in prostate cancer were subjective (objective response rate ~10%). EP has been combined with other anti-microtubules (P, VBL) and etoposide with a clinical benefit in 30–60% of patients. Overexpression of beta (III & IVa)-tubulin and tau may play a role in resistance to EP |

Drug resistance

Most of the basic research into drug resistance has involved using pairs of sensitive and resistant tumour cells derived from the same parental cell line, usually by serial passage in increasing concentrations of the drug under investigation. This is an artificial situation, which often results in resistance that is really very substantial with concentration variants in excess of 40–100-fold sometimes required to overcome such resistance. It is unclear whether this laboratory-derived resistance correlates with the types of clinical resistance that are outlined above.

Pharmacological resistance

The underlying concept of pharmacological resistance is that the dose of chemotherapy that can be safely given is insufficient to result in an effective concentration of the active drug at its target site. This may be due to:

- toxicity in other organs
- enhanced clearance of drugs
- physical barrier between bloodstream and tumour cells (many tumours have avascular centres)
- *de novo* resistance – tumour does not respond despite full-dose chemotherapy
- acquired resistance – initial response to chemotherapy, then tumour fails to respond and regrows
- combination of *de novo* and acquired.

Alteration of target or transport mechanisms

Tumour cells have the ability to mutate such that the drug is either not taken up by the cell or, having been taken up, is detoxified more rapidly than normal. Alternatively, the actual target of the drug may change by mutation such that it becomes impervious to the form of attack. Or the normal repair mechanisms that are present in all mammalian cells may become more active and repair damage as produced by a cytotoxic agent in a more efficient manner, resulting in overall resistance to the agent.

Classical multidrug resistance

'Classical' drug resistance has been the most studied form of this phenomenon in the laboratory and results from overexpression of a 170 Da glycoprotein known as P-glycoprotein (Pgp). This spans the outer cell membrane and acts as an energy-dependent drug efflux pump. Thus, as the drug enters the tumour cell, by diffusion or transport, the drug in the interior of the cell is picked up and is effluxed into the extracellular environment. This reduces the effective concentration of the drug within the cell and allows the cell to express resistance to the agent in question.

The development of this form of resistance is most commonly associated with exposure to the anti-tumour antibiotics, the anthracyclines, taxanes, and etoposide. In fact, resistance to one of this group of agents usually confers resistance to the other groups in addition, thereby leading to the phenomenon of 'multidrug resistance'.

Multidrug resistance-associated protein (MRP)

This protein is one member of a family of proteins that also act as energy-dependent pumps, in this case resulting in drug efflux or sequestration of the drug, within intracytoplasmic organelles or vacuoles. The most studied member of this family of proteins is a 190 kDa protein that has a similar substrate specificity to Pgp but is usually associated with less resistance to the taxanes. The clinical relevance of this form of resistance is less clear than with the Pgp.

Glutathione

Glutathione is the predominant cellular thiol and participates in a complex biochemical pathway that interacts with the alkylating function of some agents (including cisplatin). Glutathione overexpression in cell lines results in relative resistance to alkylating agent attack. In addition, glutathione is able to detoxify free radicals, which may be an important pathway of action for some cytotoxics, including doxorubicin. Clinical trials of glutathione depletion have been performed with somewhat equivocal results.

Failure to engage apoptosis

The common final pathway of cell death for many cytotoxics is apoptosis. This is an active process within cells, somewhat akin to 'cell suicide'. The engagement of the apoptosis programme is a complex interacting pathway. At the centre of this is p53, the so-called 'guardian of the genome'. In cells that are unable to engage apoptosis, the damage done by cytotoxics can be 'ignored' and cell division continues. This results in clinical drug resistance. Gene-therapy approaches to correct this apoptosis failure are being actively investigated.

Summary

Clinical drug resistance is a major problem in oncology and the underlying mechanisms are multifactorial. In any one patient it is unclear to what extent each mechanism contributes. Nevertheless, the potential clinical benefits of mechanisms to circumvent drug resistance are enormous. Undoubtedly, other mechanisms of drug resistance will be found as we come to understand more about the regulation of cell cycle, cell life, and cell death.

Dose intensification

Dose–response

The strategy of therapeutic dose intensification in oncology has been largely driven by experimental evidence suggesting that the drug resistance of cancer cells is often relative. Results of studies indicate that arbitrary dose reduction should be avoided, and suggest that clinicians should consider use of prophylactic antibiotics, haemopoietic growth factors, etc. in situations where neutropenia and its complications threaten to undermine timely delivery of potentially curative chemotherapy.

High-dose chemotherapy (HDC) with haemopoietic support

In the clinic, dose escalation within a 'conventional' range has an inconsistent effect on response rates and, with some exceptions, a negligible survival impact. Dose escalation is complicated by increased toxicity. Substantial advances in haemopoietic support have allowed investigation of high doses of chemotherapy in the clinic. Autografting, using either autologous marrow or cytokine-mobilized peripheral blood progenitors, is seen to facilitate administration of high doses of those drugs that are dose limited by myelosuppression.

It was also discovered that administration of these factors, either at steady state or following myelosuppressive chemotherapy, resulted in mobilization of haemopoietic progenitors from the bone marrow into the peripheral blood. These 'peripheral blood progenitors' (PBPs) could be harvested by leucopheresis, then re-infused as haemopoietic rescue following subsequent HDC. PBP autografting is superior to marrow autografting, with shortened neutropenia and thrombocytopenia, and reduced mortality and morbidity.

Historically, HDC has generally been given as a form of consolidation following conventional chemotherapy. Less frequently, it has been studied as primary treatment. It can be administered in single or in multiple cycles.

Role of HDC in the treatment of specific tumours

- Relapsed aggressive lymphoma – proven salvage treatment
- Refractory lymphoma – 10% remission
- Poor prognosis NHL – first-line treatment
- Multiple myeloma – first-line treatment
- Relapsed refractory Hodgkin's disease – first-line treatment
- Acute leukaemia – especially if no donor
- Metastatic testicular germ-cell tumours – relapse after second remission.

Accelerated chemotherapy

An alternative approach to dose intensification is to shorten the interval between cycles of conventional chemotherapy, usually though granulocyte colony-stimulating factor (G-CSF) support. Preliminary results with this approach in adjuvant chemotherapy for high-risk breast cancer have been promising but this approach is still considered experimental.

Chemo-irradiation

Chemotherapy and radiotherapy are complementary; integration of these treatment modalities underpins successful treatment of a number of tumours. Chemotherapy reduces the burden of local diseases and eradicates systemic micrometastases, but effective loco-regional tumour control in some situations requires irradiation.

Sequential combined therapy

The traditional approach to combining chemotherapy and radiotherapy has been to attempt to predict whether eradication of systemic disease or local tumour control is of most immediate concern, then deliver the appropriate treatment first; the other treatment is delayed until completion of the first. The main difficulties are the uncertain behaviour of individual tumours and the inevitable delay in delivery of one treatment. Chemotherapy as the first-line treatment has the added potential benefit that in downstaging the tumour it may reduce both the volume of tissue that requires irradiation and the radiation dose required to control the tumour.

Concurrent combined therapy

Problems are avoided by delivering chemotherapy and radiotherapy together. This approach has advantages and some disadvantages (see Table 6.2).

Ideally, cytotoxics chosen for chemo-irradiation regimens will have known activity against the tumour but will not have toxicities that overlap the effects of irradiation of the relevant region. Agents such as cisplatin and 5-FU are particularly attractive because of their radiosensitizing effects. At least *in vitro*, the interactions of chemotherapy and radiotherapy are complex and schedule dependent. An attempt must be made to minimize the normal tissue damage of radiation during combined therapy.

Table 6.2 Benefits and problems of concurrent combined therapy

Advantage	Disadvantage
No delay in either therapy	Increased toxicity
Additive cell kill by two therapies	Compromised dose of one or both treatments
Enhanced cell kill by radiosensitizing effects of chemotherapy	Large volume irradiated
Reduced likelihood of evolution of resistance to either therapy	Pharmacodynamic interactions (e.g. cell-cycle effects)

Anal and bladder carcinomas

For both these pelvic malignancies chemo-irradiation offers the possibility of organ preservation and avoidance of a stoma. There is good evidence that pelvic irradiation with concurrent 5-FU and mitomycin is the best-established therapy for anal carcinoma. The combination of pelvic radiotherapy and cisplatin-based chemotherapy has proven successful in large phase II studies in muscle-invading transitional cell carcinoma of the bladder.

Head and neck cancer and oesophageal cancer

Chemo-irradiation of intrathoracic tumours is hindered by risk of serious morbidity, in particular pneumonitis and oesophagitis. Chemo-irradiation is superior to radiation therapy alone for oesophageal cancer but local failure rates remain high. Surgery after combined treatment may be the answer to this problem.

Primary chemo-radiotherapy of head and neck cancers is widely used and can result in good response rates with some cures. This approach has some advantages over more radical surgical excision because of the possibility of organ and function preservation with resultant reduction of morbidity. Surgical salvage can then be reserved for non-responding or relapsing cases.

Rectal cancer

There is now clear evidence that combination of fluoropyrimidine-based chemotherapy with external beam radiotherapy (EBRT) leads to improved local control and enhanced survival. There remains an area of controversy over use of pre-operative chemo-radiation versus use of the same in the post-operative phase for selected patients.

Non-small-cell lung cancer

There is some controversy over the place of combined or sequential chemo-radiation in non-small-cell lung cancer (NSCLC). Clinical studies have shown modest outcome benefits but at the cost of more toxicity and morbidity.

Principles of symptom control in palliative care

Introduction

'Palliative care is an approach that improves the quality of life of patients and their families facing the problem associated with life-threatening illness, through the prevention and relief of suffering by means of early identification and impeccable assessment and treatment of pain and other problems, physical, psychosocial and spiritual.'

(World Health Organization 2008 definition of palliative care, www.who.int/cancer/palliative/definition/en/)

The majority of metastatic solid tumours in adults are incurable and the goal of treatment is to palliate symptoms and maximize quality of life. From diagnosis, many patients will have a fear of suffering and what the future may hold. Optimal management of patients with a diagnosis of cancer requires full involvement of the multidisciplinary team from the point of diagnosis – including palliative care services. The degree of involvement from each member of the team is likely to shift as the patient progresses through the course of their illness. However, the aims are:

• for the patient to benefit from the whole range of specialist medical, psychological, spiritual, and social interventions on offer that may improve their quality of life at every stage of cancer illness
• to minimize any distress caused by the apparent transition from 'active' oncological input to so-called 'terminal care'
• to try and help the patient 'live alongside their cancer' – to enable them to live as actively as possible until death
• to offer support to the patient and carers during the patient's illness and subsequently to the family in their bereavement.

Difficulties commonly identified as contributing to patient distress are treated in the following paragraphs.

'The system'

Medical professionals are all too used to the complex organization and multiple specialties potentially involved in the care of a patient from presentation, to diagnosis, to staging, to treatment. However, for the patient or carer it is often bewildering. This may be exacerbated if hospitals are split-site, if referral to tertiary centres is required, or if the diagnosis is not straightforward. Inherent limitations in communication between departments, availability of medical notes, etc. have been minimized with the development of the multidisciplinary team and the introduction of the clinical nurse specialist (CNS). The ideal is to maintain some continuity between appointments so that the patients can have a reasonable expectation that they will not have to repeat their story each time, that they have some understanding of the purpose of each visit, and that they know who to contact should they feel 'lost in the system' (usually the CNS).

Problems with information giving and breaking bad news

Poor communication and breaking of bad news are consistently mentioned by patients and families as causes of stress and dissatisfaction. Many patients leave their consultations uncertain of the precise diagnosis and prognosis, unclear about the likely therapeutic benefits of treatments, and wanting more information than has been provided. The number of patients who genuinely prefer to have little information and leave everything up to the doctor is probably <5%. If a patient is unsatisfied about the amount of information provided they are more likely to have greater difficulty adjusting to their diagnosis and subsequently have an increased risk of anxiety and depression. It is important to establish how much information the patient would like at each stage of their illness. Information giving should be tailored to the patient.

Good communication builds trust, reduces uncertainty, and allows appropriate adjustment (practical and emotional) by patient and family, thus reducing psychological morbidity. Breaking bad news is not a single, isolated event. The process is ongoing and recurring, involving telling the diagnosis, updating the patient and family on changes, and, possibly, preparing them for death.

Breaking bad news: a ten-step approach

This approach can be used as a general framework and adapted for specific situations. Remember a patient has a right but not a duty to hear bad news.

1. Preparation: know the facts. Arrange the meeting. Find out who the patient wants to be present. Arrange not to be disturbed (turn off bleeps).
2. Establish what the patient already knows. Both doctors and family generally underestimate the level of the patient's knowledge.
3. Establish whether the patient wants more information.
4. Allow denial. Denial is a defence and a way of coping. Allow the patient to control the amount of information.
5. Give a warning shot. This allows the patient time to consider their own reactions and whether they feel able to ask for more information.
6. Explain if requested. Be clear and simple. Avoid harsh statments and medical jargon. Check understanding. Be as optimistic as possible.
7. Listen to concerns. Avoid premature reassurance.
8. Encourage ventilation of feelings.
9. Summarize and make a plan: this minimizes confusion and uncertainty.
10. Offer availability. Communicating bad news is an ongoing process. Include time for questions; ideally provide written information and give details of a contact person (often a CNS) who can be available to answer any queries that arise later. Be clear about the next appointment or investigation – its time, place, and purpose.

Uncertainty

This is one of the most difficult problems for the human psyche to bear. It is a state in which most patients with cancer remain from the time that they discover sinister symptoms and undergo diagnostic tests until they complete treatment. Doctors are also faced with a dilemma when trying to offer reassurance to an anxious patient and be honest about an enig-matic disease that has an uncertain outcome. It can be especially prob-lematic when discussing clinical trials where uncertainty about the efficacy of treatment is inherent and must be discussed in order to gain informed consent.

There is often fear of potential:

- discomfort
- disfigurement
- disability
- dependency
- death.

Most patients told they have cancer will have personal experiences of rel-atives or friends previously diagnosed and treated for malignant disease. The clinician must be alert to these influences. Reassurance may be pos-sible. Misunderstandings can be clarified. Valid concerns can be acknowl-edged and addressed.

Discharge from follow-up

Paradoxically it is when treatment ends that a patient may be in greatest need of support in re-appraising their lives and coping with 'survivorship'. Patients often gain (false) reassurance from surveillance programmes and may feel unsupported when regular specialist contact ends. This problem is exacerbated by the fact that there are few adult malignancies from which patients can be given the 'all clear', and patients must cope with an ongoing risk of relapse. Sometimes this uncertainty is almost too much to cope with and on the one hand increases requests for review and more investigations, or conversely causes withdrawal and isolation.

Symptom control

For medical professionals involved in the day-to-day (and out-of-hours) management of patients with cancer, a large part of the clinical responsibility involves assessment and treatment of a range of symptoms. Symptoms may be:

- directly attributable to the cancer
- a side-effect or toxicity of palliative treatment
- physical, psychosocial, emotional, or spiritual
- due to an unrelated condition.

Therefore, each symptom requires careful assessment in order that the most appropriate management strategy can be adopted.

Pain management

Pain control is an obvious priority for patients with cancer, whether embarking on curative or palliative treatment. Approximately 80% of pain due to cancer can be relieved relatively simply with oral analgesics and adjuvant drugs in accordance with World Health Organization (WHO) guidelines, used in combination with interdisciplinary management. Inadequate pain control may exacerbate many other problems including fatigue, anorexia and nausea, constipation, depression, anxiety and hopelessness. It is also more difficult for a patient in pain to continue with demanding cytotoxic treatment and hospital visits. Relief of pain at the expense of side-effects is unacceptable to most patients; therefore a variety of treatment modalities are often required.

The commonest causes of uncontrolled cancer pain are:

- lack of sophistication in patient assessment, resulting in misdiagnosis of cause and type of pain and failure to detect general distress, which lowers the pain threshold. If pain distress is greater than pain severity and this is not identified, then the pain will never be dealt with adequately by analgesia alone. Psychological distress must be acknowledged and managed appropriately
- lack of a systematic approach to analgesia including lack of understanding of the WHO analgesic ladder, adjuvant analgesics, and titration of opioids. 'Panic prescribing' is more likely to result in unacceptable side-effects
- lack of knowledge of opioid pharmacology including failure to anticipate and prevent drug side-effects.

The ideal management of pain involves effective treatment of the underlying condition causing that pain. Hence, appropriate palliative chemotherapy, radiotherapy, or hormone therapy for the causative malignancy is the approach of first choice. In the palliative setting, a reduction in analgesic use is an established method of assessing response to treatment. However, even if the patient is embarking on a course of therapy, immediate pain control needs must be assessed as any response to oncological treatments will not be immediate.

Categories of cancer pain

The importance of taking a good history cannot be overemphasized in pain management, as it allows the medical team to assess the likely mechanism(s) of pain and therefore to select treatment accordingly.

Is the pain acute or chronic?

A diagnosis of cancer is not necessarily sufficient reason for a person to be in pain. Pain of sudden onset may suggest an acute complication of either the malignancy or the treatment for that malignancy, or of an unrelated cause. For example, a new pathological fracture potentially requiring orthopaedic fixation, an acute intra-abdominal event necessitating surgical review, mucositis due to recent or ongoing chemo and/or radiotherapy.

Conversely, chronic escalating pain may represent underlying disease progression, e.g. soft tissue or nerve root infiltration.

What is the nature of the pain?
- *Somatic*: typically localized and persistent, e.g. bone metastases, localized inflammation such as cellulitis
- *Visceral*: usually poorly localized, of variable intensity and often with associated symptoms such as nausea, e.g. liver capsular stretch due to hepatic metastases, malignant abdominal lymphadenopathy, or smooth muscle spasm causing colic (bowel, bladder renal or biliary)
- *Neuropathic*: classically described as 'shooting or burning pain' usually following a dermatomal distribution, e.g. compression of a spinal nerve root.

What is the patient's interpretation of the pain?
Pain perception has a strong affective component and is greatly influenced by mood and morale. An understanding of the patient's interpretation of his/her own pain will help to formulate a realistic management plan. For instance, do they have specific anxieties related to this new pain, perhaps it has adversely affected their level of functioning, or maybe they view it as heralding the final stages of their illness. Addressing any anger, fear, or distress will increase the likelihood of achieving satisfactory pain control.

Pharmacological pain relief

The use of the WHO analgesic ladder is based upon a number of simple principles:
- strength of analgesia depends on the *severity of pain* rather than the stage of disease
- medication should be prescribed regularly 'around the clock' with the aim of preventing pain from reoccurring. Appropriate 'as required' medication must also be available for breakthrough pain at a dose that reflects the background regularly prescribed dose
- a single drug is rarely sufficient
- initiate treatment with immediate-release formulations and then switch to sustained-release formulations once pain is controlled and the dose has stabilized
- opioids are often used in combination with non-opioids
- adjuvant analgesia is chosen according to cause and type of pain
- the WHO analgesic ladder is summarized in Fig. 7.1.

Step 1: non-opioid analgesia
Paracetamol acts centrally and is a non-opioid analgesic. It is also an antipyretic but has no anti-inflammatory action. Adverse reactions are rare at prescribed doses, i.e. up to 1 g qds, and it is well tolerated.

Non-steroidal anti-inflammatory drugs (NSAIDs) have an important role in the management of cancer pain and are often used in combination with weak or strong opioids when opioid analgesia alone fails to achieve adequate pain control. They are not however without problems, especially when used continuously for weeks or months. Gastric irritation should be considered (even more so if the patient is receiving concomitant steroids), and renal function should be monitored at regular intervals. The most frequently prescribed NSAIDs are **ibuprofen** and **diclofenac**. Some units also use **naproxen** and **flurbiprofen** and the COX-2 **celecoxib** when there is higher risk of gastrointestinal (GI) morbidity. Paracetamol can be safely used in combination with an NSAID and may have a synergistic action.

Step 2: weak opioid analgesics
The patient should continue with their regular non-opioid analgesics. If pain is not adequately controlled, then a regular weak opioid agonist can be added. This step bridges the theoretical gap between steps 1 and 3.

Codeine (methyl morphine, a pro-drug of morphine) is metabolized to low-dose morphine and thus steps 2 and 3 might be thought of as 'low-dose' morphine and 'higher-dose morphine' respectively.

Codeine is demethylated by the CYP3A3/4 and CYP2D6 hepatic enzyme systems yielding around 10% morphine. It is important to recognize that pharmacogenomics have an important role to play, with substantial interindividual variability in the analgesic response to codeine. About 10% of Caucasians lack the enzyme and therefore do not respond to codeine. Sub-therapeutic doses of codeine often found in over-the-counter preparations (<30 mg in each tablet) should be avoided.

Dihydrocodeine, unlike codeine is an analgesic in its own right and does not depend upon conversion to morphine for its analgesic activity. It does, however, have a low oral bio-availability and is therefore similar mg for mg to codeine when taken orally. (1/10 potency of morphine).

Tramadol acts centrally and works through both opioid receptors and serotonergic/noradrenergic inhibitory mechanisms similar to antidepressants. Again, as with codeine, 5–10% of Caucasians in Europe lack the CYP2D6 enzyme and in those people, tramadol has little or no analgesic activity.

Step 3: strong opioid analgesics
If pain remains uncontrolled with a combination of regular non-opioid and weak opioid analgesics, continue the non-opioid but substitute a strong opioid for the weak opioid agonist. The strong opioid of choice remains morphine administered orally.

The body's endogenous opioid system consists of three peptide families: the enkephalins, endorphins, and dynorphins. Each have different receptor affinities for the mu, kappa and delta opioid receptors. These receptors are widely distributed throughout the CNS, particularly within the periaqueductal grey matter and throughout the spinal cord. Similarly, different exogenous opioid drugs prescribed to control pain exhibit different receptor affinities for these three opioid receptors.

The differing efficacy and side-effect profiles of different opioid drugs is in part due to these differences.

WHO Analgesic Ladder

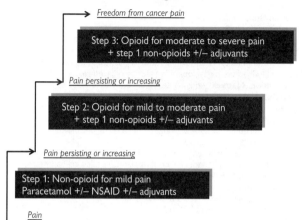

Freedom from cancer pain

Step 3: Opioid for moderate to severe pain
+ step 1 non-opioids +/− adjuvants

Pain persisting or increasing

Step 2: Opioid for mild to moderate pain
+ step 1 non-opioids +/− adjuvants

Pain persisting or increasing

Step 1: Non-opioid for mild pain
Paracetamol +/− NSAID +/− adjuvants

Pain

Fig. 7.1 The WHO analgesic 'ladder'. Adapted from a slide by Flora Watson.

Opioid titration on oral morphine

- Titration should be initiated with a 4-hourly dose of immediate-release morphine (solution or tablets).
- The starting dose should be higher than the current medication.
- If moving up from step 2 then 10 mg every 4 h and for breakthrough might be suitable.
- The frail and elderly might require titration from a lower dose, e.g. 5 mg 4-hourly.
- Increase the dose by 30–50% each day until the pain is controlled.
- Once a stable dose is achieved, convert to either a 12-hourly (bd) or 24-hourly (od) modified-release morphine preparation. This provides the continuous background analgesia and should be accompanied by a prescription for normal-release morphine available for breakthrough pain.
- This 'as required' (prn) dose should be 1/6th of the total 24-h dose.
- In renal impairment, a smaller dose less frequently maybe appropriate.
- Titration can continue once a patient has commenced modified-release morphine. The continued use of breakthrough medication is an indication that adequate pain control has not been achieved and the titration should continue in steps of 30–50% every 24–48 h. It is not good practice to simply add up the breakthrough requirements in a 24 h- period and add them into the total 24-hourly background modified-release dose. If a lot of breakthrough medication has been used, this might lead to a doubling (or more) of the daily opioid dose, which is never good practice. The risk of precipitating opioid toxicity is very high, especially if there is a degree of renal impairment.

- Common side-effects on initiating opioid therapy include:
  - nausea
  - constipation
  - drowsiness
  - dry mouth.

These are common during the titration phase and due to changing drug levels within the blood stimulating the area postrema along with decreased GI motility leading to gastroparesis (causing delayed gastric emptying) and constipation. **Nausea** tends to settle once a stable dose of morphine is achieved, but a prokinetic anti-emetic is often helpful: metoclopramide 10–20 mg, 3–4 times daily or domperidone 10–20 mg, 3–4 times daily. Occasionally a more potent dopamine antagonist is required for continual background nausea following the prescribing of opioids: haloperidol 1.5–3 mg nocte or 1.5 mg bd.

A combined stimulant and softening laxative is the most effective way to combat the opioid induced **constipation**: regular co-danthramer or co-danthrusate, the dose titrated to effect.

Drowsiness: usually improves after a few days following commencement of opioid or following titration to a stable dose.

Dry mouth: 📖 Mouthcare, p.158.

Morphine has an oral bioavailability of about 30%, undergoes extensive first-pass metabolism, and its metabolites (which are active) are excreted in the urine. Requirements vary greatly from patient to patient. It is important that the prn dose remains one-sixth to the daily morphine dose (as above). Clinical practice and evidence from trials tell us that opioid responsiveness is a continuum and no pain can be predicted as opioid unresponsive. However, certain types of pain require larger doses of opioids and can be poorly opioid responsive. Unacceptable side-effects such as sedation and hallucinations can then be reached before adequate pain control is achieved. It is in these situations where the gap between efficacy and toxicity is narrow that adjuvant analgesics become particularly important, often in the management of neuropathic pain.

Opioid toxicity

Often seen in patients with renal impairment, or severe liver disease and in whom the opioid dose has been increased by too much too quickly. Never increase the opioid dose by more than 50% at a time. It is bad practice to double a dose of opioid and there is never an indication to do this. It is very important to promptly recognize opioid toxicity and take immediate action:

- vivid dreams
- hallucinations – these often take the form of crawling insects or animals or a vague shadow in the periphery of the visual field
- drowsiness
- sometimes subtle agitation and/or confusion
- subtle paranoid delusions
- miosis (pinpoint pupils)
- muscle twitching/myoclonic jerks
- allodynia (pain caused by non-painful stimulus)
- hyperalgesia (increased sensitivity to pain) or complaints of 'pain all over'

- respiratory depression – usually only seen at doses above those required for analgesia or if the drug is accumulating, e.g. in renal impairment or severe liver failure. The use of naloxone is very rarely indicated for use in opioid toxicity as it will precipitate unacceptable pain escalation and distress. Remember that pain is the physiological antagonist to respiratory depression.

Managing opioid toxicity
- Reduce opioid dose by 30–50%.
- In renal impairment convert to short-acting (normal-release) opioid preparations to minimize the risk of accumulation.
- Check biochemistry and calcium.
- IV or subcutaneous (s/c) fluids may be indicated.
- Remember agitation and/or confusion can be misinterpreted as uncontrolled pain, leading to further opioids being administered and completing a vicious circle of opioid toxicity.

Reasons for considering switch to alternate opioid
- Poor compliance via oral route
- Intractable constipation
- Poorly responsive pain and/or intolerable side-effects.

Alternative strong opioids
- **Morphine** by s/c infusion:
  - water soluble
  - 1 g morphine sulphate requires 24 ml water for injection to dissolve
  - twice the potency of oral morphine
  - renal excretion of active metabolites
- **Diamorphine** by subcutaneous infusion:
  - much more water **and** fat soluble than morphine
  - 1 g diamorphine hydrochloride dissolves in 1.6 ml of water for injection, making it the drug of choice for small volume subcutaneous infusions
  - greater fat solubility compared to morphine explains increased potency, penetrating the blood–brain barrier much more rapidly, gaining access to brain and spinal cord
  - three times the potency when administered s/c compared with oral morphine
  - renal excretion of active metabolites
- **Fentanyl**:
  - extremely lipid soluble with totally different drug distribution and pharmacokinetics compared to morphine
  - 100–150 times the potency compared to oral morphine
  - lipid solubility permits transdermal administration. Controlled-release transdermal patches are useful for stable controlled pain
  - may cause less constipation and sedation
  - opioid toxicity may be more subtle and difficult to spot
  - the first patch requires cover with an alternative opioid at least over the first 12 h
  - less toxic in renal impairment
  - affected by significant liver function impairment and CYP-450 drug interactions
  - renal excretion of inactive metabolites

- **Alfentanil**:
  - similar to fentanyl
  - highly lipid soluble and suitable for continuous s/c infusion
  - 30 times the potency of oral morphine
  - 10 times the potency of s/c diamorphine
  - similar to fentanyl in renal and liver impairment.
  - renal excretion of inactive metabolites
- **Oxycodone**:
  - similar molecule to morphine
  - different receptor profile
  - an alternative opioid when morphine poorly tolerated or intolerable morphine side-effects
  - twice the potency of oral morphine
  - CYP-450 metabolism (potential drug interactions)
  - renal excretion of active metabolites
- **Hydromorphone**:
  - structurally very similar to morphine,
  - 7.5 times as potent as oral morphine
  - possibly less toxic in renal impairment
  - renal excretion of (possibly) active metabolite
- **Methadone**:
  - oral alternative to morphine with similar toxicity profile
  - relative analgesic potency hard to predict.
  - no active renal metabolites; safe in all but the severest renal failure
  - predominantly excreted faecally
  - extensively metabolized in the liver and affected by cytochrome p450 drug interactions
  - likely to accumulate in severe liver disease
  - complicated pharmacokinetics and different dosing schemes make this a drug requiring experienced specialist supervision.

Opioid potencies relative to oral morphine and 24-h equianalgesic doses of opioids

Fentanyl '25' patch provides 25 µg fentanyl per hour or 600 µg every 24 h. Potencies are given in Table 7.1.

Table 7.1 Opioid potencies and doses

Opioid	Potency (relative to oral morphine)	24 h dose
25 µg/h fentanyl patch	100–150×	1 patch
Oral morphine	1×	90 mg
s/c Morphine	2×	45 mg
s/c Diamorphine	3×	30 mg
Oral oxycodone	2×	45 mg
Oral hydromorphone	7.5×	12 mg
s/c Alfentanil	30×	3 mg

Adjuvant analgesics

The use of adjuvant analgesics should be considered at every stage in pain management. Adjuvants are not primarily analgesics themselves, but when combined with analgesics, aim to improve pain control, often allowing opioid dose reduction with fewer side-effects. This may widen the gap between efficacy and toxicity. Appropriate selection of therapy requires an understanding of the mechanism of pain, e.g.:

- somatic
- visceral
- neuropathic
- mixed.

It is important to give each selection an appropriate trial of efficacy but also to be prepared to withdraw ineffective medication. Otherwise, the patient could easily accumulate a vast array of tablets, requiring a complex timetable of administration without clear symptomatic benefit, but with a greatly increased risk of adverse side-effects.

Steroids

Indicated for:

- intra-cranial pressure (ICP)
- nerve root, spinal cord or cauda equina compression
- distension of the liver capsule (due to metastatic disease or subcapsular haemorrhage)
- soft tissue infiltration.

Dexamethasone up to 16 mg/day may be indicated initially, although the dose should be reviewed regularly and reduced to the minimum effective dose as soon as possible. Common side-effects or symptoms seen when maintaining too high a dose for too long:

- proximal myopathy affecting both upper and lower limbs
- fluid retention
- gastric irritation (from indigestion to haematemesis or perforation)
- insomnia and mood swings
- hyperglycaemia or deterioration in diabetic control
- iatrogenic Cushing's syndrome.

Dexamethasone has fewer mineralocorticoid-related effects, whilst prednisolone has less glucocorticoid activity.

Other adjuvant drugs include:

- **tricyclic antidepressants** (TCAs): useful in neuropathic pain, e.g. amitriptyline or imipramine 10–25 mg nocte cautiously titrated upwards aiming for 75–100 mg daily if tolerated (lower starting dose for the frail and elderly). Anticholinergic side-effects include sedation, confusion, dry mouth, blurred vision, postural hypotension, constipation, and urinary retention
- **anticonvulsants**: gabapentin is the only drug licensed for all types of neuropathic pain. Alternative drugs include sodium valproate, pregabalin and carbamazepine. Anticonvulsants can be used instead of TCAs or in combination if either agent on their own affords insufficient pain control
- **NMDA** (N-methyl D-aspartate) receptor antagonists: ketamine used for severe neuropathic pain refractory to combined strong opioid,

antidepressant and anti-epileptic. Central sensitization and wind-up pain characterized by hyperalgesia and allodynia

- **smooth muscle relaxants**: hyoscine butyl bromide for colic of bowel, urinary tract, or biliary tract etc.
- **benzodiazepines**: for skeletal muscle spasm or neuropathic pain
- **bisphosphonates**: there is evidence from randomized placebo-controlled trials that bisphosphonates reduce pain due to skeletal metastatic disease in breast, prostate, and lung cancer and reduce bone-related complications such as pathological fractures. They also have a role in multiple myeloma. Analgesic effect takes up to 2 weeks to develop. Their role in other malignancies remains to be established. Treatment is currently intravenous (e.g. pamidronate or zoledronic acid on a 3–4 weekly schedule) although work continues to develop an oral agent with equivalent efficacy. Renal function and serum Ca^{2+} (risk of hypocalcaemia) need to be monitored.

Other interventions

Anaesthetic techniques

- **Peripheral nerve block** e.g. intercostal nerve block for painful rib metastasis or peripheral lung tumour/mesothelioma infiltrating chest wall.
- **Coeliac plexus block** for pancreatic cancer pain or other advanced upper GI malignancy.
- **Brachial plexus block** for malignant axillary disease from e.g. breast cancer, metastatic melanoma or pancoast tumour infiltrating the brachial plexus. The placement of a brachial plexus catheter could allow continous infusion of analgesia.

Indications for spinal opioids

- Poor pain control despite escalating opioid requirements
- Opioid switch already tried or not appropriate
- Unacceptable or intolerable systemic opioid side-effects.

Indications for epidural or intrathecal analgesia

- Pathological hip/pelvic fractures in patients unsuitable for surgical fixation
- Intractable low back pain with metastatic disease affecting the lumbo-sacral spine
- Advanced pelvic malignancy involving any of the pelvic organs
- Recurrent rectal tumours causing intractable pain and/or tenesmus
- Upper abdominal pain (coeliac plexus pain) can be managed with thoracic epidural initially prior to consideration of coeliac plexus block
- Early referral to the pain team or a specialist anaesthetist should be considered.

Neurosurgical techniques

- Spinal cord decompression/laminectomy, +/– stabilization
- Open anterolateral cordotomy
- Percutaneous cervical cordotomy
- Implanted intrathecal pump
- Neuromodulation – implanted spinal cord stimulator.

Orthopaedic surgery

- Fixation of pathological fractures, hip nailing, hemi-arthroplasty, girdlestone, pelvic stabilization, humeral intramedullary wiring
- Vertebroplasty with injection of cement into a collapsed vertebral body for bone pain

Important practice point

DO NOT FORGET TO REDUCE SYSTEMIC OPIOID DOSE BY 30–50% FOLLOWING SUCCESSFUL NERVE BLOCK OR FIXATION OF UNSTABLE FRACTURE (to prevent opioid toxicity).

Palliative radiotherapy

External-beam radiotherapy can be effective in reducing pain due to local tumour effects, e.g. from skeletal metastases. However, it must be remembered that the maximum benefit of radiotherapy can take several weeks to develop. Indeed, radiotherapy may initially exacerbate pain. Pain control must be adequately addressed whilst the patient is undergoing treatment and in the subsequent weeks.

Bone-targeted radioisotopes, e.g. strontium-89, can be considered for diffuse pain from osteoblastic metastases unresponsive to conventional analgesia. The radioisotope is absorbed at areas of high bone turnover. It can take up to 3 months to derive any analgesic benefit, and myelosuppression can be a significant toxicity.

Supportive care

There are many other interventions that complement the medical approach to pain control and may have therapeutic benefit. These include:
- transcutaneous electrical nerve stimulation (TENS)
- occupational therapy
- physiotherapy
- acupuncture, aromatherapy, or reflexology
- relaxation therapies, including massage and hypnosis
- patient education and psychological support
- daycare can provide a framework and environment for some or all of the above as well as other creative therapies through raising self esteem and distracting the focus away from unpleasant symptoms.

Nausea and vomiting

Nausea and/or vomiting occur in up to 70% of patients with advanced cancer.

Nausea is an extremely unpleasant sensation with patients rating it often as bad as pain.

Vomiting is the forceful expulsion of gastric contents co-ordinated within the medulla of the brainstem. Surprisingly, nausea and vomiting can exist as separate entities. Not every patient with nausea vomits, nor does every vomiting patient have nausea.

As with pain control, appropriate management requires a thorough assessment so that a probable cause can be suspected which then fits with the underlying neuropharmacological mechanism. A logical choice of anti-emetic can then be made (Fig. 7.2). Particular attention should be paid to the history with regard to reduced appetite, early satiety, retching, and small- or large-volume vomiting.

Mechanisms

There are many neurotransmitters, receptors, and neural pathways involved in nausea and vomiting connecting the central nervous system (CNS) with the periphery. The optimal choice of anti-emetic therefore requires an understanding of the potential mechanism(s) of nausea and the site(s) of action of the anti-emetic selected (Fig. 7.2).

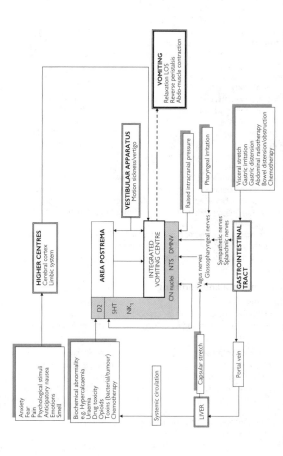

Fig. 7.2 Diagram of the neural mechanisms controlling vomiting. D₂, dopamine 2 receptors; 5HT, 5-hydroxytryptamine receptors; NK1, neurokinin 1 receptors; NTS, nucleus of the tractus solitarius; DMNV, dorsal motor nerve of vagus; CN, cranial nerve.

Neuroanatomy and description of receptors

- The **cerebral cortex** and **limbic system** respond to pain and various emotional stimuli and will affect the threshold for nausea and vomiting within the vomiting centre. The receptors of relevance within these neural pathways include GABA (gamma-amino butyric acid) receptors, 5-HT (serotonin) and the neurokinin-1 (NK_1) receptor which selectively binds the emetogenic tachykinin, substance P.
- **The area postrema** (AP) lies in the wall of the fourth ventricle and is outside the blood–brain barrier. This allows it to respond to drugs, toxins, and changes within both plasma and cerebrospinal fluid (CSF) biochemistry. The main receptors in this area are dopamine (D_2) receptors, the $5HT_3$ serotonin subtype and the (now ubiquitous) NK_1 receptor already mentioned.
- **The vomiting centre** (VC) lies within the medulla of the brainstem and within the blood brain barrier. The most important receptors here include muscarinic acetylcholine receptors (ACh_m), histamine (H_1) receptors, $5-HT_2$ serotonin receptor subtype and again, the NK_1 receptor as above. The vomiting centre receives afferent impulses from the other parts of the system and is in close proximity to other important brainstem nuclei including the **nucleus of the tractus solitarius and the dorsal motor nucleus of the vagus.** These nuclei contain a large quantity of both serotonin (5-HT) and NK_1 receptors.
- The connections between the **vestibular apparatus** (contained within the bony labyrinths) and the vomiting centre and area postrema contain both ACh_m and H_1 receptors.
- There are many pathways and receptors within the **GI tract**, but most importantly the $5-HT_3$ and $5-HT_4$ serotonin receptor subtypes, ACh_m and D_2. The latter three receptors are involved in the regulation of GI motility.

Causes of nausea and vomiting

Area postrema

Drugs, biochemical derangement or blood-borne toxins will stimulate the AP. Serum biochemistry including a corrected calcium and renal function should be checked.

Common metabolic causes

- ↑Ca^{2+} may be accompanied by dehydration, constipation, abdominal pain, and confusion. Alternatively, nausea/vomiting may be the only sign.
- Uraemia also causes nausea, often in the absence of other clinical signs.
- Hyponatraemia caused by advanced malignant disease or diuretic therapy.
- Secretion of inappropriate antidiuretic hormone (SIADH):
  - caused by specific malignancies
  - drugs – antidepressants, carbamazepine
  - chemotherapy
  - head injury.
- Opioids will cause gastric stasis and also stimulate the AP.
- Antibiotics, cytotoxic agents, and alcohol can cause damage or irritation of the GI mucosa and stimulate the AP.

- Cytotoxic chemotherapy can cause acute and/or delayed emesis and anticipatory nausea and vomiting.

Vomiting centre
- **Raised ICP** from brain tumours, metastatic disease, or other intracranial pathology. The history may be suggestive, e.g. early morning headaches associated with vomiting. Fundoscopy looking for papilloedema should be performed.
- **Pharyngeal irritation** due to a productive cough. Treat the cause if appropriate with antibiotics and aid expectoration with mucolytics such as a saline nebulizer.
- **Liver capsular stretch** can cause nausea and vomiting as well as pain. Steroids (dexamethasone) can often help with both.
- **Motion sickness**.

GI causes
- **(Sub)acute obstruction**, high index of suspicion particularly if the patient is known to have intra-abdominal malignant disease. A history detailing the timing and nature of any vomiting (e.g. shortly after eating/ hours after eating/unaltered food/faeculent vomitus/recent bowel habit/any flatus/associated pain, etc.) will guide in establishing the likely level of obstruction. Examination of the abdomen including a rectal examination and an abdominal X-ray (AXR) are needed. Computerized tomography (CT) scan and small bowel series may assist diagnosis of remediable causes.
- **Inoperable bowel obstruction:** dictated by performance status, fitness for anaesthesia, and the nature of the bowel obstruction. Laparotomy is not indicated in cases of widespread intraperitoneal carcinomatosis with multiple sites of obstruction.
- **Squashed stomach**: as above, caused by intra-abdominal pathology limiting the free and normal distension of the stomach. Significant ascites, large tumour masses, or liver metastases can cause delayed gastric emptying as well as early satiety. The use of a prokinetic anti-emetic taken 20–30 min before mealtimes combined with an anti-flatulent antacid containing dimeticone after meal times can help significantly.

Other causes
- Pain, fear, and anxiety can all precipitate nausea and vomiting and lower the threshold of the vomiting centre for emesis.
- Radiotherapy may also cause sickness, particularly if the CNS or small bowel are within the radiation field.

Drug profiles
- **Metoclopramide** and **domperidone**: both are dopamine antagonists and prokinetic anti-emetics with weak central action within the AP. Not always effective for biochemical or drug-induced nausea, but especially useful to aid gastric emptying. Metoclopramide works both by countering the dopamine inhibition of motility and stimulating motility as a 5-HT$_4$ agonist. Domperidone, however, works only by blocking the dopamine inhibition. Domperidone does not cross the blood–brain barrier and so does not cause extra-pyramidal side-effects.

- **Haloperidol:** Potent dopamine receptor antagonist useful for treating AP mediated nausea refractory to metoclopramide or domperidone. Watch for extra-pyramidal side-effects.
- **Cyclizine:** the drug of choice for vomiting centre or vestibular apparatus-mediated nausea and vomiting. Antihistamine and anticholinergic activity. First choice for nausea and vomiting caused by raised intracranial pressure, motion sickness, liver capsular stretch, or pharyngeal irritation. Should not be combined with metoclopramide as its anticholinergic action will negate the pro-motility effect of the metoclopramide.
- **Levomepromazine:** phenothiazine with useful broad-spectrum anti-emetic profile. Blocks D_2, ACh_m, H_1, $5-HT_2$ serotonin receptor subtype as well as α_2 receptors. This last receptor is responsible for the risk of postural hypotension at higher doses, especially when fluid intake has been marginal because of refractory nausea and vomiting.
- **Lorazepam:** short-acting benzodiazepine that can be administered sublingually. Particularly useful as an adjuvant anti-emetic for anxiety and anticipatory nausea and vomiting.
- **Dexamethasone:** fluorinated corticosteroid often used as part of anti-emetic regime given with chemotherapy. It acts as an adjuvant anti-emetic with other drugs. Its mechanism of action is possibly by reducing the permeability of the blood–brain barrier and the AP to emetogenic substances and by reducing GABA and leu-enkephalin release within the brainstem.
- **Ondansetron/granisetron:** Specific $5-HT_3$ serotonin receptor subtype antagonists. Narrow spectrum and specifically developed to treat acute nausea and vomiting associated with both chemo- and radiotherapy. Less effective with delayed nausea and vomiting. **NOT** to be used as an anti-emetic when other drugs have failed. Can cause significant constipation.
- **Aprepitant:** New NK_1 receptor antagonist developed specifically to treat the delayed emesis sometimes seen with highly emetogenic chemotherapy regimens. It is reported as having a broad spectrum of action and may have a wider role in the management of nausea and vomiting in the future.

Choice of drug (see Table 7.2)

- A first-line anti-emetic is selected subject to identifying the most likely cause and is administered via a suitable route.
- If vomiting prevents oral administration other options include subcutaneous, sublingual, buccal, rectal, intravenous, and intramuscular routes.
- Continuous subcutaneous administration via a syringe driver guarantees drug administration in the vomiting patient.
- Anti-emetics should be prescribed regularly.
- Second-line or combination therapy should be introduced if symptoms persist after 24 h.
- Reversible causes of nausea and vomiting should be addressed separately, e.g.:
  - correcting hypercalcaemia
  - optimizing hydration

- stopping emetogenic drugs wherever possible
- draining ascites
- managing bowel obstruction appropriately, etc.
- It should be remembered that nausea and vomiting in patients with cancer is often multifactorial. If the causes are not clear, or first-line therapy has failed, then levomepromazine is an appropriate subsequent choice of anti-emetic as it acts at many different receptor sites. Its broad spectrum of activity means it is frequently effective even when combinations of specific anti-emetics have been unsuccessful. Its anxiolytic and sedative effect can also be advantageous in this group of patients although doses above 25 mg/24 h can frequently cause sedation and postural hypotension.
- Inoperable bowel obstruction is often treated on a surgical ward by 'drip and suck', deploying an uncomfortable nasogastric (NG) tube and IV fluids.
- A more conservative approach can be successful using a combination of broad-spectrum anti-emetic such as levomepromazine and the anticholinergic (antisecretory and antimotility) drug hyoscine butylbromide (Buscopan®).
- Sometimes an empirical trial of subcutaneous dexamethasone can also be added to the regime.
- Octreotide (a somatostatin analogue) can be useful in cases refractory to the above management.
- A venting gastrostomy may have to be considered in high duodenal or jejunal obstruction. This is essentially a feeding tube used in reverse, and is very effective for refractory nausea and vomiting.

Table 7.2 Selection of anti-emetics

Causes of nausea/vomiting	Anti-emetic	Class of drug	Example dose schedule	Common side-effects
Chemotherapy				
Acute	Acute emesis (<24 h)			
	Ondansetron	5-HT$_3$ antagonist	8 mg bd PO	Constipation
	Dexamethasone	Corticosteroid	2–4 mg bd PO for 1–3 days	Agitation/insomnia, gastric irritant
Delayed	Delayed emesis (>24 h)			
	Metoclopramide	Peripherally acting prokinetic and AP anti-emetic	10–20 mg qds PO	Restlessness, extrapyramidal effects
	Aprepitant	NK$_1$ antagonist	3 day chemo pack or 80 mg od PO	Gi side-effects, headache dizziness
Anticipatory	Lorazepam	Benzodiazepine	1–2 mg prn, max 4 mg/24 h	Sedation
Drugs, e.g. opioids, metabolic – (whilst correcting the cause)	Haloperidol	Dopamine antagonist	1.5–3 mg nocte PO or 0.5–1.5mg bd PO	Sedation, extrapyramidal effects
	Levomepromazine	Dopamine antagonist, antimuscarinic, antihistamine and 5-HT$_2$ antagonist	6.25–12.5mg nocte PO or 6.25mg bd PO	Sedation, blurred vision, risk of urinary retention postural hypotension
Gastric irritation including radiotherapy	Lansoprazole	Proton pump inhibitor	30 mg od–bd PO	Constipation
	Ondansetron	5-HT$_3$ antagonist	8 mg bd PO	
	Cyclizine	Antihistamine and anticholinergic	50 mg tds PO/s/c	Drowsiness, dry mouth, blurred vision, risk of urinary retention

Indication	Drug	Class	Dose	Side effects
Raised intracranial pressure	Dexamethasone	Corticosteroid	Up to 16 mg/24 h	Agitation/insomnia, gastric irritant
	Cyclizine	Antihistamine and anticholinergic	50mg tds PO or 150mg/24hrs/s/c	
Gastric stasis/subacute bowel obstruction	Metoclopramide or	Prokinetic	10–20 mg qds PO/IV/s/c	Agitation. Discontinue if colicky pain develops. Central effects less likely with domperidone
	Domperidone	Prokinetic	10–20 mg qds PO or as rectal suppository	
Pharyngeal irritation, liver capsular stretch, motion sickness	Cyclizine	Antihistamine and anticholinergic	50 mg tds or 150 mg/24 h s/c	Drowsiness, dry mouth, blurred vision, risk of urinary retention
Obstruction	Cyclizine	Antihistamine and anticholinergic	50 mg tds or 150 mg/24 h s/c	Drowsiness, dry mouth, blurred vision, risk of urinary retention
	Haloperidol	Dopamine antagonist	2–3 mg bd or 2–5 mg/24 h s/c	Sedation, extrapyramidal effects
	Dexamethasone	Corticosteroid	2–8 mg bd s/c	Agitation/insomnia, gastric irritant
	± Hyoscine butylbromide	Antispasmodic antisecretory	Up to 100 mg/24 h s/c	Dry mouth, blurred vision urinary retention
	±Octreotide	Somatostatin analogue	Up to 1000 µg/24 h s/c	Constipation
	Levomepromazine	Broad-spectrum phenothiazine anti-emetic	6.25–25 mg/24 h s/c	As other page

Hiccup

- Hiccup is a pathological respiratory reflex, part of a symptom complex originating and integrated within closely related brainstem nuclei and also the respiratory and vomiting centres.
- It is characterized by spasm of the diaphragm, resulting in sudden inspiration followed by abrupt closure of the glottis.
- Over 90% of hiccups are thought to be caused by gastric distension.
- Gastroparesis as a consequence of opioid therapy can cause hiccup.
- Also caused by pathology around or involving the diaphragm:
  - disease around the lower oesophageal sphincter
  - the crura of the diaphragm
  - subphrenic abscess
  - lower lobe consolidation or empyema
  - disease infiltration of the diaphragm or phrenic nerve(s).
- Phrenic nerve infiltration can occur anywhere along the course of the nerve, including mediastinal disease involvement causing spasm of the diaphragm.
- Other causes include brain tumours and uraemia.

Management
- Correct the correctable
- Promote GI motility and gastric emptying
- Drain empyaema or pleural effusion
- Drain sub-diaphragmatic collection
- Stenting of obstructing lower oesophageal tumour
- Drain ascites.

Traditional remedies
- These rely on pharyngeal stimulation which acts as a gating mechanism through negative feedback to the brainstem.
- Raising the partial pressure of carbon dioxide (pCO_2) in the blood through breath holding will raise the threshold for continued hiccuping. Rebreathing from a brown paper bag will have the same effect.
- Startling the patient often causes neck hyperextension, which in turn stimulates (via stretching) the pharynx.
- A couple of drams of alcohol ingested promptly.
- A couple of heaped teaspoonfuls of granulated sugar.
- Dry bread or biscuit.
- Rubbing the roof of the mouth at the junction of the soft and hard palate quickly and repetitively to and fro with a cotton bud.

Medical treatments
- Saline nebulizer.
- Enhance GI motility and encourage stomach emptying with metoclopramide 10–20 mg or domperidone 20 mg, 20–30 min before meal times, PO tds.
- Finish each meal with an anti-foaming ant-flatulant antacid containing dimeticone, e.g. Asilone®.
- Relaxation of diaphragmatic spasm, consider baclofen or nifedipine.

- For phrenic nerve involvement, treat similarly to neuropathic pain. Steroid with an anti-neuropathic pain adjuvant such as gabapentin or sodium valproate maybe helpful.
- Central depression of the hiccup reflex in the brainstem with midazolam, or levomepromazine.
- (The use of chlorpromazine and haloperidol should be thought of as a last resort.)

Constipation

Causes

There are many potential causes of constipation in patients with malignancy.

- Drugs, particularly the more water-soluble opioid analgesics, drugs with either anticholinergic action or anticholinergic side-effects, which include a number of the common anti-emetics as well as the 5-HT$_3$ antagonists. Constipation is also associated with some forms of chemotherapy, e.g. vinca alkaloids.
- Dehydration due to inadequate fluid intake or secondary to vomiting, diuretic therapy, etc.
- Anorexia: reduced oral intake or change in dietary content.
- Immobility/general weakness and 'can't push'.
- Hypercalcaemia, particularly if accompanied by nausea and vomiting, dehydration, and abdominal pain.
- Spinal cord compression.
- Intestinal obstruction. Intrinsic compression due to malignancy, intraperitoneal disease causing stricture, or adhesion or extrinsic compression from pelvic tumour. Post-surgery or post-radiotherapy adhesions.

Presentation

- Decreased frequency, difficulty with bowel evacuation, or no bowel movements at all
- Nausea and vomiting (may be accompanied by other symptoms and signs of bowel obstruction)
- Abdominal pain, often colicky
- Overflow diarrhoea: the passage of fluid stool around faecal impaction. Highly likely if the diarrhoea follows an episode of untreated constipation and suggested by a history of passing or leaking very loose stool
- Urinary retention
- Acute confusional state possibly accompanying infection or hypercalcaemia.

Assessment

- History: to help identify precipitating factors or potentially reversible causes. This should include details of current home care package around the practical issues of toileting
- Examination, including rectal examination
- AXR only required to exclude obstruction or pseudo-obstruction if suspected
- Bloods: routine biochemistry including serum Ca^{2+}.

Management

Non-pharmacological

- Increase fluid and dietary fibre intake if at all possible. Obtain dietary advice
- Mobilize
- Maximize privacy and dignity.

Pharmacological

- **Prophylaxis**: when prescribing an opioid always consider prescribing a combined softener and stimulant laxative from the outset. Fentanyl patches may be less constipating than morphine due to the highly fat-soluble nature of the drug and entirely different drug distribution within the body. Conversion to transdermanl fentanyl might be considered if pain is stable.
- **Osmotic agents**: these osmotically active compounds, within the bowel lumen are not absorbed and retain water, softening the bowel content, increasing stool volume, and stimulating peristalsis. These include magnesium, citrate, and phosphate salts, and polyethylene glycol (Movicol®) as well as sugars that are not absorbed, such as lactulose and sorbitol. Lactulose (a synthetic disaccharide) is commonly prescribed and causes unpleasant side-effects of abdominal colic, bloating, and flatulence due to its breakdown and gas production within the bowel by the gut flora.
- **Other softeners**: these include poloxamer and docusate; the former is found in co-danthramer and the latter in co-danthrusate or on its own as the stool softener, docusate. Docusate does not have the disadvantages of lactulose described above, working more as a surface wetting agent and enhancing the penetration of water into the stool.
- **Stimulant agents**: senna is a naturally occurring anthranoid laxative derived from plant extracts. Synthetic anthranoids include danthron found in co-danthramer and co-danthrusate. Along with the phenolics such as bisacodyl and sodium picosulfate, they exert their effects by stimulating both secretion and motility via the enteric nervous system comprising Auerbach's and Meissner's plexus. Stimulant laxatives are contraindicated in intestinal obstruction. Dantron is licensed only for use in the palliative setting and is particularly effective in opioid-induced constipation. Patients must be warned that their urine may become discoloured.
- **Bulking agents**: useful in patients who are otherwise well and able to eat and drink relatively normally. Require a fluid intake of 2–3 l per day, e.g. ispaghula husk. It is neither effective nor recommended to combat opioid-induced constipation.
- Rectal preparations, e.g.:
  - glycerine suppositories to soften, lubricate, stimulate, and facilitate the passage of hard stool from a loaded rectum
  - an arachis oil enema to soften stool at night prior to a high-phosphate enema the following morning to stimulate evacuation
  - bisocodyl stimulant suppositories or liquid are particularly useful to restore a pattern of bowel evacuation following spinal cord compression
  - a range of osmotic micro-enema preparations are available such as Micolette® or Micralax®.

Diarrhoea

The passage of abnormally loose stool; usually combined with increased frequency of bowel movement.

Causes and management

- Exclude pathogens, especially bacterial, viral, fungal; NB *C. diff* or Norwalk virus/Norovirus.
- Exclude overflow diarrhoea, most frequently caused by prescription of opioid therapy without a laxative. Requires rectal examination and intervention if indicated.
- Too much laxative.
- Bowel resection.
- Post-radiotherapy diarrhoea:
  - loperamide
  - codeine
  - morphine
  - local steroid foam enemata
  - ondansetron
  - octreotide.
- Consider fistula – diversion procedure/colostomy may be appropriate management.
- Malabsorption of pancreatic insufficiency – Creon®.
- Bacterial overgrowth within blind loop following surgical reconstruction after major surgery (Whipples/Roux-en-Y):
  - probiotics to encourage friendly bacteria – yoghurt drinks
  - metronidazole.
- Carcinoid syndrome:
  - ondansetron
  - octreotide.
- Cholegenic diarrhoea:
  - colestyramine.
- Candidal overgrowth causing secretory diarrhoea:
  - fluconazole.
- Autonomic neuropathy or post-lumbar sympathectomy:
  - clonidine.
- Drug induced – chemotherapy, misoprostol, non-steroidal anti-inflammatory drug (NSAID), antibiotics, laxatives:
  - stop causative drug if possible.

Loperamide is a peripheral opioid receptor agonist with no central action and hence no analgesic activity; 2 mg is equivalent to codeine 30 mg or 15–30 mg of morphine. Loperamide may, however, be more effective as it is longer acting:

- loperamide should be used alone initially
- then codeine alone
- then in combination
- and then loperamide and morphine could be tried as a combination.

Drugs may be lost from the bowel prematurely if transit time is very short and diarrhoea severe. Opioid via continuous subcutaneous infusion maybe necessary to guarantee absorption and evaluate efficacy.

Correct the correctable wherever possible.

Cachexia and anorexia

Cachexia
- Involuntary increase in basal energy expenditure culminating in loss of both lean muscle and adipose tissue.
- Affects >85% of patients with advanced cancer.
- Often associated with anorexia. However, cachexia differs from starvation (in which muscle mass tends to be spared) because the associated loss of fat and lean body mass cannot be reversed by simply increasing calorific intake.
- Most commonly seen in patients with advanced solid tumours, particularly affecting the lungs or GI tract.
- The underlying causative mechanisms are unknown, although circulating cytokines such as tumour necrosis factor clearly play a role, causing metabolic abnormalities such as protein breakdown, lipolysis, and increased gluconeogenesis.
- Thought of as a chronic inflammatory state, the enormity of which relates directly to the degree and rate of weight loss.
- A major cause of symptoms towards the end of life, with multiple associated physical, psychological, and social co-morbidities. Often distressing to both the patient and their carers.

Anorexia
- Reduced or absent appetite for food.
- May be associated with the fatigue and cachexia of advanced malignancy without any other specific cause.
- However, assessment requires consideration of potentially reversible causes that may benefit from intervention, e.g.:
  - inadequate pain control
  - nausea
  - constipation
  - depression
  - metabolic abnormalities, e.g. hypercalcaemia, uraemia
  - infection, e.g. oral thrush
  - obstruction/ascites.

Management
Correct reversible causes. Interventions usually do not influence cachexia.

Non-pharmacological
- Dietary advice: small, frequent meals. Eat when hungry. High-calorie, low-volume foods. Small amounts of alcohol as an appetite stimulant.
- Education: try to minimize any stress related to food. Encourage carers not to pressurize. Promote enjoyment of food.
- Activity: maximize any potential for exercise.

Pharmacological
- **Supplements**: high-protein, high-calorie, e.g. Ensure®.
- **Enteral/parenteral feeding** is occasionally appropriate during active anti-cancer therapy. It is rarely appropriate in the latter stages of progressive disease.
- **Corticosteroids** may stimulate appetite, reduce nausea, and help in general by promoting a sense of well-being. They do not, however, increase lean body mass. The use of potent, fluorinated corticosteroids, e.g. dexamethasone, should be considered only in the short term as they will decrease muscle mass, cause proximal myopathy, cushingoid facies, and problems with upper GI irritation. Change to low-dose prednisolone 10–20 mg daily maintenance for those with a better prognosis, or consider change to progestogen.
- **Progestogens** aid appetite and are more appropriate than steroids in the longer term, although evidence for useful weight gain is limited, e.g. megestrol acetate 160 mg od.
  - Increased risk of thromboembolism.
  - Combinations of megestrol and ibuprofen have been shown to improve quality of life and weight gain.
  - Similarly, medroxyprogesterone has been combined with celecoxib and found to stabilize weight and help generally with symptom control
  - Neither combination increases lean body mass, but they increase both fat and total body water (not oedema) and so lead to weight gain. Inclusion of the NSAID probably helps by dampening down the chronic inflammatory response driving the weight loss.
- **EPA (eicosapentanoic acid)** is one of the omega-3 essential fatty acids and can help dampen down the acute inflammatory response as well as protect muscle against proteolysis-inducing factor. It is found in fish oil capsules and Prosure®. Pure EPA capsules can be obtained from most health food stores.

Respiratory symptoms

Causes of breathlessness in malignant disease

We become conscious of being short of breath when it is necessary to increase the rate and/or depth of respiration to keep pace with the body's gas exchange requirements for O_2 consumption and CO_2 production. Dyspnoea becomes frightening and unpleasant when gas exchange is insufficient to support a given task.

Shortness of breath (SOB) in patients with metastatic malignancy is commonly multifactorial in origin. The patient must be fully assessed for potentially reversible causes.

Pulmonary
- Lung tumour
- Pneumonia
- Pleural effusion – (if recurrent consider pleurodesis)
- Lymphangitis carcinomatosa
- Obstruction of large airways (see 📖 Chapter 33, 'Stridor') ± distal collapse
- Concomitant chronic obstructive pulmonary disease (COPD).

Cardiovascular
- Pericardial effusion
- Congestive cardiac failure
- Pulmonary emboli.
- Superior vena caval obstruction (see 📖 Chapter 32)
- Anaemia
- Arrhythmias.

Chest wall and diaphragm
- Muscle weakness/fatigue
- Carcinoma en-cuirasse, i.e. restrictive malignant infiltration of the chest wall
- Lytic bone metastases/pathological fracture(s) affecting the ribs
- Pleurisy
- Infiltration of phrenic nerve at any point along its course from the emerging nerve roots or throughout the mediastinum or at the diaphragm.

Ventilation–perfusion mismatch
A large proportion of the above causes of SOB are due to ventilation–perfusion mismatch. The majority of useful gas exchange takes place at the lung bases. Frequently, pathology interferes with this process:
- pleural effusion
- empyema
- basal consolidation
- multiple metastases
- lung tumour and basal collapse
- poor basal expansion due to paralysis of the diaphragm (e.g. phrenic nerve infiltration in mesothelioma) or splinting of the diaphragm due to abdominal cause of distension.

Decreased compliance/increased airways resistance
- Pulmonary fibrosis
- Consolidation
- Tumour
- Pulmonary oedema
- Lymphangitis carcinomatosa
- Exophytic endobronchial tumour
- Reversible airways obstruction/COPD.

Psychological
- Anxiety/fear

Management of breathlessness
- Reversible causes of SOB as above should be treated accordingly. Correct the correctable.
- A multidisciplinary approach is helpful, with consideration given to non-pharmacological strategies such as breathing exercises, physiotherapy, relaxation therapy, and massage. Patients should be helped to adjust their expectations.
- Treat pain.
- Non-drug measures: controlled breathing exercises, companionship, reassurance, relaxation, and distraction therapies.
- **Drug palliation to relieve SOB**:
  - **opioids** – decrease respiratory panic and the distressing sensation of SOB. They reduce anxiety and are analgesic. They also decrease the sensitivity of the respiratory centre to a raised pCO_2, reducing excessive respiratory drive; e.g: morphine sulphate 2.5 mg/4 hourly PO
  - **benzodiazepines** are anxiolytic, sedative, and muscle relaxants. Concerns about respiratory depression are usually unfounded, e.g. lorazepam 0.5–2 mg PO prn
  - **O_2** can be beneficial for correcting hypoxia. Can also relieve SOB even when oxygen tension is normal, possibly through a cooling effect on the face or as a placebo (similar effect using a fan or a breeze from an open door or window). Beware if the patient has coexisting COPD (no more than 28% oxygen should be administered).

Cough
- Protective reflex for clearing the airways
- Some drugs exacerbate cough (e.g. Ramipril®).

Management
- Treat the cause, e.g: antibiotics for chest infection.
- Aid expectoration with saline nebulizers, bronchodilators.
- Soothing cough syrup – simple linctus to coat the pharynx – 10–15 ml 4-hourly and as required.
- Can be combined with low-dose oramorph as a soothing cough suppressant (5 mg oramorph with 10–15 ml simple linctus) 2–4-hourly as required.
- Refer for laser ablation if endobronchial tumour is cause of continued large-airway irritation/obstruction.

- 1–2% nebulized lidocaine starting at initially low concentration 2–2.5 ml mixed with 2–2.5ml normal saline. NB remind patient and carers of risk of aspiration 1–2 h after administration.
- Involvement of the recurrent laryngeal nerve by malignant infiltration within the mediastinum:
  - hoarse voice ± 'bovine' cough (often difficulty in clearing the airway as cough poorly effective)
  - ear, nose, and throat (ENT) referral for injection of paralysed vocal cord or thyroplasty procedure if appropriate.

Pruritus

- Pruritis or itch is an unpleasant and/or annoying sensation that provokes the urge to scratch.
- Overlap of C-fibre afferent nerve function with pain.

Causes of pruritus

- Drug reactions: e.g. antibiotics
- Infestation: lice, scabies
- Histamine released through mast cell degranulation:
  - dermatitis
  - allergy
  - anaphylaxis
  - opioid
- Cupitch syndrome (cutaneous pain and itch) often seen in metastatic manifestation of skin metastases in breast cancer en cuirasse. Inflammatory mediators including prostaglandins sensitize the cutaneous nerve endings
- Skin cancers or metastatic deposits
- Cholestatic jaundice
- Uraemia
- Opioids (especially via spinal route)
- Haematological
- Paraneoplastic.

Management

Skin management first, drugs second:
- moisturiser and skin care for dry skin
- menthol 1% in aqueous cream
- treat infestations
- consider stenting bile duct in cholestatic jaundice (if appropriate).

Drug therapies to consider

General points:
- **naltrexone** should not be used if patient on opioid therapy for pain management
- the majority of causes of itch in malignant disease or during its oncological management will not respond to **antihistamines**
- **thalidomide** can cause severe, irreversible peripheral neuropathy in long-term use
- **haematological** causes includes lymphoma, iron-deficiency anaemia, polycythaemia vera.

Aetiology and drug therapies to consider

- *Skin causes/allergies/drug reactions*
  - antihistamines
- *Opioid-induced itch*
  - try alternative opioid
  - ondansetron
- *Uraemia*
  - ondansetron

- naltrexone
- mirtazapine
- thalidomide
- *Cholestatic*
  - ondansetron
  - naltrexone
  - paroxetine/sertraline
  - danazol
- *Haematological*
  - cimetidine
  - mirtazapine
- *Paraneoplastic*
  - paroxetine
  - mirtazapine
  - thalidomide
- *Unknown or other*
  - paroxetine
  - mirtazapine
  - thalidomide
  - doxepin.

Lymphoedema

A chronic, progressive, incurable condition characterized by swelling (often non-pitting), and associated with chronic skin changes. It can lead to profound physical and psychological morbidity often with significant impairment of function. Damage to the lymphatics due to malignant disease or as a consequence of treatment is called secondary lymphoedema:

- tumour infiltration of lymphatics
- surgery damaging lymphatics or excision of lymph nodes during block dissection
- radiotherapy
- failure of lymph drainage, blockage, surgery, or scarring causes an excessive accumulation and stagnation of protein-rich interstitial fluid
- affects most commonly the limbs but can affect any part
- often non-pitting.

Pathogenesis of lymphoedema

- Stasis of protein-rich tissue fluid
- Impaired immune function as fluid neither circulating nor reaching the lymph nodes
- Impaired macrophage function
- Protein, debris, and inflammatory factors accumulate
- Excellent culture medium for bacteria and/or fungi
- Recurrent infection eventually leads to fibrosis with irreversible swelling and thickening of the tissues and skin
- Fibrin deposition within tissues and blood vessels leads to poor perfusion and oxygenation causing further damage
- Increasing protein increases osmotic pressure, tending to draw in even more fluid
- Uninterrupted cycles of recurrent infection can lead to end-stage lymphoedema (elephantiasis)
- **Before embarking upon lymphoedema management, exclude other causes of a swollen limb. It may be appropriate to manage extrinisic venous compression or deep vein thrombosis by stenting and/or anticoagulation.**

Prevention of lymphoedema

- This is the best strategy.
- Patient education and information is vital.
- Referral to a specialist lymphoedema service if available.
- Massage and exercise techniques.
- Advice on minimizing risk of infection/trauma, e.g. gardening gloves when gardening, avoiding sunburn.
- Avoid insect bites if at all possible.
- Avoid venepuncture or blood pressure measurement on the affected limb.
- Plan an exercise programme during air travel.

Treatment of acute inflammatory episodes

- Early intervention essential.
- Refer to local lymphoedema service regarding local antibiotic protocols (poor tissue penetration in lymphoedema).

The cause of an acute inflammatory episode is often a streptococcus, and treatment should be continued for a minimum of 2 weeks. IV antibiotics are often required and often long-term prophylaxis is required.

Management

- Aim to prevent progression by preventing acute inflammatory episodes and containment of the oedema. Left unchecked, there will be continous inexorable progression towards limb swelling and skin changes (elephantiasis).
- Lymphorrhoea should be managed promptly with skin care and padded bandaging. Remember increased risk of infection with compromise of skin integrity.
- Prophylactic use of athletes foot powder or the prompt treatment of fungal infections as even small breaks in the skin between the toes act as a portal of entry for infection.
- Daily skin care.
- Self-massage and exercise.
- Specialist fitted gradient compression garments.
- Refractory oedema may require pressure bandaging to reshape the limb before maintenance compression garments can be fitted.
- Meticulous attention to skin care and hygiene of the affected area. Particular attention to between the fingers, toes and skin folds, which should be washed and dried thoroughly.
- There is no drug therapy yet available for the treatment of lymphoedema.

Mouthcare

Good oral hygiene is essential for patients who are about to embark upon cancer therapies or those further on in their disease journey who need to keep up their calorie intake and communicate with those around them. Mouth problems can be a cause of significant psychological morbidity and possible social isolation.

Those at risk
- Frail elderly
- Terminally ill
- Undergoing chemo- and/or radiotherapy especially of head and neck tumours
- On drugs with anticholinergic side-effects
- Immunosuppressed or immunocompromised patients
- Those with oropharyngeal pathology
- Patients with dysphagia
- Patients with tracheostomies
- Periodontal disease and/or tooth caries
- On steroids
- Bacterial, fungal, or viral infections.

Aim of therapy
- To clean the teeth, gums, tongue, and oral cavity
- Treat infections
- Protect the mucosa
- Maintain neutral or alkaline pH of oral cavity
- Encourage maximum from own saliva – protective, cleansing with neutral to alkaline pH and natural buffers to protect the mouth from huge swings in pH and neutralize the continuous production of bacterial acids
- Natural saliva is best
- Aim for clean, moist mouth, nothing beats saliva.

Cleaning principles
- Meticulous attention to tooth and gum hygiene, with sodium bicarbonate or triclosan-containing fluoride toothpaste.
- Removal of debris with simple warm water, saline, or dilute sodium bicarbonate solution.
- Soft baby toothbrush useful to help clear the tongue of coating and debris.
- Daily or twice-daily rinse with chlorhexidine mouthwash.
- Apply water-soluble lubricating jelly or oral balance gel to mouth and lips.
- Angular cheilitis is common and troublesome and often of fungal or bacterial aetiology. Hydrocortisone creams containing antifungals or antibacterials are helpful.
- Dentures pose a significant risk to the gums for recurrent infection and mechanical trauma. They should be cleaned daily and soaked in Milton solution or chlorhexidine solution overnight.

Specific treatments
- **Bacterial infections** as above and use regular chlorhexidine mouthwash. Tetracycline or doxycycline solutions can also be used.
- **Fungal infections:** common cause of sore mouth. Prophylaxis can be with nystatin suspension, but only active on mucosal contact with no systemic absorption. Heavily coated mouths should be cleaned as above prior to treatment. Systemic alternative fluconazole 50 mg od for 7 days. Miconazole sugar-free oral gel can be used instead of nystatin and can be applied with a soft baby tooth brush to the tongue and oral cavity.
- **Viral infections**: in severe herpetic stomatitis, systemic therapy with aciclovir is indicated. Solitary lesions may be treated locally with aciclovir cream.

Chemo-radiotherapy mucositis
- Often associated with anthracycline, fluorouracil and methotrexate chemotherapy.
- As above, prevention through oral hygiene far better than remedial treatment.
- Benzydamine oral rinse has mild local anaesthetic and anti-inflammatory effect. Often stings if used undiluted.
- For a generally painful mouth consider mucosal protectants which can be mixed at the bedside with analgesics or anti-inflammatories.
- Raspberry mucilage (obtained as special order from Nova Laboratories) can be combined with baby soluble aspirin and soluble prednisolone tablets to provide a soothing anti-inflammatory mouth rinse.
- Polyvinylpyrrolidine and sodium hyaluronate (Gelclair®) can also be mixed with oramorph or the anti-inflammatories as above.
- A more discrete collection of painful ulcers at the gingival margin or sulcus can be treated with the application of Adcortyl in Orabase® paste.
- Single painful apthous ulcers can be treated with the local application of hydrocortisone oral pellets.
- Folinic acid rescue for methotrexate-induced mucositis.
- Palifermin: human keratinocyte growth factor used before and after myeloablative therapy and autologous haematopoietic stem-cell support for haematological malignancies.

The dry mouth
- There are many preparations for the dry mouth but none are as effective as natural saliva.
- Can anticholinergic drugs be stopped?
- Regular meals and drinks to encourage normal salivary flow.
- Frozen fruit juices stimulate saliva and are pleasant, e.g. fruit pastille lollies.
- Sugar-free chewing gum containing xylitol (anti-bacterial) is helpful. Low-tack gum for denture wearers.
- Aqueous lubricating jelly or oral balance gel.

- Atomized water spray, small ice chips, soda water, and cider mixed 50:50.
- Saliva replacement:
  - Saliva Orthana® (mucin based) more like real saliva than other cellulose-based products
  - Saliva natura light oral spray containing natural extracts of the *Yerba santa* plant which mimic the mucoprotective and buffering actions of natural salivary glycoproteins
  - Salinum® saliva substitute containing linseed extract and polysaccharide gel-forming substances
- **Pilocarpine hydrochloride** (salivary stimulant) 5 mg tds taken at mealtimes. Prophylactic use whilst receiving radiotherapy to head and neck. Continued for 4–6 weeks following completion of treatment. NB contraindicated in uncontrolled asthma and COPD, hepatic and renal impairment, and closed-angle glaucoma.

Altered taste

Cause
- Commonly linked with poor oral hygiene and candida infection
- Dry mouth lacks saliva as solvent for taste
- Coated tongue blocks taste buds
- Number of drugs and chemotherapeutic agents cause altered or reduced taste (dysgeusia or hypogeusia)
- Paraneoplastic phenomenon

Management
- Treat oral candidiasis
- Mouthcare and clean tongue
- Stimulate saliva production
- Vitamin and zinc supplements can be helpful.

Control of psychological distress

Assessment of psychological problems and the provision of psychological support must be an integral part of the package of care for patients with malignant disease. Presentation may be in the form of:

- denial/confusion
- anger
- anxiety
- sadness/depression
- sense of loss
- alienation
- seemingly poor control of physical symptoms
- attention-seeking and manipulative behaviour

All healthcare professionals should be aware of the frequency with which psychological problems are overlooked. Time must be set aside for mental state assessment. Cues from patient or carer should be heeded. Standardized clinical tools to measure psychological morbidity and quality-of-life may be helpful, e.g.:

- Hospital Anxiety and Depression Scale (HADS)
- Functional Assessment of Cancer Therapy (FACT)
- Functional Living Index – Cancer (FLIC)
- European Organization for Research and Treatment Quality-of-Life Questionnaire (EORTC QLQ-C30).

Management

- Self-help: patients should be given control over their management and helped to set realistic goals and develop coping strategies.
- Informal support: the sharing of experiences, the ventilation of feelings in a supportive environment, and the exchange of information about the physical, psychological, and social consequences of cancer and its treatment can help to reduce the sense of alienation and isolation sometimes associated with cancer, e.g. Cancer BACUP, Cancerlink, local cancer support groups. Many patients draw spiritual and practical support from their religious community.
- Formal support: access to trained counsellors is often available through primary care services or hospital-based cancer information centres. Palliative care specialist nurses are also trained in assessing the need for and offering psychological support and usually have access to psychologists and/or psychiatrists if additional help is required.
- Psychological therapies: cognitive behavioural therapy and brief psychotherapeutic interventions can be effective for more significant levels of anxiety or depression.
- Psychiatric interventions: medical staff should be able to recognize when referral to a liaison psychiatrist and also when drug therapy (antidepressant or anxiolytic) is required. Psychotropic medication benefits around 25% of cancer patients suffering significant anxiety and depression.

Symptom control at the end of life

Assessment

Although death may be imminent it is important that changes in a patient's mental state are adequately assessed. This is because there may be potentially reversible causes of distress and agitation that the patient may benefit from having specifically addressed. These include:

- inadequate pain control
- urinary retention or the need to have their bowels open
- nausea
- breathlessness
- fear of the unknown and the future and spiritual issues
- side-effects of medication
- unfinished business or family conversations
- dealing with family conflict.

However, symptom assessment at this stage should be achieved with minimal disruption to the patient in terms of examinations and investigations. The priority is to optimize the patient's physical and psychological comfort and to facilitate a dignified and peaceful death. Removing the medicalized barriers to family communication such as oxygen masks, and bandaged IV infusion cannula and tubing interfering with ability to hold a relative's hand.

Prescribing in the terminal phase

- Discontinue all non-essential medication. In practice this usually means discontinuing everything except analgesia, anxiolytics, anticholinergics for respiratory secretions, and possibly anti-emetics. If the patient is unconscious and has entered the terminal phase it is usually not necessary to continue corticosteroids.
- Avoid the oral route. Continuous subcutaneous infusion via a syringe driver is often the route of choice and does not necessarily require admission, although it will require significant support from the primary care services or community palliative care team.
- Intravenous medication should also be avoided if at all possible. Cannulation is intrusive and painful.
- Adequate prn doses: the ideal is for the subcutaneous infusion to achieve optimal symptom control without the need for additional doses. It remains essential to ensure that 'as required' (prn) doses are available so that the nursing team has ready access to them should any signs of distress develop.
- **Opioids**: these should be continued if they have been part of the patient's medication previously but converted to the equivalent subcutaneous dose (see 📖 p.130). The prn dose should be 1/6 of the total 24-hour dose. If the patient is opioid naïve but seems in pain then a small dose of diamorphine or morphine can be introduced, e.g. 5–10 mg s/c over 24 h with 2.5 mg s/c available as the prn dose. Review regularly and titrate as required.
- **Anxiolytics**, e.g. midazolam starting at 5–10 mg s/c over 24 h with 2.5–5 mg s/c available as a prn dose. This needs frequent review as

often many patients may need significantly greater doses. Occasionally agitation persists despite escalating midazolam doses.

- Always check for a simple reversible cause of agitation such as urinary retention, and catheterize if necessary.
- Levomepromazine can be added for its sedating properties, typically starting with a stat dose of 6.25–12.5 mg s/c, adding 12.5–25 mg s/c over 24 h and titrating as required.
- Haloperidol, e.g. 2.5–5 mg s/c, can also be useful for distress.
- **Anti-emetics** are often being co-prescribed with opioids and can be continued as necessary.
- **Respiratory tract secretions**: these are frequently more upsetting for the relatives than for the patient. The conscious patient is more likely to be distressed by the dry mouth that is an inevitable side-effect of the pharmacological intervention for respiratory tract secretions. If the patient is unconscious then simple methods such as appropriate positioning and gentle suction may be effective. Anti-cholinergic agents should usually be reserved for the unconscious, actively dying patient.
- Remember that anti-cholinergics will reduce the production of subsequent secretions, but the current secretions within the airways will have to dry during respiration or be removed by gentle suctioning.
- **Hyoscine hydrobromide** 400 µg s/c stat can be tried or incorporated into the syringe driver (usual dose 0.8–2.4 mg over 24h) It crosses the blood–brain barrier, is anti-emetic, causes sedation, and can cause delirium.
- **Hyoscine butylbromide** is also effective (10–20 mg prn and 20–120 mg s/c over 24 h) but does not cross the blood–brain barrier and so although it is anti-secretory and anti-spasmodic, it lacks anti-emetic activity nor is it sedating.
- **Glycopyrronium** (200 µg s/c stat and 600–1200 µg over 24 h) again, does not cross the blood–brain barrier.
- Side-effects of all three relate to their antimuscarinic action.
- **Explanation and communication**:
  - it is essential that the relatives (and the patient if conscious) understand the aims behind what is being done and what is now past the point of being appropriate
  - the balance between adequate pain control and possible sedation must be explained
  - the relatives should be kept informed of what is happening at every stage when the patient is too unwell to engage in conversation. All goals and aims are explained and will help reduce their inevitable upset and anxiety.
  - the contents and purpose of the subcutaneous infusion should be clarified.
  - the relatives must be reassured that the needs of the patient will continue to be reviewed and adjustments made accordingly. Time spent at this stage will hopefully help the relatives to understand and subsequently grieve without anger, suspicion, or unanswered questions about those final hours.
- Involvement of specialist palliative care services, either hospital based or community based. Advice on difficult symptoms may be invaluable, as are the additional skills in managing the needs of relatives before, during, and following the patient's death.

Integrated care pathway

Increasingly, hospitals are formalizing the care of the dying patient and their family by implementing an integrated care pathway for the use of the multidisciplinary team. This is in accordance with National Institute for Health and Clinical Excellence (NICE) guidelines in England and through the 'Living and Dying Well' Government initiative in Scotland, and may provide a framework for addressing aspects of physical, social, psychological, and spiritual care in the latter stages of life and after the patient's death. Further research is ongoing.

Further reading

Bennett M (2006) *Neuropathic pain. Oxford pain management library*. Oxford: Oxford University Press.

Fallon M, Hanks G (2006) *ABC of palliative care*, 2nd edn. Oxford: Blackwell Publishing BMJ Books.

Forbes K (2007) *Opioids in cancer pain. Oxford pain management library*. Oxford: Oxford University Press.

Lo B, Ruston D, Kates LW, et al. (2002) Discussing religious and spiritual issues at the end of life: a practical guide for physicians. *J Am Med Assoc* **287**, 749.

McQuay H, Moore A (1998) *An evidence-based resource for pain relief*. Oxford: Oxford University Press.

Quigley C (2004) Opioid switching to improve pain relief and drug tolerability. *Cochrane Database Syst Rev* (3), CD004847.

Twycross R, Wilcock A (2001) *Symptom management in advanced cancer*, 3rd edn. Oxford: Radcliffe Medical Press.

Twycross R, Wilcock A (2007) *PCF3. Palliative care formulary*, 3rd edn.

Twycross R, Greaves MW, Handwerker H, et al. (2003) Itch: scratching more than the surface. *QJM* **96**, 7–26.

Yosipovitch G, Greaves MW, Schmelz M. (2003) Itch. *Lancet* **361**, 690–4.

Late effects of chemotherapy and radiotherapy

Introduction

- Recent decades have seen significant advances in oncological treatments for many paediatric malignancies and some adult tumours, e.g. germ cell cancer, lymphomas.
- The focus has always been to optimize the chance of a cure.
- For the first time, there are long-term survivors after treatment for advanced malignancy.
- Additionally, adjuvant or neoadjuvant chemotherapy has an expanding role in the management of many resected or potentially resectable solid tumours, e.g. breast, colorectal.
- For those managing curable cancers, the challenge is to maximize rates of cure while minimizing long-term toxicity from the treatment.
- It is important for the medical profession as a whole to be aware of the potential long-term consequences of treatment for cancer because:
  - studies have shown that a significant proportion of adult survivors of childhood cancers either are unable to confirm their diagnosis of malignancy or misclassify their treatment
  - many potential toxicities have the potential to detract significantly from future quality of life and some may even shorten life expectancy.
- Surveillance for complications of therapy needs to be continued for many decades.

Endocrine and metabolic dysfunction

Pituitary dysfunction

- Common after whole-brain radiotherapy, >90% become growth hormone (GH) deficient, potentially affecting bone density, cardiovascular risk, and sense of well-being.
- Adrenocorticotrophic hormone (ACTH) insufficiency (causing adrenal failure), thyroid dysfunction, and gonadal failure can also occur.
- Continued surveillance needed for ≥10 years. Initial investigations: serum GH and insulin-like growth factor (IGF-1) ± thyroid-stimulating hormone (TSH), thyroxine (T_4), ACTH, follicle-stimulating hormone (FSH), testosterone/oestrogen.
- Replacement therapy is an established treatment in children (in the absence of active malignancy) but is more controversial in adults.

Adrenal failure

- Most common cause of adrenal insufficiency is suppression of hypothalamic–pituitary–adrenal function by prolonged administration of synthetic glucocorticoids.
- The cortisol-producing parts of the adrenal gland atrophy in the absence of ACTH stimulation.
- Mineralocorticoid production usually remains near normal.
- Recovery is usual but occasionally adrenal failure is permanent
- Initial investigation: early-morning cortisol, Synacthen® test.
- Symptoms are typically non-specific, including chronic malaise and anorexia.
- Presentation with adrenal crisis is rare but patients may require additional supplementation at times of physiological stress, e.g. sepsis.

Primary thyroid dysfunction

- Common after total body or cranio-spinal irradiation or radiotherapy to the neck, e.g. cumulative incidence of ~30% in patients treated for Hodgkins's disease by 20 years post-radiotherapy.
- Subclinical syndrome may persist for years before development of overt hypothyroidism.
- Typically an insidious-onset multisystem disorder with symptoms that can include fatigue, weight gain, cold intolerance, constipation, and depression
- Annual screening with thyroid function tests (TFTs) recommended in high-risk patients.
- Treatment should usually begin once the TSH is elevated, even if T_4 levels are normal, to avoid overstimulating the gland.

Metabolic syndrome

- Quartet of insulin resistance, dyslipidaemia, hypertension, and abdominal obesity.
- Observed in up to 50% of long-term survivors of childhood bone marrow transplants.
- Potential risk of premature cardio- and cerebrovascular events.
- Long-term monitoring should probably include serum lipids and fasting blood glucose.

Fertility issues

- Patients should always be alerted to the risk of infertility.
- ~30% treated for childhood cancers become infertile. Treatment in adulthood can also cause infertility.

Causes of gonadal dysfunction:

- **Direct involvement by tumour**, e.g. 5% incidence of contralateral carcinoma in situ in testicular tumours.
- **Surgery**, e.g. removal of gonad.
- **Radiotherapy affecting pituitary/gonadal function**, e.g. total body irradiation tends to cause infertility in men and women. Lower doses may produce transient oligospermia in men. Radiotherapy is more damaging to ovarian tissue than chemotherapy – a dose- and age-dependent effect.
- **Chemotherapy**: effects vary greatly depending on the agent, e.g. high risk of gonadal dysfunction particularly with alkylating agents (e.g. cyclophosphamide) and cisplatin. In women, the number of maturing follicles appears to decrease the most, while primordial follicles can appear unaffected.

Effects of age

- The older a woman, the more likely treatment is to precipitate the menopause, e.g. adjuvant anthracycline or cyclophosphamide chemotherapy for breast cancer in a 40 year old → ~70% chance of inducing the menopause, in a 25 year old → ~10%. This probably represents their greater reserve of oocytes.
- Effects are not consistent; women of a similar age receiving similar treatment may experience very different effects on ovarian function.
- The prepubertal testis seems less susceptible to the effects of chemotherapy than the mature adult testis.

Effects of gender

- e.g. post-chemotherapy-containing alkylating agents for Hodgkin's disease: ~90% of men are infertile; ~50% of women will have an early menopause but will not necessarily have been infertile.

Fertility vs sexual function

- Important to differentiate when discussing risks of treatment with patients.
- Spermatogenesis is more likely to be disrupted than testosterone production so men may be infertile without loss of libido or erectile function.

Strategies for preservation of gonadal function

Men

- Sperm-retrieval techniques:
  - from ejaculated sperm (straightforward to arrange for adults)
  - testicular/epididymal retrieval in combination with intracytoplasmic sperm injection (ICSI) – see 📖 p.171
  - conception rates using stored sperm are ~30%

- certain diagnoses (e.g. Hodgkin's, testicular cancer) may be associated with abnormal pre-treatment testicular function

Women

- Oophoropexy: a surgical procedure to move the ovaries beyond a planned radiotherapy field – mixed results only. Probably limited by effects of scatter radiation or surgically induced alterations in ovarian blood supply.
- Ovarian suppression: gonadotrophin-releasing hormone (GnRH) analogues to reduce ovarian function reversibly during treatment with chemotherapy have little supporting evidence in humans.
- Storage of ovarian tissue/oocytes: increasingly available following recent reports of successful pregnancies. Ovarian tissue can be retrieved without the need for ovarian stimulation. Ovarian hyperstimulation following an (o)estrogen receptor (ER)-positive tumour is to be avoided if at all possible.

Alternative strategies for fertility preservation

- Natural conception: may occur, sometimes unexpectedly. Menstrual function and fertility may return to normal even years after completing treatment.
- Storage of frozen embryos: possible. Generally requires the woman to have a partner, to delay treatment, and undergo ≥1 cycle of *in vitro* fertilization (IVF) (preceded by ovarian hyperstimulation).
- ICSI: a single sperm is injected directly into the cytoplasm of a mature oocyte. Appropriate particularly if the spermatozoa are limited in number or quality.
- Donor eggs.

Organ-specific problems

Cardiac
- Anthracycline exposure (e.g. doxorubicin, epirubicin):
  - most commonly associated with long-term cardiovascular complications, particularly dilated cardiomyopathy
  - risk is dose dependent – cumulative doses should be calculated (empiric guidelines for maximum lifetime doses: doxorubicin 550 mg/m^2, epirubicin 900 mg/m^2. Local guidelines should be followed and these figures should not preclude careful clinical monitoring)
  - risk also increases with age, if there is pre-existing cardiac disease, or in the presence of other cardiotoxic therapies, e.g. trastuzumab
  - prior or concurrent radiotherapy has an additive effect. This is significant because chemotherapy for breast cancer typically includes an anthracycline, and chest wall radiotherapy is also commonly used in this group of patients
  - effects can be seen many years later
  - evidence suggests that infusional treatment is associated with a lower risk of cardiotoxicity than bolus therapy. In reality, most protocols use bolus doses (no need for long line, fewer admissions etc.)
  - monitoring via echocardiography or multigated acquisition (MUGA) scanning is appropriate – abnormal septal movement is usually observed before any decline in ejection fraction
  - initial management is usually with an angiotensin-converting enzyme (ACE) inhibitor and referral to a cardiologist.
- Trastuzumab (Herceptin®):
  - monoclonal antibody targeting a specific epitope of the HER2 protein
  - can cause treatment-related cardiomyopathy. This can range from an asymptomatic reduction in left ventricular function to congestive cardiac failure
  - preliminary evidence suggests this cardiotoxicity is reversible
  - regular surveillance echocardiograms are recommended for women receiving treatment.

Pulmonary
- Bleomycin (e.g. to treat germ cell tumours):
  - can cause pulmonary fibrosis
  - symptoms include dyspnoea, a non-productive cough, and chest pain
  - risk factors include ↑ age, ↑dose, renal insufficiency (80% bleomycin is renally excreted) and high doses of inspired O$_2$ (anaesthetists should be made aware of prior bleomyin therapy)
  - treatment with bleomycin should be discontinued immediately the diagnosis is suspected
  - presentation may be acute or many months after treatment.

Renal

- Several drugs used in oncology have the potential to cause chronic impairment of renal function, e.g.:
  - cisplatin
  - aminogycloside antibiotics (frequently used in neutropenic sepsis)
  - non-steroidal anti-inflammatory drugs (NSAIDs).

Neurological

Oxaliplatin can cause an acute transient neurotoxicity, typically experienced as pain or numbness in the feet, hands, or around the mouth, and frequently exacerbated by cold.

Many chemotherapy drugs can cause a cumulative symmetrical sensory neuropathy which is frequently dose limiting.
- Examples include:
  - cisplatin (usually at cumulative doses >400 mg/m^2) and oxaliplatin (cumulative dose >640 mg/m^2)
  - the taxanes
  - vincristine.
- Patients may complain of:
  - intermittent pins and needles
  - numbness in the finger-tips or toes
  - discomfort walking ('like walking on cotton wool or cobblestones')
  - difficulty performing fine tasks, such as doing up buttons or holding a pen.
- If treatment is continued, the neuropathy may become chronic.
- In some circumstances, temporary cessation of the causative agent may allow recovery of the neuropathy to such an extent that it permits reintroduction of the drug, e.g. intermittent oxaliplatin in colorectal carcinoma.
- Symptoms may continue to worsen even after ceasing therapy. Recovery can be slow but occurs to some extent in most patients.

Ears

Several treatments can also damage hearing permanently, typically causing high-frequency sensorineural loss ± tinnitus. Examples include:
- platinum agents
- high-dose radiotherapy
- amoniglycoside antibiotics.

Ocular

- Cataracts can be a consequence of radiotherapy or the use of high-dose steroids.
- Radiotherapy-induced Sjögren's syndrome is a recognized phenomenon.

Skeletal

- Treatment-related reduction in bone mineral density is being increasingly recognized as a significant long-term complication.
- Induction of premature menopause will also put the patient at risk of osteoporosis. Vitamin D and calcium supplements can minimize bone loss. At-risk patients should have bone densitometry and consideration of biphosphonate therapy.
- Prolonged use of exogenous steroids can also cause osteopenia.

Secondary malignancies

- Risk factors for development of secondary malignancies include:
  - specific treatments previously received, e.g. alkylating agents, topoisomerase II inhibitors, radiotherapy
  - ↑ inherent genetic risks, e.g. predisposing genetic polymorphisms, *BRCA1/2* carrier
  - field changes, due to carcinogen exposure, e.g. cigarette smoking and risk of lung, head and neck, or urothelial cancers
  - other persisting environmental factors such as smoking.
- 5–10% of all childhood cancer survivors develop second malignancies.
- The peak incidence of secondary myeloid malignancies occurs 2–10 years after treatment. Prognosis is poor. Secondary solid malignancies typically occur 10–20 years after treatment for the primary diagnosis.
- The risk of a testicular cancer survivor treated with radiotherapy developing a second solid malignancy is reported to be 2–3 times the rate in the general population. The incidence of leukaemia is also greater in those patients treated with etoposide-containing chemotherapy regimes.
- Successful treatment for Hodgkin's disease is associated with an increased incidence of leukaemias, non-Hodgkin's lymphomas, and solid tumours, e.g. lung, breast, and thyroid cancers. A UK screening programme for breast cancer has been introduced for women previously treated with mantle radiotherapy for Hodgkin's disease.

Neuropsychological consequences

The long-term neuropsychological sequelae of the treatment for cancer cannot be underestimated.

Problems related to specific treatments

- Cranial irradiation in a young child is associated with:
  - impairment in short-term memory, attention span, and information processing
  - often preservation of verbal IQ, therefore the child may give the appearance of coping well.
- Cognitive dysfunction following adjuvant chemotherapy for breast cancer has been extensively studied. Although some studies have suggested an association (particularly with high-dose adjuvant chemotherapy) this has not yet been conclusively proven.

Problems related to the process of treatment

Cancer therapies are often intensive, debilitating, and protracted. Survivors may experience:

- social isolation – time away from work or school
- problems integrating back into the peer group
- difficulties accepting alterations in appearance or ability
- psychological consequences of adapting to long-term effects, e.g. changes in sexual function and employability
- practical consequences that may impact on quality of life, e.g. difficulty in arranging life insurance or taking out a mortgage.

Further reading

Anderson FS, Kunin-Batsan AS (2008) Neurocognitive late effects of chemotherapy in children: the past 10 years of research on brain structure and function. *Pediatr Blood Cancer* **52**, 159–64.

Anderson B, Sawyer DB (2008) Predicting and preventing the cardiotoxicity of cancer therapy. *Expert Rev Cardiovasc Ther* **6**, 1023–33.

Fossa SD, Vassilopoulou-Sellin R (2008) Long-term sequelae after adult-onset cancer. *J Cancer Surviv* **2**, 3–11.

Skylar CA, Mertens AC, Mitby P, *et al.* (2006) Premature menopause in survivors of childhood cancer: a report from the childhood cancer survivor study. *J Natl Cancer Inst* **98**, 890.

Stava CJ, Jimenez C, Vassilapoulou-Sellin R (2007) Endocrine sequelae of cancer and cancer treatment. *J Cancer Surviv* **1**, 261–74.

Wasilewski-Masker K, Kaste SC, Hudson MM, *et al.* (2008) Bone mineral density deficits in survivors of childhood cancer: long-term follow-up guidelines and review of the literature. *Pediatrics* **121**, e705–13.

Hormone therapy

Introduction

Hormones have been implicated in the aetiology and growth of many malignant tumours (including vaginal, ovarian, thyroid, pancreatic, gastro-intestinal (GI) cancers, melanomas, and meningiomas). The best evidence that hormones promote the growth of cancers relates to sex steroid hormones and cancers of their target organs, namely oestrogens and progestins in breast and endometrial cancer and androgens in prostatic cancer. In general, the aim of hormone therapy for cancer is to deplete the circulating level of the hormone promoting tumour growth, or to block binding of the hormone to its receptors within the tumour cell. Both can result in tumour regression in response to reduction of hormone-dependent tumour cell proliferation and induction of cell death (apoptosis).

Principles of hormone therapy for cancer

- Either remove or reduce hormone driving cell proliferation or block binding of hormone to cell receptor
- Results in inhibition of cell proliferation and/or programmed cell death

The effects of endocrine therapy are generally confined to normal target organs for the hormone, and there are few side-effects outside these organs. This accounts for the tolerability of these treatments in comparison with cytotoxic chemotherapy. In addition, tumour responses to hormone therapy may be durable even in advanced disease. However, some cancers arising in hormone-dependent organs are resistant to endocrine therapy, either at presentation or on relapse, and become increasingly unresponsive during the course of treatment and disease progression. Thus, most patients with breast and prostate cancers die with hormone-independent disease.

Hormone-responsive cancers

- Sex hormones:
  - breast, prostate, endometrial cancer
- Renal cancer, meningioma
- Peptide hormones:
  - thyroid, neuroendocrine cancers, carcinoid tumours

Types of endocrine therapy

Ablation of endocrine glands

In men and pre-menopausal women, the major sites of sex hormone synthesis are the gonads. Castration decreases circulating testosterone in males by over 95% and oestrogens in pre-menopausal women by 60% (relative to follicular phase levels). These endocrine effects produce clinical benefits in about 80% of men with metastatic prostate cancer and in 30–40% of unselected pre-menopausal women with advanced breast cancer. Oophorectomy is not beneficial in post-menopausal women because the post-menopausal ovary produces relatively little oestrogen.

Hypophysectomy and adrenalectomy have been used in post-menopausal women with advanced breast cancer, the adrenal being one source of post-menopausal oestrogen. These produce benefit in about one-third of cases, but the procedures have significant morbidity and lack specificity, removing other classes of hormones in addition to the sex steroids. The irreversible nature of surgical ablation of endocrine organs, when all patients cannot be guaranteed benefit, has provided the impetus to develop alternative pharmacological therapies that are specific, reversible, and self-limiting. Thus, if therapy proves ineffective, drug withdrawal allows hormone levels to return to normal with amelioration of side-effects.

Agonists/supraphysiological doses of hormone

The gonadotrophins luteinizing hormone (LH) and follicle-stimulating hormone (FSH) provide the stimulus for gonads to produce steroid hormones; in turn their synthesis and release from the pituitary is regulated by the hypothalamic factor gonadotrophin-releasing hormone (GnRH) (or LH-releasing hormone, LHRH). Highly potent agonist analogues of GnRH have been synthesized by introducing incorrect amino acids into the native peptide. When administered for short periods they cause a rapid release of gonadotrophins, but in the long term these agonists downregulate and desensitize the pituitary receptors. As a result, circulating gonadotrophins fall, the trophic drive to the gonads is abolished, and circulating sex hormones are reduced to castration levels. Depot formulations of LHRH agonists are available so that a single injection can maintain effective medical castration over prolonged periods. The use of GnRH analogues in pre-menopausal women with breast cancer and men with prostate cancer has produced anti-tumour effects equivalent to surgical castration.

A similar mechanism of action underpins the response seen in hormone-dependent cancers following use of pharmacological doses of steroid hormones such as:
- oestrogen (diethylstilbestrol)
- progestogens (medroxyprogesterone and megestrol)
- androgens.

Lower physiological doses of the same hormones may accelerate tumour growth.

While downregulation of steroid hormone receptors occurs in target organs, other non-specific effects can occur, and these agents may be associated with, e.g. thromboembolic disease. Also, tumour flare may occur at the start of treatment. Despite this they are of clinical benefit, e.g. high-dose progestogens for advanced endometrial and breast cancer.

Inhibition of steroid-producing enzymes

This approach is illustrated by inhibitors of aromatase activity. The aromatase enzyme converts androgens to oestrogens and is the last step of the synthetic cascade. It is the main source of oestrogen in post-menopausal women. Its inhibition represents the most specific method of blocking oestrogen production. Because oestrogen biosynthesis can occur in non-endocrine tissue such as adipose tissue and malignant tumours themselves (particularly in post-menopausal women), aromatase inhibitors have the potential to suppress oestrogen levels beyond that achievable by adrenalectomy.

Two major types of aromatase inhibitors have been developed:

- **steroidal or type I inhibitors** – interfere with the attachment of androgen substrate to the catalytic site
- **non-steroidal type II inhibitors** – interfere with the enzyme's cytochrome p450.

Early type II inhibitors such as aminoglutethimide were neither potent nor specific, inhibiting other steroid-metabolizing enzymes that had a similar cytochrome p450 prosthetic group, so that steroid replacement therapy was required. The current generation of triazole drugs (anastrozole, letro-zole) are 2000-fold more potent than amino-glutethimide and have dif-ferential affinity towards aromatase cytochrome p450 with highly selective inhibition of oestrogen biosynthesis. These drugs can reduce circulating oestrogens in post-menopausal women to undetectable levels, without influencing other steroid hormones.

Among type I inhibitors, exemestane is thought to act as 'suicide' inhibitors, blocking aromatase irreversibly through their own metabolism into active intermediates by the enzyme; oestrogen biosynthesis can only be resumed when aromatase molecules are synthesized *de novo*.

Steroid hormone antagonists

These agents block hormone-mediated effects usually at the level of their receptors. Antagonists for oestrogens, progestins, and androgens have been developed. The most extensive experience relates to the use of the anti-oestrogen, tamoxifen, in the treatment of breast cancer. Tamoxifen binds to the oestrogen receptor and blocks the effects of endogenous oestrogens. Responses are more likely to occur in tumours that are oestrogen receptor positive.

Tamoxifen incompletely blocks the trophic actions of oestrogen and can demonstrate partial agonist activity, especially when endogenous oestrogens are low. This explains its positive effects protecting against osteoporosis, but also unwanted stimulation of endometrial proliferation, which can give rise to polyps and, rarely, endometrial cancer. More potent 'pure' anti-oestrogens have therefore been developed, such as fulvestrant, which completely blocks the transcriptional activity of the oestrogen receptor. This drug produces clinical responses in some patients with breast cancer who are resistant to tamoxifen.

Anti-androgens such as flutamide and bicalutamide have clinical efficacy in the treatment of prostatic cancer. Anti-progestins such as RU-486 and onapristone have been used against breast and endometrial cancer.

Steroid sex hormone therapy treatment options

- Castration (surgical or medical)
- Synthetic pathway blockade (e.g. aromatase inhibition)
- Steroid receptor blockade
- Combination therapy

Single-agent versus combination hormone therapy

In the same way that combination chemotherapy has proved superior to single-agent therapy in many cancers, combined hormone treatments might be predicted to produce improved response rates. In fact for most hormone combinations toxicity is increased with no improvement in treatment outcome. However, there are exceptions to this rule.

Breast cancer

- Castration plus tamoxifen is superior to either alone in advanced pre-menopausal disease.
- Tamoxifen plus aromatase inhibitor is of no benefit over aromatase inhibitor alone in advanced disease or adjuvant therapy.
- Sequential substitution of one hormone treatment by another can result in second and third responses when the previous treatment has failed in advanced disease.

Prostate cancer

- Castration plus anti-androgen has failed to produce clear benefits compared with castration alone.
- Sequential addition of anti-androgen to castration can result in second response when disease is progressing post-castration.

Predictors of response

Given that hormone therapy is not effective in all tumours, indiscriminate application of treatment exposes patients with resistant cancer to the side-effects of endocrine-deprivation therapy and delays other potentially beneficial treatment such as chemotherapy.

Currently no biomarker correlates absolutely with response to endocrine therapy. For breast cancer the most widely used predictor is the oestrogen receptor (ER). Between 60% and 75% of breast cancers are ER positive by biochemical assay or immunohistochemistry; two-thirds of ER-positive advanced breast cancers respond to hormone manipulation, compared with <10% of ER-negative tumours. The highest response rates are in tumours expressing both ER and progesterone receptors (PRs), and the majority of ER-negative responding cancers are PR positive.

The value of other markers such as the progesterone receptor in endometrial cancer is less clear, and measurement of the androgen receptor in prostatic cancer has not proved useful.

Previous response to hormone manipulation and disease-free interval are useful clinical predictors for response to second-line endocrine therapy. Although progression on one hormone therapy does imply relative resistance to further endocrine manipulation, response rates to second-and third-line therapy fall progressively (for advanced breast cancer to 30–40% second-line, 20–30% third-line).

Resistance to hormone therapy

Resistance to hormone therapy may be primary, i.e. no response to initial hormone therapy, or acquired, i.e. disease progresses during treatment after initial response. Several possible mechanisms are listed.

Primary resistance

- Mutation has resulted in hormone-independent proliferation in the tumour with, or without, loss of the hormone receptor.
- Hormone-dependent pathway is present but unresponsive to treatment, e.g. mutated receptor.
- Hormone-independent stimulation of pathway, e.g. 'cross-talk' from other growth factor receptors (there is good laboratory evidence of epidermal growth factor receptor (EGFR) and ER cross-talk in breast cancer).

Acquired resistance

- Clonal selection of the above pathways
- Increased production of hormone receptor or hormone
- Increased affinity of receptor for hormone
- Altered hormone–receptor interaction, responds to hormone antagonists as agonists (clinical evidence comes from observed responses to withdrawal of tamoxifen in advanced breast cancer, and withdrawal of anti-androgens in advanced prostate cancer)
- Induction of metabolic enzymes, reducing intracellular levels of hormone antagonist.

Controversies

Duration of adjuvant therapy

If hormone-deprivation therapy is not cytotoxic but cytostatic, therapy would need to be given indefinitely. The counter-argument is that resistance may be accompanied by a change in tumour phenotype induced by the continued presence of the drug. Discontinuation of the first adjuvant treatment followed by another non-cross-resistant regime might be more effective. Such approaches have been explored in ER-positive early breast cancer, with tamoxifen and aromatase inhibitors. Although switching from tamoxifen to an aromatase inhibitor after 2–3 years of adjuvant tamoxifen has been shown to reduce the risk of recurrence of breast cancer compared with five years of adjuvant tamoxifen alone, it remains uncertain how this approach compares with five or more years of aromatase inhibitor only, in terms of both cancer recurrence and late toxicities, e.g. osteoporosis.

Chemo-endocrine therapy

If endocrine therapy is an effective systemic treatment, and combination chemotherapy is beneficial, there is good reason to use chemo-endocrine therapy. However, hormone therapy, by suppressing tumour cell growth, may give protection from chemotherapeutic agents that are most effective against replicating cells. This has been demonstrated to be clinically relevant in the adjuvant therapy of breast cancer. In general, these treatment modalities are best given sequentially rather than concurrently, with endocrine therapy started after completion of chemotherapy.

Biological and targeted therapies

Introduction

- Conventional chemotherapies are limited by their non-specific toxic effects on normal tissues, particularly those that are rapidly proliferating.
- The ideal goal is to develop strategies of anti-neoplastic treatment which specifically kill malignant cells, do not induce tumour resistance, and minimize the damage to the rest of the body.
- Greater understanding of the molecular differences between normal tissue and tumour cells allows targeting of these differences.
- One approach is to produce anti-tumour effect through the activation of host defence mechanisms or the administration of natural substances with similar effects – targeted biological agents.
- 'Immune surveillance theory of cancer':
  - introduced by Burnet in the 1960s
  - provides the background for the growing area of cancer immunotherapy – involving the use of immune-mediated agents, such as recombinant cytokines, cellular, or humoral products and vaccines
  - suggests that immune system cells continuously patrol the body, eliminating newly mutated malignant cells and protecting against the development of cancer
  - this vigilance would only be circumvented if the immune system was depressed or if malignant cells became more aggressive
  - supported by the observation that host immunologic responses appeared occasionally to affect the natural course of a disease – for instance in metastatic melanoma and renal cell carcinoma.
- This chapter is inevitably complex. It will also inevitably become outdated more rapidly than other areas of the handbook. The aim of the chapter is to introduce the principles of biological therapies, explain some of the rationale behind new therapies, and give selected examples. Many treatments remain restricted to the context of clinical trials. National Institute for Health and Clinical Excellence (NICE) guidance is included where appropriate, but the reader is advised to consult current guidelines via the website (www.nice.org.uk/guidance).

Active immunotherapy

The immunization of the patient with materials that elicit an immune reaction capable of eliminating/delaying tumour growth. It includes the administration of non-specific stimulators of the immune system. Two examples are described below:

Bacillus Calmette–Guérin (BCG)

- The anti-neoplastic effect of the live attenuated form of *Mycobacterium bovis*, bacillus Calmette–Guérin (BCG), was reported by Pearl in 1929. Subsequently, Mathe and co-workers suggested a survival benefit in animals with haematological malignancies treated with BCG.
- The immunotherapeutic action of BCG includes activation of macrophages, T- and B-lymphocytes and natural killer (NK) cells. It induces local type II immunological responses via interleukins (IL-4, IL-1, IL-10). Bacterial surface glycoproteins attach to epithelial cells and act as antigens.
- Clinical studies that followed did not confirm any effectiveness of BCG systemic administration in patients with various malignancies (lymphocytic leukaemia, melanoma, lung cancer).
- Currently there are only two applications of BCG in cancer patients:

Intravesical instillation of BCG for the treatment of patients with superficial bladder cancer

- Most effective intravesical agent for the prophylaxis of Ta and T1 superficial bladder cancer, with a 38% reduction of recurrence rate.
- Only approved intravesical treatment for CIS (carcinoma *in situ*), with an average complete response rate of 72% (vs < 50% for chemotherapy).
- Exact mechanism of anti-tumour action is unclear, although multiple local inflammatory effects have been documented.
- Side-effects of treatment include dysuria, haematuria, mild fever, urinary frequency and, rarely, sepsis.

Intralesional injection into cutaneous melanoma metastases

- Observed association between BCG vaccination in early childhood and a lower incidence of malignant melanoma in later life.
- Multiple clinical trials examining adjuvant BCG in early-stage melanoma, or oral BCG and intralesional BCG in s/c melanoma deposits.
- Mixed results – but objective response to intralesional BCG appears most likely in patients with solely cutaneous metastases.

Cytokines

- Soluble proteins that mediate the interactions between the cells and their extracellular environment, in both an autocrine and paracrine manner.
- Exert their biological effect in a wide range of tissues, but mainly on cells of the haematopoietic and immune lineage.
- A given cytokine can both promote and inhibit tumour growth. How the cytokine will act depends on its concentration, the type of the tumour, and factors relating to the stage of disease.
- Several cytokines promise to be of therapeutic importance in oncology and are described below.

Interferons

- Family of proteins produced by the immune system in response to viral infection.
- Anti-viral, anti-microbial, anti-proliferative, and immuno-modulatory activity.
- Anti-tumour effects include direct cytostatic activity, modulation of oncogene expression, and enhancement of the cytotoxic activity of NK cells, macrophages and T-cells.
- Interferon-α (IFN-α):
  - **hairy cell leukaemia** – treatment of choice with a 90% response rate in the peripheral blood and 40% normalization of the bone marrow
  - **chromic myeloid leukaemia** – previous role as first-line in the management of chronic myeloid leukaemia (CML) (now replaced by imatinib – see 📖 p.197) was based on studies reporting 50–75% haematological remission rates. Monotherapy increases the median survival from 3 to 5 years, while its combination with other treatment modalities increases the response rate further
  - **renal cell carcinoma** – partial response rates of 10–20% can be seen with the typical duration of response being 6–8 months. Occasional complete responses are also reported
  - **malignant melanoma** – monotherapy has moderate anti-tumour activity but when combined with chemotherapy (e.g. dacarbazine), response rates are as high as 20%. A potential role in the adjuvant treatment of early-stage melanoma remains to be clarified
  - **carcinoid tumours** – see 📖 Cancers of the small intestine, p.342.
- Interferon-β and interferon-γ:
  - not in routine clinical use although both are also believed to exert some anti-tumour effect.
- Side-effects of the interferons include 'flu-like symptoms (>90%), anorexia, fatigue, ↑LFTs (liver function tests), myelosuppression, and depression (>15%).

Interleukins

- Interleukin-2 (IL-2):
  - a lymphokine produced by activated T-cells, which enhances the proliferation of lymphoid cells and the migration of lymphocytes from the peripheral blood
  - anti-tumour activity includes the capacity to lyse fresh tumour cells, the regression of distant metastases in murine models, and the *in vivo* release of other members of the cytokine family
  - **renal cell carcinoma** – systemic administration of high doses of IL-2, alone or in combination with lymphokine-activated killer (LAK) cells, activated *ex vivo*, can induce a durable partial or even complete response in a minority (~10%) of patients with metastatic renal cell carcinoma. Predictors of response appear to include good performance status, longer time since nephrectomy and low disease burden. IL-2 is the immunotherapy of choice in the USA for patients with relapsed renal carcinoma
  - **metastatic melanoma** – a similar low response rate (<15%); synergy with concomitant dacarbazine has been reported

• IFN-α enhances IL-2 lymphocyte proliferation and IFN-α/IL-2 combination therapy is undergoing clinical assessment in patients with renal cell carcinoma and melanoma.

• Toxicity is dose dependent and includes 'flu-like symptoms, drowsiness, and anaemia. More serious adverse events including neuropsychiatric disturbances, capillary leak syndrome, severe ↓blood pressure (BP), and arrythmias are also common (toxic fatalities in up to 10% of patients).

Tumour necrosis factor (TNF)

• An important mediator of the inflammatory response – involved in stress conditions, cachexia, and endotoxin shock.

• Mainly produced by monocytes, activated macrophages, and T-cells.

• Induces expression of major histocompatibility complex (MHC) class I and II antigens, as well as adhesion molecules responsible for leukocyte migration and accumulation.

• Clinical trials in several malignancies, mostly in patients with advanced melanoma and sarcoma. Disappointing with poor response rates <5%.

• Systemic administration is limited by toxicity including acute fever, ↑LFTs, central nervous system (CNS) toxicity (including encephalopathy), and impaired renal function.

• Loco-regional administration (intraperitoneally, intravesically, intralesionally) seemed more promising and led to trials of TNF-α administered via isolated limb perfusion (in combination with melphalan and IFN-γ ± hyperthermia) in patients with recurrent sarcoma and in-transit melanoma. Prospective randomized trials failed to support initial encouraging retrospective data.

Erythropoietin (recombinant human)

• A hematopoietic cytokine usually administered subcutaneously.

• Evidence from many randomized double-blind placebo-controlled trials supports its use in patients with anaemia and (non-myeloid) cancer-related fatigue.

• Improvements in haemoglobin (Hb) (to ≥12 g/dl) correlate with improvements in quality-of-life parameters, independently of chemotherapy regime and tumour response. Transfusion requirements fall.

• Generally well tolerated, side-effects include injection site pain and hypertension.

• Conflicting evidence exists in patients receiving curative radiotherapy for head and neck squamous cell carcinoma – erythropoietin treatment has been associated with poorer loco-regional progression-free survival, although methodological issues make these data difficult to interpret.

Granulocyte colony-stimulating factor (G-CSF)

- A cytokine secreted mainly by macrophages, monocytes, endothelial cells, and fibroblasts.
- Promotes myelopoiesis – the primary target cells appear to be late myeloid progenitors.
- Also affects the function and life span of mature neutrophils.
- Subcutaneous (s/c) G-CSF administration shortens the period of neutropenia following myelosuppressive chemotherapy. In potentially curable tumours, e.g. germ cell tumours, childhood malignancies, acute leukemia, adjuvant treatment of breast cancer etc., dose reduction or delay in chemotherapy due to neutropenia is to be avoided. Treatment with G-CSF can support neutrophil production on the days subsequent to chemotherapy when the bone marrow is most affected.
- Current European guidelines recommend primary prophylaxis with s/c G-CSF if the risk of febrile neutropenia associated with the regime is ≥20%.
- Secondary prophylaxis following an episode of febrile neutropenia is also appropriate as an alternative to dose reduction.
- Use during established febrile neutropenia has been examined in several studies. No consistent correlation between a reduction in duration of neutropenia and clinical benefit (mortality from infection or improvement in overall survival) has been demonstrated.
- Clearer role in some treatments for haematological malignancies, including patients undergoing haematopoietic stem cell transplantation.
- Side-effects: bone pain is the most common (up to 30%) but can usually be managed with simple analgesia.
- In most other adult oncology patients in the UK receiving chemotherapy with palliative intent, chemotherapy dose reduction is the preferred option following an episode of neutropenia.

Adoptive immunotherapy

The cell-mediated immune response is crucial in the rejection of alloge-neic and syngeneic tumours.

This prompted the use of cells with anti-tumour activity in patients with malignancies – an approach known as **adoptive immunotherapy**.

Several strategies have been applied to generate cells with reactivity to tumours. These include:

- production of lymphocyte-activated killer (LAK) cells:
  - incubate human peripheral blood lymphocytes with IL-2 to produce cells that can lyse fresh tumour cells
  - the exact mechanism of recognition and destruction of tumours by LAK cells is not fully understood
  - work in animal models initially suggested that the benefit of IL-2 was maximized by the addition of LAK cells. However, subsequent clinical trials in patients with metastatic renal cell carcinoma and melanoma failed to reveal any therapeutic advantage in the addition of LAK cells, compared to IL-2 monotherapy
- isolation of tumour-infiltrating lymphocytes (TILs):
  - isolated from human tumours
  - can recognize tumour-associated antigens
  - these have been administered to patients with advanced melanoma, in combination with IL-2. Response rates of 25–35% have been reported, including in some patients previously treated with IL-2
  - a resource-consuming treatment modality and it is unlikely that any clinical benefit will outweigh the use of IL-2 alone.

Small-molecule inhibitors

Increased understanding of the mechanisms of signal transduction and intracellular signal amplification in tumour cells has led to identification of key families of proteins with critical roles in cell division and cell death.

Tyrosine kinase inhibitors

Tyrosine kinases (TKs) can be divide into:
- receptor tyrosine kinases (RTKs):
  - e.g. epidermal growth factor (EGF) and Her2/neu receptors
  - family of cell surface receptors
  - activity of these receptors controls intracellular signal transduction, cellular proliferation, apoptosis etc.
  - physiological binding to the extracellular domain of the receptor activates the intracellular tyrosine kinase domain, initiating a cascade of downstream events
- non-receptor tyrosine kinases:
  - e.g. c-ABL
  - found at intracellular locations, e.g. in the cytosol
  - mutation and aberrant function of these also has a role in oncogenesis.

Genes encoding TKs are usually under tight inhibitory control. However, in many malignancies it is known that this control is lost. This may result in:
- upregulation:
  - e.g. ~30% of breast cancers over-express the RTK Her2/neu as described in 🕮 Monoclonal antibodies, p.202.
- constitutive activation of the TK domain:
  - e.g. BCR-ABL, the non-receptor fusion TK observed in chronic myeloid leukaemia (CML) described below.

Much interest has focused on mechanisms of inhibiting TKs:

Direct inhibition by small molecule TK inhibitors (TKI)
- Molecules with specific activitiy
  - e.g. erlotinib inhibits EGFR (see next section), and lapatinib specifically inhibits the Her2/neu and EGFR pathways and has a potential role in progressive metastatic breast cancer in patients previously treated with trastuzumab.
- Broad-spectrum inhibition of several pathways:
  - e.g. sunitinib – a TKI whose multiple targets include KIT, platelet-derived growth factor (PDGF), and vascular endothelial growth factor (VEGF) – see 🕮 p.199.

Indirect inhibiton of the TK signaling cascade by antibody binding to the receptor or ligand cascade
- See 🕮 Monoclonal antibodies, p.202.

Aim is to produce treatments with greater specificity for malignant cells in the hope of minimizing toxicity to normal tissue.

Spectrum of side-effects observed with TKI includes effects probably due to inhibition of TK activity in normal tissues, e.g. acneiform rash after erlotinib and cetuximab, cardiomyopathy after trastuzumab.

Small-molecule inhibitors of tyrosine kinases
Imatinib (Glivec®)
- Orally administered specific Abl tyrosine kinase inhibitor.
- Common side-effects include oedema/effusions, nausea, diarrhoea, rashes and myelosuppression.

Role of imatinib in CML
- Approved for use as first-line treatment in patients with CML.
- CML is a clonal disorder of haematopoesis invariably associated with a specific genetic translocation – t(9;22) – also known as the Philadelphia (Ph) chromosome.
- The translocated gene product is an abnormal fusion protein BCR-ABL, unique to the leukaemic cells, which possesses constitutively active non-receptor tyrosine kinase activity.
- Cells expressing BCR-ABL have primary mitogenic activity, stimulate cellular growth in the absence of cytokine stimulation, demonstrate resistance to apoptosis, and possess defects in normal cellular adhesion.
- Randomized phase III trial of imatinib versus IFN-α plus cytarabine in previously untreated patients confirmed that imatinib was associated with significantly improved rates of complete haematological response (97 vs 69%) and complete cytogenetic response (76 vs 14%), although an improvement in overall survival has yet to be demonstrated.
- Also evidence supporting its use in patients in the chronic phase of illness after failure of treatment with IFN-α (when complete haematological response rates of 95% have been reported) and in the accelerated and blast phases of the illness.

Role of imatinib in the treatment of gastrointestinal stromal tumours (GISTs)
- >80% of GISTs have a mutation in the KIT proto-oncogene, leading to constitutive activation of the c-kit receptor tyrosine kinase. Remainder usually possesses a mutation in a related RTK e.g. PDGFR.
- Imatinib is active against the mutant tyrosine kinase isoforms.
- Mutation testing may allow selection of patients likely to benefit from imatinib, or requiring higher-dose imatinib or an alternative TKI, and hence improve targeting of treatment.
- Metastatic or unresectable disease:
  - early trials suggest it is a well-tolerated treatment with radiological response rates of ~50% and 2-year survival rates of >70% in a group of patients for whom there previously was no therapeutic option
  - despite the high response rates, complete responses are rare (<10%) and most patients eventually become resistant to therapy probably via the acquisition of additional KIT mutations. The median time to progression is around 2.5 years
  - approved by NICE for treatment of patients with KIT-positive GIST tumours that either are unresectable or have metastasized
  - continuous treatment is recommended with reassessment of response every 12 weeks.
- Adjuvant treatment:
  - a large (~600 patients) randomized phase III trial reported that treatment with imatinib following resection of a GIST is associated

with significantly fewer instances of disease relapse (3 vs 27%) – the trial was prematurely halted and patients in the placebo arm were offered treatment with imatinib
- however, the long-term impact on overall survival is not known and adjuvant imatinib is not yet standard therapy in the management of resected GIST tumours.

Inhibition of the EGFR pathway

Gefitinib (Iressa®)
- A small-molecule TKI, which specifically targets the EGFR tyrosine kinase domain.
- Orally administered and generally well-tolerated.
- Studied in many solid tumours.
- Early-phase trials in non-small-cell lung cancer (NSCLC) were particularly encouraging and prompted larger phase III studies which have shown no benefit from the addition of gefitinib to standard chemotherapy in terms of response rate, time to progression, or overall survival.
- Ongoing clinical trials in a number of tumour types.
- First-line treatment with gefitinib is superior to chemotherapy in Asian non-smokers, particularly patients with mutated EFGR.

Erlotinib (Tarceva®)
- Another orally available selective inhibitor of the EGFR TK.
- Studied in many solid tumours with some encouraging results.
- The most significant side-effects are diarrhoea and a diffuse acneiform rash, occurring in over two-thirds of patients, which can be disfiguring and distressing.

Role of EGFR TKIs in NSCLC:
- in a randomized placebo-controlled trial in patients with advanced NSCLC who had already failed first- or second-line therapy, the use of erlotinib was associated with an increased median survival (6.7 vs 4.7 months), despite an objective response rate of only 9%. Improvement in symptom control was also reported
- phase III trials of standard first-line chemotherapy in combination with erlotinib have failed to demonstrate a benefit from the addition of the TKI. However, it has been suggested that these studies were inadequately designed to reveal benefit to specific patient subgroups
- ongoing trials aimed at examining any role of erlotinib as first-line monotherapy in carefully selected patients
- certain clinical parameters correlate with response to treatment, including:
  - female sex
  - adenocarcinoma
  - never smoked
  - Asian ethnicity
- the optimal molecular marker to predict response to treatment is not yet established:
  - upregulation of EGFR (either protein over-expression or gene amplification) is predictive of response to treatment, as are specific activating mutations in the TK domain of the EGFR

- k-ras mutations are associated with resistance
  - erlotinib approved in the USA as second- or third-line treatment
  - approved by NICE for use as second-line treatment in specific circumstances (2009).
- **Role of erlotinib in pancreatic cancer:**
  - randomized phase III data to suggest that the addition of erlotinib to standard palliative gemcitabine chemotherapy increases overall survival (23 vs 17% at 1 year), although the increase in median survival was only 2 weeks
  - approved for use in the USA. Not used in the UK outside of the context of clinical trials.

Inhibition of the VEGF pathway

Sunitinib

- A multi-targeted small-molecule kinase inhibitor which inhibits the VEGF receptor TK as well as other TKs associated with the PDGF receptor and the *c-kit* oncogene.
- **Role of sunitinib in metastatic renal cell carcinoma:**
  - important role in patients not deemed suitable for treatment with high-dose IL-2
  - in a phase III trial of 750 previously untreated patients randomized to treatment with either sunitinib or IFN-α, sunitinib was associated with improvements in median progression-free (11 vs 5 months) and overall survival (26.4 vs 21.8 months)
  - ↑BP can occur in almost one-quarter of patients, with clinically severe hypertension in ~6%. Oedema, proteinuria and cardiac toxicity have also been reported
  - phase II data suggest that combination with chemotherapy, such as doxorubicin, may produce additional benefit. Phase III trials awaited
  - licensed for single-agent use in advanced renal cell carcinoma and approval for first-line use in the UK in patients with advanced/metastatic renal cell carcinoma in certain circumstances (NICE guidance 2009).

Sorafenib

- Multi-targeted small-molecule kinase inhibitor which inhibits multiple kinases including those associated with the PDGF receptor and fibroblast growth factor receptor-1. Also inhibits C-raf and B-raf and blocks the intracellular domain of the VEGF receptor.
- Administered orally.
- **Role of sorafenib in metastatic hepatocellular carcinoma:**
  - in a randomized multicentre phase III trial of >600 patients with hepatocellular carcinoma, monotherapy with sorafenib in addition to supportive care was associated with longer overall survival (10.7 vs 7.9 months)
  - generally well tolerated with the main side-effects being diarrhoea and hand and foot syndrome. Hypertension and cardiac toxicity have also against its use in 2009

- phase II data suggest that combination with chemotherapy, such as doxorubicin, may produce additional benefit. Phase III trials and comparison with single-agent sorafenib awaited
- licensed for single-agent use in unresectable hepatocellular carcinoma. Under consideration by NICE (further guidance expected 2010).

- **Role of sorafenib in metastatic renal cell carcinoma:**
  - constitutive activation of the B-raf pathway has been observed in up to 50% of renal cell cancers
  - in a trial involving >900 previously treated patients randomized to either supportive care or sorafenib, treatment with sorafenib was associated with a significantly longer progression-fee survival (5.5 vs 2.8 months). Overall survival is difficult to compare in this trial as patients in the supportive care arm were offered sorafenib after the interim analysis
  - there is currently insufficient data to support the use of sorafenib first-line
  - licensed for use and can be prescribed in the UK. Currently not approved for use in the UK in patients with metastatic renal cell carcinoma under NICE guidance (2009).

mTOR inhibition

Temosirolimus

- An intravenously administered analogue of rapamycin which acts as a completivve inhibitor of the mTOR kinase.
- mTOR kinase is the mammalian target of rapamycin and plays a critical role in several transduction pathways necessary for cell cycle progression and cellular proliferation.

- **Role of temosirolimus in metastatic renal cell carcinoma:**
  - data from a randomized phase III trial involving the first-line treatment of poor-prognosis patients suggests temosirolimus is associated with an increase in median overall survival when compared to single-agent IFN-α (10.9 vs 7.3 months). Treatment with temosirolimus was also better tolerated.

- **Potential role of temosirolimus in other malignancies:**
  - temosirolimus may also have a role in the treatment of mantle cell lymohoma and Kaposi's sarcoma.

Monoclonal antibodies

- The development of hybridoma technology and the resulting tumour-associated monoclonal antibodies (mAbs) offers new prospects for strategies of targeted biological therapies.
- Some of the applications of mAbs in oncology are in diagnosis, e.g. immuno-histochemistry, radio-immunodetection.
- Recently, evidence supporting the use of specific mAbs in the therapy of solid malignancies has emerged.
- New biological response-modifying agents can be added to chemotherapy regimes and seem to improve results.
- They have entered the mainstream in terms of management options in breast and colorectal cancer.

Trastuzumab (Herceptin®)

- A humanized mAb, administered intravenously, that binds to the HER2/neu protein, a cell surface growth factor receptor, discussed earlier in the section on tyrosine kinase inhibitors.
- Binding to the HER2/neu protein inhibits signal transduction, hence inhibiting cellular growth and reducing malignant potential.
- Generally well tolerated and does not appear to increase most side-effects of standard chemotherapy. However, clinically significant cardiomyopathy can occur (~4%) and a higher proportion (up to 15%) may have asymptomatic left ventricular dysfunction. Routine echocardiograms are suggested in patients commencing treatment or those on long-term maintenance, particularly if pre-treated with anthracyclines.

Role of trastuzumab in breast cancer

- ~20% of breast cancers overexpress HER2/neu (C-erbB-2), a transmembrane glycoprotein with tyrosine kinase activity.
- HER2 overexpression appears to be associated with a more aggressive form of the disease, is strongly predictive of response to trastuzumab, and should be assessed in all patients to select those appropriate for treatment. It is usually confirmed via either:
  • strong immunohistochemical staining (3+) for the gene product
  • fluorescence in situ hybridization (FISH) analysis confirming gene amplification.
- Expression rates in the primary tumour were generally believed to represent expression rates in subsequent metastases. However, discordance has been reported in up to 20% of cases and retesting on relapse should be considered.
- Approved by NICE in the adjuvant treatment of HER2-positive breast cancer and for the treatment of HER2-positive metastatic disease.
- **Adjuvant treatment:**
  • the addition of trastuzumab to adjuvant chemotherapy for HER2-positive disease significantly reduces the likelihood of relapse and death. This has been confirmed in several large randomized trials including the multinational HERA trial involving >5000 women with HER2-positive disease. One year of treatment with trastuzumab in addition to standard adjuvant therapy was associated with a 36% reduction in disease recurrence after an average of 24 months'

follow-up. Cardiac toxicity was the main treatment-related side-effect. The results of long-term follow-up and the outcome after two years' treatment with trastuzumab are awaited, as are the results of trials using a shorter duration of treatment.

- **Metastatic disease:**
  - response rates to monotherapy in selected patients with relapsed breast cancer overexpressing HER2/neu who have already failed at least one line of treatment for metastatic disease are ~15% and may be as high as 26% in previously untreated patients. Response rates in patients not expressing the Her2/neu protein are as low as 0%. Clear randomized evidence of synergy between trastuzumab and several standard cytotoxic agents used in the treatment of metastatic breast cancer (MBC) including doxorubicin, alkylating agents, and vinorelbine. For example, response rates (RR) and time to progression (TTP) in patients with MBC (with previous anthracycline exposure) treated with the combination of paclitaxel and trastuzumab were significantly greater than in those receiving paclitaxel alone (RR 38 vs 16%, TTP 6.9 vs 3 months).

Potential role of trastuzumab in other cancers

- Trials are ongoing in other solid tumours known to overexpress HER2, which include advanced gastric carcinomas, salivary duct tumours, and some bladder cancers.

Cetuximab (Erbitux®)

- A human/mouse chimeric monoclonal antibody, administered intravenously, that binds to the epidermal growth factor receptor (EGFR).
- Causes inhibition of the EGFR signalling pathway.
- Adverse effects of treatment with cetuximab include hypersensitivity reactions (~3%) and an acneiform rash (possibly due to high levels of EGFR expression in the basal layer of the epidermis).

Role of cetuximab in colorectal carcinoma (CRC)

- ~80% of all CRCs are positive for EGFR expression on immunohistochemistry.
- Stimulation of the EGFR is believed to have a role in the proliferation of CRC cells and possibly in the development of metastases.
- However, there is no correlation between the intensity of EGFR staining and clinical response to treatment. The EGFR status of the primary tumour is insufficient for predicting response to treatment for subsequent metastatic disease.
- Emerging data suggest that upregulation of other genes in the EGFR signalling pathway, e.g. the EGFR ligand epiregulin, may be more relevant in predicting clinical response to cetuximab. Activating k-RAS mutations (observed in ~45% of metastatic CRC) may be associated with resistance.
- Evidence supports its role in patients with metastatic CRC who have failed treatment with irinotecan. In this group, the response rate to cetuximab alone is 11% but the objective response rates when irinotecan is continued in addition to commencing cetuximab are significantly greater at 23%. A benefit in progression-free survival (1.5 vs 4.1 months) is also seen although effects on overall survival are still to be confirmed.

- It is not yet known whether promising early data on combining oxaliplatin-based regimes with cetuximab will translate into clinically useful therapy.
- Recent NICE approval given in UK for use in down-staging of liver metastatis in CRC.

Role of cetuximab in head and neck cancer

- High levels of EGFR expression in head and neck cancer correlate with an aggressive and treatment-resistant phenotype, although the molecular mechanism of this association is not understood.
- Cetuximab has been shown to have some efficacy as monotherapy in advanced disease, based on relatively small trials which report modest response rates up to <25% of typically short duration (<2 months).
- Evidence supporting its role as a radio-sensitizing agent is stronger. A randomized multinational trial involving >400 patients with loco-regionally advanced squamous cell carcinoma treated with radiotherapy with or without weekly cetuximab showed that cetuximab was associated with better median survival (49 vs 29 months) and better loco-regional control (50 vs 41%) without apparent exacerbation in side-effects usually associated with radiotherapy.
- Approved in the UK (NICE guidance issued 2008) for use in combination with radiotherapy in locally advanced squamous cell head and neck cancer in fit patients for whom platinum-based chemotherapy is inappropriate.
- Approved in the USA as monotherapy in platinum-resistant disease.

Potential role of cetuximab in NSCLC

- There is now randomized Phase III evidence to suggest that the addition of cetuximab increases the response rate (36 vs 29%) and overall survival (11.3 vs 10.1 months) in patients treated with platinum doublet chemotherapy, with subgroup analysis suggesting certain groups may benefit more.

Bevacizumab (Avastin®)

- A monoclonal antibody targeting vascular endothelial growth factor (VEGF), a growth factor implicated in cellular proliferation, and the primary factor controlling angiogensis.

Role of bevacizumab in CRC

- Metastatic disease:
  - studied in combination with several standard chemotherapy regimes including 5-fluorouracil (5-FU), leucovorin, irinotecan, and oxaliplatin
  - use of bevacizumab first-line: a randomized, placebo-controlled phase III trial examined the addition of bevacizumab to IFL (irinotecan/leucovorin (LV)/5-FU) in chemo-näve patients and demonstrated an increase in objective response rate from 35% to 45%, with a statistically significant increase in both progression-free survival (6.2 to 10.6 months) and median survival (15.6 to 20.3 months). There are also data suggesting bevacizumab increases disease response, progression-free, and overall survival in patients treated with first-line 5-FU/leucovorin or combination oxaliplatin/5-FU regimes

- use of bevacizumab second-line: reported increase in median survival in patients treated with FOLFOX4 (oxaliplatin/LV/5-FU) from 10.7 to 12.5 months
- there is insufficient evidence to support continuing treatment with bevacizumab with second-line chemotherapy, if it was a component of first-line treatment
- no molecular marker yet exists that predicts response to treatment
- adverse effects: associated with delayed wound healing, gastrointestinal (GI) perforation, fistula formation (all <1%), hypertension, proteinuria, and an increased incidence of serious arterial thromboembolic events, including fatal episodes
- licensed for use in metastatic carcinoma of the colon or rectum, in combination with 5-FU/folinic acid with or without irinotecan, and can be prescribed in the UK. However has not been approved by NICE (2009).
- Adjuvant treatment :
  - One negative trial reported. Results from USA based study awaited.

Role of bevacizumab in metastatic breast cancer (MBC)
- There are phase III data to support the fact that the addition of bevacizumab to a taxane in the first-line treatment of MBC improves response rates (e.g. from 21% to 36%) and progression-free survival, although data on overall survival are missing.
  - The combination of paclitaxel and bevacizumab is approved for use in the USA in HER2-negative disease but is not used in the UK outside the context of a clinical trial.

Role of bevacizumab in metastatic renal cell carcinoma
- A randomized trial involving almost 650 patients receiving either IFN-α monotherapy or IFN-α plus bevacizumab found that addition of bevacizumab was associated with an increase in progression-free survival (5.4–10.2 months) and an increase in response rate (13–31%).
- Further trials awaited.

Role of bevacizumab in NSCLC
- There are data from randomized phase III trials to suggest that bevacizumab given to fit patients with non-squamous NSCLC in combination with platinum doublet chemotherapy is associated with improvements in objective response rates (35 vs 15% in one trial) and progression-free survival . However, data on overall survival have been inconsistent and may be dependent on the chemotherapy regime used. Cautious patient selection excluded any patients felt to be at risk of haemorrhage or arterial thrombosis.
- Currently not approved by NICE (2009).

Potential role of bevacizumab in recurrent malignant gliomas
- Evidence from a phase II trial suggests some benefit from treatment with bevacizumab after progression following treatment with temozolomide. Further results awaited.

Tumour vaccines

Virally induced tumours

- Hepatitis B virus (HBV) vaccine is a widely used and effective vaccine against hepatocellular carcinoma.
- Studies are in progress to develop vaccines against Epstein–Barr virus (EBV), which is closely linked to the development of Burkitt's lymphoma, non-Hodgkin's lymphomas, and nasopharyngeal carcinoma.
- The NHS now offers a vaccination programme against the human papilloma viruses (HPV), strains 16 and 18, which are responsible for 70% of cervical cancer – see 📖 Chapter 2 'Aetiology and epidemiology'. The programme will initially target girls aged 12–13 years (commencing 2008) with plans for a 'catch-up' programme to include older teenage girls commencing shortly afterwards.

Non-virally induced tumours

- The concept of a vaccine for a non-virally induced tumour is more complex. The theory is that tumour cells or tumour cell extracts are used as cancer vaccines intending to enhance a humoral or cell-mediated immune response (i.e. B- or T-cell mediated) to relevant tumour-specific antigens rather than to induce prophylactic immunity.
- The antibodies produced may kill the tumour cells by complement fixation or antibody-dependent cellular cytotoxicity, while the activation of cytotoxic T-cells that recognize antigens on the tumour cell surface may induce specific cytolysis.
- Immunization strategies rely on the efficient presentation of tumour antigens on either the MHC class I or II molecules of specialized antigen-presenting cells, such as dendritic cells. Unfortunately, it is believed that many neoplastic cells employ tactics that minimize their risk of immune recognition, e.g. loss or downregulation of MHC class I molecules. Co-administration of appropriate epitopes with dendritic cells may be one method of optimizing antigen presentation, to maximize the T-cell response.
- Several vaccines for melanoma, colorectal, breast, prostate, and lung cancers are currently under clinical evaluation. Preliminary data support the concept that active immunization will be effective for patients with high-risk recurrent disease, after surgical removal of the tumour, when the tumour burden is small.
- Most clinical trials to date have been in patients with advanced, extensive disease, refractory to conventional therapies, who are probably already immunosuppressed.

Conclusion

Positive results in phase II trials are often followed by disappointing results at phase III level. Even if phase III data remain positive it can be difficult to translate this into a valid clinical role for a new drug. Establishing the optimal use of a new drug with proven activity, in the context of competing treatments, is complex. A cost–benefit analysis is an inevitable requirement. Many trials are not yet mature enough for us to be confident about long-term side-effects – an area of increasing relevance now that we are seeing long-term survivors of malignant disease. Only a selection of drug targets and a selection of drugs has been included in this section. The number of potential targets, and consequently the number of targeted biological agents under investigation, is constantly expanding and numerous clinical trials are under way at any one time.

Further reading

NICE updates its guidance regularly (www.nice.org.uk/guidance).

Baldo P, Cecco S, Giacomin E, *et al.* (2008) mTOR pathway and mTOR inhibitos as agents for cancer therapy. *Curr Cancer Drug Targets* **8**, 647–65.

Baxevanis CN, Perez SA, Papamichail M (2008) Combinatorial treatments including vaccines, chemotherapy and monoclonal antibodies for cancer therapy. *Cancer Immuno Immunother* **58**, 317–24.

Dy GK, Adjei AA (2008) Systemic cancer therapy: evolution over the last 60 years. *Cancer* **113(7 Suppl)**, 1857–87.

Flaherty KT (2008) The future of tyrosine kinase inhibition: single-agent or combination? *Curr Oncol Rep* **10**, 264–70.

Nielsen DL, Anderson M, Kamby C (2009) HER2-targeted therapy in breast cancer. Monoclonal antibodies and tyrosine kinase inhibition. *Cancer Treat Rev* **35(2)**, 121–36.

Part 3

Clinical trials, cancer prevention, and screening

Clinical trials

Methodology in cancer

Introduction

Clinical trials can be classified as:
- phase I studies
- phase II studies
- phase III studies.

In addition, some phase III studies are sometimes referred to as phase IV or post-marketing studies.

No study should be started without a protocol that describes in detail:
- aim of the study
- patient eligibility criteria
- screening and follow-up studies
- treatment
- criteria to score toxicity and activity.

In addition, rules for informed consent procedures should be specified. Trials of any sort should have approval by a properly constituted ethics committee.

All of these criteria have been specified in guidelines produced by the International Conference for Harmonisation for Good Clinical Practice (ICH-GCP). They are also now embedded in EU legislation on the conduct of all trials of new therapeutics.

Phase I studies

Phase I studies are human toxicology studies. Their endpoint is **safety** and they usually include 15–30 patients. They are designed to define a feasible dose for further studies. These studies begin at a dose that is expected to be safe in man. Dose escalation is usually between cohorts, and infrequently in individual patients. It can be:
- according to the Fibonnaci method (dose is escalated in decreasing percentages of the previous dose, i.e. 100%, 66%, 50%, 33%, 25%)
- according to pharmacokinetics (pharmacokinetically guided dose escalation or PGDE), using a method that combines statistics with the experience and expectations regarding side-effects (continuous reassessment method)
- variation on these methods.

The aim of the phase I study is to describe the side-effects that limit further dose escalation (dose-limiting toxicities or DLTs) and to recommend a dose for further studies with the drug or the new administration method (maximal tolerated dose or MTD).

Phase II studies

In phase II studies, anti-tumour activity of a new drug or method is the endpoint. There are various statistical designs, including 14–60 patients on average. With the emergence of drugs that create tumour dormancy rather than cell kill, the endpoint of time to progression becomes important. This is the time from the start of treatment until the first evidence of tumour progression. In addition, phase II studies can provide information on side-effects related to cumulative drug dose.

Phase III studies

Phase III studies have either time to progression or survival time as the endpoint. Phase III studies always include randomization against a standard form of therapy or no treatment when no standard therapy exists. Secondary endpoints such as toxicity, pharmaco-economics, and quality of life are often included. Phase III trials can involve between 50 and several thousand patients. The number of patients is dependent on the size of difference expected/clinically important. Cancer trials have often been criticized in the past for being too small to find realistic differences between therapies. Breast cancer studies involving many thousands of patients have been able to define the long-term benefits of hormone therapy and paved the way for larger-scale trials in other common tumours. In the modern era many large-scale cancer trials are performed in order that the true level of benefit of a new approach can be proven and to allow for regulatory approval of new agents.

Quality of life

Introduction

Most cancer treatments produce unwanted toxicities that interfere with the patient's quality of life. In many cancers the benefits of new treatments over existing approaches have been modest. As new cancer treatments are developed, a common problem is the comparison of a novel intensive treatment regimen against a relatively less toxic standard. In such circumstances, if the survival gain from the new treatment is reliably established but of modest magnitude, then it may be questioned whether the gain is worthwhile for individual patients. In weighing up the risks and benefits of all treatments, it is important to consider many aspects, such as:

- duration of treatment
- length of hospital stay
- number of clinic visits
- short- and long-term toxicities
- less clinical aspects (perhaps less well-appreciated) summarized as quality of life (QoL).

Assessing health-related QoL

Several questionnaires for completion by patients have been developed. The European Organisation for Research and Treatment of Cancer (EORTC) Quality of Life Study Group has developed a core questionnaire, the EORTC QLQ-C30, to which are added disease-specific modules. A patient who scores high for global health-status/QoL is deemed to have high QoL.

Difficulties in QoL assessment

- Compliance declines as patient becomes terminal.
- Compliance may also be poor if the patient feels well.
- Surrogate, relative, nurse, physician can fill in form?

There are important challenges in reporting QoL outcomes in clinical trials. These include the description of compliance, summarizing longitudinal data in a complete yet clinically meaningful way, balancing the multiple endpoints under consideration, and, perhaps most importantly, relating the findings with regard to QoL to other treatment outcomes such as patient survival and treatment-related toxicity.

Attempts have been made to integrate QoL and survival data into quality-adjusted life years (QALYs). The duration of survival is adjusted according to periods of different levels of QoL before summing to give the overall survival time for analysis. The final QALY can then be used for a comparison between treatments, embracing both survival effects and changes in QoL.

Further reading

Eisenhauer EA, Therasse P, Bogaerts J, et al. (2009) New response evaluation criteria in solid tumours: revised RECIST guidelines (version 1.1). *Eur J Cancer* **45**, 228–47.

Cancer prevention

Prevention strategies: introduction

Chemoprevention is the use of chemical agents or dietary compounds to reduce the incidence of cancer. The chemical compounds could be trace elements or hormones or other medicaments; the dietary compounds could be fibre, nutrients, vitamins, etc. This field of medical oncology brings together the disciplines of:
• epidemiology
• carcinogenesis
• toxicology
• pharmacology
• molecular biology
• genetics.
Burkitt observed that colorectal cancer was almost unknown in numerous tribes in Africa, possibly due to their high-fibre diet. Similarly, a number of studies associated breast cancer with obesity, and numerous studies have subsequently attempted to explore the relationship between fat in the diet and the onset of breast cancer.

There are numerous other risk factors for breast cancer including many that have an endocrine basis:
• delayed puberty
• history of nulliparity
• lack of breast feeding
• contraceptive pill in early life
• hormone replacement therapy around the menopause.
Manipulation of the risk of breast cancer through endocrine therapy is therefore a tempting therapeutic target.

Biochemical alterations have been shown in population studies of cancer patients' blood. Low levels of retinoids such as vitamin A and carotene and elements like selenium have been associated with cancer, again providing hypotheses to support cancer-prevention trials.

Having understood the cancer process and the predisposing factors, it is easier to identify which patient group might be at highest risk of specific cancers and might benefit most from an intervention such as change of diet or addition of a medication.

Cancer: genetic and environmental risks

Genetic risks

Patients with certain genetic defects are more likely to get cancer – either they have overexpressed oncogenes such as *K-ras* or a mutated tumour suppressor gene such as *p53* or *Rb*.

Environmental risks

- A number of environmental factors are known to cause pre-malignant lesions, e.g. chewing tobacco frequently causes leucoplakia, which may progress to oral cancer.
- Smoking and lung cancer: cigarette smoking remains the most important avoidable environmental carcinogen worldwide (see ☐ Smoking-related cancers, p.218).
- Viruses have been incriminated in the aetiology of:
  - hepatoma (hepatitis viruses)
  - Burkitt's lymphoma (Epstein–Barr virus, EBV)
  - nasopharyngeal carcinoma (EBV)
  - cervical carcinoma (human papilloma virus 16).
- Vaccines are available against each of these agents. Vaccination against hepatitis B is commonplace in the West and in the UK, vaccination of school children against the papilloma virus for cervical cancer began in 2008.
- *Helicobacter pylori* has been linked to gastric carcinoma, and early claims of eradication of the organism by antibiotics and subsequent protection from cancer are being validated.
- The association of ultraviolet light with skin cancer is well established, as is the increase of malignant melanoma in the UK (approximately 10% per annum).

Overall it is considered about 50% of all new cancer cases and cancer deaths worldwide are preventable. In developing countries the most important preventable risk factors are smoking (30%), poor diet, obesity, and lack of exercise (combined) (30%).

Smoking-related cancers

- Tobacco smoke contains upwards of 4000 chemicals, and of these about 55 are known to be carcinogens. These agents cause DNA gene mutations. Nicotine *per se* does not cause cancer but causes the addiction to tobacco and hence the exposure to the carcinogens.
- Tobacco use causes 30% of all deaths in the Western world, and an estimated 10 million deaths each year worldwide.
- Smoking causes about 90% of lung cancers, with a clear dose–response relationship between the risk of developing cancer and cigarette consumption.
- Passive smoking is now well recognized to be a danger and a cause of smoking-related cancers.
- Male lung cancer deaths have now decreased, whereas in females lung cancer deaths are increasing and this reflects smoking patterns.
- Smoking is the major cause of cancers of the larynx, mouth, tongue, pharynx, oesophagus, and lung. Smoking is also a factor in the development of cancer of the pancreas, kidney, stomach, colon, bladder, and cervix.
- In an effort to stop exposure to passive smoking, many countries have banned smoking in workplaces, restaurants, bars, and other public areas. Smoking in such public areas has been banned in the UK since 2007.

Cancer prevention: diet

This is a controversial area with conflicting data in the literature. Dietary modifications are difficult to promote in populations.

Dietary fat

Dietary fat promotes tumour growth in animal models and, conversely, energy restriction appears to reduce the incidence of tumours.

Excess dietary fat is associated with cancer of the breast, colon, endometrium, and prostate. Dietary studies are fraught with methodological problems but, nonetheless, there are increasing case control and cohort studies to point towards an association of excess fat in the diet with breast and colon cancer in particular. The data showing the relationship between a high-fat diet and prostate cancer are conflicting.

Dietary fibre

Diets with increased fibre tend to reduce colonic transit time and bind some potentially carcinogenic chemicals.

Randomized controlled trials of dietary manipulation are extremely difficult and are dogged by poor compliance.

In over a dozen case studies, meta-analysis indicates an inverse relationship between fibre intake and colon cancer. These are mostly retrospective studies. Prospective studies have produced conflicting data, in particular the huge Nurses' Health Study.

- There is no evidence that increasing fibre in the diet inhibits the development of colorectal adenomas.
- Evidence that increased fibre in the diet inhibits the development of colorectal cancer is uncertain and data are conflicting.
- Similarly, while high-fibre diets may reduce the risk of breast and stomach cancer, the data are unclear.

Fruit and vegetable consumption

Again data are conflicting and the Nurses' Health Study revealed no association between the consumption of fruit and vegetables during over 1.5 million person years of follow-up.

- Some studies have found an inverse association between fruit and vegetable consumption and stomach cancer but, again, data are conflicting.
- There appears to be little association between fruit and vegetable consumption and breast cancer.
- High consumption of fruit and vegetables may be protective for men and women, who have never smoked, in the development of lung cancer.

Folate

- Folate may reduce carcinogenesis through DNA repair and DNA methylation.
- In animals, folate deficiency increases intestinal carcinogenesis.
- A diet rich in folate may lower the risk of colorectal cancer and the precursor adenoma.
- Several studies have shown that folate supplementation can decrease colorectal cancer risk.

Carotenoids

These are antioxidants and promote cell differentiation. β-carotene has been investigated and the data are conflicting.

In some cancers early data are encouraging (aspirin in colorectal cancer prevention), whereas in lung cancer vitamin supplementation has no proven role.

Clinical trials of cancer prevention

The rules in prevention trials in normal people are very different from classical cancer therapeutic trials. During the trials of tamoxifen given as an adjuvant therapy in early breast cancer it was observed that the incidence of second primary breast cancer in the contralateral breast was lower in women treated with tamoxifen compared with placebo. This led to the hypothesis that tamoxifen might be a cancer-preventive agent as well a cancer therapy. There followed a series of trials leading to the landmark publication of the Breast Cancer Prevention Trial (BCPT) from the United States in 1998, which showed that tamoxifen could halve the number of breast cancers observed in normal women at high risk. However, in two further trials in different patient populations, no proven benefit in terms of survival was observed. The role of tamoxifen in the prevention of breast cancer in high-risk individuals is not clear and the British view is that the side-effects of venous thrombosis/embolism and risk of endometrial cancer outweigh the benefits. While tamoxifen and raloxifene decrease breast cancer incidence, there is no overall effect on survival. Such trials have highlighted problems inherent in chemoprevention studies.

- Which healthy individuals should be invited to participate in such trials?
- How should these individuals be identified/contacted?
- When should the drug be started and how long continued?
- Side-effects that are quite acceptable in cancer patients may be unacceptable in healthy subjects.

Phase I/II clinical trials

The main objective of early clinical trials of chemopreventive agents is to establish tolerability and side-effects of candidate compounds. One major difference from conventional cytotoxic agents is that the duration of administration of the preventive agent will be much longer than for a cytotoxic, so chronic side-effects are at least as important as acute side-effects. For phase I studies:

- a major side-effect would include either fatality or problems requiring intervention by a physician or long-term disability. Major side-effects would automatically rule out any further development of a chemopreventive agent
- minor side-effects may preclude chronic dosing with the agent. The route of administration is usually oral.

A phase II trial will frequently be of longer duration and may have more than one dose level. It may be randomized with a placebo control to clarify toxicities.

- A crucial component in assessment of the agent at this stage is compliance, which may require pharmacokinetic confirmation.
- Duration may be 1–5 years and the sample size could be anything from 100 to >1000 volunteers or potential patients.
- The use of surrogate endpoints is extremely important for cost-efficient studies, although there are few biomarkers that are of proven value (e.g. development of carcinoma *in situ* or other precancerous lesion).
- Ease of recruitment is important because 'high risk' may be clear to a physician but not so clear to a normal individual.

Phase III clinical trials

Randomized placebo-controlled phase III studies of chemopreventive agents need to be large and lengthy. As it is costly, in terms of time and resources, to test each new agent with the classical phase III design, two solutions are being tested. One is the concentration on high-risk groups of individuals and the other is the development of intermediate biomarkers.

The Euroscan trial investigated people who had been cured of one smoking-related cancer in the lung, head, or neck. Second cancers are known to occur in at least 15% of these patients.

- The primary endpoint was the appearance of a second smoking-related cancer, genotypically different from the first, anywhere in the aerodigestive tract.
- 'Ex-patients' were randomized to receive retinol or N-acetyl cysteine.
- Retinol induces differentiation and inhibits malignant transformation in preclinical models.
- N-acetyl cysteine has been used widely in chronic bronchitis and works in a totally different way from retinol. It is a potent antioxidant and increases intracellular glutathione. It has been shown in laboratory animals to be an anti-carcinogen.
- In order to test the possible benefits in combining chemopreventive agents, the 3rd arm of the Euroscan trial received both agents and the 4th arm neither.
- This allows two questions to be answered with half the number of patients.
- Nonetheless, the study requires 2500 individuals to be randomized.

Summary

Chemoprevention is in its infancy. New methodologies are being evaluated and new surrogate endpoints and novel candidate interventions are emerging rapidly from the revolution in molecular biology and genetics. It is an extremely promising and exciting branch of oncology.

Cancer chemoprevention

Principles of chemoprevention

Many human cancers are preventable, because their causes have been identified in the human environment. Minimization of exposure towards carcinogens in the environment (primary prevention) is an effective strategy in cancer prevention, e.g. smoking avoidance or cessation. However, most environmental factors that initiate or promote cancer remain to be identified and, once identified, the avoidance of such factors may necessitate difficult lifestyle changes.

Epidemiological data suggesting that cancer is preventable by intervention with chemicals are based on:

- time trends in cancer incidence and mortality
- geographic variations and effect of migration
- identification of specific causative factors
- lack of simple patterns of genetic inheritance for the majority of human cancers.

Chemopreventive agents

Epithelial carcinogenesis proceeds via multiple, discernible steps of molecular and cellular alterations, culminating in invasive neoplasms. These events can be separated into three distinct phases:

- **initiation** which is rapid; involves direct carcinogenic damage to DNA; and the resulting mutation is irreversible
- **promotion** follows initiation and is generally reversible; involves the clonal expansion of initiated cells induced by agents acting as mitogens for the initiated cell
- **progression** results from promotion in the sense that cell proliferation caused by promoters allows cellular damage inflicted by initiation to be further propagated.

During tumour progression, genotypically and phenotypically altered cells gradually emerge. Both promotion and progression phases are prolonged. Depending on which phase of carcinogenesis they affect, chemopreventive agents can be divided into tumour-'blocking' agents, which interfere with cancer initiation, and tumour-'suppressing' agents, which inhibit promotion or progression (Table 12.1). Blocking agents, such as oltipraz, that prevent metabolic activation of carcinogens or their subsequent binding to DNA, probably reduce the accumulation of initiating mutations.

Altered states of cell and tissue differentiation are characteristic of pre-malignant lesions long before they become invasive. It may be possible to reverse abnormal differentiation with a hormone-like non-toxic agent. Two other approaches to the control of pre-neoplastic lesions are to block their expansion with non-toxic agents that suppress cell replication, or to induce an apoptotic state in these cells.

Although in the past, cancer chemopreventive agents have been discovered serendipitously or developed empirically, recent advances in understanding of the molecular biology of carcinogenesis offers hope for more rational drug design.

Table 12.1 Mechanisms of tumour suppression and examples of cancer chemopreventive agents

Mechanism	Examples
Scavenging oxygen radicals	Polyphenols (curcumin, genistein), selenium, tocopherol (vitamin E)
Inhibition of arachidonic acid metabolism	N-acetylcysteine, NSAIDs (sulindac, aspirin), polyphenols, tamoxifen
Modulation of signal transduction	NSAIDs, retinoids, tamoxifen genistein, curcumin
Modulation of hormonal/growth factor activity	NSAIDs, retinoids, curcumin tamoxifen
Inhibition of oncogene activity	Genistein, NSAIDs, monoterpenes (D-limonene, perillyl alcohol)
Inhibition of polyamine metabolism	2-Difluoromethylornithine, retinoids, tamoxifen
Induction of terminal differentiation	Calcium, retinoids, vitamin D_3
Induction of apoptosis	Genistein, curcumin, retinoids, tamoxifen

NSAIDs = non-steroidal anti-inflammatory drug.

The role of surgery in cancer prevention

Prophylactic surgery to prevent cancer in selected patients is of benefit in the following diseases:

- multiple endocrine neoplasia type II and familial medullary cell thyroid carcinoma, in particular the relatives of patients who have the MEN 2B and 2A syndrome. Prophylactic thyroidectomy is recommended under the age of 5 years
- in patients with Barrett's oesophagus, especially with high-grade dysplasia, there may be a role for prophylactic oesophageal resection (with the advent of powerful proton pump inhibitors this role is less clear except in very high-grade dysplasia or carcinoma *in situ*)
- hereditary diffuse gastic cancer – there may be a role for preventative total gastrectomy
- ulcerative colitis of over 10 years in the patient with total colitis, and who has dysplasia; this may warrant a total colectomy although this is now less frequent with the advent of regular surveillance colonosocopy
- hereditary colorectal cancer:
  - familial adenomatous polyposis coli. After the diagnosis of this condition (with over 100 adenomas) total colectomy with a pouch procedure is now accepted practice to prevent the inevitable development of colorectal carcinoma
  - hereditary non-polyposis colorectal cancer (HNPCC) accounts for 5% of all colorectal cancers. There is currently no consensus regarding surgery and most units use colonoscopic surveillance
- the 5–10% of patients with hereditary breast carcinoma, and who carry the *BRCA1* gene; these individuals have a lifetime risk of 60–85% of getting breast cancer. Some of these patients may opt for bilateral mastectomy and breast reconstruction
- women who carry a mutation in *BRCA1* and *BRCA2* genes – these individuals are at a high risk of developing ovarian cancer. The lifetime risk lies between 60% and 85% and, after counselling, some of these women will opt for laparoscopic prophylactic oophorectomy
- patients with a maldescended testis – have a higher chance of developing testicular cancer of more than 20 times the general population
  - 10% of testicular tumours arise from undescended testes
  - orchidopexy is generally recommended within the first year or two of life. However, this does not abolish the risk of developing future testicular cancer
  - it is generally agreed that in the post-pubertal boy a non-palpable undescended testicle should be excised.

Further reading

Benamouzig R, Chaussade S (2004) Calcium supplementation for preventing colorectal cancer – where do we stand? *Lancet* **364**, 1197–9.

Chan A (2007) Can aspirin prevent colorectal cancer? *Lancet* **369**, 1577–8.

Doll R, Peto R, Boreham J, Sutherland I (2004) Mortality in relation to smoking: 50 years observations on male British doctors. *BMJ* **328**, 1519–28.

Fisher B, Constantino JP, Wickerham DL, et al. (1998) Tamoxifen for prevention of breast cancer – report of NSABP-1 study. *J Int Cancer Inst* **90**, 1371–88.

Fountoulakis A, Zafirellis KD, Dolan K, et al. (2004) Effect of surveillance of Barrett's oesophagus on the clinical outcome of oesophageal cancer. *Br J Surg* **91**, 997–1003.

Hartmann LC, Scharo DJ, Woods JE, et al. (1999) Efficacy of bilateral prophylactic mastectomy in women with a family history of breast cancer. *N Engl J Med* **340**, 77–84.

Holmes MD, Stampfer MJ, Colditz GA, et al. (1999) Dietary factors and survival of women with breast cancer. *Cancer* **86**, 826–35.

Jamrozik K (2005) Estimate of deaths attributable to passive smoking among UK adults: database analysis. *BMJ* **330**, 812–15.

McTiernan A (2003) Behavioural risk factors in breast cancer – can risk be modified? *Oncologist* **8**, 326–34.

Marrett LD, De P, Airia P, Dryer D (2008) Cancer in Canada in 2008. *Can Med Assoc J* **179**, 1163–70.

Norat T, Lukanova A, Ferrari P, et al. (2002) Meat consumption and colorectal cancer risk – dose response meta-analysis of epidemiological studies. *Int J Cancer* **98**, 241–56.

Osborne M, Boyle P, Lipkin M (1997) Cancer prevention. *Lancet* 349(**Suppl 2**), S1127–30.

Potter JD (1999) Fiber and colorectal cancer – where to now? *N Engl J Med* **340**, 223–4.

Slatore CG, Littman AJ, Au DH, et al. (2007) Long term use of supplemental multivitamins, Vit C, Vit E and folate does NOT reduce risk of lung cancer. *Am J Respir Care Med* **177**, 524–30.

Turner N, Jones AL (2008) Management of breast cancer Part I. *BMJ* **337**, 107–10.

Wands JR (2004) Prevention of hepatocellular carcinoma. *N Engl J Med* **351**, 1567–70.

Willet WC, Stampfer MJ, Colditz GA, et al. (1990) Relationship of meat, fat and fibre intake to the risk of colon cancer in a prospective study amongst women. *N Engl J Med* **323**, 1664–72.

Population screening for cancer

Screening for cancer

Principles

The strongest evidence that early detection of cancer increases the chance of cure comes from randomized trials of screening. This has led to public awareness campaigns to persuade individuals to seek advice regarding suspicious symptoms at an early stage. There is, however, no evidence as yet that this strategy of encouraging early self-referral does improve survival.

Screening is the process whereby asymptomatic individuals are tested in order to detect a disease that has yet to be symptomatic. For this to be effective in a population there are certain criteria that must be met by the disease in question, the screening test, and the screening programme.

The disease
- Its natural history is well understood
- It has a recognizable 'early' stage
- Treatment at an early stage is more successful than at a later stage
- It is sufficiently common in the target population to warrant screening.

The test
- Sensitive and specific
- Acceptable
- Safe
- Inexpensive.

The programme
- Adequate facilities for diagnosis in those with a positive test
- High quality of treatment for screen-detected disease
- Screening repeated at intervals if the disease is of insidious onset
- Benefit must outweigh physical and psychological harm
- Benefit must justify financial cost.

It is crucial that treating the disease to be screened at an early stage is more effective than treating at a later stage. To justify a screening programme, one cannot compare the outcome of screen-detected disease with that of symptomatic disease, because three biases operate in favour of screen-detected disease.

- **Lead-time bias** arises from the fact that, if early diagnosis advances the time of diagnosis of a disease, then the period from diagnosis to death will lengthen irrespective of whether or not treatment has altered the natural history of the disease. If patients die of their cancer at the same age at which this event would have occurred without screening, no benefit has been afforded by screening. Screening will only be of value if it improves the survival curve of a screened population compared with unscreened.
- **Length bias** operates as slow-growing tumours are more likely to be detected by screening tests when compared to fast-growing tumours, which are more likely to present with symptoms before a screening test can be applied or between tests. Thus, screen-detected tumours will tend to be less aggressive and associated with a relatively good prognosis.

- **Selection bias** results from the characteristics of individuals who accept an invitation to be screened. Such a person is more likely to be health conscious than one who refuses or ignores screening and may therefore be more likely to survive longer, irrespective of the disease process.

Screening

In screening, it is also important to have a target population to avoid large numbers of fruitless tests in individuals at low risk of cancer. In screening for the common cancers, where the incidence is highly age dependent, the age range should be that in which the disease is relatively common and in which the patients are likely to be fit enough for curative treatment.

There are other predictors of risk, and family history is becoming important in this respect, particularly as it is now possible to detect specific genetic mutations from blood samples and to use these to screen close relatives. Examples of this are mutations in the *APC* gene in familial adenomatous polyposis, in the DNA mismatch repair genes in hereditary non-polyposis colorectal cancer, and in the *BRCA1* and 2 genes in familial breast and ovarian cancer.

A screening test must be acceptable and safe, so that it will be adopted by the target population. It must also be sensitive and specific. Sensitivity is the proportion of individuals with the disease who have a positive test, and specificity is the proportion of individuals without the disease who have a negative test.

Screening programmes

When a screening programme is established, it is important that the diagnostic facilities are adequate. Similarly, treatment of early disease must be associated with minimal morbidity and mortality.

It must also be remembered that screening may cause psychological harm and, along with any physical morbidity caused by investigation and treatment, this represents part of the cost of screening. The benefits gained through cancer screening must outweigh such morbidity, and society must make a decision whether or not the health gain justifies these and the financial costs.

Randomized trials have been done in breast and colorectal cancer, and in both instances screening has been shown to significantly reduce cancer mortality. In the former condition, the screening test studied was the mammogram, and efficacy of screening proved highly dependent not only on the quality of the imaging but also on the quality of the reporting. In colorectal cancer, the test investigated was the faecal occult blood test, followed by colonoscopy when positive.

The breast cancer screening programme has involved 3-yearly mammography since 1986 of women between 50 and 64 years. In 2009, the upper age has increased to 70 years in most areas. While it is accepted that mammographic screening reduces mortality by up to 35% according to the Cochrane Review, 2000 women need to be screened for 10 years to prevent one death from breast cancer. There is current debate about the cost-effectiveness of beginning breast cancer screening under the age of 50 years. This is discussed in detail on pages 286–288.

Cervical cancer screening is performed in the UK by family doctors, using a cervical smear for women who are aged 21 years and above who are sexually active. While this has been introduced in a non-controlled fashion, in the absence of clinical trials, it is thought that the decrease in mortality from cervical cancer is largely due to screening. In the US the interval between screening, using the cervical smear, is between 1 and 3 years.

Colorectal cancer screening

Over the age of 50 years in the US, faecal occult bloods yearly, with flexible sigmoidoscopy every 5 years and colonoscopy every 10 years, is currently recommended. If faecal occult bloods are positive, then colonoscopy is required. Those at high risk of colorectal cancer should have screening earlier and more frequently.

In 2005 in the UK, colorectal cancer screening was approved in principle by the government, following the publication of several trials that have demonstrated benefit. This is now being rolled out in most areas of England and Scotland in 2009. The data show that the cost of this programme is approximately £20 000 per year of life saved. In Scotland, screening is offered 2-yearly to each person aged 50–74 years. In England the age for screening is 60–74 years.

Newer techniques, including virtual colonoscopy, using computerized tomography (CT) scan, are non-invasive. In expert hands, lesions down to 5 mm can be detected. It may find a role in screening in the next 5–10 years. It has been estimated that 2500 lives will be saved each year in the UK by 2025 by bowel cancer screening.

Other national screening programmes are not yet proven. Prostatic screening by prostate-specific antigen (PSA) is not recommended. There are some early encouraging data on CT lung cancer screening.

Further reading

Agrawal J, Syngal S (2005) Colon cancer screening strategies. *Curr Opin Gastroenterol* **21**, 59–63.

Berry DA (1998) Benefits and risks of screening mammography for women in their forties – a statistical appraisal. *J Natl Cancer Inst* **90**, 1431–9.

Elmore JG, Barton MB, Moceri VM, et al. (1998) Ten year risk of false positive screening mammograms and clinical breast examinations. *N Engl J Med* **338**, 1089–96.

Goodman GE (1992) The clinical evaluation of cancer chemoprevention agents: defining and contrasting phase I, II and III objectives. *Cancer Res (Suppl)* **52**, 2752–7.

Harris R, Lohr KN (2002) Screening for prostate cancer—an update of the evidence for the US Preventative Services Task Force. *Ann Intern Med* **137**, 917–29.

Kmietowicz Z (2009) Screening for bowel cancer is set to save 2500 lives a year in UK. *BMJ* **338**, 9.

Mayor S (2004) England to start national bowel cancer screening programme. *BMJ* **329**, 1061.

Meyskens Jr FL (1992) Biomarker intermediate endpoints and cancer prevention. *J Natl Cancer Inst Monogr* **13**, 177–81.

Peto J, Gilham C, Fletcher O, Matthews FE (2004) The cervical cancer epidemic that screening has prevented in the UK. *Lancet* **364**, 249–56.

Shaheen NJ, Indomi JM, Overholt BF, Sharma P (2004) What is the best management strategy for high grade dysplasia in Barrett's oesophagus? A cost-effective analysis. *Gut* **53**, 1736–44.

Sporn MB (1993) Chemoprevention of cancer. *Lancet* **342**, 1211–12.

Turner NS, Jones AL (2008) Management of breast cancer – Part I. *BMJ* **337**, 107–10.

Van Schoor G, Broeders MJM, Paap E, et al. (2008) A rationale for starting breast cancer screening under age 50. *Ann Oncol* **19**, 1208–1209.

Wilson DD, Weissfeld JL, Fuhrman CR, et al. (2008) The Pittsburgh Lung Screening study (PLUSS). *Am J Respir Crit Care Med* **178**, 956–61.

Winawer S, Fletcher R, Rex D, et al. (2003) Colorectal cancer screening and surveillance – clinical guidelines and rational – update on new evidence. *Gastroenterology* **124**, 544–60.

Part 4

Specific types of cancer

Thoracic cancer

Lung cancer

Epidemiology
The statistics are a stark reminder of the cost of this largely preventable disease.
- Second most common cancer in UK (breast cancer commoner), 14% of all cancers.
- In 2001 there were 37 450 new lung cancers in UK, affecting 22 700 men and 14 750 women.
- Lung cancer is the most frequent cause of cancer deaths in both men and women in the UK and US.
- In 2002 there were 33 600 deaths from lung cancer in UK; 160 000 deaths in the US.
- Incidence and mortality rate are falling in men in these countries, but rising in women in UK (Table 14.1).
- Worldwide the incidence is continuing to rise, particularly in developing countries, as cigarette smoking becomes more prevalent.
- Survival rates remain dismal with 5-year survival 6–7% in the UK, <15% in the US.

Table 14.1 Lung cancer incidence figures

Sex	UK incidence by year (age-adjusted, per 100 000 population)	
	1980	2000
Male	113	69
Female	28	36

Aetiology
- 80–90% of lung cancers are due to smoking.
- Risk of lung cancer relates to the number of cigarettes smoked, the number of years of smoking, early age starting to smoke, and the type of cigarette (greater risk with unfiltered and high-nicotine).
- Less than 10% of lung cancers occur in never smokers, usually women.
- Passive smoking.
- Asbestos.
- Previous radiotherapy to the chest.
- Rarely, inhalation of radon gas, polycyclic aromatic hydrocarbons, nickel, chromate, or inorganic arsenicals.

Screening and prevention
- Lung cancer is a preventable disease.
- Currently 30% of the adult population of the UK smokes.
- Health education has had some success in reducing tobacco consumption in men.
- However, smoking in women and adolescents is increasing in the UK.
- Stopping smoking reduces the risk of developing lung cancer.
- Nicotine replacement therapy can improve smoking cessation rates.

- Screening with chest X-ray and sputum cytology does not reduce mortality from lung cancer.
- Clinical trials are currently testing whether regular spiral computerized tomography (CT) scan of the chest might be a useful screening tool for lung cancer, e.g. in smokers.
- The UK ban on smoking in public and work places from 2007 may in the longer term decrease lung cancer rates with less passive smoking.

Pathology

There is evidence that lung cancers may arise in pluripotent stem cells in the bronchial epithelium, and this would certainly offer an explanation for the mixed histology that is fairly commonly seen. The 1999 World Health Organization (WHO) pathological classification is as follows:

1. squamous cell carcinoma (30%)
2. small-cell carcinoma (SCLC, 15–20%)
3. adenocarcinoma (40%):
   a. acinar
   b. papillary
   c. bronchioloalveolar
   d. mucinous
   e. mixed
4. large-cell neuroendocrine carcinoma
5. mixed carcinomas:
   a. adenosquamous
   b. mixed small-cell and non-small-cell
6. carcinomas with pleomorphic, sarcomatoid, or sarcomatous elements:
   a. carcinomas with spindle and/or giant cells
   b. pleomorphic carcinoma
   c. spindle cell carcinoma
7. giant-cell carcinoma:
   a. carcinosarcoma;
   b. pulmonary blastoma
8. carcinoid tumour
9. carcinomas of salivary gland type:
   a. mucoepidermoid carcinoma
   b. adenoid cystic carcinoma
10. unclassified carcinomas.

For the purposes of management, lung cancers are grouped as non-small cell (NSCLC) or small cell (SCLC), but within the former certain patterns of disease do relate to histological subtype. For example, squamous cancers typically arise in proximal segmental bronchi and grow slowly, disseminating relatively late in their course. Adenocarcinomas are often peripheral in origin, and even small resectable lesions carry a risk of occult metastases. Common sites of metastatic spread include the regional lymph nodes, bone, liver, adrenal, lung, central nervous system (CNS), and skin.

However, the risk of dissemination is greatest in SCLC, where it is estimated that >90% of patients have either overt or occult metastases at presentation. These aggressive tumours, derived from neuroendocrine cells, most frequently arise in large airways but can, rarely, present as a small peripheral nodule. The latter presentation may be indicative of a different pathology with an inherently better prognosis.

Genetics

The majority of clinically apparent lung cancers have more than 20 genetic alterations, acquired in a stepwise fashion. These may disrupt cell cycle regulation and cause genomic instability, but also result in failure to undergo apoptosis, invasion of normal tissues, and dissemination to other tissues. Examples of the relevant genes include:

- oncogene activation:
  - epidermal growth factor receptor (EGFR) overexpression, leading to stimulation of this proliferative pathway (70% of SCLCs and 40% of adenocarcinomas)
  - point mutation of *RAS* or *MYC*, activating signal transduction pathways
- tumour suppressor gene inactivation:
  - *p53* alteration is frequent (more than 80% SCLC, 50% NSCLC)
  - *BCL2* high expression in SCLC protects against apoptosis
- angiogenesis – tumor progression and metastasis:
  - vascular endothelial growth factor (VEGF) receptor – high levels of VEGF expression are detected in 50% of all lung cancers
- telomerase activation occurs in 100% of SCLCs and 80% of NSCLCs.

Genetic predisposition to development of lung cancer

- Family history of lung cancer increases risk x2.5 even when smoking is taken into account.
- Likely mechanisms include genetic variation in the enzymes responsible for carcinogen metabolism and detoxification, and DNA damage repair.
- Rarely, germline mutation of *Rb* or *p53*.

Presenting symptoms and signs

Typically, presentation is late, symptoms such as persistent cough and dyspnoea being attributed to smoking. Small adenocarcinomas in the periphery of the lung may be asymptomatic, picked up on chest X-ray or CT scan done for coincidental indication.

- Persistent cough, haemoptysis, dyspnoea
- Recurrent chest infections
- Pleural effusion
- Chest pain (constant, progressive)
- Hoarse voice (vocal cord palsy)
- Wheeze, stridor
- Superior vena cava obstruction
- Horner's syndrome, arm or hand pain, and neurological deficit (apical cancer)
- Fatigue
- Anorexia, weight loss
- Paraneoplastic syndromes (see 📖 Chapter 28)
- Symptoms from metastatic disease.

Investigations (see Fig. 14.1)

After physical examination and chest X-ray, patients with suspected lung cancer require further imaging with CT scan (chest and abdomen) and a tissue diagnosis, obtained by the least invasive route:

- sputum cytology
- fine needle aspiration (FNA) cytology from palpable disease, most commonly supraclavicular fossa (SCF) nodes
- bronchoscopy with direct biopsy, brushings/washings for cytology, or transbronchial biopsy of lung, or lymph node (e.g. under endoscopic ultrasound control)
- pleural aspirate cytology or pleural biopsy
- FNA or core biopsy lung lesion
- FNA or core biopsy metastatic disease, e.g. liver
- mediastinoscopy and lymph node biopsy;
- video-assisted thoracoscopy (VATS) and biopsy
- rarely, open lung biopsy.

Other important assessments include performance status (see Table 14.2), pulmonary function tests, full blood count (FBC), biochemical profile. Patients with symptoms suggestive of metastatic disease may require bone scan or CT brain.

Table 14.2 Performance status scales, National Institute for Health and Clinical Excellence (NICE) guidelines

WHO (Zubrod) scale	Karnofsky scale
0 Asymptomatic	100 Asymptomatic
1 Symptomatic but ambulatory (able to carry out light work)	90 Normal activity, minor symptoms
	80 Normal activity, some symptoms
2 In bed <50% of day (unable to work but able to live at home with some assistance)	70 Unable to work, cares for self
	60 Occasional assistance with needs
3 In bed >50% of day (unable to care for self)	50 Considerable assistance
	40 Disabled, full assistance needed
4 Bedridden	30 Needs some active supportive care
	20 Very sick, hospitalization needed
	10 Moribund
	0 Dead

Reproduced from Detterbeck FC, et al. (2001) Diagnosis and treatment of lung cancer: an evidence-based guide for the practicing clinician. Philadelphia: WB Saunders, p. 40, with permission from Elsevier.

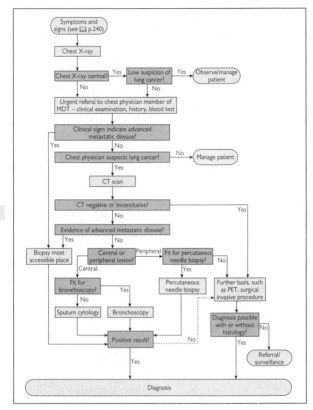

Fig. 14.1 Diagnosis of lung cancer. MDT, multidisciplinary team; PET, positron emission tomography. Reproduced with permission of National Clinical Guidelines Centre – Acute and Chronic Conditions. © 2005.

Non-small-cell lung cancer (NSCLC)

Staging (see Table 14.3, Fig. 14.2)

The following assessments are required:
- clinical examination (particular attention to cervical, SCF, axillary lymph adenopathy, soft tissue masses, e.g. chest wall)
- bronchoscopy:
  - movement of vocal cords
  - site of endobronchial tumour in relation to carina and major bronchial divisions
  - extrinsic compression of bronchi
- CT chest and abdomen:
  - size and site of primary tumour
  - relationship to lung fissures, mediastinum, chest wall
  - mediastinal or other lymphadenopathy
  - metastatic disease, in particular lung, pleura, liver, adrenal, bone
  - CT brain and isotope bone scan performed if clinical suspicion of metastatic disease.

PET scanning

Fluorodeoxyglucose positron emission tomography (FDG-PET) scanning has greater sensitivity and specificity than CT scan for staging NSCLC, and is recommended for pre-operative assessment. It is also commonly used to exclude metastatic disease in patients being considered for radical non-surgical treatment.

Multidisciplinary team meetings

Key to the optimal management of lung cancers is the multidisciplinary discussion of each case, with input from radiologists and pathologists, as well as chest physician, thoracic surgeon, and clinical and medical oncologists.

Treatment modalities

Surgery
- Complete surgical removal of NSCLC offers the best possibility of a cure.
- Appropriate for patients with stage I–II disease who are fit for surgery (see 🕮 Surgery for NSCLC, p.248).

Chemotherapy
- Systemic treatment improves symptoms from advanced disease, and has a modest survival benefit.
- Appropriate for patients with stage III–IV disease particularly with good performance status.
- Developing role prior to surgery and as adjuvant therapy for stage II disease.

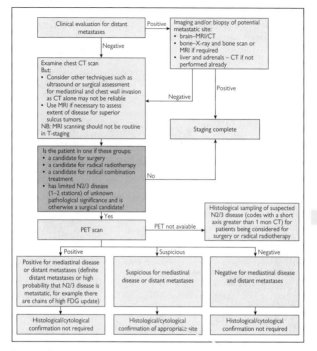

Fig. 14.2 Staging of non-small-cell lung cancer. CT, computerized tomography; FDG, fluorodeoxyglucose; MRI, magnetic resonance imaging; PET, positron emission tomography. Reproduced with permission of National Clinical Guidelines Centre – Acute and Chronic Conditions. © 2005.

Radiotherapy
- Effective local treatment, giving prompt symptom relief from advanced disease especially involving large airways.
- Can be curative in stage I–II and, infrequently, stage III.

Table 14.3 TNM staging of lung cancer (2009 revision)

T1	Tumour 3 cm or less in diameter, surrounded by lung or visceral pleura, distal to the main bronchus
T2	Tumour 3–7 cm diameter; or involving main bronchus 2 cm or more distal to carina; or invading visceral pleura; or associated with atelectasis which extends to the hilum but does not involve the whole lung
T3	Tumour >7 cm; or invading chest wall, diaphragm, mediastinal pleura, or pericardium; or tumour in main bronchus <2 cm distal to carina; or atelectasis of the whole lung; or separate tumour nodule in the same lobe
T4	Tumour invading mediastinum, heart, great vessels, trachea, oesophagus, vertebra, or carina; or separate tumour nodule in a different ipsilateral lobe
N0	No regional node metastases
N1	Ipsilateral peribronchial or hilar node involvement
N2	Ipsilateral mediastinal or subcarinal nodes
N3	Contralateral mediastinal nodes; scalene; or supraclavicular nodes
M0	No distant metastases
M1	Metastatic disease either malignant pleural effusion or distant metastasis

Stage grouping

I	T1–2 N0
II	T1–2 N1; or T3 N0
IIIa	T1–2 N2; or T3 N1–2
IIIb	T4 any N M0; or any N3 M0
IV	Any M1

Surgery for NSCLC

- Surgical removal of NSCLC offers the best possibility of cure.
- Every patient with non-metastatic NSCLC should be considered for surgical treatment.
- However, advanced stage and significant co-morbidity will preclude this option in the majority.
- In UK only 11% are NSCLC resected; in the US – 21%.
- Aim of surgical treatment is cure, in patients where this is not possible, suitable non-surgical treatments should be considered.

Before embarking on surgery, all cases should undergo careful and detailed pre-operative assessment to confirm the following:

- histological/cytological confirmation of diagnosis
- operable stage of disease (I–II):
  - no evidence of metastasis on PET scan
  - commonly requires pathological staging of the mediastinum by mediastinoscopy and lymph node biopsies;
  - lymph nodes that appear normal size on CT (<1 cm diameter) may contain cancer (~15%); enlarged lymph nodes commonly reactive (45%)
  - in presence of pleural effusion, aspirated fluid for cytology and pleural biopsy should be negative for cancer cells before proceeding with operation
- fitness for surgery:
  - age alone is unimportant, but need to take into account performance status, weight loss, and co-morbidities that may exclude surgery as a feasible option
  - pulmonary function tests, spirometry, and gas transfer, taking account of predicted values and extent of surgery planned
  - cardiac assessment; may require exercise testing and at least an ECHO.

Thoracotomy and major lung resection carry significant risks of morbidity and mortality. Surgery for lung cancer should be carried out promptly in a unit with the appropriate level of experience and expertise. In the majority of patients, general anaesthesia with use of a double-lumen endotracheal tube is desirable to allow one-lung ventilation during thoracotomy. With specialization increasing resections are being done thoracoscopically.

Surgical resection

- This may require lobectomy, bi-lobectomy, or pneumonectomy, removing all cancer with clear margins of surrounding normal tissue.
- Wedge resection is not recommended because of the risk of incomplete resection, but may be appropriate occasionally in patients with small tumours and poor lung function. This can usually be done with minimal invasive techniques.
- Operation should include regional lymph node sampling.
- Involvement of chest wall, pericardium, or diaphragm can be dealt with by *en bloc* dissection along with the primary, but survival benefit of such extensive surgery is limited by the high risk of systemic relapse.
- The role of extended lymphadenectomy (mediastinal) is unproven.
- Limited segmental resection performed through the thoroscope is technically possible, but long-term outcome is uncertain.

Post-operative management

Patients should be nursed in an intensive care or high-dependency unit with adequate monitoring of:
- electrocardiogram (ECG)
- blood pressure (BP)
- central venous pressure
- respiratory rate
- oxygen saturation.

Adequate pain control is essential following thoracotomy and can be provided by:
- thoracic epidural anaesthesia (now routine)
- intravenous opiates administered by patient-controlled analgesia (PCA)
- intercostal nerve block prior to wound closure.

Routine postoperative ventilation is no longer needed.

Oxygen therapy is required in the early post-operative stage, preferably through a nebulizer, and in patients with significant airways obstruction, a bronchodilator should be added. Regular chest physiotherapy is essential.

Post-operative complications

Early (within days)
- Haemorrhage (e.g. after dissection of pleural adhesions) may result in a haemothorax
- Respiratory failure:
  - opiate-induced respiratory depression
  - pneumothorax with, or without, surgical emphysema
  - atelectasis due to retained bronchial secretions
- Prolonged air leak following lobectomy
- Cardiac arrhythmias, particularly atrial fibrillation
- Sepsis:
  - chest infection
  - wound infection
  - empyema
- Broncho-pleural fistula (particularly on the right following pneumonectomy).

Late (within weeks to months)
- Post-thoracotomy pain
- Late broncho-pleural fistula with empyema.

Results of lung resection

Post-operative mortality rate should be less than 3% following lobectomy and less than 5% following pneumonectomy. Five-year survival is influenced by a number of factors, the most important of which is pathological staging, (see Table 14.4). Overall 5-year survival for patients undergoing resection may be as high as 40%, approaching 70% in cases without nodal involvement (N0). However, when mediastinal nodes are involved (N2) only 15% of patients will survive 5 years.

Table 14.4 5-year survival after surgery for NSCLC

Stage	Five-year survival
I	60–80%
II	25–40%
IIIa	10–30%
IIIb and IV	<5%

Further reading

Gajra A, Newman N, Gamble GP, et al. (2003) Impact of tumour size on survival in stage 1A, non small cell lung cancer: a case for subdividing stage 1A disease. *Lung Cancer* **42**, 51–7.

Sawada S, Komori E, Yamashita M, et al. (2007) Comparison in prognosis after VATS lobectomy and open lobectomy for stage I lung cancer. *Surg Endosc* **21**, 1607–11.

Chemotherapy of NSCLC

Older studies with alkylating agents in advanced NSCLC showed decreased survival with chemotherapy, and until the 1980s no systemic treatments were available with objective response rates in excess of 20%. Over the last 15 years there has been significant progress in this area, and increasing use of chemotherapy in most stages of the disease.

Metastatic disease

Tumour response and survival

Cisplatin-based chemotherapy with 1980s regimens such as MVP (mitomycin, vinblastine, cisplatin) and MIC (mitomycin, ifosfamide, cisplatin) produced significant benefits in stage IV disease.
- Symptom relief and improved quality of life in >50%.
- Objective response rate of 20–30%:
  - little benefit and increased toxicity in patients with performance status 2 or worse.
- Modest impact on survival:
  - median survival increased by 2 months compared with no chemotherapy
  - 1-year survival 25% (without chemotherapy 15%).
- Toxicities of treatment include nausea, vomiting, lethargy, myelosuppression, sepsis, thromboembolism, and neuropathy.

During the 1990s, several new drugs demonstrated anti-tumour activity in NSCLC as single agents and in combination with carboplatin or cisplatin (see Tables 14.5 and 14.6).
- These drugs included docetaxel, gemcitabine, paclitaxel, and vinorelbine.
- Doublet regimens (one new drug plus platinum complex) proved superior to MVP/MIC in terms of response rate and survival.
- None of the new chemotherapy regimens appeared superior to the others.
- Doublet therapy with the combination of either cisplatin or carboplatin and one of gemcitabine/vinorelbine/paclitaxel/docetaxel is now accepted as standard therapy for advanced NSCLC (approved by NICE June 2001).
- Little evidence to justify >4 cycles of chemotherapy.
- Single-agent chemotherapy with agents such as gemcitabine or vinorelbine can be of modest benefit in patients with advanced disease and performance status 2.

Recent advances in chemotherapy for NSCLC

Since 2000 significant progress has been made in the systemic treatment of NSCLC:
- second-line treatment of advanced disease is feasible and of modest benefit in patients with good performance status
- single-agent chemotherapy with docetaxel or pemetrexed has similar response rate, the latter with less toxicity

- some evidence that selection of first-line chemotherapy may be rationalized according to histological subtype of NSCLC, e.g. cisplatin + pemetrexed particularly effective in large-cell carcinoma
- targeted therapies have been demonstrated to be of benefit both as single agents, e.g. second- or third-line therapy, and in combination with first-line doublet chemotherapy
- **EGFR-targeted therapies**:
  - oral tyrosine kinase inhibitors, e.g. erlotinib or gefitinib
  - appear to be most active in adenocarcinomas, non-smokers, females, Japanese, EGFR mutations
- **VEGFR-targeted therapies**:
  - bevacizumab licensed for use in combination with platinum doublet chemotherapy as first-line treatment for advanced disease
  - tyrosine kinase inhibitors in trial.

Quality of life

Although cytotoxic regimens produce objective tumour response rates of the order of 20–50% in advanced NSCLC, symptom improvement can be achieved in a greater proportion of patients.

- Cough, haemoptysis, and pain are relieved in 70%.
- Anorexia in 40%.
- Dyspnoea in 30%.

Table 14.5 New single agents for NSCLC, results in stage IIIB–IV

Drug	Number of patients	1-year survival (%)	Median survival (weeks)	Response rate (%)
Vinorelbine	621	20	32.5	24
Gemcitabine	572	21	40.6	39
Paclitaxel	317	26	37.3	41
Docetaxel	300	26	41	52
Topotecan	119	13	38	35

Data from Bunn PA Jr, Kelly K (1998) New chemotherapeutic agents prolong survival and improve quality of life in non-small cell lung cancer: a review of the literature and future directions. *Clin Cancer Res* **4**, 1087–100.

Table 14.6 New platinum-based combination therapies for NSCLC

Drug combination	Number of patients	Response rate (weeks)	Median survival (%)	1-year survival (%)
Paclitaxel + C	333	46	38	40
Vinorelbine + P	328	41	38	35–40
Paclitaxel + P	286	42	42	36
Docetaxel + P	255	35	35	58
Gemcitabine + P	245	47	57	61
Topotecan + P	22	22	32	26

P = cisplatin; C = carboplatin.

Data from Bunn PA Jr, Kelly K (1998) New chemotherapeutic agents prolong survival and improve quality of life in non-small cell lung cancer: a review of the literature and future directions. *Clin Cancer Res* **5**, 1087–100.

Stage III disease

About 30% of NSCLC patients present with locally advanced disease but no evidence of metastases. This is a heterogeneous group, with an overall poor prognosis, but includes some patients who may have durable responses to appropriate radical therapy. In general, responses to chemotherapy are more frequent in localized compared with metastatic disease, but the benefits of chemotherapy are again limited to patients with good performance status.

The same cisplatin or carboplatin chemotherapy doublets are used with the following principles:

- response to chemotherapy should improve symptoms, reduce loco-regional disease prior to local therapy, and reduce microscopic metastatic disease
- platinum-based combination chemotherapy followed by radiotherapy gives better survival rates than radiotherapy alone (3-year survival 13–23 % versus 6%)
- a commonly used regimen for patients with performance status 0–1 is 4 cycles of a platinum-based doublet followed by radiotherapy to residual chest disease
- patients with progressive disease or serious toxicity on chemotherapy require prompt treatment with radiotherapy
- poor performance status patients may be treated with palliative radiotherapy only
- selection and co-ordination of appropriate therapy require close co-operation of medical and radiation oncologists within the multidisciplinary team.

Chemo-radiotherapy

Cisplatin, and some of the new drugs like gemcitabine and the taxanes, are potent radiosensitizers and there is increasing interest in concomitant delivery of chemotherapy and radiotherapy to take advantage of potential synergy. There is evidence that concurrent radiotherapy is more effective than sequential, but toxicity (in particular oesophagitis and pneumonitis) remains a problem, and an optimum chemotherapy regimen and fractionation schedule for radiotherapy is yet to be determined.

Surgery for locally advanced disease

Where stage III disease appears resectable by pneumonectomy (e.g. stage IIIA disease, where only ipsilateral mediastinal nodes are involved), surgery cures less than 10% of patients, because of a combination of unresected loco-regional disease and occult systemic disease. Chemotherapy improves survival over surgery alone by around 5% at 5 years. Several small studies have suggested a survival advantage for pre-operative chemotherapy (with or without radiotherapy) in stage III disease. Five-year survival rates up to 40% have been reported, but this has been achieved in small, selected groups of patients. Two recent randomized studies have shown significantly improved relapse-free and overall survival for patients given cisplatin-based treatment before and after surgery.

Overall, the data are not dissimilar from those seen with chemotherapy followed by radiotherapy in unresectable disease, and it is not clear if surgery has a role in this situation. On the other hand, only 5–15% of patients undergoing neo-adjuvant therapy have a pathological complete response at surgery, demonstrating the importance of further local treatment if cure is the aim. Large phase III trials of chemo-radiotherapy pre-surgery, and of chemotherapy followed by radiotherapy or surgery, are in progress to help clarify this issue.

Adjuvant chemotherapy

Thirty to forty per cent of patients with stage II NSCLC relapse after surgery only, with systemic metastatic disease. The meta-analysis of adjuvant chemotherapy trials in NSCLC showed a 5% improvement in 5-year survival for patients treated with a cisplatin-based regimen after surgical resection. This benefit held for patients across stages IB–IIIA. Recent results with platinum-based doublet chemotherapy (e.g. cisplatin vinorelbine or carboplatin paclitaxel) suggest particular benefit as adjuvant therapy after surgery for stage II–IIIA disease.

While neo-adjuvant strategies offer potential downstaging of disease, increasing the likelihood of a complete resection and theoretical reduction in risk of tumour dissemination at surgery, no studies have yet shown pre-operative chemotherapy to be superior to post-operative adjuvant therapy.

Conclusion

Chemotherapy for inoperable NSCLC now offers benefits similar to those obtained with chemotherapy in SCLC in terms of survival. Results of adjuvant treatment also suggest that a survival benefit comparable to that observed in breast and colorectal cancer can be achieved. Grounds for the previous nihilistic view of NSCLC chemotherapy are diminishing, but patients still need to be entered into clinical trials wherever possible in order to build on this progress.

Radiation therapy for NSCLC

External beam radiotherapy is used as the local treatment for thoracic disease in the majority of NSCLC patients, and local tumour control rates and duration correlate with the dose of radiotherapy given.

Radical radiotherapy

- Radical radiotherapy is indicated:
  - for patients with stage I–II NSCLC who are unfit for surgery
  - for stage IIIA and IIIB disease that can be encompassed in a feasible volume (determined by both the tumour volume and the pulmonary function of the patient) in patients with good performance status.
- Patients with inoperable NSCLC have a 20–30% chance of surviving 2 years after radical radiotherapy.
- The cost of radical treatment includes:
  - frequent hospital attendances
  - acute toxicities, e.g. lethargy, oesophagitis
  - late toxicities, e.g. lung fibrosis.
- Patient selection is crucial to minimize risk of prolonged side-effects in patients destined to die of systemic disease within 12 months of diagnosis.

Dose and fractionation

- Standard international dose is 60–66 Gy in 30–33 fractions over 6 weeks.
- Attempts to increase tumour dose by giving an increased number of fractions of size <2 Gy given over 6–7 weeks (hyperfractionation without acceleration) have not shown any benefit.
- However, the CHART regimen (Continuous Hyperfractionated Accelerated RadioTherapy) has shown significant benefits compared with conventional fractionation and is recommended for use in the UK:
  - 54 Gy in 36 fractions over 12 days
  - gave a 9% survival advantage at 2 years compared with 60 Gy in 30 fractions in a UK trial in stage I–III NSCLC
  - costs of this treatment included inconvenience for patients and staff, increased acute toxicity with grade 3 in 20%, but no increase in late toxicity
  - no trial has compared these regimes with shorter 3–4 week schedules (e.g. 50–55 Gy in 15–20 fractions), which remain popular in the UK
  - CHART is logistically difficult to deliver (treatment 8 am, 2 pm, 8 pm, including weekends) but is available in some UK centres
  - modification to exclude weekends, CHARTWEL, delivers 60 Gy in 40 fractions over 17 days
  - this regimen has shown promising results and can be delivered safely after chemotherapy.

Treatment volume

No randomized trials have examined what volume should be irradiated. The standard in most of the world has been the primary tumour and hilar and mediastinal lymph nodes, with a 1–2 cm margin. Retrospective comparisons have not demonstrated any advantage over volumes encompassing tumour and radiologically involved lymph nodes only. In dose escalation studies with conformal therapy, adjuvant nodal irradiation constrains the radiation dose delivered to the primary tumour. Omitting uninvolved nodal groups does not appear to increase local relapse rate.

Chemo-radiation

The Non-Small Cell Lung Cancer Collaborative Group Overview suggested a 2% increase in 5-year survival when cisplatin-based chemotherapy is added to radical radiotherapy. The Radiation Therapy Oncology Group (RTOG) 88–08 study reinforces these conclusions, with a 4-year survival advantage of 5% with combined therapy.

Chemotherapy delivered synchronously with radiotherapy has not yet been shown to increase survival in randomized trials, and certainly adds to toxicity. A recent review of the RTOG database reported a significant increase in morbidity in combined regimes. Over one-third of patients receiving chemotherapy and hyperfractionated radiotherapy experienced severe oesophagitis. Nonetheless, the promising results of phase II studies with this approach warrant further investigation, planned in the form of the SOCCAR (Sequential or Concurrent Chemotherapy and Radiotherapy) study in the UK.

Recent developments

- Long-term loco-regional control of NSCLC remains poor, even with intensive regimens e.g. CHART.
- High risk of systemic relapse in patients in whom long-term control of the loco-regional disease is achieved.
- The benefit of chemotherapy prior to CHART are being tested in the INCH (INduction chemotherapy and CHart) study.
- With improved 3D planning of radiotherapy using conventional (2Gy/ fraction/day) fractionation, dose escalation with conformal therapy may be safely achieved.
- Using normal tissue complication probabilities to estimate a 'safe' dose of radiotherapy, up to 92.4 Gy has been delivered to small volumes encompassing inoperable T1–T2N0 tumours with excellent control rates without significant morbidity.
- Hypofractionated high-dose radiotherapy (e.g. 66 Gy/24 fractions) shows promise in this setting:
  - short-course treatment less demanding on patients and treatment facilities
  - stereotactic radiotherapy, the logical extension of this approach, similarly shows promise for small inoperable tumours (e.g. 50 Gy/5 fractions).
- As local control of loco-regional disease improves, relapse with metastatic disease becomes an increasing problem, in particular brain metastases:
  - increasing use of FDG-PET scanning in patients receiving radical medical treatment may reduce the number of relapses from occult metastases
  - trials of prophylactic cranial irradiation are under way in patients receiving chemo-irradiation for stage III NSCLC.
- Increasing use of FDG-PET scanning may reduce the number of patients with occult metastatic disease receiving radical radiotherapy.

Post-operative radiotherapy

A meta-analysis of randomized trials of post-operative radiotherapy for completely resected NSCLC has shown impaired survival following irradiation in patients with N0 and N1 disease. There is evidence that radiotherapy affords an improvement in local control for patients with N2 disease. The best results have been reported with 50 Gy in 25 daily fractions.

Palliative radiotherapy

For many patients with advanced NSCLC, radiation therapy is a key component in alleviating symptoms from thoracic disease, in particular:
- haemoptysis
- chest pain
- cough
- large airway obstruction or stridor
- superior vena cava (SVC) obstruction.

Radiotherapy can also improve systemic symptoms such as anorexia and weight loss, and produces useful palliation for many metastatic sites including lymph nodes, bone, brain, and soft tissue.

In the UK, Medical Research Council (MRC) trials have shown equivalent survival and symptom control for 1-, 2-, and 10-fraction regimes, establishing the shorter courses as the treatment of choice for symptom control in advanced NSCLC, particularly in patients with poor performance status. However, these short schedules are associated with chest pain and flu-like symptoms in up to 40% of patients. A transient reduction in peak expiratory flow rates may occur. Most patients receiving the two-fraction regimen suffer at least moderate but short-lived oesophagitis.

Another MRC trial has shown that higher-dose palliative therapy (39 Gy in 13 daily fractions) offers a modest survival advantage for good performance status patients with locally advanced NSCLC, compared with 2 fractions, but at the cost of greater toxicity in particular oesophagitis. The selection of an appropriate radiotherapy regimen requires individual assessment.

Outcomes of radiotherapy treatment

The key prognostic factors are the TNM staging and the patient's performance status. When these are controlled for, treatment-related factors such as chemotherapy and radiotherapy dose can provide modest survival benefits.

Radical radiotherapy
- Stage I–II, 20–30% 5-year survival
- Stage III, chemotherapy plus radiotherapy, 25% 2-year survival, 15% 5-year survival

Palliative radiotherapy
- Median survival in MRC trials of short course radiotherapy 6 months; 4 months in poor-performance patients
- After high-dose palliative radiotherapy (39 Gy/13 fractions) median survival 9 months, 36% 1-year survival, 12% 2-year survival

Small-cell lung cancer (SCLC)

Introduction
- SCLC accounts for 15–20% of all lung cancers.
- Staging and management are quite distinct from NSCLC because:
  - almost all SCLCs demonstrate rapid growth and early dissemination
  - >90% have systemic disease at presentation
  - surgery is inappropriate in the vast majority – less than 10% are operable
  - chemotherapy is the key primary treatment and has an important impact on survival.

Staging and prognostic factors
A much simplified staging system is used for SCLC, as the vast majority of patients are initially treated with chemotherapy irrespective of disease extent. A two-stage system was drawn up by the Veterans Administration Lung Group:
- **limited-stage disease:** tumour confined to one hemithorax and regional lymph nodes, and can be covered by tolerable radiotherapy fields
- **extensive-stage disease**: disease beyond these bounds.

Within these broad categories, subgroups may be defined according to one or more of the following prognostic factors.
- performance status
- sex (females have better prognosis)
- lactate dehydrogenase (LDH)
- alkaline phosphatase
- Serum Na$^+$ (hyponatraemia carries a poor prognosis).

Chemotherapy for SCLC

Prior to the introduction of systemic treatment with chemotherapy in the 1970s, the outlook for patients diagnosed with this disease was dreadful, with a median survival of 6 weeks for patients with extensive disease and 3 months for those with limited disease. Combination chemotherapy leads to objective response in the majority, with improved survival times, and is now the standard primary treatment for both stages of disease.

Principles of treatment

- Etoposide plus cisplatin or carboplatin (EP or EC) has been established as best first-line treatment (see Table 14.7).
- These regimens have demonstrated superior response rates and tolerability compared with older anthracycline regimens, e.g. cyclophosphamide, doxorubicin, vincristine (CAV).
- Etoposide platinum chemotherapy is compatible with concomitant thoracic irradiation.
- Standard chemotherapy treatment comprises 4 cycles of EP or EC.
- No benefit from maintenance treatment or increased dose intensification or high-dose chemotherapy.
- Disease is reassessed by chest X-ray each cycle and by CT scan at the end of chemotherapy.
- During chemotherapy, particular risks are:
  - neutropenic sepsis. Prophylactic broad-spectrum antibiotics, e.g. ciprofloxacin, reduce the risk of serious infection. Greatest risk in poor-performance status patients
  - deep vein thrombosis (DVT) and thromboembolic disease.
- Objective response rate 80% all patients:
  - complete responses in 30–40% patients with limited-stage disease, 10–20% with extensive disease.
- Despite this, almost all patients relapse after chemotherapy only.
- Consolidation radiotherapy to the chest can prevent this in some patients, particularly those with limited disease and complete response to chemotherapy.
- High risk of central nervous system (CNS) relapse after chemotherapy, and this can be reduced by prophylactic cranial irradiation.

Specific problems of SCLC

- Poor performance status:
  - unlike NSCLC, patients with performance status 2–3 may benefit from chemotherapy, if previously fit and deterioration is due to recent rapid tumour progression.
- SVC obstruction is relatively common with locally advanced right-sided central tumours/mediastinal lymphadenopathy:
  - initial treatment with chemotherapy is appropriate for most and leads to prompt resolution of SVC obstruction in the majority.
- Paraneoplastic syndromes are not uncommon:
  - e.g. secretion of inappropriate antidiuretic hormone (SIADH), ectopic adrenocorticotrophic hormone (ACTH), neuromuscular syndromes.

Table 14.7 Commonly used combination regimens in SCLC

EP	Etoposide	100 mg/m² IV days 1–3 q 3 weeks
	Cisplatin	60–80 mg/m² IV day 1 q 3 weeks
CAE	Etoposide	50 mg/m² IV days 1–5 q 3 weeks
	Doxorubicin	45 mg/m² IV day 1 q 3 weeks
	Cyclophosphamide	1000 mg/m² IV day 1 q 3 weeks
CAV	Cyclophosphamide	1000 mg/m² IV day 1 q 3 weeks
	Doxorubicin	50 mg/m² IV day 1 q 3 weeks
	Vincristine	2 mg/m² IV day 1 q 3 weeks

- Elderly patients:
  - 25% of patients with SCLC are >70 years
  - there is good evidence to support the use of primary chemotherapy in these patients if there are no other contraindications to treatment.
- CNS disease at presentation. Chemotherapy may be given as initial treatment in fit patients or after initial cranial radiotherapy.
- Surgery:
  - in general, resection is not recommended for SCLC
  - rarely, patients present following resection of a small peripheral tumour, without evidence of regional lymphadenopathy or metastasis
  - if SCLC is treated by primary surgery, systemic relapse rate is high, and adjuvant chemotherapy with four cycles of EP or EC is recommended.

Second-line chemotherapy

This cancer can remain chemosensitive at relapse after primary chemotherapy ± radiotherapy. Treatment options with response rates of around 20% include:
- CAV
- topotecan
- taxanes.

Despite the chemosensitivity of this disease, only limited progress has been made with regard to long-term survival after relapse (see Table 14.8). Currently, clinical trials are evaluating the potential benefits of, e.g.:
- drugs that interfere with autocrine growth-factor loops and signal transduction pathways
- angiogenesis inhibitors
- tumour vaccines.

Table 14.8 Outcome of chemotherapy for SCLC

Stage of disease	Median survival (months)	1-year survival	3-year survival
Limited	18–24	50–70%	20–30%
Extensive	8–10	20%	
Relapsed[a]	6		

[a] Limited to patients who remain fit to receive chemotherapy for relapsed disease.

Radiotherapy for SCLC

Background

- The primary treatment for most patients with SCLC is combination chemotherapy:
  - more than 90% have systemic disease (either overt or microscopic) at presentation
  - highly chemosensitive disease.
- However, many patients with SCLC benefit from radiotherapy:
  - highly radiosensitive disease
  - post-chemotherapy irradiation of the thorax (TI) improves the relapse-free and overall survival of patients with localized disease
  - palliative radiotherapy is effective treatment in patients relapsing after, resistant to, unfit for, or refusing chemotherapy.

Thoracic irradiation

- 60% of relapses after chemotherapy are in the thorax.
- TI reduces risk of loco-regional recurrence by 50% and improves survival by 5% at 3 years in limited stage disease.
- The optimum schedule remains uncertain (see Table 14.9).
- Conventionally, treatment is restricted to patients with limited-stage disease who have a complete response or good partial response to chemotherapy.
- The target volume includes all sites of disease at presentation.
- Mediastinal lymph nodes traditionally were irradiated even if of normal size because of the high risk of microscopic involvement.
- Recently, the best results reported have been with radiotherapy delivered early, and concurrently, with chemotherapy.
- Concurrent chemo-irradiation poses certain problems:
  - no way of restricting treatment to chemotherapy responders
  - increased toxicity, in particular, oesophagitis, which may require nasogastric tube feeding
  - patient selection is essential so that only patients with a realistic chance of long-term survival are exposed to this treatment.

Prophylactic cranial irradiation (PCI)

- SCLC has a high propensity for brain metastases:
  - 20% have brain involvement at diagnosis
  - 80% have brain involvement at death.
- The blood–brain barrier limits access of chemotherapy to the CNS, which is a so-called 'sanctuary site'.
- The outlook for CNS disease is very poor:
  - only 50% achieve palliation with treatment with chemotherapy or radiotherapy
  - median survival is only 3 months.
- Because of these risks and the radiosensitivity of SCLC, prophylactic cranial radiotherapy has been evaluated since the 1980s.
- Low-dose PCI halves the risk of brain metastases in patients in complete remission after chemotherapy, with a 5% improvement in 3-year survival.

- PCI is recommended in patients for whom thoracic irradiation is appropriate, but is given at the end of chemotherapy in an effort to minimize CNS toxicity.
- The optimum treatment regimen is uncertain.
- Examples include 25–30 Gy/10 fractions, 36 Gy/18 fractions.
- Following PCI, 30% of patients complain of somnolence 2–3 months after treatment, which is self-limiting.

Palliative radiotherapy

- A short course of irradiation to either the primary tumour or metastases can provide useful symptom control even in frail patients.
- The choice of dose and radiation schedule is similar to that used in NSCLC using the lowest effective dose and number of fractions.
- In most situations, a single fraction or up to 5 fractions of treatment is appropriate and effective.

Table 14.9 Thoracic irradiation – examples of treatment regimens

Timing of radiotherapy	Dose (Gy)	Number of fractions	Fractions/ day
Post-chemotherapy	50	25	1
	40–45	15	1
Concomitant with cycles 1 or 2 chemotherapy	45	30	2
	50	25	1

Recent advances in SCLC management

- PCI has now been shown to provide benefit in patients with both limited- and extensive-stage disease.
- Dose escalation is being explored for TI with 3D conformal radiotherapy limited to the primary tumour and lymph nodes >1 cm at presentation.
- TI may also have benefits following chemotherapy for extensive-stage disease.

Further reading on lung cancer

British Thoracic Society (2001) British Thoracic Society guidelines on the selection of patients with lung cancer for surgery. *Thorax* **56**, 89–108.
Clinical Oncology Information Network (COIN) guidelines on the non-surgical management of lung cancer http://www.rcr.ac.uk/index.asp?PageID=667 (accessed 27 June 2009).
Herbst RS, Heymach JV, Lippman SM (2008) Lung cancer. *New Engl J Med* **359**, 1367–80.
Non-small Cell Lung Cancer Collaborative Group (1995) Chemotherapy in non-small cell lung cancer: a meta-analysis using updated data on individual patients from 52 randomised clinical trials. *BMJ* **311**, 899–909.
Scottish Intercollegiate Guidelines Network (SIGN) (2005) *SIGN guidelines no 80. Management of patients with lung cancer.* http://www.sign.ac.uk/pdf/qrg80.pdf (accessed 26 June 2009).
Simon GR, Wagner H (2003) Lung cancer guidelines: small cell lung cancer. *Chest* **123**, 2595–715.

Mesothelioma

Malignant pleural mesothelioma (MPM) is an aggressive tumour arising from the serosal lining of the chest and characterized by poor survival rates.

Epidemiology

- Rare, around 2200 cases each year in the UK
- Incidence expected to rise to 2500 in the next decade and fall thereafter
- Peak age 60–70 years
- Male: female ratio 5:1.

Aetiology

- Caused by asbestos exposure in the vast majority.
- 90% have an occupational history of exposure; high risk in, e.g., builders, shipyard workers.
- Non-occupational exposure leads to increased risk in the partners of these at-risk workers, e.g. washing their overalls.
- All types of asbestos fibre are implicated.
- Prolonged latent period after exposure, so that clinical presentation is often 30–40 years later.
- Rarely caused by other agents:
  - erionite fibres (Turkey);
  - thorium dioxide.

Prevention

Recognition of the hazards of asbestos and improved protection of workers at risk should result in a falling incidence of mesothelioma after 2020.

Pathology

- Mesothelioma arises from the parietal or visceral pleural and grows diffusely within the pleural space, commonly associated with pleural effusion, and often leads to encasement of the lung by solid tumour.
- Tumour invades directly into lung and mediastinum, and may cross the diaphragm to involve peritoneum.
- Metastatic spread to other organs, e.g. liver in advanced disease.
- Malignant mesothelioma has 3 distinct histological subtypes:
  - epithelial (around 50%)
  - sarcomatous
  - mixed.
- Malignant tumours may be localized or diffuse and are more commonly associated with asbestos exposure and symptoms such as chest pain and dyspnoea.
- Differentiation from other intrathoracic malignancies such as pulmonary adenocarcinoma or metastatic pleural disease requires the assistance of an experienced pathologist.
- Primary mesothelioma of the peritoneum is rare, associated with heavy exposure and ingestion of asbestos.

Clinical presentation

Late presentation is common, with only insidious development of the classic symptoms:

- non-pleuritic chest pain
- dyspnoea

- systemic symptoms of fatigue, weight loss, sweating, and fever.

Physical examination frequently demonstrates finger clubbing and signs of pleural effusion or solid pleural tumour. Signs of advanced disease may include:

- palpable chest wall mass
- hoarse voice, vocal cord palsy
- SVC obstruction
- Horner's syndrome
- ascites due to extension of tumour into peritoneum.

Occasionally early disease, which is asymptomatic, is picked up on chest X-ray for another cause.

Investigations

- Laboratory results in mesothelioma are usually unremarkable.
- No serological tumour marker reproducibly identified.
- Radiological appearances are often non-specific:
  - pleural effusion/thickening on chest X-ray
  - 20% have associated pulmonary fibrosis (asbestosis)
  - CT scan demonstrates extent of pleural mass and effusion, and encasement of lung
  - MRI provides superior definition of tissue planes, e.g. in mediastinal or transdiaphragmatic extension.
- Histological diagnosis should be obtained in the majority of cases, using the least invasive technique:
  - aspiration cytology (30% positive)
  - blind biopsy
  - ultrasound or CT-guided biopsy
  - thoracoscopy and biopsy (80% positive)
  - each of these procedures carries a risk of implantation of tumour in the chest wall.

Staging

The TNM classification (Table 14.10) is not commonly used, but staging is vital if patients are considered for surgery. The Brigham staging system (Table 14.11) provides an alternative straightforward method, based on key disease characteristics, that stratifies survival.

Accurate pre-operative pathological staging is best achieved by thoracoscopy for pleural evaluation, mediastinoscopy for mediastinal nodal involvement, and laparoscopy to rule out peritoneal seeding or diaphragmatic involvement when indicated.

Management

Without treatment, the average patient with MPM survives less than 1 year from the time of diagnosis. Patient selection is crucial for the appropriate use of treatment such as surgery and chemotherapy, and all patients should be discussed at a thoracic multidisciplinary meeting.

Surgery

- For the vast majority of patients, the extent and spread of disease at presentation precludes complete surgical removal of the disease.
- Perhaps 5% of patients present with localized disease for which radical surgery with extrapleural pneumonectomy (EPP) may be followed by prolonged survival – in the rare patient where this is possible, 46%

5-year survival is reported, if margins are negative for tumour, but overall long-term results are poor – median survival 9.4 months.
- The mortality of EPP has fallen from 31% in 1970 to 3.8% in specialized centres in 2000.
- Pleurectomy and decortication control effusions in 80% if patient is fit. Thoracoscopy is useful in obtaining tissue for diagnosis and for pleurodesis.

Pleurodesis

Talc pleurodesis is effective in many patients in delaying the reaccumulation of the pleural effusion.

Radiotherapy

- Early irradiation of chest drain/biopsy/thoracoscopy wounds prevents the development of chest wall tumours (e.g. 21 Gy/3 fractions).
- Short-course palliative radiotherapy for painful chest disease/masses.

Chemotherapy

- Objective responses in 10–20% patients with advanced disease treated with, e.g. cisplatin, carboplatin, ifosfamide, mitomycin.
- Improved results are reported with the anti-folate pemetrexed in combination with cisplatin or carboplatin (response rate 20–40%), with median survival of 12 months.

Palliative care

Symptom control is often difficult, in particular, pain and dyspnoea, and early involvement of specialist palliative care services may be beneficial.

Compensation and notification

Patients may be entitled to claim compensation in two ways:
- a claim for Industrial Injuries Disablement Benefit from the Department of Social Security (via the Benefits Agency)
- a common law claim for damages from the firm/firms where exposure to asbestos occurred.

All deaths of patients with mesothelioma must be notified to the coroner (procurator fiscal in Scotland).

Table 14.10 TNM staging system for malignant pleural mesothelioma

Stage	Description
T1	Ipsilateral parietal pleural
T2	Ipsilateral lung, diaphragm, confluent involvement of visceral pleura
T3	Endothoracic fascia, mediastinal fat, focal chest wall, non-transmural pericardium
T4	Contralateral pleura, peritoneum, rib, extensive chest wall or mediastinal invasion, myocardium, brachial plexus, spine, malignant pericardial effusion
N1	Ipsilateral bronchopulmonary or hilar nodes
N2	Subcarinal, ipsilateral mediastinal nodes
N3	Contralateral mediastinal or ipsilateral/contralateral neck nodes
M1	Distant metastasis

Table 14.11 Brigham staging system for malignant pleural mesothelioma

Stage	Description
I	Disease completely resected within the capsule of the parietal pleura without adenopathy; ipsilateral pleura, lung, pericardium, diaphragm, or chest wall disease limited to previous biopsy sites
II	All of stage I with positive resection margins and/or intrapleural adenopathy
III	Local extension of disease into the chest wall or mediastinum, heart, or through diaphragm into peritoneum; or with extrapleural lymph node involvement
IV	Distant metastatic disease

Treatment outcome

- Overall median survival is poor, 8–14 months.
- Better prognosis with epithelioid pathology.
- Single-centre results from Boston USA, in carefully selected patients undergoing radical surgery followed by chemotherapy and radiotherapy, are better, particularly in patients in whom early disease is excised with clear pathological margins:
  - median survival 17 months
  - 2-year survival 36%
  - 5-year survival 14%.

Further reading

British Thoracic Society (2001) BTS statement on malignant mesothelioma in the United Kingdom. *Thorax* **56**, 250–65.

Pistolesi M, Rusthoven J (2004) Malignant pleural mesothelioma. *Chest* **126**, 1318–20.

Robinson BWS, Musk AW, Lake RA (2005) Malignant mesothelioma. *Lancet* **336**, 379–408.

Sterman DH, Albelda SM (2005) Advances in the diagnosis, evaluation and management of malignant pleural mesothelioma. *Respirology* **10**, 266–283.

Sugarbaker DJ, Garcia JP (1997) Multimodality therapy for malignant pleural mesothelioma. *Chest* **112(Suppl)**, 272S–275S.

Sugarbaker DJ, Flores RM, Jaklitsch MT, *et al.* (1999) Resection margins, extrapleural nodal status and cell type determine postoperative long-term survival in trimodality therapy of malignant pleural mesothelioma – results in 183 patients. *J Thorac Cardiovasc Surg* **117**, 54–63.

Thymic tumours

Tumours derived from the thymus (thymomas) comprise approximately 20% of all mediastinal tumours and are the most common tumour in the anterior mediastinum (less common pathologies include lymphoma and teratoma).

Epidemiology

Thymomas occur at any age but are rare before the age of 20 and peak between 40 and 60 years, with similar frequency in both sexes. The incidence varies somewhat in different countries, more frequent in the Far East. The average in Europe is around 0.5 new cases per year per 100 000.

Aetiology

Cause is unknown.

Pathology

Most thymomas are slow-growing 'low-grade' malignant tumours. It is believed that they derive from epithelial elements, but the tumours retain the capacity for production of T-cells. The T-cells are generally of normal phenotype.

According to the relative abundance of epithelial and lymphocytic cells, histological subgroups have been described:

- epithelial
- lymphocytic
- mixed.

These cellular characteristics have no clear influence on prognosis. In contrast, the gross appearance of the resected tumour is related to clinical prognosis. The presence or absence of an intact capsule is of key importance, and local invasion remains the most consistent factor in predicting outcome.

The following classification is of practical benefit:

- encapsulated thymoma – benign cytology and biological behaviour (50%)
- invasive thymoma – benign cytology but capable of local invasion and, rarely, distant metastasis (40%)
- thymic carcinoma (10%) – demonstrates cytological and biological features of cancer.

However, recurrent disease can occur after complete excision of a histologically bland thymoma. Metastatic spread can involve pleura, lung, lymph nodes, and other viscera.

Clinical presentation

- 30% diagnosed with an asymptomatic mediastinal mass.
- 40% have local symptoms, e.g. chest pain, cough, dyspnoea, SVC obstruction.
- 30% have paraneoplastic syndromes, most associated with an immunological phenomenon.

- Myasthenia gravis is the commonest paraneoplastic effect; occurs in 15–25% of patients with thymoma:
  - antibodies target acetylcholine receptor
  - 10–25% of patients with myasthenia have a thymoma.
- Red-cell aplasia occurs in 5% of thymomas:
  - in 30%, low platelets or low white-cell count also
  - 30–50% of patients with red-cell aplasia have a thymoma.
- Hypogammaglobulinaemia occurs in 5–10% of thymomas.

Investigations
- Imaging by CT or MRI is essential to stage and plan therapy.
- No specific tumour markers.
- CT-guided core biopsy preferred to FNA cytology.

Management and staging
- 90% present with localized disease for which surgery is the preferred treatment.
- Thymectomy performed through a median sternotomy although bilateral anterolateral thoracotomy, with transverse sternotomy (clam shell approach), is better for advanced tumours.
- Modern surgical techniques allow complete resection of invasive thymomas, e.g. including lung resection, SVC removal and reconstruction, but debulking alone is of little benefit.
- Video-assisted thorascopic approaches are increasingly used.
- Complete resection gives 85% 5-year survival.
- Operative mortality is now less than 2%.
- Staging of disease is based on the surgical findings and radiology:
  - I – tumour confined within intact capsule
  - II – pericapsular growth into the mediastinal fat tissue
  - III – invasive growth into the surrounding organs
  - IV – disseminated disease.
- In stage I disease, adjuvant treatment is not recommended.
- Post-operative radiotherapy is recommended for stages II and III, particularly where excision has been incomplete, and for local recurrence of thymoma:
  - 50–60 Gy in 20–30 fractions.

Chemotherapy
- Malignant thymoma is chemosensitive, with objective response rates in advanced disease 40–60%.
- Most regimens include an anthracycline and cisplatin, e.g. CAP (cyclophosphamide, doxorubicin, and cisplatin).
- Indications for chemotherapy include:
  - metastatic disease
  - bulky recurrent disease
  - recurrence post-radiotherapy
  - pre-operative treatment of locally advanced disease.

Treatment outcomes

- Overall survival rates are good (see Table 14.12).
- Patients with autoimmune disorders such as myasthenia are diagnosed with relatively small tumours.
- However, thymectomy leads to remission in paraneoplastic syndromes in only 30–50%.
- Patients with persistent symptoms, e.g. myasthenia, require ongoing medical treatment with anti-cholinesterases and/or immuno-suppressants.

Table 14.12 Treatment outcomes for thymoma

Stage of disease	Recurrence rate	10-year survival
I	4%	88%
II	14%	70%
III	26%	57%
IV	46%	38%

Further reading

Lee HS, Kim ST, Lee J (2007) A single institutional experience of thymic epithelial tumours over 11 years: clinical features and outcome and implications for future management. *Brit J Cancer* **97**, 22–28.

Lequaghe C, Grudice G, Massone PPB (2002). Clinical and pathologic predictors of survival in patients with thymic tumours. *J Cardiovasc Surg* **43**, 269–74.

Sperling B, Marschall J, Kennedy K (2003). Thymoma: a review of the clinical and pathological findings in 65 cases. *Can J Surg* **46**, 37–42.

Breast cancer

Introduction

Much effort has been invested in this, the most common solid tumour occurring in women. The study of breast cancer has rewarded us with lessons in the application of many aspects of oncology including:

- population screening
- organ conservation
- medical genetics
- adjuvant therapy
- meta-analyses
- clinical guidelines.

The benefits of this industry are now visible, with a significant fall in breast cancer deaths over the last decade.

Epidemiology

Key facts about breast cancer
- Commonest female cancer in Europe (200 000 cases per year)
- 20% of all malignancies
- Incidence is increasing by 1% per year
- Rate of increase is increasing especially in low-risk populations
- Lifetime risk in UK is 1 in 9 women
- Risk of breast cancer correlates with income per capita
- Mortality in Western Europe and USA, 15–25 per 150 000 women
- In UK 41 000 new breast cancers diagnosed per year
- Currently 13 000 breast cancer deaths per year
- Breast cancer mortality rate in UK is one of the highest in world
- However, since the 1980s, UK breast cancer mortality has fallen by about 20%, in response to improvements in diagnosis and treatment
- Male breast cancer is rare: 300 cases per annum in UK.

Aetiology
Several risk factors have been identified by epidemiological studies.

Age
- Breast cancer is very rare before the age of 20 years and rare below 30 years.
- Incidence of breast cancer doubles every 10 years until the menopause.
- After 50 years, the rate of increase slows and in some countries plateaus.

Geography
- 7-fold variation in incidence between high- and low-risk countries.
- Low rates in the Far East.
- Migrants from low-incidence countries assume the risk in the host country within two generations.

Age at menarche and menopause
- Early menarche and late menopause increase the risk.
- Ovarian ablation before 35 years reduces the risk of breast cancer by 60%.
- Menopause after the age of 55 years doubles the risk.

Age at first pregnancy
- Nulliparity and late age at first pregnancy increase the risk.
- A woman whose first pregnancy is at 30 years has double the risk of breast cancer compared with first pregnancy at <20 years.

Family history
- Genetic predisposition accounts for around 10% of female breast cancers, and 20% of male.

Exogenous oestrogens
- Use of oral contraceptives for >4 years before first pregnancy increases the risk of pre-menopausal breast cancer.
- The use of unopposed oestrogens in hormone replacement therapy (HRT) for 10–15 years is associated with an increase in breast cancer.
- Combined HRT preparations also increase the risk, but the magnitude of effect is uncertain.
- Prenatal exposure to diethylstilboestrol increases the risk in women over 40 years of age.

Diet
- Associations have been shown with high dietary fat intake, obesity, and alcohol consumption.

Benign breast disease
- Previous breast surgery for severe atypical epithelial hyperplasia is associated with a four-fold increase in risk.

Radiation
- Exposure to ionizing radiation at an early age, e.g. treatment of Hodgkin's disease.
- Mammographic screening is associated with a decrease in breast cancer deaths but the effects of screening younger women (less than 50 years) are uncertain.

Male breast cancer
- Peak incidence 10 years later than in women.
- It may occur in association with Klinefelter's syndrome.

Genetics of breast cancer

- 5–10% of female breast cancer is due to inheritance of a mutated copy of either *BRCA1* or *BRCA2*.
- Women who inherit a mutated copy of either gene have an elevated lifetime risk of breast cancer – up to 87% by the age of 70 years.
- Particular risk of pre-menopausal breast cancer, often before the age of 40 years.
- Associated risk of ovarian cancer (greater with *BRCA1*).
- Male carriers are at risk of prostate cancer and, for *BRCA2* carriers, breast cancer.
- Some ethnic groups are at particular risk for carriage of these mutations (estimated 2% of US Ashkenazi Jews).
- Other genes contribute less often to familial breast cancer:
  - hypothesized that ataxia–telangiectasia heterozygotes are at risk, but this is as yet unproven
  - risk associated with mutation in *PTEN* (Cowden disease), *MSH1* or *MSH2* (hereditary non-polyposis colorectal cancer (HNPCC)), and p53 (Li–Fraumeni syndrome).

The management of hereditary breast cancer is essentially that of non-hereditary disease. Less clear is how to manage asymptomatic female members of these families and the contralateral breast of the index cases. Published guidelines define groups of women at moderate and high risk, recommending referral to medical genetic clinics for the latter group for counselling, advice on risks, consideration of testing for mutations of *BRCA1* and *BRCA2*, and referral for appropriate further management. Women at moderate risk are offered annual mammography and review in a breast clinic between ages 40 and 50 years.

Currently, the following options are open to women at moderate and high risk.

Prophylactic surgery

- Bilateral subcutaneous mastectomy (usually with immediate reconstruction) reduces the incidence of breast cancer in these women but its impact on survival is uncertain. This reduces the risk of breast cancer by 95% (not 100%).
- May be offered in conjunction with prophylactic oophorectomy.

Screening

- Magnetic resonance imaging (MRI) has been shown to be superior to mammography in women under 50 years at high risk of breast cancer because of their family history.
- Annual MRI of both breasts recommended for:
  - carriers of mutated *BRCA1* or *BRCA2* aged 30–50 years
  - carriers of mutated *p53* aged greater than 20 years
  - women with a 10-year risk of breast cancer >8% from age 30–39 years
  - women with a 10-year risk of breast cancer >20% from 40–49 years.

Breast cancer-prevention trials
- Four clinical trials of tamoxifen have demonstrated that this drug reduces the incidence of oestrogen receptor-positive breast cancer by about 50%.
- As yet there is no evidence that it reduces breast cancer mortality in women with a family history of breast cancer, and it is not recommended for routine use in the UK.

Risk assessment for women with a family history of breast cancer (examples)

- Women at population risk: <3% develop breast cancer aged 40–50 years, <17% lifetime risk:
  - only one first- or second- degree relative with breast cancer diagnosed ages <40 years
  - and no family history of bilateral breast cancer, ovarian cancer, male breast cancer
- Women at moderate risk: 3–8% develop breast cancer aged 40–50 years, 17–30% lifetime risk:
  - only one first-degree relative with breast cancer diagnoses <40 years
  - or one first-degree relative with male breast cancer
  - or one first-degree relative with bilateral breast cancer diagnosed <50 years
  - or two first-degree relatives with breast cancer at any age
  - or one first- or second-degree relative with breast cancer at any age and one first- or second-degree relative with ovarian cancer
  - or three first- or second-degree relatives with breast cancer at any age
- Women at high risk: >8% develop breast cancer aged 40–50, 30% lifetime risk
  - two first-degree relatives with breast cancer diagnosed aged <50 years
  - or three first- or second- degree relatives with breast cancer aged <60 years
  - or four first- or second-degree relatives with breast cancer at any age
  - or one relative with ovarian cancer and a first- or second-degree relative on the same side with breast cancer aged <50 years
  - or two relatives with ovarian cancer
  - or one relative with bilateral breast cancer aged <50 years

Further reading

National Institute for Health and Clinical Excellence (NICE) (2006) Clinical Guideline 41. Familial Breast Cancer: classification and care of women at risk of familial breast cancer in primary, secondary, and tertiary care. London: NICE.

Ore S (2008) Who should have breast magnetic resonance imaging evaluation? *J Clin Oncol* **26**, 703–11.

Turner NC, Jones AL (2008) Management of breast cancer. *BMJ* **337**, 107–10.

Pathology

- Breast cancer is more common in the left breast.
- Around 50% arise in the upper outer quadrant.
- Commonest pathology is ductal carcinoma.

Ductal carcinoma *in situ* (DCIS)

- 90% of breast carcinomas arise in the ducts of the breast.
- Begin as atypical proliferation of ductal epithelium that eventually fills and plugs the ducts with neoplastic cells.
- As long as the tumour remains within the confines of the ductal basement membrane, it is classified as DCIS.
- Localized DCIS is impalpable but often visible on mammography as an area of microcalcification.
- Not all DCIS will inevitably progress, but the probability of development of invasive cancer is estimated at 30–50%.

Lobular carcinoma *in situ*

- These pre-invasive lesions carry a risk not only of ipsilateral invasive lobular carcinoma but also of contralateral breast cancer.
- Typically are neither palpable nor contain microcalcification.

Invasive ductal carcinoma

- This accounts for 75% of breast cancers.
- The malignant cells are associated with a fibrous stroma that can be dense (scirrhous carcinoma).
- Tumour invades through breast tissue into the lymphatics and vascular spaces, to gain access to the regional nodes (axillary and, less often, internal mammary) and the systemic circulation.
- Systemic spread can involve almost any organ, but most commonly bone, lung or pleura, liver, skin, and CNS.
- The histological grade (I–III) of the tumour is assessed from three features and predicts tumour behaviour. The features are:
  - tubule formation
  - nuclear pleomorphism
  - mitotic frequency.
- Oestrogen and progesterone receptor status is commonly assessed by immunocytochemistry.
- Other biological markers (e.g. HER2) are of value both as a predictor of prognosis and as a guide to therapy, assessed by immunocytochemistry or fluorescence *in situ* hybridization (FISH).

Oestrogen receptor-positive breast cancer

- 60–70% of breast cancers express the nuclear oestrogen receptor (ER).
- This conveys a better prognosis compared with ER-negative tumours, which have a higher risk of spread to lymph nodes and distant sites at presentation.

HER2-positive breast cancer

- Amplification of the growth factor receptor gene *HER2* occurs in 25–30% of breast cancers.

- Associated with aggressive behaviour, high risk of lymph node involvement, and haematogenous spread.

Triple negative breast cancer
- These tumours do not express ER, progesterone receptor (PR), or HER2.
- Account for 15% of breast cancers.
- More common in premenopausal women and in association with *BRCA1*.
- Most express epidermal growth factor receptor (EGFR).
- Paradoxical high risk of early relapse but relative sensitivity to chemotherapy.

Ductal carcinoma of special type

A number of pathological variants are identified with relatively good prognosis, namely medullary carcinoma, tubular carcinoma, and mucinous carcinoma. Paget's disease of the breast is ductal carcinoma of the ducts with involvement of the skin of the nipple and areola. All have an underlying invasive ductal carcinoma.

Invasive lobular carcinoma

Lobular carcinomas account for 5–10% of breast cancers. About 20% develop contralateral breast cancer. Unusual patterns of spread are recognized, including propensity for spread to the peritoneum, meninges, ovaries, and uterus.

Table 15.1 Histological types of breast malignancy

- Invasive ductal carcinoma
  - no special type
  - combined with other type
  - medullary carcinoma
  - mucinous carcinoma
  - Paget's disease

- Invasive lobular carcinoma

- Mixed lobular and ductal carcinoma

- Sarcoma (various)

- Lymphoma

- Metastases (e.g. breast cancer, small-cell lung cancer)

Prognostic factors

Survival after a diagnosis of breast cancer is dependent upon:
- eradication of the primary tumour
- eradication of any loco-regional disease, particularly involved axillary, internal mammary, or supraclavicular fossa lymph nodes
- successful treatment of any systemic micrometastases.

Currently macroscopic metastatic disease is incurable but is often compatible with several years of good quality life especially if the disease is confined to bone.

The most important independent prognostic factors are:
- tumour size
- number of histologically positive axillary lymph nodes
- tumour grade
- these are commonly combined in the Nottingham Prognostic Index (NPI).

Other prognostic factors include:
- hormone receptor status (oestrogen and progesterone receptors)
- HER2neu overexpression
- histological subtype
- lymphovascular invasion
- proliferative index.

Nottingham prognostic Index (NPI) calculation

NPI = (0.2 × pathological tumour size (cm) + grade (1–3) + axillary node score)

Axillary node status	Score
No lymph nodes positive	1
1–3 lymph nodes positive	2
>3 lymph nodes positive	3

NPI	Prognosis
<3.41	Good
3.41–5.4	Intermediate
>5.4	Poor

Gene expression profiling

Three gene expression-based prognostic cancer tests are licensed for the prediction of prognosis and treatment benefit for women with early-stage breast cancer. Two use real-time reverse transcriptase polymerase chain reaction (RT-PCR) to examine gene profiles of 21 and 70 genes; the third uses DNA microarray technology to evaluate two genes. All require pathological review of specimens to check tumour content and evaluate RNA quality. Such approaches should pave the way to the individualization of therapy for women with breast cancer, but at present further clinical trials are ongoing to clarify how best such assays be integrated into standard clinical practice.

Breast cancer screening

- There have been at least 7 randomized controlled trials of mammographic screening over the last 30 years.
- The Health Insurance Plan (HIP) study of New York and the Two Counties Study from Sweden both showed a 30% reduction in mortality in the >50-year-old age group who were screened with mammography.
- Meta-analysis of all the published trials confirms a significant benefit for the over-50s.
- None of the trials published so far have shown a mortality benefit for women under the age of 50 years.
- 2 meta-analyses report a 14% but non-significant reduction in mortality in younger women.
- Screening the under-50 age group remains a controversial area, and in the UK a current trial is recruiting over 200 000 women to address this question.

Imaging modality

- Aim of screening for breast cancer is to identify pre-invasive disease or invasive disease before dissemination (through the lymphatics or blood).
- No evidence that simple breast self-examination is an effective means of screening for breast cancer.
- X-ray mammography is the most sensitive technique for detecting breast cancer and is also the most specific.
- Mammography is most sensitive once involution of the breast tissue has occurred (i.e. post-menopausal women).
- Mammography is less sensitive in women with dense breasts – that is, those with predominantly glandular tissue or residual stromal tissue.
- Breast ultrasound, useful for assessment of focal abnormalities, is also useful in detecting impalpable lesions.
- Telediaphanography (infrared scanning of the breast tissue) has both low sensitivity and low specificity for malignancy and is not used routinely.
- MRI with dynamic intravenous contrast is a very sensitive technique but variable specificity has been reported. It has a role in young women with a family history of breast cancer.

Mammographic technique

- The breast is compressed to flatten the breast tissue to reduce movement, overlapping shadows, and radiation dose.
- The uniform thickness of the tissue improves image quality and contrast.
- Low-energy radiation is passed through the breast, resulting in a high-contrast image.
- The image is recorded on X-ray film at present, but in the future will be digitally recorded, with display on a high-resolution computer screen.

- Two views of each breast are performed – one in the lateral oblique position diagonally across the chest, the other in the cranio-caudal position.
- Compression of breast tissue lasts only a few seconds, but 7% of women find the examination very painful, and a large proportion find it uncomfortable.

Radiation dose

- Low radiation dose (72 mGy per examination).
- The radiation risk is 1–2 excess cancers per million women screened after a latent period of 10 years in the post-menopausal age group but is higher in women under 30 years.
- Dose to the breast 75 times that of a chest X-ray.

Organization of the UK Breast Screening Programme

In the UK, women aged 50–70 years are invited through their general practitioner (GP), to attend either a breast screening centre or a mobile van for mammography every 3 years. Women aged over 70 years are not routinely called for screening, but are encouraged to make their own appointments at breast screening units every 3 years. The under-50 age group will not be invited unless the UK Centre for Cancer Care and Research (CCCR) Age Trial, screening 40–49-year-olds, is completed and demonstrates a significant benefit.

The mammograms are read by a consultant radiologist (double reading is now the usual practice). If an abnormality is seen that is thought to be suspicious, the woman is recalled to an assessment clinic at the breast screening centre. A clinical examination is performed at the recall visit with further X-rays, an ultrasound examination, and a fine needle biopsy for cytology or core biopsy if appropriate. Women diagnosed with cancer are referred promptly to a breast surgeon who will arrange appropriate treatment.

- An average of 73% of women accept the invitation to be screened.
- 4.5% of women are recalled for further tests.
- 10 cancers per 1000 women screened are found.
- A rigorous quality control system monitors performance in all breast screening centres annually.

Interval cancers

These are cancers that occur in the interval between two screening episodes. They fall into five categories:

- **true interval cancer** – appears in the 3-year interval and was not present on the previous screening mammogram
- **false negative** – the lesion was present on the previous screening mammogram
- **technical** – cancer was not on the film due to its position
- **mammographically occult** – cancer is not visualized on either the screening mammogram or at the time of diagnosis
- **unclassifiable** – no mammogram taken at the time of diagnosis.

There are currently 712 interval cancers per 10 000 women screened in the first 2 years after screening and 13 interval cancers appear in the third year.

- Many European countries offer screening every 2 years.
- A large UK trial is currently examining the costs and benefits of more frequent screening.

Screening for high-risk groups

- Women at moderate–high risk of breast cancer because of their family history should be offered annual breast MRI between ages 40 and 50 years.

Features of screen-detected breast cancer

The reduction in breast cancer deaths resulting from mammographic screening is attributed to:

- diagnosis and effective treatment of asymptomatic pre-invasive disease (DCIS)
- diagnosis and effective treatment of early invasive breast cancer, which would otherwise not present until systemic spread had occurred. A number of studies have found good evidence to support this, including the following observations:
  - 10–20% screen-detected lesions are non-invasive
  - >30% screen-detected invasive cancers are <10 mm
  - <20% are grade 3
  - 70–80% node negative.

Further reading

Moss SM, Cuckle H, Evans A, et al. (2006) Effect of mammographic screening from age 40 years on breast cancer mortality at 10 years followup – a randomised controlled trial. *Lancet* **368**, 2053–60.

NHS Breast Screening Programme. http://www.cancerscreening.nhs.uk/breastscreen/index.html (accessed 26 June 2009)

Nystrom L, Andersson I, Bjurstam N, et al. (2002) Long-term effects of mammography screening: Updated overview of the Swedish randomised trial. *Lancet* **359**, 909–19.

Van Goethem M, Tjalma W, Schelfont K (2006) Magnetic resonance imaging in breast cancer. *Eur J Surg Oncol* **32**, 901–10.

Presentation and staging

The most common presentations include the following (see Table 15.2):
- abnormal screening mammogram:
  - now accounts for around 25% of cases
  - microcalcification, mass lesion, distortion
- breast lump or thickening
- axillary tumour
- breast skin changes: dimpling, puckering, erythema
- nipple changes: inversion, discharge, rash (Paget's disease).
- persistent breast tenderness or pain
- infrequently, symptoms from metastatic disease, e.g. bone pain, spinal cord compression
- worrying symptoms are highlighted by the GP's 'red flag' referral letter and should be seen within two weeks.

Investigations

The diagnosis of breast cancer is made by 'triple assessment':
- full clinical examination:
  - including calliper measurement of any lump in either breast, and clinical assessment of tumour including fixity to adjacent skin and pectoral muscle
  - lymphadenopathy, in particular axillae and supraclavicular fossae (SCF) (although clinical assessment of the axillary lymph nodes correlates poorly with pathological spread to the nodes). If nodes are palpable, a fine needle aspiration (FNA) should be done with ultrasound guidance
- bilateral mammography usually combined with ultrasound
- FNA cytology and/or core biopsy:
  - impalpable lesions will require stereotactic or ultrasound-guided FNA or biopsy
  - core biopsy is the preferred diagnostic test, avoiding the risk of false positives cytology, and allowing differentiation between carcinoma *in situ* and invasive cancer in the majority.

This combined approach to assessment has >90% sensitivity and specificity.
- In a few cases where there is still uncertainty, excision biopsy of the breast lesion may be required. This is now unusual.
- The axilla is staged surgically in patients with invasive disease, usually with sentinel node biopsy.
- Pre-operative assessment of the axilla by ultrasound-guided biopsy of enlarged or abnormal lymph nodes is recommended.
- No serum tumour markers have been found to be useful.
- In the absence of locally advanced disease (see below) or symptoms/ signs of metastatic disease, routine radiological investigation such as chest X-ray, bone scan, or computerized tomography (CT) scan have not been found to be of benefit.

Table 15.2 Indications for referral to breast clinic

- Screen-detected breast cancer

- Breast lump:
    - any new discrete lump
    - new lump in pre-existing nodularity
    - asymmetrical nodularity persisting after menstruation
    - abscess/inflammation which does not settle after one course of antibiotics
    - persistent or recurrent cyst

- Pain:
    - associated with a lump
    - intractable pain that interferes with the patient's life and fails to respond to simple measures (well-supporting bra, simple analgesics, abstention from caffeine, evening primrose oil)
    - unilateral persistent pain in post-menopausal women

- Nipple discharge:
    - in any woman age >50 years
    - in younger women if blood-stained, persistent single duct, or bilateral, sufficient to stain clothes

- Nipple retraction, distortion, or eczema

- Change in breast contour

TNM staging system

Recent changes have been made in the staging system to take account of improvements in the pathological assessment of this disease. Pathological assessment of the extent of disease may differ considerably from clinical staging. See Table 15.3.

Table 15.3 TNM staging system

T stage	
Tis	*In situ* disease only
T1	≤2 cm
T1mic	≤0.1 cm
T1a	>0.1 to 0.5 cm
T1b	>0.5 to 1 cm
T1c	>1 to 2 cm
T2	>2 to 5 cm
T3	>5cm
T4	Any size of tumour with involvement of chest wall or skin
T4a	Direct extension into chest wall
T4b	Direct extension into skin, with oedema, ulceration or nodules
T4c	Both chest wall and skin involvement
T4d	Inflammatory breast cancer
N stage	
Nx	Lymph node status has not been assessed
N1	Mobile axillary lymphadenopathy
pN1mi	Micro-metastasis, >0.2 mm ≤2 mm
pN1a	1–3 positive axillary nodules
pN1b	Internal mammary nodes with micro-metastasis
pN1c	1–3 positive axillary nodes and internal mammary micro-metastasis
N2a	Fixed axillary lymph nodes
pN2a	4–9 positive axillary nodes
N2b	Internal mammary nodes clinically apparent
pN2b	Internal mammary nodes positive, clinically apparent, negative axillary nodes
N3a	Infraclavicular lymphadenopathy
pN3a	≥10 positive axillary nodes or positive infraclavicular node
N3b	Internal mammary and axillary lyphadenopathy

Table 15.3 (Cont'd)

N stage	
pN3b	Positive axillary and internal mammary nodes
N3c	Supraclavicular lymphadenopathy
pN3c	Supraclavicular node positive
M stage	
M1	Positive evidence of distant metastasis

Management of non-invasive (*in situ*) breast cancer

DCIS and lobular carcinoma *in situ* (LCIS) are rarely symptomatic, although extensive pre-invasive disease may present with a mass or thickening of breast tissue. The former is often diagnosed during screening.

Management options

Simple mastectomy
- *In situ* breast cancer was rarely diagnosed before the advent of mammographic screening.
- Standard treatment until the 1980s was mastectomy.
- Following mastectomy, relapse rates are very low (2–3%).
- Loco-regional recurrence and metastatic disease are attributed to undiagnosed micro-invasive cancer.
- Axillary surgery/staging is not indicated because of the low risk of positive nodes. If the DCIS is multifocal and widespread, some surgeons would biopsy lower axillary nodes.
- Mastectomy remains standard treatment for large *in situ* cancers and for multifocal disease (with breast reconstruction if desired).

Wide excision alone
- With the increased diagnosis of small localized non-invasive cancers by mammographic screening, breast-conserving surgery has been adopted for the majority. Because the lesion is usually screen-detected and impalpable, the lesion (often micro-calcification) is localized first by the radiologist. A specimen X-ray is essential to ensure complete excision of the abnormality.
- Cavity wall shavings for pathology are increasingly routine.
- However, 20–30% develop local recurrence within 5 years.
- Highest risk of recurrence is with high-grade DCIS and excision margin involved or <1 mm clear – excision margin of 1 cm is now preferred.
- Half of the recurrences are non-invasive, but the rest contain invasive cancer.
- Sentinel node biopsy in DCIS is not routinely indicated.

Wide excision and post-operative radiotherapy
- Three large randomized studies have now confirmed the benefit of radiotherapy in this setting.
- Whole breast is irradiated – 50 Gy/25 fractions.
- Risk of recurrence <10% at 5 years.

Adjuvant hormone therapy
- Results of two large clinical trials are contradictory.
- Tamoxifen 20 mg daily taken for 5 years reduces the frequency of recurrence of DCIS by about 30%, but there is uncertainty with regard to recurrence of invasive cancer.
- Clinical trials with aromatase inhibitors are under way.

The management of LCIS is controversial. Many were managed by wide local excision and post-operative radiotherapy, but problems include:
• LCIS is commonly missed on mammograms
• risk of multifocal ipsilateral disease
• risk of contralateral disease.
Most breast specialists now view LCIS as a risk marker, and local excision alone is adequate therapy. Some units simply follow-up LCIS when diagnosed on a CORE biopsy.

For all patients with early breast cancer, the key to selection of the optimum treatment is multidisciplinary discussion including radiology, pathology, surgery, and oncoloy input. Appropriate treatment options can then be presented to the patient to help them decide their individual preference.

Further reading

Barnes NLP, Bundred NJ (2007) Treatment of ductal carcinoma in situ. In: Dixon JM, ed. *Breast Surgery* , 3rd edn. Edinburgh: Elsevier, pp. 149–66.

Van la Parra RF, Ernst MF, Barneveld PC, *et al.* (2008) The value of sentinel lymph node biopsy in ductal carcinoma in situ (DCIS) and DCIS with microinvasion of the breast. *Eur J Surg Oncol* **34**, 631–5.

Management of early invasive breast cancer

Early breast cancer is defined as disease that can be completely removed by surgery, that is T1–3, N0–1 tumours. The management of this disease comprises the following:
- surgical treatment of the breast and axilla
- pathological assessment and staging to direct adjuvant therapy
- adjuvant therapy:
  - chemotherapy
  - radiotherapy
  - endocrine therapy
- follow-up.

Again, multidisciplinary discussion and planning of treatment is essential to optimize treatment outcomes.
- Consensus guidelines do not recommend routine staging investigations such as chest X-ray, liver ultrasound, bone scan, or CT imaging of the chest and abdomen.
- However, individuals at high risk of metastatic disease should be identified by the multidisciplinary team and imaged accordingly.
- Similarly breast MRI can improve loco-regional staging in selected cases.

Breast surgery
- All patients require complete removal of the primary tumour by either wide local excision or mastectomy.
- Halsted mastectomy was the operation most extensively applied to breast cancer patients during the first half of the 20th century, but it has gradually been replaced by a variety of less radical operations.
- Total mastectomy and axillary dissection is a less mutilating operation preserving the pectoralis major muscle and its neurovascular bundle. Seroma and numbness of the axillary skin are common sequelae. Lymphoedema is unusual (5%) unless radiotherapy is given to the axilla post-operatively.
- Quadrantectomy, introduced at the beginning of the 1970s, is a breast-conserving operation that removes the primary cancer with a margin of 2.0 cm of normal breast tissue. Infrequently performed now because of poor cosmesis.
- Wide local excision removes the tumour mass with a limited margin of normal tissue (0.5–1 cm) – this is now the most commonly performed procedure for early breast cancers but must be followed by radiotherapy to prevent local recurrence.
- Breast-conserving surgery alone was followed by local recurrence of breast cancer in up to 30% of patients.
- Several large randomized trials comparing breast-conserving surgery followed by breast radiotherapy with mastectomy alone have demonstrated similar local control rates and survival.
- Wide local excision followed by breast irradiation is the preferred treatment for the majority of T1–2 breast cancers.

- Breast conservation may not be appropriate, e.g.:
  - multifocal disease
  - large tumour in a small breast
  - where breast irradiation would be contraindicated
  - recurrent tumour after previous surgery.
- Some patients simply prefer mastectomy, not least because of the possible avoidance of radiotherapy (not always).
- Irrespective of the choice of local treatment, it should result in a local recurrence rate of <10% after 10 years' follow-up.
- Breast reconstruction can be offered after mastectomy, either at the time of primary surgery or at a later date – transverse rectus abdominis muscle (TRAM) flap, latissimus dorsi flap, and implants all have a role. These are well described recently by Cordeiro (2008). Generally primary (immediate) reconstruction is best carried out either by a plastic surgeon or, increasingly, by a full-time onco-plastic breast surgeon.
- Breast conservation or immediate reconstruction is now feasible, with good cosmetic results in some patients who would previously have required mastectomy through oncoplastic surgical techniques.
- Patients with Paget's disease are usually best served with a mastectomy.

Axillary surgery

- Clinical assessment of axillary nodes is inaccurate, palpable mobile lymphadenopathy is associated with reactive lymph node changes as commonly as metastasis.
- At least 30% of positive nodes are impalpable.
- Ultrasound examination of the axilla and biopsy of abnormal nodes improves the accuracy of pre-operative assessment.
- Aim of axillary surgery:
  - provide pathological staging of axillary lymph nodes
  - clear the axilla of disease so that radiotherapy is not required to treat positive nodes.
- Axillary clearance:
  - complete staging of the axilla
  - provides regional control of the disease unless nodes are fixed or extracapsular spread of cancer beyond the lymph node
  - problem of overtreatment particularly for small low-grade cancers with low probability of positive nodes
  - side-effects lymphoedema, arm pain, stiff shoulder, sensory deficit. Must preserve lateral thoracic nerve and thoracodorsal nerve.
- Axillary lymph node sampling (less frequently done – superceded by sentinel node biopsy):
  - minimum of four lymph nodes sampled from the lower axilla
  - patients with positive sample may then be treated by axillary clearance, or axillary radiotherapy
  - less morbidity for node-negative patients than axillary clearance
  - equivalent local control rates and survival compared with clearance.

- Sentinel node biopsy:
  - aim is the identification and removal of the first draining lymph node for careful pathological examination
  - should allow node-negative patients to avoid axillary clearance
  - sentinel node-positive patients may then be treated by axillary clearance (usually) or axillary radiotherapy (less often)
  - dye and radiolabelled colloid injected around the tumour and nipple (usually both techniques together are used)
  - any blue-stained node or nodes with radioactivity count >10 times background is excised (there may be more than one sentinel node)
  - UK ALMANAC (Axillary Lymphatic Mapping Against Nodal Axillary Clearance) trial shows advantages of sentinel node biopsy over axillary node sampling and clearance. There is less morbidity but there is a definite learning curve. Many breast units in the UK are now trained, and routinely use sentinel node biopsy
  - the role of frozen section and imprint cytology while the patient is anaesthetized is currently being evaluated
  - the prognostic impact of isolated tumour cells (<0.2 mm) and micrometastases (over 0.2 mm and less than 2 mm) in the sentinel node is controversial – the former is currently considered node 'negative' and the latter node 'positive', and may require chemotherapy.

Further reading

Cordeiro PG (2008) Breast reconstruction after surgery for breast cancer. *N Eng J Med* **359**, 1590–601.

Salem AA, Douglas-Jones AG, Sweetland HM, Mansel RE (2006) Intraoperative evaluation of axillary sentinel lymph nodes using touch imprint cytology. *Eur J Surg Oncol* **32**, 484–7.

Zavagno G, Del Bianco P, Koussis H (2008) Clinical impact of false negative sentinel lymph nodes in breast cancer. *Eur J Surg Oncol* **34**, 620–5.

Loco-regional radiotherapy

- Breast irradiation reduces the risk of local recurrence after breast-conserving surgery from about 30% to <10% at 10 years.
- In addition to the 75% reduction in the local recurrence rate, it is estimated that for every four local recurrences prevented, one cancer-related death at 10 years is avoided.
  - Breast irradiation is recommended for all patients after wide local excision for invasive breast cancer.
  - The whole breast is treated with tangential fields to a dose of 50 Gy in 25 fractions (or an equivalent dose-fractionation regimen).
  - Care taken to minimize the volume of lung and heart irradiated, most centres now using CT planning.
  - Boost of 10–15 Gy is commonly delivered to the tumour bed, using electrons or ^{192}Ir implant.
  - Post-operative irradiation of the breast now accounts for a large proportion of the work of most radiotherapy departments, and efforts are being made to reduce this.
  - Risk-adjusted strategies are under investigation, e.g. no radiotherapy in women >70 years who have undergone wide local excision for ER-positive T1N0 breast cancer.
  - Accelerated partial breast irradiation, e.g. high-dose-rate brachytherapy, intensity-modulated radiotherapy (IMRT), or intra-operative radiotherapy (IORT) are also under investigation.
- Post-mastectomy radiotherapy to the chest wall reduces the risk of loco-regional recurrence:
  - recommended for patients with 4 or more positive axillary nodes and for patients with T3 node-positive disease
  - there is a modest survival benefit.
- Axillary radiotherapy:
  - certainly indicated after a lymph node sampling that is positive
  - generally should be avoided after axillary clearance because of the high risk of lymphoedema and brachial plexopathy
  - supraclavicular fossa may be irradiated after axillary clearance if 4 or more nodes positive.

In general, radiotherapy should begin as soon as possible after surgery. However, enhanced normal tissue damage can result when radiotherapy and adjuvant chemotherapy are given together, and radiotherapy is often postponed until completion of chemotherapy.

Adjuvant systemic therapy

Despite effective local therapy with surgery and radiotherapy, many women with 'early breast cancer' harbour occult micro-metastases, and if untreated these give rise to overt metastatic disease, which leads to the eventual death of the patient. There is now a large body of evidence that effective systemic treatment directed against micro-metastatic disease at the time of diagnosis of breast cancer conveys a significant survival benefit in the majority of women.

- The risk of micro-metastatic disease correlates well with the recognized prognostic factors, simply summarized by the NPI.
- Similarly, the potential gains from systemic therapy in terms of improved survival are greatest in patients with poor prognosis.
- There have been many trials among women with operable breast cancer, examining the effects of systemic treatment, either endocrine manoeuvres or chemotherapy or both, on the survival of these patients.
- The basis of all these therapies is the reduction or eradication of microscopic systemic metastatic disease in women in whom all macroscopic local tumour has been effectively removed.
- In 1992 the Early Breast Cancer Trialists' Collaborative Group published an overview of 133 randomized trials involving 75 000 women with early breast cancer.
- This has had major impact, setting standards of care for adjuvant therapy for this disease, with regular revisions published to keep pace with clinical research. It was most recently updated in 2005.

Adjuvant chemotherapy (see Table 15.4)
Combination chemotherapy reduces recurrence and mortality in all groups of women.
- Age <50 years:
  - node-negative, 5.7% increase 10-year survival
  - node-positive, 12.4% increase 10-year survival.
- Age 50–69 years:
  - node-negative, 6.4% increase 10-year survival
  - node-positive, 2.3% increase 10-year survival.
- Chemotherapy should therefore be considered in all but very good prognosis pre-menopausal breast cancer and post-menopausal women with intermediate or poor prognosis breast cancer.
- Until recently, 'standard' adjuvant regimens included six months of CMF (cyclophosphamide, methotrexate, 5-fluorouracil) or 12 weeks of AC (Adriamycin® (doxorubicin), cyclophosphamide).
- Similar benefits from the shorter anthracycline regimen, but this was unsuitable for some patients with, e.g. past history of cardiac disease.
- Published in 2006, positive results established the epirubicin CMF regimen as the new gold standard for the UK, with a 7% improvement in 5-year survival compared with 6 months' treatment with CMF (82% versus 75%).

- Other regimens that have demonstrated superiority to CMF include six cycles of FEC (5-fluorouracil, epirubicin, cyclophosphamide) and 4 x AC followed by 4 x paclitaxel or docetaxel.
- Other trials are exploring the benefits of combinations including docetaxel, capecitabine, and gemcitabine.
- HER2-positive breast cancer has a relatively poor prognosis, despite adjuvant chemotherapy, but several large co-operative trials have demonstrated significant survival benefits when the monoclonal antibody trastuzumab is given in addition to adjuvant chemotherapy.
- Clinical trials with trastuzumab are currently addressing several unresolved questions:
  - duration of adjuvant therapy
  - optimal timing with chemotherapy
  - cardiotoxicity particularly in combination with anthracyclines.
- Estimates of benefit from adjuvant chemotherapy with different regimens may be calculated for individual patients available via www.adjuvantonline.com.

Table 15.4 Examples of adjuvant chemotherapy regimens

CMF 6 cycles over 6 weeks			
Cyclophosphamide	100 mg/m^2	d1–14	q 4/52
	oral		
	or		
	600 mg/m^2 IV	d1&8	q 4/52
Methotrexate	40 mg/m^2 IV		
5-fluorouracil	600 mg/m^2 IV	d1&8	q 4/52
AC 4 cycles over 12 weeks			
Doxorubicin	60 mg/m^2	d1	q 3/52
Cyclophosphamide	600 mg/m^2	d1	
EpiCMF 8 cycles over 28 weeks			
Epirubicin	100 mg/m^2	q 3/52	4 cycles
then			
CMF	As above	q 4/52	4 cycles
FEC 6 cycles over 6 weeks			
5-fluorouracil	500 mg/m^2 IV	d1	q 3/52
Epirubicin	100 mg/m^2 IV	d1	q 3/52
Cyclophosphamide	500 mg/m^2 IV	d1	q 3/52

Table 15.4 (Cont'd)

FEC 3 cycles followed by docetaxel 3 cycles over 18 weeks

FEC as above followed by:

Docetaxel	100 mg/m²	d1	q 3/52

TAC 6 cycles over 18 weeks

Docetaxel	75 mg/m²	q 3/52	4 cycles
Doxorubicin	75 mg/m²		
Cyclophosphamide	500 mg/m²	q 4/52	4 cycles

Adjuvant endocrine therapy

- 60% of breast cancers are ER-positive.
- Adjuvant hormone therapy confers survival benefits in these patients, in some cases greater than with chemotherapy.
- Toxicity is less than for chemotherapy, mainly menopausal symptoms.
- No benefit in ER-negative breast cancer.
- For pre-menopausal women ovarian ablation provides a 10.6% improvement in 10-year survival: node negative 6.8%, node positive 13%.
- Tamoxifen 20 mg daily for 5 years improves survival in both pre-and post-menopausal women:
  - 10-year survival improved by 5% node-negative, 11% in node-positive patients
  - reduced risk of contralateral breast cancer and osteoporosis
  - however, risk of thromboembolic disease and increased incidence of endometrial cancer (×2.5).
- Several clinical trials suggest aromatase inhibitors may be superior to tamoxifen as adjuvant therapy in post-menopausal women:
  - improved relapse-free survival
  - reduced risk of thromboembolic disease and endometrial cancer; optimum duration of therapy remains uncertain.
- Endocrine therapy may result in long-term health problems in breast cancer survivors, e.g. osteoporosis, and efforts to prevent these are under investigation (routine bone densitometry, prophylactic bisphosphonate therapy)
- Interaction with chemotherapy:
  - tamoxifen given simultaneously with chemotherapy reduces its benefit
  - adjuvant hormone therapy should only be commenced after completion of chemotherapy.

Neo-adjuvant therapy

Primary chemotherapy or hormone therapy for operable breast cancer provides early systemic treatment and allows assessment of the response to treatment; by definition this is impossible with adjuvant therapy. Its disadvantages are the delay in definitive local surgery and the risk of overtreatment with chemotherapy in the absence of pathological staging (e.g. post-menopausal, ER-positive, node-negative tumour).

Several large randomized trials (e.g. NSABP-B18 and B27) have shown no difference in survival when pre- and post-operative chemotherapy were compared. Pre-operative treatment can downstage the primary tumour and, in some women, facilitates breast-conserving surgery where mastectomy would otherwise be required.

Adjuvant and neo-adjuvant therapy are compared in Table 15.5.

Table 15.5 Comparison of adjuvant and neo-adjuvant therapy

	Adjuvant therapy	**Neo-adjuvant therapy**
Advantages	Pathological staging available for patient selection Immediate surgical removal of all macroscopic disease	Tumour response is visible to both clinicians and patients Reduction in tumour volume can facilitate breast conservation Lack of response gives opportunity to change chemotherapy
Disadvantages	No visible benefit in individual patients No means of assessing efficacy of treatment regimen in individual patients Mastectomy required for many tumours >3cm diameter	Risk of overtreatment particularly low-risk post-menopausal women Disease progression may occur prior to surgery (clinical trials have shown this is a rare event)

Further reading

Early Breast Cancer Trialists' Collaborative Group (1992) Systemic treatment of early breast cancer by hormonal, cytotoxic or immune therapy – Parts I and II. *Lancet* **339**, 1–15, 71–85.

Early Breast Cancer Trialists' Collaborative Group (1998) Tamoxifen for early breast cancer: an overview of the randomized trials. *Lancet* **351**, 1451–67.

Early Breast Cancer Trialists' Collaborative Group (1998) Polychemotherapy for early breast cancer: an overview of the randomized trials. *Lancet* **352**, 930–42.

Early Breast Cancer Trialists' Collaborative Group (2000) Favourable and unfavourable effect on long-term survival of radiotherapy for early breast cancer: an overview of the randomized trials. *Lancet* **355**, 1757–70.

Early Breast Cancer Trialists' Collaborative Group (2005) Effects of chemotherapy and hormonal therapy for early breast cancer on recurrence and 15 year survival: an overview of the randomized trials. *Lancet* **365**, 1687–717.

NICE (2009) *Clinical Guideline 80. Early and locally advanced breast cancer: diagnosis and treatment.* London: NICE.

Management of locally advanced breast cancer

Locally advanced disease is defined by the presence of infiltration of the skin or the chest wall or fixed axillary nodes, i.e.:
- T4a–d
- N2–3.

The probability of metastatic disease is high (>70%) but long-term survival is possible and the median survival of these patients exceeds 2 years.

At presentation, in addition to mammography and core biopsy, staging investigations should include:
- chest X-ray
- isotope bone scan
- liver ultrasound or CT scan – increasingly MRI is used for staging.

Local control of the tumour and the prevention of tumour fungation are of major importance to the quality of life of these women irrespective of the presence of metastases. A combination of primary systemic treatment and radiotherapy is commonly used.

Many of these patients are elderly and have indolent ER-positive disease that responds well to endocrine therapy. First-line therapy in this group should be with one of the aromatase inhibitors (anastrozole, letrozole, or exemestane), which have been shown to be superior to tamoxifen in advanced breast cancer. Following maximal response, radical radiotherapy is delivered to the breast, axilla, and supraclavicular fossa.

Younger patients and patients with ER-negative disease are treated with primary chemotherapy, usually an anthracycline-based combination. In some patients with a good response to systemic treatment, surgery may be feasible, followed by loco-regional radiotherapy. Hormone therapy is started after chemotherapy for ER-positive tumours:
- pre-menopausal – ovarian suppression (luteinizing hormone-releasing hormone (LHRH) agonist) and tamoxifen
- post-menopausal – aromatase inhibitor.

Promising results have been reported in HER2+++ locally advanced breast cancer treated with primary chemotherapy plus trastuzumab.

Prognosis

Table 15.6 summarizes the 10-year survival rates according to the stage of disease at presentation. Although many women with metastatic breast disease survive 5 years, despite progress in all aspects of treatment, this stage of disease remains incurable.

Table 15.6 Treatment outcomes: breast cancer survival rates

Stage	10-year survival[a]
0	>95%
I	75–95%
IIA	45–85%
IIB	40–80%
IIIA	10–60%
IIIB	0–35%
IIIC	0–30%
IV	0.5%

[a]Wide range of survival rates, individual prognosis determined by TNM stage, grade, ER status, and treatment, e.g. chemotherapy.

Management of metastatic breast cancer

Between 15% and 20% of patients present with metastatic breast cancer, and currently around 50% of patients with operable breast cancer relapse with metastatic disease. Despite advances in the systemic treatment of breast cancer, metastatic breast cancer is incurable with current therapies. Principles of its management include the following:

- aim of treatment is palliation
- however, 20% survive 5 years, so key aims also include extension of life and maintenance of its quality
- ER-positive bone disease commonly demonstrates indolent growth, with prolonged survival
- ER-negative visceral disease has worse prognosis
- response to chemotherapy may be quicker than to hormone therapy, response to hormones often more durable
- common sites of spread include lung and pleura, liver, bone, brain, lymph nodes and skin
- rarer sites include the peritoneum (lobular carcinoma), choroid, pituitary.

Endocrine therapy

Treatment with tamoxifen, ovarian ablation, progestins, or aromatase inhibitors will provide an objective response or prevent disease progression in ~30% of women with advanced disease, and in 50–60% of those with ER-positive tumours. It is preferred over chemotherapy in older patients, and for non-visceral metastatic disease.

Disease that responds to endocrine therapy and then progresses has a 25% response rate with second-line treatment; the response to a third agent is 10–15%. Randomized studies now suggest that the first-line treatment with best response rate and longest progression-free interval is not tamoxifen but:

- pre-menopausal – ovarian suppression (LHRH agonist) plus tamoxifen
- post-menopausal – aromatase inhibitor (anastrozole, letrozole, or exemestane)
- these treatments are also effective in patients who relapse during or after adjuvant tamoxifen
- subsequent second-, third- and fourth-line therapy with agents to which the patient has not previously been exposed can be of benefit:
  - megestrol acetate (progestin)
  - fulvestrant (anti-oestrogen).

Chemotherapy (see Table 15.7)

Advanced breast cancer is moderately chemosensitive. Active agents include:

- anthracyclines (doxorubicin, epirubicin)
- alkylating agents (cyclophosphamide)
- anti-metabolites (5-fluorouracil (5-FU), capecitabine, methotrexate, gemcitabine)
- taxanes (docetaxel, paclitaxel)
- vincas (vinorelbine)
- platinum complexes (carboplatin, cisplatin).

Table 15.7 Example of chemotherapy regimens for advanced breast cancer

FAC		
5-FU	500 mg/m^2	3 weekly
Doxorubicin	50 mg/m^2	
Cyclophosphamide	500 mg/m^2	
EC		
Epirubicin	75 mg/m^2	3 weekly
Cyclophosphamide	600 mg/m^2	
Taxanes		
Docetaxel	75–100 mg/m^2	3 weekly
or		
Paclitaxel	175 mg/m^2	3 weekly
	or	
	90 mg/m^2	weekly
Other agents		
Vinorelbine	25 mg/m^2 day 1 & 8	3 weekly
Capecitabine	1250 mg/m^2 PO bd	3 weekly
Trastuzumab	4 mg/m^2 loading dose	Week 1
	2 mg/ m^2	Week 2 onwards weekly
	or	
	8 mg/m^2 loading dose	Week 1
	6 mg/ m^2 weekly	Week 4 onwards 3 weekly

Vinorelbine, capecitabine, and trastuzumab may be used as a single agent or in combination, e.g. with paclitaxel or docetaxel.

Combination chemotherapy is the preferred treatment for patients with visceral metastatic disease:
• liver and lung, rather than soft tissue, pleura, and bone
• ER-negative tumours.

Combinations such as FAC (5-FU, doxorubicin, cyclophosphamide) produce response rates of 40–60%, with a median time to progression of around 8 months. Despite the toxicity of such combinations (alopecia, nausea, mucositis, lethargy, myelosuppression), clinical trials have shown that the quality of life of women improves as they respond to treatment. Patients who have previously received anthracycline-based adjuvant chemotherapy may be treated with a taxane instead when they develop metastatic disease.

Following disease progression, 25–50% of women respond to second-line chemotherapy, e.g. with a taxane. In patients who remain fit for further chemotherapy, 3rd- and 4th-line treatment may result in tumour response.

Although phase II studies have suggested that high-dose chemotherapy may produce durable remissions from metastatic breast cancer, no survival benefit has yet been proven for such treatment.

Targeted therapy

Trastuzumab

Between 25% and 30% of breast cancers overexpress HER2, a growth factor receptor, associated with poor-prognosis disease. Trastuzumab (Herceptin®) is a recombinant monoclonal antibody against HER2, administered intravenously weekly or three weekly. This drug has significant benefits in the treatment of HER2-positive advanced breast cancer, either as a single agent after failure of other chemotherapy regimens (response rate 10%), or more effectively in combination with chemotherapy. When trastuzumab is given in combination with taxanes in the first-line treatment of metastatic breast cancer, it improves both the response rate and the survival time. However, combination with anthracyclines is contraindicated because of cardiotoxicity. Similar promising results are reported with trastuzumab in combination with other cytotoxics, e.g. capecitabine.

Lapatinib

In patients refractory to trastuzumab, the receptor tyrosine kinase inhibitor lapatinib, which inhibits EGFR and HER2, has shown positive results in combination with capecitabine.

Other agents

A variety of growth factor recceptor tyrosine kinase inhibitors and anti-angiogenesis agents including bevacizumab are under investigation in the setting of metastatic breast cancer refractory to conventional endocrine therapy.

Radiotherapy

Low-dose radiotherapy (e.g. 20 Gy/5 fractions) provides effective palliation for:
• painful bone metastases
• soft tissue disease
• spread to brain or choroid.

Bisphosphonates

These drugs have important roles in patients with bone metastases from breast cancer:
• treatment and prevention of malignant hypercalcaemia
• healing of osteolytic metastases
• reducing bone pain
• delaying progression of bone disease with reduced requirement for radiotherapy and reduced fractures.

Prolonged treatment is recommended, starting from the time of diagnosis of bone metastases and continuing even in the face of progressive disease. Osteonecrosis of the jaw (ONJ) is a rare but serious toxicity of bisphosphonates, particularly when given continuously over a long period for metastatic disease, and may be precipitated by dental extractions. Ongoing trials are exploring:

- prophylactic treatment with these agents hoping to prevent the future development of bone metastases in women with high-risk early breast cancer
- monitoring biomarkers of bone turnover, such as collagen cross-links, to determine the optimum frequency/dose/duration of therapy.

Bisphosphonates for bone metastases from breast cancer
- Zoledronate 4 mg 15 min IV infusion 4-weekly
- Pamidronate 90 mg 2 h IV infusion 4-weekly
- Ibandronate 6 mg 2 h IV infusion 4-weekly
- Ibandronate 50 mg daily oral
- Clodronate 1600 mg daily oral

Further reading
NICE (2009) *Clinical Guideline 81. Advanced Breast Cancer: diagnosis and treatment.* London: NICE.

Colorectal cancer

Introduction

- Colorectal cancer is the fourth commonest cancer worldwide.
- Affects men and women almost equally.
- Environmental factors (diet) play a major role in the aetiology of the disease.
- A minority of cases (<8%) are associated with genetic predisposition syndromes such as familial adenomatous polyposis (FAP) and hereditary non-polyposis colorectal cancer (HNPCC).
- Almost always adenocarcinoma.
- Loco-regional lymph nodes tend to be involved before the development of disseminated disease.
- In rectal cancer there is also a propensity for the tumour to infiltrate laterally into the peri-rectal fat and lymph nodes.

Colorectal cancer: surgery

- Surgery is the mainstay of curative therapy for colorectal cancer.
- Curative resection requires excision of the primary tumour and its lymphatic drainage with an enveloping margin of normal tissue.

Pre-operative preparation

- Precise **site** and local **extent** of the tumour should be known before laparotomy or laparoscopic resection. In the latter, the site of the tumour must be carefully marked with ink via the colonoscope before laparoscopic resection; knowledge of distant spread is helpful.
- Full colonoscopy or proctosigmoidoscopy and air-contrast barium enema (in the absence of obstruction or perforation) are required.
- The liver is imaged with computerized tomography (CT) and/or ultrasound examination; CT and endo-anal ultrasound imaging of the pelvis may offer additional information of the depth of invasion of rectal cancers. Magnetic resonance imaging (MRI) of pelvis to stage rectal cancer is useful.
- Peri-operative antibiotics and thromboembolic prophylaxis are mandatory.

Principles in primary resection

- Bowel segment and its lymphatic field are excised intact.
- If an anastomosis is planned, it is fashioned without tension, ensuring a good lumen, secure apposition, and good blood supply.
- Minimally invasive colon cancer surgery is now commonplace. While there is a distinct learning curve, the benefits in the short term are proven and early long-term data show no adverse impact on survival.

Rectal cancer

- Total excision of the mesorectum is considered essential (TME). This involves removal of the rectum itself together with a sleeve of surrounding tissue contained within the mesorectal fascia. This has been shown to reduce local relapse rates.
- A proximal limit of 5 cm clearance and distal limit of 2 cm clearance is adequate. There is now increasing evidence that rectal cancer surgery should be done in high-volume units by specialists.

Post-operative care

- There is now clear evidence that the routine use of the enhanced recovery programme leads to speedier recovery and (perhaps) fewer post-operative complications.

Local excision

- Pre-op assessment with MRI and endoanal ultrasound is essential.
- 5% of rectal cancers may be removed by non-radical transanal surgery. In specialized centres, transanal endoscopic microsurgery has a role in very selected patients.
- Particularly appropriate in small, low, well-differentiated cancers on the posterior wall.

- If the pathologist reports incomplete excision, spread through the rectal wall, or poorly differentiated carcinoma, radical surgery may be required to obtain local extirpation of tumour, if the patient is fit.

Surgery of recurrent cancer

- Local recurrence occurs most commonly in rectal cancer, usually outside the bowel lumen. This is less common with adequate TME. If investigations suggest that a recurrence is isolated and potentially resectable, further surgery should be considered.
- Metastases confined to one lobe of the liver or less than four in both lobes may warrant resection, as there is up to a 30% chance of cure. Laparoscopic liver resection of secondaries is routine in specialized centres.
- Repeat liver resection of further colorectal secondaries is helpful in selected patients. In a few centres this is being done laparoscopically.

Further reading

Baatrup G, Elbrand H, Hesselfeldt P (2007) Rectal adenocarcinoma and transanal endoscopic microsurgery. *Int J Colorectal Dis* **22**, 1347–52.

den Dulk M, van de Velde CJ (2008) Time to focus on the quality of colon cancer surgery. *Lancet Oncol* **9**, 815–16.

Hendry PO, Hausel J, Nygnen J, et al. (2009) Determinant of outcome after colorectal resection within an enhanced recovery programme. *Br J Surg* **96**, 197–205.

Hogan AM, Kennelly R, Winter DC (2009) Volume–outcome analysis in rectal cancer – a plea for enquiry, evidence and evaluation. *Eur J Surg Oncol* **35**, 111–12.

Liang Y, Li G, Chen P, Yu J (2008) Laparoscopic versus open colorectal resection for cancer: a meta analysis of result of randomised controlled trial on recurrence. *Eur J Surg Oncol* **34**, 1217–24.

The Colon Cancer Laparoscopic Group (2009) Survival after laparoscopic surgery versus open surgery for colon cancer: long term outcome of a randomised clinical trial. *Lancet Oncol* **10**, 44–52.

Tythenleigh MG, Warren BF, Mortensen NJ (2008) Management of early rectal cancer. *Br J Surg* **95**, 409–23.

Adjuvant chemotherapy of colorectal cancer

Rationale

Half of the patients undergoing apparently curative resection of bowel cancer are destined to relapse and eventually die with either locally recurrent or distant metastatic disease. This is due to the presence of residual micro-metastases invisible at the time of surgery. The aim of adjuvant chemotherapy is to eradicate these micro-metastases and thereby prevent future relapse.

Indications

Adjuvant chemotherapy is an exercise in risk reduction. Questions to be considered after a potentially curative operation are the following:
- what is the probability of micro-metastases?
- will adjuvant therapy prevent/delay relapse?
- what are the side-effects?

Multidisciplinary team discussion is essential.

The risk that the patient has micro-metastases is estimated, after surgery, by examining the pathological features of the primary cancer.
- Dukes' C cancers, which have spread to the nearby lymph nodes, carry a much higher risk (around 50%). There is good evidence that this risk is reduced by adjuvant chemotherapy, which is now offered routinely in most centres unless there is a strong contraindication.
- Dukes' B cancers, which have breached the muscle layers but not spread to lymph nodes, carry an intermediate risk of around 30%. There is evidence to support the use of adjuvant chemotherapy in these patients, the absolute survival benefit being between 3% and 5%.
- Rectal cancer, which accounts for nearly 40% of bowel cancers, presents some special considerations. A relative lack of a barrier to lateral spread and increased technical difficulty of surgery in the pelvis combine to make local recurrence a particular problem. Radiotherapy, targeted to the pelvis either before or after surgery, reduces local recurrence rates. Adjuvant therapy for rectal cancer may therefore include both radiotherapy and chemotherapy aimed, respectively, at local and systemic micro-metastases.

Chemotherapy used in adjuvant setting

- Until recently the standard was 5-fluorouracil (5-FU) given in combination with folinic acid, by bolus intravenous injection for a total period of 6 months.
- Addition of oxaliplatin to 5-FU and folinic acid has been shown to result in superior survival at the cost of some (mainly short-lived) extra toxicity. This regimen (FOLFOX) has become a standard in many countries in those patients who are deemed suitable for such therapy.
- New studies are investigating the addition of agents that target epidermal growth factor (EGF) or vascular endothelial growth factor (VEGF) receptors.

- 5-FU is also a radiosensitizer. For patients with rectal cancer, pre- or post-operative pelvic radiotherapy is sometimes given concurrently with chemotherapy to harness this effect. This may be followed by a more prolonged course of standard adjuvant chemotherapy aimed at distant micro-metastases.

Side-effects

The clinical activity of 5-FU and its side-effects are both critically dependent upon the dose and schedules used, and vary considerably from patient to patient. The side-effect profile should, for most patients, be quite easily tolerable and consistent with continuing normal activity, including work. Treatment is feasible even in the elderly.

Common side-effects

- Nausea and vomiting
- Oral mucositis
- Diarrhoea
- Red, painful palms and soles
- Peripheral neuropathy (when oxaliplatin is included).

Chemotherapy for advanced colorectal cancer

- Defined as disease that is outwith the possibility of curative resection.
- Mostly this is defined by the presence of metastatic disease.
- Poor prognosis and in most cases the aim of therapy is palliation though modest prolongation of survival has been achieved by application of modern chemotherapy agents.
- The median survival time for such patients without further therapy is of the order of 6 months.
- In most cases therapy is based on chemotherapy but this does not preclude the use of combined modalities such as localized radiotherapy or ablative techniques for liver metastases.
- Small proportion of patients have so-called pauci-metastatic disease, in other words, disease that is potentially resectable or could be made so by volume reduction using chemotherapy (downstaging). These highly selected patients should be identified and treated within a multidisciplinary team setting with a view to surgical resection and potential cure of the disease.

First-line chemotherapy (see Table 16.1)

5-FU is still the most widely used single agent. There is no consensus as to the optimal dosing and scheduling of this drug. However, most authorities now accept that infusional regimens result in better response with less toxicity. Biochemical modulation by the use of concurrent folinic acid (leucovorin) also seems to improve response rates. Response rates of between 10% and 50% have been quoted for regimens combining 5-FU/folinic acid (FA).

This variability is probably a reflection of patient selection as much as efficiency of the chemotherapy employed. Various regimens have been able to demonstrate survival improvements of about 6 months over patients treated with best supportive care alone. Different regimens have differences in the toxicity profile, with bolus tending to cause more marrow toxicity, and protracted infusion causing more diarrhoea and hand–foot syndrome (see Table 16.2).

Oxaliplatin is a platinum analogue that is active in colorectal cancer. Synergy with fluoropyrimidines has been demonstrated in clinical trials. Combination studies with 5-FU-based regimens versus the same regimen without oxaliplatin have confirmed a higher response, with some studies also showing survival benefits. A striking feature of these studies is the numbers of patients who are 'downstaged' by the combination therapy and then go on to have salvage surgery with some achieving long-term remission. Even though there are no prospective studies, this combination is often used in patients with pauci-metastatic disease. In the last few years the introduction of a number of new agents into this therapy area has dramatically changed how this disease is treated.

Table 16.1 Commonly used regimens in first-line treatment of advanced colorectal cancer

Regimen	Mode	5-FU	Leucovorin	Ralitrexed	Duration	Interval
Mayo	Bolus	425 mg/m^2	20 mg/m^2	–	Daily for 5 days	4–5 weeks
DeGramont	Bolus/infusion	400 mg/m^2 bolus, 600 mg/m^2, 46 h	200 mg/m^2	–	2 days	2 weeks
Lokich	Continuous infusion	300 mg/m^2 per day	–	–	8–12 weeks	–
Tomudex®	Bolus	–	–	3 mg/m^2	15 min	3 weeks

Table 16.2 Toxicities of commonly used regimens in first-line treatment of advanced colorectal cancer

	Mayo	DeGramont	Lokich	Tomudex
Nausea/vomiting	+	+	+	+
Diarrhoea	+++	+	+	
Mucositis	+++	+	+	+
Myelosuppression	++	+	+	+
Alopecia	–	–	–	–
Hand–foot syndrome	–	–	++	–

Irinotecan is a topoisomerase inhibitor. The drug has shown single agent activity in first- and second-line use. In combination with FU/FA, first-line trials confirmed improved response and overall survival such that this combination became an accepted standard of care. However, the combination does have the potential to cause severe toxicity such as diarrhoea and neutropenia. As a result there is no current consensus as to the optimal regimen for therapy of advanced colorectal cancer.

Capecitabine is an orally administered pro-drug of 5-FU. In advanced colorectal cancer it has shown improved response over a 5-FU regimen, and equivalent survival. The convenience to the patient of replacing infusional regimens of 5-FU with oral medication is an important factor. Studies combining capecitabine with irinotecan or oxaliplatin have shown favourable results, and larger-scale comparative studies are under way.

Although other oral fluoropyrimidines have been developed none are as widely used as capecitabine.

Combinations of the agents listed above have been tested in a large number of clinical trials. Consensus exists that combination therapy offers higher response rates at the cost of some increase in subjective toxicity. Since in most cases the aim of therapy is palliation, a number of important issues arise:

- which combination is best?
- which sequence of agents?
- optimum duration of therapy?
- continuous or intermittent exposure to treatment?

These and other questions will form the basis of clinical research in this area for some time to come.

Second-line chemotherapy

Irinotecan was the first agent to show real activity in patients who had relapsed following 5-FU or progressed while on this therapy.

Oxaliplatin has not been tested as extensively as a single agent in second line therapy. However, addition of oxaliplatin into a regimen of 5-FU where the patient has 'failed' has shown some promise.

The optimal sequencing of these agents is not yet clear.

Novel cytotoxic agents

Avastin® (bevacizumab) is an anti-angiogenic compound targeted at VEGF. Recent randomized trials in combination with IFL (irinotecan, 5-FU, leucovorin) have shown superior survival for the combination arms. The drug has now been licensed in the US and Europe – full integration of this agent awaits further clinical trials in various combinations and schedules.

Erbitux® (cetuximab) is a monoclonal antibody that targets the EGF receptor. The drug has shown activity both as a single agent and in combination with cytotoxic drugs, particularly irinotecan. It seems likely it will be integrated into colorectal therapy in the near future.

Radiotherapy in colorectal cancer

- In colonic cancer, radiotherapy is limited to the palliative situation in most circumstances.
- The rectum is immobile and fixed within the pelvis and therefore a suitable target for radiotherapy.
- Radiotherapy has been used in both the pre-operative and post-operative setting in this disease.
- In the pre-operative situation there are a group of patients (10–15%) who present with large fixed or tethered tumours that are non-resectable. Only half of this group will have distant metastases at presentation. The conversion rate to resectability is 35–75%, with a dose of 50–60 Gy given over a 5-week period.

Anal cancer

Introduction

- 3–5% of all large bowel malignancies.
- Most anal tumours arise from the epidermal elements of the anal canal lining (squamous cell – 85% of anal tumours), though some arise from the glandular mucosa of the uppermost part of the anal canal or from the anal ducts and glands (adenocarcinomas – 10% of anal tumours).
- Malignant melanoma of the anus is very rare (<5% of anal tumours) and carries a poor prognosis.

Anal squamous cell carcinoma

Epidemiology
- Rare cancer, around 250 UK cases per annum.
- Male to female 1:3.
- Usually >50 years.
- Areas with a high incidence of anal cancer also tend to have a high incidence of cervical, vulval, and penile tumours.

Aetiology
- HPV infection
- Receptive anal intercourse
- Sexually transmitted disease, >10 sexual partners
- Previous cervical, vulval, or vaginal cancer
- Immunosuppression after solid organ transplant
- HIV infection
- Cigarette smoking.

Pathology and natural history
- Included within the category of epidermoid tumours are:
  - squamous cell carcinomas
  - basaloid (or cloacogenic) carcinomas
  - mucoepidermoid cancers.
- Anal sphincter and the recto-vaginal septum, perineal body, and the vagina are common sites of direct invasion.
- Lymph node spread occurs initially to the peri-rectal group of nodes and thereafter to inguinal, haemorrhoidal, and lateral pelvic lymph nodes.
- 10% of patients will present with inguinal lymph node involvement, but this rises to approximately 30% when the primary tumour is greater than 5 cm in diameter.
- Blood-borne spread tends to occur late and is usually associated with advanced local disease. The most common sites of metastases are the liver, lung, and bones.

Clinical presentation
- Symptoms of epidermoid anal cancer:
  - pain
  - bleeding
  - itch
  - discharge
  - mass
- Later symptoms:
  - faecal incontinence
  - ano-vaginal fistula

Approximately one-third of patients with anal carcinoma have enlarged inguinal lymph nodes on presentation, but less than half this number have metastatic nodes. Often the nodes are secondarily infected or reactive.

Investigation and staging
- Careful examination under anaesthetic with biopsy of lesion, documentation of length, site, and extent of primary tumours.
- Fine needle aspiration (FNA) cytology: enlarged inguinal lymph nodes.
- Computerized tomography (CT) or magnetic resonance imaging (MRI) scan: abdomen and pelvis.
- Staging commonly uses the TNM system (see Table 17.1).

Management
Over the last 20 years, treatment of this cancer has moved from surgery (abdominoperineal resection) to organ-conserving therapy, and chemo-irradiation is now a standard treatment for the majority (T2–4, and all node-positive patients).

Randomized trials such as ACT 1 (Anal Cancer Trial) have demonstrated a 20% improvement in local control with chemo-irradiation compared with radiotherapy alone. The current UK ACT 2 study compares 2 versus 4 cycles of 5-fluorouracil (5-FU) plus mitomycin versus cisplatin with concomitant pelvic radiotherapy.
- Most recurrence is loco-regional.
- Small lesions at the anal margin may still best be treated by local excision alone, obviating the need for protracted courses of non-surgical therapy. The most recent development is sentinel node biopsy of the inguinal nodes and it has been well demonstrated in a recent German study to be efficient and practical.
- An important role for the surgeon is in treatment after failure of primary non-surgical therapy, either early or late. The appearance of the primary site can be misleading after radiotherapy. A proportion of patients develop complications such as radio-necrosis, fistula, or incontinence, following radical radiation or combined therapy.

Treatment outcomes
- 60–70% 5-year survival
- 70–80% anal preservation
- Prognosis depends on T size, lymph node status (node-positive 50% 5-year survival).

Further reading
Gretschel S, Warnick P, Bembenek A, *et al.* (2008) Lymphatic mapping and sentinel lymph node biopsy in epidermoid carcinoma of the anal canal. *Eur J Surg Oncol* **34**, 890–4.

Table 17.1 TNM staging of anal cancer

Cancer of the anal canal

T: primary tumour

Tis	Carcinoma *in situ*
T1	Tumour 2 cm or less in greatest dimension
T2	Tumour >2 cm but not >5 cm in greatest dimension
T3	Tumour >5 cm in greatest dimension
T4	Tumour invading adjacent organ(s) (vagina, prostate, pelvic wall)

N: regional lymph nodes

N0	No regional lymph node metastasis
N1	Metastases in perirectal lymph node(s)
N2	Metastases in unilateral internal iliac and/or inguinal lymph node(s)
N3	Metastases in perirectal and inguinal lymph nodes and/or bilateral internal iliac and/or inguinal lymph nodes

Cancer of the anal margin

T: primary tumour

Tis, T1, T2, T3	Identical to cancer of the anal canal
T4	Tumour invades deep extradermal structures (cartilage, skeletal muscle, or bone)

N: regional lymph nodes

N0	No regional lymph node metastases
N1	Regional lymph node metastases

Rarer tumours

Adenocarcinoma

Adenocarcinoma in the anal canal is usually a very low rectal cancer that has spread downwards to involve the canal, but true adenocarcinoma of the anal canal does occur, probably arising from the anal glands that arise around the dentate line and pass radially outwards into the sphincter muscles. This is a very rare tumour; although it is radiosensitive, it is still usually treated by radical surgery.

Malignant melanoma

This tumour is excessively rare, accounting for just 1% of anal canal malignant tumours. The lesion may mimic a thrombosed external pile due to its colour, though amelanotic tumours also occur. It has an even worse prognosis than at other sites. As the chances of cure are minimal, radical surgery as primary treatment has been all but abandoned.

Practical points

- Rectal bleeding and anal pain are common – a high degree of suspicion is required to diagnose anal cancer correctly.
- Multifocal anal and genital disease may co-exist – be sure to examine the anal and genital areas.
- Examination under anaesthetic is essential for adequate staging and also permits a generous biopsy.
- Biopsy or needle aspiration of enlarged inguinal lymph nodes is essential prior to treatment.
- Local excision may be appropriate for small anal margin cancers.
- Chemo-irradiation is the treatment of choice for most anal squamous carcinomas.

Upper gastrointestinal cancer

Oesophageal cancer

Incidence and aetiology

- Carcinoma of the oesophagus is the eighth commonest cancer in Western countries.
- Accounts for approximately 5% of cancer-related deaths in Western countries.
- Incidence increases with age, with an 8-fold increase between the age ranges 45–54 years and 65–74 years.
- Is approximately 2.5 times as common in males compared with females.
- Significant change in the incidence of the two most common histological subtypes over the past half century.
- There has been a striking rise in incidence of adenocarcinoma of the lower oesophagus and gastro-oesophageal junction, and this is now the most common subtype in the UK.
- Aetiological factors vary with geographical region and with histological subtype.
- Risk factors for squamous cell carcinomas include smoking, excess alcohol consumption, dietary factors, betel-nut chewing, achalasia, Plummer–Vinson's syndrome, and tylosis palmaris.
- Risk factors for adenocarcinomas include gastro-oesophageal reflux disease, Barrett's oesophagus (especially high-grade dysplasia), obesity, and dietary factors.

Diagnosis and staging

- Early symptoms may be subtle and non-specific.
- Common clinical presentations include dysphagia, weight loss, anorexia, retro-sternal discomfort, odynophagia, regurgitation of food, anaemia.
- Endoscopy and biopsy are the diagnostic investigations of choice.
- Staging investigations may include computerized tomography (CT) scanning, endo-oesophageal ultrasound (EUS), positron emission tomography (PET) scanning, bronchoscopy, and laparoscopy.
- CT scanning can detect distant metastatic disease and also local infiltration of adjacent structures, including the aorta and trachea.
- EUS can give more accurate regional TNM staging, particularly in detecting lymph node metastases.
- PET with ^{18}F-fluorodeoxyglucose can improve detection of distant metastases.
- Laparoscopy is important for patients with lower oesophageal or gastro-oesophageal adenocarcinomas, to detect peritoneal, liver, and coeliac lymph node metastases.
- Bronchoscopy may be necessary in addition to CT scanning and EUS to clarify if there is involvement of the trachea or main bronchi by tumour.
- Staging follows the TNM system (see Table 18.1).

Table 18.1 TNM staging of oesophageal cancer

T: primary tumour

Tx	Primary tumour cannot be assessed
T0	No evidence of primary tumour
Tis	Carcinoma *in situ*
T1	Tumour invades lamina propria or submucosa
T2	Tumour invades muscularis propria
T3	Tumour invades adventitia
T4	Tumour invades adjacent structures

N: regional lymph nodes

Nx	Regional lymph nodes cannot be assessed
N0	No regional lymph node metastases
N1	Regional lymph node metastases

M: distant metastases

Mx	Distant metastases cannot be assessed
M0	No distant metastases
M1	Distant metastases

For tumours of the lower thoracic oesophagus

M1a	Metastases in coeliac lymph nodes
M1b	Other distant metastases

For tumours of the mid-thoracic oesophagus

M1a	Not applicable
M1b	Non-regional lymph node metastases, or other distant metastases

For tumours of the upper thoracic oesophagus

M1a	Metastases in the cervical lymph nodes
M1b	Other distant metastases

Stage grouping

Stage 0	Tis	N0	M0
Stage I	T1	N0	M0
Stage IIA	T2	N0	M0
	T3	N0	M0
Stage IIB	T1	N1	M0
	T2	N1	M0
Stage III	T3	N1	M0
	T4	Any N	M0
Stage IVA	Any T	Any N	M1a
Stage IVB	Any T	Any N	M1b

Treatment

- A multidisciplinary team approach including surgeons, gastroenterologists, radiologists, oncologists, pathologists, dieticians, and specialist nurses, is recommended.

Resectable tumours

- Operative mortality is now less in specialized centres (5%).
- Surgical approaches include trans-thoracic oesophagectomy and trans-hiatal oesophagectomy (often reserved for less fit patients).
- Minimally invasive oesophagectomy is practised in selected centres but is not yet in widespread use – there is a steep learning curve. Post-operative recovery may be faster but complications are significant in early studies. One recent study (2008) reported a mortality of 1% but almost 50% complication rate. Mean disease-free survival was 33 months.
- Post-operative adjuvant therapy is difficult to deliver after major oesophageal surgery.
- Neither chemotherapy, radiotherapy, or chemo-radiotherapy has a survival advantage when administered post-operatively.
- The UK MRC OE02 study (n = 802 patients) demonstrated a significantly greater overall survival for patients who received two courses of pre-operative chemotherapy with cisplatin (80 mg/m^2 on day 1) and 5-FU (1 g/m^2/day) by continuous infusion (days 1–4) at 3-week intervals compared with surgery alone.
- Median survival was significantly improved with pre-operative chemotherapy (16.8 months) compared with surgery alone (13.3 months).
- There was no increase in peri-operative morbidity and mortality in patients treated with pre-operative chemotherapy.

Locally advanced unresectable disease

- Combined modality approaches incorporating cisplatin-based chemotherapy in addition to radiation are superior to radiotherapy alone for patients with locally advanced oesophageal cancer.
- Combined modality treatment results in a significantly better median survival (14 months) compared with radiotherapy alone (9.3 months), and a significantly better 5-year survival (26% versus 0%).

Metastatic disease

- Many patients have metastatic disease at presentation or develop metastases after treatment for localized disease.
- The combination of cisplatin and 5-FU is one of the most commonly used regimens for advanced disease.
- Epirubicin in addition to cisplatin and 5-FU in the ECF schedule has been the standard in the UK for adenocarcinomas of the oesophagus or gastro-oesophageal junction.
- Other methods of treatment may be required to palliate the symptoms of local disease, including palliative radiotherapy, endoscopic stenting, and laser therapy.

Further reading

Bancewicz J, Clark PI, Smith DB, *et al.* (2002) Surgical resection with or without preoperative chemotherapy in oesophageal cancer: a randomised controlled trial. *Lancet* **259**, 1727–33.

Berrisford RG, Wajed SA, Sanders D (2008) Short term outcomes following totally minimally invasive oesophagectomy. *Br J Surg* **95**, 602–10.

Herskovic A, Martz K, al-Sarraf M, *et al.* (1992) Combined chemotherapy and radiotherapy compared with radiotherapy alone in patients with cancer of the oesophagus. *N Engl J Med* **326**, 1593–8.

Law S, Wong J (2005) Current management of oesophageal cancer. *J Gastrointest Surg* **9**, 291–310.

Mariette C, Piessen G, Triboulet J-P (2007) Therapeutic strategies in oesophageal carcinoma: role of surgery and other modalities. *Lancet Oncol* **8**, 545–53.

Ott K, Lordick F, Molls M (2009) Limited resections and free jejunal graft interposition for squamous cell carcinoma of the cervical oesophagus. *Br J Surg* **96**, 258–60.

Patterson-Brown S (2007) Surgical volume and clinical outcome. *Br J Surg* **94**, 523–4.

Gastric cancer

Incidence and aetiology

- The second commonest cause of death from cancer worldwide.
- Almost 10 000 deaths per year in the UK.
- Significant rise in Western countries in gastro-oesophageal junction and proximal stomach cancers.
- *Helicobacter pylori* infection is associated with a 3–8-fold increase in incidence of gastric cancer.
- Barrett's oesophagus has been associated with an increase in gastro-oesophageal junction tumours.
- Other risk factors include reduced gastric acid production (e.g. as in pernicious anaemia, previous gastric surgery), infection with Epstein–Barr virus, and dietary factors.

Diagnosis and staging

- The most common clinical manifestations include weight loss, anorexia, abdominal discomfort, indigestion, anaemia, early satiety, nausea and vomiting.
- The majority of gastric tumours (>90%) are adenocarcinomas, which are further divided into intestinal and diffuse types.
- Diagnosis is usually by endoscopy and biopsy.
- Staging investigations include CT scanning, endoscopic ultrasound (EUS), and laparoscopy.
- Laparoscopy, with cytological assessment of peritoneal cavity washings, is recommended to detect peritoneal metastases, and also allows assessment of direct fixation of tumour to adjacent structures.
- Staging follows the TNM system (see Table 18.2).

Treatment

Operable disease

- Surgical resection can give long-term survival in patients who have a complete macroscopic and microscopic tumour clearance (Ro resection).
- Best results are achieved in patients with T1N0 or T1N1 tumours; 70% of such patients are alive at 5 years. However, under 5% present with T1 tumours. Hospital mortality should be less than 5% in specialized centres.
- Type of operation will depend on the site of the tumour; oesophago-gastrectomy may be required for cancers of the oesophago-gastric junction (OGJ) and proximal stomach, total gastrectomy for mid-gastric tumours, and partial gastrectomy may be adequate treatment for tumours in the distal stomach.

Table 18.2 TNM staging of gastric cancer

T: primary tumour	
Tx	Primary tumour cannot be assessed
T0	No evidence of primary tumour
Tis	Carcinoma *in situ*: intra-epithelial tumour with invasion of the lamina propria
T1	Tumour invades lamina propria or submucosa
T2	Tumour invades muscularis propria or subserosa
T2a	Tumour invades muscularis propria
T2b	Tumour invades subserosa
T3	Tumour penetrates serosa without invasion of adjacent structures
T4	Tumour invades adjacent structures
N: regional lymph nodes	
Nx	Regional lymph nodes cannot be assessed
N0	No regional lymph node metastases
N1	Metastases in 1–6 regional lymph nodes
N2	Metastases in 7–15 regional lymph nodes
N3	Metastases in more than 15 regional lymph nodes
M: distant metastases	
Mx	Distant metastases cannot be assessed
M0	No distant metastases
M1	Distant metastases

Stage grouping

Stage 0	Tis	N0	M0
Stage IA	T1	N0	M0
Stage IB	T1	N1	M0
	T2a/b	N0	M0
Stage II	T1	N2	M0
	T2a/b	N1	M0
	T3	N0	M0
Stage IIIA	T2a/b	N2	M0
	T3	N1	M0
	T4	N0	M0
Stage IIIB	T3	N2	M0
Stage IV	T4	N1/N2/N3	M0
	T1/T2/T3	N3	M0
	Any T	Any N	M1

- In Japan, patients routinely undergo extensive lymphadenectomy, whereas in Western countries most patients have more limited lymph node resection. Medical Research Council (MRC) and Dutch studies have compared R1 dissection (lymph nodes within 3 cm of the tumour) to R2 dissection (more extensive lymphadenectomy). In both studies post-operative mortality was significantly higher with R2 resection and no survival advantage has been observed. Consequently, R2 resection is not used as standard treatment at present.
- Minimally invasive gastrectomy is *not* widely practised.
- Limited gastric resection may be suitable for selected patients with early gastric cancer (EGC). A few Japanese centres are performing endoscopic mucosal resection of EGC. Recent data from Japan have shown that pylorus-preserving gastrectomy in over 600 patients is safe (no deaths, 3% major complications) with 5-year survival of 96% in EGC.
- Non-randomized series from Japan have shown that extended lymphadenectomy (D2 resection) improves disease-free survival in selected patients compared to historical controls; this has not been shown in European studies.
- Several adjuvant chemotherapy studies have used a number of regimens, and only one small study has shown an improved survival. A meta-analysis of over 2000 patients treated in adjuvant chemotherapy trials concluded that there was no survival benefit.
- Post-operative radiation, combined with concurrent 5-fluorouracil (5-FU)-based chemotherapy, can improve the 3-year overall survival rate (50%) compared with surgery alone (41%).
- The standard of care in the UK is peri-operative ECF chemotherapy, based on the results of the MAGIC (MRC Adjuvant Gastric Infusional Chemotherapy) study. Peri-operative chemotherapy yielded a statistically significant improvement in progression-free and overall survival (5-year survival 36% versus 23%).

Advanced (inoperable) disease
- Most patients in Western countries have locally advanced (inoperable) or metastatic disease at presentation.
- Combination chemotherapy regimens can improve survival in advanced disease compared with best supportive care.
- Recently, a randomized trial in the UK has compared four regimens in advanced gastric cancer in a 2 × 2 design. Capecitabine was equivalent to infusional 5-FU. The combination of epirubicin, oxaliplatin, and capecitabine gave a further improvement in overall survival, and it is likely that oxaliplatin will be increasingly used in the UK in the future.
- Other agents with activity in advanced gastric cancer include etoposide, irinotecan, and the taxanes (e.g. docetaxel).
- The addition of docetaxel to cisplatin and 5-fluorouracil improves overall survival compared with cisplatin and 5-fluorouracil. However, this regime is also associated with significant increase in toxicity.

- Current developments are exploring the use of molecularly-targeted therapies.
- Patients with dysphagia from inoperable tumours of the OGJ and cardia may benefit from the insertion of rigid or expandable metal stents. Bleeding from intraluminal tumours can be reduced by ablation of the tumour with endoscopic laser treatment. There remains a role for palliative surgery to bypass gastric outlet obstruction (increasingly via the laparoscope). Palliative bypass with gastrojejunostomy for malignant gastric outlet obstruction is not always successful – mortality can be as high as one-third in some series, and 20% of patients post-operatively cannot tolerate a normal diet.

Further reading

Allum WH (2008) Gastric cancer in Europe. *Br J Surg* **95**, 406–408.

Cunningham D, Allum W, Stenning S, *et al.* (2006) Perioperative chemotherapy versus surgery alone for resectable gastroesophageal cancer. *N Engl J Med* **355**, 11–20.

Cunningham D, Starling N, Rao S, *et al.* (2008) Capecitabine and oxaliplatin for advanced esophagogastric cancer. *N Engl J Med* **358**, 36–46.

Dicken BJ, Bigam DL, Cass C, *et al.* (2005) Gastric adenocarcinoma – review and considerations for future directions. *Ann Surg* **241**, 27–39.

MacDonald JS, Smalley SR, Benedetti J, *et al.* (2001) Chemoradiotherapy after surgery compared with surgery alone for adenocarcinoma of the stomach or gastro-oesophageal junction. *N Engl J Med* **345**, 725–30.

Medino-Franco H, Abarco-Perez C, Espana-Gomez N, *et al.* (2007) Morbidity-associated factors after gastrojejunostomy for malignant gastric outlet obstruction. *Am Surg* **73**, 871–5.

Morita S, Katai H, Saka M, *et al.* (2008) Outcome of pylorus-preserving gastrectomy for early gastric cancer. *Br J Surg* **95**, 1131–5.

Saidi RF, ReMine SG, Dudrick S, *et al.* (2006). Is there a role for palliative gastrectomy in patients with Stage IV gastric cancer? *World J Surg* **30**, 21–7.

Webb A, Cunningham D, Scarffe H, *et al.* (1997) Randomised trial comparing epirubicin, cisplatin and fluorouracil versus fluorouracil, doxorubicin and methotrexate in advanced oesophagogastric cancer. *J Clin Oncol* **15**, 261–7.

Cancers of the small intestine

Incidence and pathology
- Account for less than 10% of all gastrointestinal (GI) tumours.
- Approximately 65% of all small bowel tumours are malignant.
- Adenocarcinomas constitute 40% of all malignant small bowel tumours.
- Carcinoid tumours make up 30% of all small bowel malignant tumours.
- Increased risk associated with Peutz–Jeghers syndrome and with von Recklinghausen's neurofibromatosis.

Adenocarcinoma
- Same staging system as for colon cancers is usually used.
- Patients with a primary small bowel carcinoma should be monitored for the development of a second malignant tumour, most commonly in the colon.
- Most commonly (80%) arise in the proximal small bowel.
- Clinical presentations most frequently include abdominal pain, anaemia, and jaundice (due to biliary obstruction).

Carcinoid tumours
- Approximately 90% of small bowel carcinoid tumours arise in the ileum and appendix.
- Tumours with metastatic potential are invariably >2cm in diameter.
- An intense desmoplastic reaction around the primary tumour can lead to small bowel obstruction.
- The 'carcinoid syndrome', due to the secretion of vasoactive amines, occurs in about 5–15% of patients.
- Clinical manifestations of the carcinoid syndrome including flushing, diarrhoea, bronchial constriction, and right-sided valvular heart disease.

Lymphoma
- Primary small bowel lymphoma represents approximately 1% of all GI malignancies.
- Are usually of intermediate or high grade.

Treatment
Adenocarcinoma
- Surgical resection is the treatment of choice for operable small bowel tumours.
- 5-year survival after resection of small bowel adenocarcinomas is approximately 65%.
- Laparoscopic small bowel resection for tumour is not yet widely practised.
- Few trials of chemotherapy have been performed due to the relative rarity of this disease.
- The regimens most frequently used are based around 5-FU.
- Adjuvant chemotherapy regimens and the use of chemotherapy for inoperable disease are usually similar to the treatment principles of colon cancer.

Carcinoid tumours
- Operable disease is resected where possible, along with local node excision.
- Somatostatin analogues are effective in controlling symptoms in patients with the carcinoid syndrome.
- Combination chemotherapy regimens are usually favoured for the management of faster-growing disease, aggressive and atypical carcinoid tumours.
- Radionuclide therapy, e.g. with ^{131}I-MIBG (meta-iodobenzylguanidine), is of increasing interest in patients with a positive tracer scan.
- Hepatic artery embolization may be used to palliate painful, refractory liver metastases.

Further reading

Landry CS, McMasters KM, Scoggins CR (2008) Proposed staging system for gastrointestinal carcinoid tumours. *Am Surg* **74**, 418–22.
Robertson RG, Geiger WJ, Davis NB (2006) Carcinoid tumours. *Am Fam Physician* **74**, 429–34.

Cancer of the pancreas

Incidence and aetiology

- Around 7000 new cases per year diagnosed in the UK.
- Fourth commonest cause of cancer-related deaths, accounting for approximately 5% of all cancer deaths in the UK.
- Associated with smoking, and with dietary factors including high consumption of saturated fats.
- Increased risk of developing pancreatic cancer for patients with chronic pancreatitis.
- Familial syndromes associated with an increased risk of pancreatic cancer including hereditary non-polyposis colon cancer, the familial atypical mole/malignant melanoma syndrome, hereditary pancreatitis, familial adenomatous polyposis, and familial breast/ovarian cancer syndrome associated with *BRCA2* mutations.

Diagnosis, pathology, and staging

- The majority of pancreatic cancers are ductal adenocarcinomas (90%).
- Approximately 75% arise in the head of the pancreas, 15% in the body, and 10% in the tail.
- Clinical manifestations depend on the anatomical location of the primary tumour. The classical presentation of carcinomas arising in the head of the pancreas is with obstructive jaundice, often in association with weight loss, anorexia, and abdominal pain radiating through to the back.
- Investigations may include CT scanning. Endoscopic retrograde cholangiopancreatography (ERCP) (if there is obstructive jaundice), EUS, laparoscopy.
- EUS can give additional information on the relationship of the pancreatic mass to vascular anatomy prior to surgical resection, and can also allow fine needle aspiration (FNA) of the pancreatic mass to establish a cytological diagnosis.
- Laparoscopy is used to detect small deposits that are not visualized by conventional imaging techniques in patients who are potentially candidates for surgical resection.
- Staging is according to the TNM classification (see Table 18.3).

Treatment – exocrine pancreas cancer

Resectable disease

- Resection is possible in only 10–15% of cases.
- Outcome is related to hospital volume, with operative mortality of <2% in high-volume centres.
- Whipple's procedure is the most common surgical management for resectable disease (with/without pylorus preservation).

Surgical resection is the only chance of cure, but survival remains poor after surgery alone: median survival is 13–18 months, 5-year survival of 10–20%. Current trend is away from total pancreatectomy. Pylorus-preserving pancreatectomy decreases the long-term sequelae and the role of extended radical pancreatectomy is now limited. A trial from Johns Hopkins, published in 2000, showed no advantage in morbidity (2%) nor in survival (5-year survival, 7%). Pylorus-preserving pancreaticoduodenectomy is now the preferred option with fewer side-effects and equal survival data.

Table 18.3 TNM staging of exocrine pancreatic cancer

T: primary tumour

Tx	Primary tumour cannot be assessed
T0	No evidence of primary tumour
Tis	Carcinoma *in situ* (including pancreatic intra-epithelial neoplasia III)
T1	Tumour limited to the pancreas, <2 cm in greatest dimension
T2	Tumour limited to the pancreas, >2 cm in greatest dimension
T3	Tumour extends beyond the pancreas, but without involvement of the celiac axis or the superior mesenteric artery
T4	Tumour involves the coeliac axis or the superior mesenteric artery (unresectable)

N: regional lymph nodes

Nx	Regional lymph nodes cannot be assessed
N0	No regional lymph node metastases
N1	Regional lymph node metastases

M: distant metastases

Mx	Distant metastases cannot be assessed
M0	No distant metastases
M1	Distant metastases

Stage grouping

Stage 0	Tis	N0	M0
Stage 1A	T1	N0	M0
Stage IB	T2	N0	M0
Stage IIA	T3	N0	M0
Stage IIB	T2	N1	M0
Stage III	T4	N0	M0
Stage IV	Any T	Any N	M1

- In selected patients, vascular resection and reconstruction are appropriate.
- A few centres in Europe suggest resection of involved caval nodes is beneficial but this has not achieved widespread acceptance.
- The role of laparoscopic resection for pancreatic cancer is unclear, but technically is feasible.
- Post-operative complications include bronchopneumonia, pancreatic fistulae, sepsis, abscess and haemorrhage – but the mortality rate is less than 8% in specialist centres (some centres 2%).

- The ESPAC-1 (European Randomized Adjuvant Study Comparing Radiotherapy, 6 Months Chemotherapy and Combination Therapy versus Observation in Pancreatic Cancer) trial demonstrated a significant benefit from the use of adjuvant (post-operative), chemotherapy using six cycles of 5-FU and folinic acid administered in a modified Mayo clinic schedule.
- The benefits of post-operative chemotherapy have been confirmed in a subsequent meta-analysis of five randomized controlled trials.

Localized unresectable disease
- Combined modality treatment with chemo-radiotherapy is commonly used, but more so in North America than in the UK.
- Two randomized studies have consistently shown that 5-FU-based chemoradiation has a survival advantage compared to radiotherapy alone.

Advanced disease

- Gemcitabine is an accepted standard of care for palliation of patients with advanced disease who have adequate performance status. Gemcitabine has a superior clinical benefit response (24%) compared to 5-fluorouracil (4%) and a modest, but significant, improvement in median overall survival (5.65 months versus 4.41 months), and in 1-year survival (18% versus 2%) compared with 5-fluorouracil.
- The addition of erlotinib, an epidermal growth factor receptor (EGFR) tyrosine kinase inhibitor, to gemcitabine resulted in a statistically significant improvement in overall survival compared with gemcitabine.
- Many patients with advanced disease are not fit enough for palliative chemotherapy.
- Palliation includes pain control, nutritional support, and palliative stenting for biliary obstruction.

Further reading

Baxter NN, Whitson BA, Tuttle TM (2007) Trends in the treatment and outcome of pancreatic cancer in United States. *Ann Surg Oncol* **14**, 1320–6.

Burris HA 3rd, Moore MJ, Andersen J, et al. (1997) Improvements in survival and clinical benefit with gemcitabine as first-line therapy for patients with advanced pancreatic cancer: a randomized trial. *J Clin Oncol* **15**, 2403–13.

Iqbal N, Lovegrove RE, Tilney HS, et al. (2008) A comparison of pancreaticoduodenectomy with extended pancreaticoduodenectomy – a meta analysis of 1909 patients. *Eur J Surg Oncol* **35**, 79–86.

Kleeff J, Michalski CW, Friess H, et al. (2007) Surgical treatment of pancreatic cancer – the role of adjuvant and multimodal therapies. *Eur J Surg Oncol*, **33**, 817–23.

Moore MJ, Goldstein D, Hamm J, et al. (2007) Erlotinib plus gemcitabine compared with gemcitabine alone in patients with advanced pancreatic cancer: a phase III trial of the National Cancer Institute of Canada Clinical Trials Group. *J Clin Oncol* **25**, 1960–6.

Neoptolemos JP, Stocken DD, Friess H, et al. (2004) A randomized trial of chemoradiotherapy and chemotherapy after resection of pancreatic cancer. *N Engl J Med* **350**, 1200–10.

Cancer of the biliary tract and gall bladder

Incidence and aetiology

- Accounts for approximately 3% of all GI cancers worldwide.
- There is a geographical variation in incidence, with high-risk areas including north-east Thailand, Japan, Korea, and Eastern Europe.
- In Western countries, the most frequent predisposing factor is primary sclerosing cholangitis (lifetime risk of 9–23%).
- Other risk factors include industrial toxins (dioxin, polyvinylchloride), chronic infection with liver flukes, hepatolithiasis, hepatitis C, smoking, alcohol consumption, and anatomical factors such as choledochal cysts and abnormal pancreatico-biliary duct junction.

Diagnosis, pathology, and staging

- The most common tumours are adenocarcinomas.
- Presenting clinical signs vary with the anatomical location of the primary tumour and include obstructive jaundice, pruritis, and abdominal pain, while weight loss and anorexia usually occur later for bile duct tumours. Gall bladder cancers usually present with pain, anorexia, weight loss and jaundice.
- Investigations include ultra-sound scan, CT scanning, and ERCP. For bile duct cancers, magnetic resonance imaging (MRI) is useful to determine the extent of invasion into hepatic parenchyma, local lymph node involvement, and vascular involvement.
- The Bismuth classification is a commonly used surgical classification of biliary tumours. The TNM system is used for extra-hepatic bile duct cancer and for gall bladder cancers.

Treatment

Bile duct cancer

- Surgical resection is the only potentially curative treatment. However, most patients (approximately 80%) present with inoperable disease.
- Should be resected if there are no distant metastases and no irreparable involvement of the hepatic artery and portal vein.
- The results of surgery are good, with microscopically curative resections possible in over 75% of the patients, and 5-year survival of approximately 50% in the best series.
- The resectability rate of hilar cholangiocarcinoma is 15–33% in the West, while in Japan it is 52–92%. Usually hilar tumours require resection also of the adjacent caudate lobe (frequently involved in tumour). Resection of a short segment of the portal vein is feasible.
- For cholangiocarcinoma of the distal common bile duct, usually a pylorus-preserving Whipple procedure is performed.
- There is no proven benefit to adjuvant chemotherapy or radiotherapy, and adjuvant therapy is not recommended outside of a clinical trial.
- Palliation includes endoscopic or percutaneous biliary stenting, and palliative chemotherapy. Gemcitabine monotherapy is the most commonly used chemotherapy regimen in the UK, and combination studies of gemcitabine with cisplatin are ongoing.

Gall bladder cancers
- If an unsuspected gall bladder carcinoma is found on histological assessment after cholecystectomy, a second, radical, surgical procedure should be performed for T2 tumours.
- Radical resection is the only chance of cure for patients in whom a diagnosis of gall bladder cancer has been made on imaging.
- Prophylactic surgery should be considered in patients with a porcelain gall bladder (25% have cancer) and patients with polyps over 1 cm in size (risk of malignancy is significant).
- Should be treated with radical surgery (resection of segments 4 and 5, bile duct, and lymphadenectomy). Laparoscopic port site recurrences may be as high as 15–20%.
- For unresectable tumours, surgical or radiological biliary drainage is performed according to the same principles as for the palliative treatment of cholangiocarcinoma.
- Palliative treatment of inoperable disease includes chemotherapy. Activity has been observed with gemcitabine monotherapy, and with a combination of cisplatin plus 5-FU (with or without epirubicin).

Outcome

The 5-year survival rate for stage I tumours is 90% and for stage II tumours is 80%. The results of surgery for more advanced disease have improved in centres performing very extensive resections, where a 5-year survival rate of 40% for stage III tumours has been obtained.

Further reading

Borg CM, Benjamin IS (2007) Malignant lesions of the biliary tract. In: Garden OJ, ed. *Hepatobiliary and Pancreatic Surgery*, 3rd edn. Philadelphia: Saunders Elsevier, pp. 219–48.

Hepatocellular carcinoma

Incidence and aetiology

- Fifth most common cancer worldwide.
- More than 500 000 cases diagnosed annually worldwide.
- Highest incidence (over 100 cases per 100 000 people) is in parts of Southern Africa and the Far East.
- Incidence is increasing in Europe and North America.
- More than 80% of cases arise in patients with cirrhosis of the liver.
- Risk factors include infection with hepatitis B (especially in Africa and Asia), infection with hepatitis C, ingestion of aflatoxin B1 from contaminated food, alcohol-induced liver disease, and haemochromatosis.

Diagnosis and staging

- Diagnosis is by FNA biopsy or by non-cytological means using criteria as defined by EASL (European Association for the Study of the Liver) or AASLD (American Association for the Study of Liver Diseases).
- Staging includes anatomical staging by CT and or MRI scanning to determine the size, number and location of the hepatic tumour(s), vascular involvement, portal vein involvement by tumour, and/or thrombus, and the presence of extra-hepatic disease.
- Staging also includes assessment of the synthetic function of the liver, as the degree of impairment of liver function, invariably due to the pre-disposing non-malignant liver disease, may influence treatment decisions.

Treatment

- Liver resection with a clearance of 1 cm (recent data show less clearance gives equal results) is the treatment of choice for patients with hepatocellular carcinoma (HCC) in the absence of cirrhosis and if the tumour is resectable.
- Most common reasons for irresectability are bilobar or multifocal disease and liver failure associated with cirrhosis.
- Resection of small tumours (<2 cm T1) produced 70% 5-year survival in one large series of 318 patients. Operative mortality in experienced hands should be less than 5%.
- Multicentric tumours are most common in patients with cirrhosis, and resection of the primary tumour may leave other undetected deposits.
- The limitations of hepatic resection due to compromised liver function in patients with cirrhosis can be overcome by transplantation using standard selection criteria.
- However, surgery can only be performed in about 15% of patients, and the 5-year survival is only approximately 33–50% after potentially curative resection in the West. However 5-year survival of 70% has been reported in Japan.
- There are, as yet, no convincing data from large randomized trials to recommend any adjuvant therapy after surgical resection.

- Percutaneous ablative therapies, including percutaneous ethanol injection (PEI) or radiofrequency ablation (RFA), have been used in early unresectable HCC.
- Two out of seven randomized controlled trials have shown a survival benefit for trans-arterial chemo-embolization (TACE) compared with conservative management, confirmed by a meta-analysis of these seven studies.
- Most patients are not suitable for surgery, percutaneous ablation or TACE, or develop progressive disease after these interventions.
- The multi-targeted tyrosine kinase inhibitor, sorafenib, significantly improves median overall survival
- Sorafenib is a new standard of care in advanced HCC. Other targeted therapies are currently being evaluated.

Further reading

Capussotti L, Ferrero A, Vigano L, *et al.* (2009) Liver resection for HCC with cirrhosis. *Eur J Surg Oncol* **35**, 11–15.

Llovet JM, Burroughs A, Bruix J (2003) Hepatocellular carcinoma. *Lancet* **362**, 1907–17.

Llovet JM, Ricci S, Mazzaferro V, *et al.* (2008) Sorafenib in advanced hepatocellular carcinoma. *N Engl J Med* **359**, 378–90.

Roxburgh P, Evans TRJ (2008) Systemic therapy of hepatocellular carcinoma: are we making progress? *AdvTher* **25**, 1089–104.

Shimada K, Sakamoto Y, Esaki M (2007) Analysis of prognostic factors affecting survival after initial recurrence and treatment efficacy for recurrence in patients undergoing potentially curative hepatectomy for hepatocellular carcinoma. *Ann Surg Oncol* **14**, 2337–47.

Van Dam RM, Hendry PO, Coolsen MME, *et al.* (2008) Initial experience with a multimodal enhanced recovery programme in patients undergoing liver resection. *Br J Surg* **95**, 969–75.

Gastrointestinal stromal tumours

These are rare tumours, incidence 10–20 per million, of which 20–30% are malignant. It is now recognized that they are the commonest GI sarcomas, the majority arising in the stomach, but around one-third originate in small bowel, and a few in large bowel, omentum, or the oesophagus.

Their particular interest is that the majority have a gain of function mutation in the *KIT* proto-oncogene, which can be demonstrated by immunohistochemistry using CD117. This has led to the rational development of targeted therapy using the tyrosine kinase inhibitor imatinib. Previous attempts to treat these tumours with 'sarcoma chemotherapy' such as doxorubicin or ifosfamide had been unsuccessful with response rates <10%.

Epidemiology and aetiology
- Median age 60 years
- Male:female 1:1
- Vast majority sporadic
- No known risk factors
- Rarely familial with germline mutation of *KIT* and multiple GI stromal tumours.

Pathology and natural history
- Spindle cell tumour, previously mistaken for leiomyosarcoma
- Difficult to grade or predict behaviour according to pathology
- Typically grow parallel to the lumen of the stomach/bowel
- May ulcerate overlying mucosa
- May grow very large without dissemination
- Present with abdominal fullness, bleeding/anaemia, obstruction
- High risk of local recurrence after surgery
- Rarely spread beyond the abdomen
- Metastasis to liver and peritoneum
- Endoscopic ultrasound FNA gives good diagnostic accuracy for gastric stromal tumours.

Treatment
- Surgery is the best treatment for non-metastatic disease. Laparoscopic resection for intermediate-sized gastric stromal tumours is safe in experienced hands.
- Surgery should also be considered for local recurrence and for resectable metastatic disease, e.g. in liver:
  - median disease-free survival after resection of primary tumour is 5 years.
- Unresectable/advanced disease is treated with imatinib:
  - 50% demonstrate objective response, and a further 20–30% stable disease.
- >50% progression-free survival after two years of therapy.
- In some patients, disease progression may be reversed by increasing the imatinib dose.
- Role of imatinib in adjuvant therapy currently being explored in clinical trials.

Further reading

Okubo K, Yamao K, Nakamura T (2004) Endoscopic ultrasound-guided fine needle aspiration biopsy for the diagnosis of gastrointestinal stromal tumours in the stomach. *J Gastroenterol* **39**, 747–53.

Robin BP, Heinrick MC, Conless CC (2007) Gastrointestinal stromal tumour. *Lancet* **369**, 1731–41.

Chapter 19

Endocrine cancers

Thyroid cancer

Epidemiology and aetiology

- Thyroid cancer accounts for ~1% of all malignancies in the UK and 0.5% of all cancer deaths.
- In UK there are ~1800 new cases/year (2005 data-Office for National Statistics, published 2008).
- Female-to-male ratio is 3:1.
- Preponderance in 4th and 5th decades – median age of presentation is 47 years.
- Relatives of patients with thyroid cancer have a 10x ↑ risk.

Differentiated (papillary including follicular) carcinomas

- 70–75% of thyroid cancers are papillary carcinomas, i.e. differentiated epithelial tumours.
- The only well-established risk factor is previous head and neck irradiation, particularly in early childhood.
- ~5% have ≥1 affected first-degree relative.
- Few rare inherited syndromes, e.g. familial adenomatous polyposis, Gardner's syndrome.

Anaplastic (undifferentiated) carcinomas

- ~5% of all thyroid cancers.
- Typically in older population than that with differentiated tumours; mean age at presentation is 65 years. Females > males.
- >1 in 5 will have a previous history or co-existing diagnosis of differentiated carcinoma.
- Up to 50% have a history of multinodular goitre.

Medullary carcinoma

- 3–5% of all thyroid cancers.
- Typically in 5th–6th decades of life.
- Slight female preponderance only.
- 75% of cases are sporadic.
- 25% of cases are familial, tending to occur in younger age groups, i.e. 3rd decade. If there is more than one case within the family always consider the possibility of familial disease, e.g.:
  - multiple endocrine neoplasia (MEN) type 2a and b
  - isolated familial medullary thyroid cancer.

Pathology and genetics

Differentiated (papillary including follicular) carcinomas

- Typically unencapsulated ± cystic components.
- Papillae consisting of a few layers of tumour cells surrounding fibrovascular core. Follicles and colloid are usually absent.
- ~50% contain calcified psammoma bodies – scarred remnants of tumour papillae.
- >50% of sporadic cases have somatic gene rearrangements, e.g. of the *RET* oncogene → chimeric proteins with tyrosine kinase activity that contribute to the development of malignancy. No germline mutations identified so far.

Several histological subtypes, most of which are rare. Examples include:
- follicular variant:
  - most common subtype (~15%)
  - microscopically small to medium-sized follicles with near total absence of papillae
  - prone to haematogenous spread but less likely to show lymphatic invasion
- tall-cell variant:
  - ~1% of papillary cancers
  - more aggressive than common-type papillary tumours – higher incidence of local invasion and distant metastases at presentation.

Anaplastic (undifferentiated) carcinomas
- Undifferentiated tumour of the thyroid follicular epithelium

Medullary
- Unencapsulated neuroendocrine tumour arising from the parafollicular C-cells (the cell of origin of calcitonin).
- Variable histological appearances within a single tumour.
- 80% show amyloid deposition; 98% are calcitonin positive.
- MEN type 2 – autosomal, dominantly inherited syndromes arising from different mutations in the *RET* proto-oncogene.
  - MEN type 2a – 100% get medullary thyroid cancer, ~50% develop phaeochromocytomas, and ~30% get hyperplasia of the parathyroid glands
  - MEN type 2b – medullary carcinoma of the thyroid, which is often bilateral, more aggressive, and occurs at an earlier age. Also Marfanoid appearance, phaeochromocytomas but normal parathyroid hormone (PTH)
  - Familial medullary thyroid cancer – variant of MEN type 2a with similar high risk of medullary carcinoma without the other associated diseases.
- 50% of sporadic cases have somatic *RET* gene mutations too.

Other
- Lymphoma
- Metastases, e.g. from breast or colon cancer.

Screening and prevention

Medullary carcinoma

- Prophylactic thyroidectomy at an early age often appropriate if known carrier of predisposing gene mutation, e.g. in MEN 2.
- Screening with serum calcitonin:
  - problematic
  - supranormal serum calcitonin response to intravenous calcium suggests C-cell hyperplasia or overt medullary carcinoma but can get false positives, e.g. in autoimmune thyroid disease.
- Screening now usually by molecular analysis for germline *RET* gene mutations; ~7% of apparently 'sporadic' cases are also positive for germline mutations in the *RET* proto-oncogene, with significant implications for family members.

Presentation

Differentiated (papillary and follicular) carcinomas

- Incidental microcarcinomas (<1 cm) are a common finding at autopsy.
- Commonest clinical presentation is with a painless lump in the neck, i.e. solitary thyroid nodule.
- Clinical regional lymph node involvement at diagnosis more common in children (~50%) than in adults. However, occult nodal involvement in 40–90% of adults.
- 2–10% have disseminated disease at presentation, most commonly pulmonary or bony metastases.
- Most patients are clinically and biochemically euthyroid:
  - Graves's disease/toxic nodular goitre may co-exist
  - Carcinomas synthesizing functioning T3/T4 (tri-iodothyronine/ thyroxine) rare.

Anaplastic (undifferentiated) carcinoma

- Rapidly enlarging neck mass that may be painful.
- Confluent bilateral lymphadenopathy.
- 90% have regional or distant spread at diagnosis.
- Commonest sites of metastases are lungs and bones.
- ± Superior vena cava obstruction and/or Horner's syndrome.

Medullary carcinoma

- Painless lump in the neck, i.e. solitary thyroid nodule (>75%).
- Usually unilateral.
- 20% have locally advanced disease at presentation, e.g. symptoms of upper aerodigestive tract compression.
- ~50% have clinically detectable cervical lymph node involvement at diagnosis and 15% have distant metastases.
- Large tumours may have an associated paraneoplastic syndrome, e.g. Cushing's syndrome due to corticotrophin secretion.

Investigations

- Investigation of patients with suspected thyroid cancer, and their subsequent management, should be co-ordinated by a specialist multidisciplinary team with expertise and interest in the management of thyroid cancer.
- The team will usually comprise a surgeon, endocrinologist, oncologist, pathologist, radiologist, medical physicist, biochemist, specialist nurse.
- Depending on the clinical situation the following investigations may be considered:
  - full blood count and liver function tests
  - renal function: especially if considering iodine-131 therapy
  - thyroid function tests
  - calcitonin: produced by C-cells. Its role in the initial diagnostic evaluation of patients remains controversial due to the frequency of falsely high serum levels. Once a diagnosis of medullary carcinoma is confirmed, a baseline level will establish whether the tumour is capable of hypersecreting calcitonin to assist with post-operative monitoring
  - high-resolution thyroid ultrasonography and fine needle aspiration (FNA): false-negative rate varies from 0% to 5% and the false positive rate is also usually <5%. Note: FNA cannot distinguish follicular adenoma from follicular carcinoma; if FNA report states 'follicular lesion' then at least a thyroid lobectomy is essential. FNA, in the hands of an experienced cytologist, can diagnose papillary, medullary, and anaplastic cancer.
- If high risk of local disease extension (e.g. presentation with hoarseness, stridor, dysphagia, or haemoptysis) consider:
  - computerized tomography (CT) scan neck/mediastinum – assess for laryngeal involvement, invasion of the great vessels, etc.
  - magnetic resonance imaging (MRI) scan neck – evaluate any soft tissue invasion
  - CT chest/liver
  - skeletal scintigraphy – if there is any suspicion of bony disease. The typical appearances are lytic lesions.

Staging

Differentiated (papillary) carcinomas

The staging system for differentiated carcinoma of the thyroid is based on the 'TNM system':

- **T,** primary tumour. Generally reflects the size of the tumour invasion beyond the thyroid capsule (T4)
- **N,** involvement of regional lymph nodes
- **M,** absence (0) or presence (1) of distant metastases or inability to assess for their presence (X).

The American Joint Committee on Cancer staging system from 2002 is given as an example (see Tables 19.1 and 19.2).

Anaplastic (undifferentiated) cancer

These tumours have a very poor prognosis – all are effectively stage IV.

Medullary carcinoma

Staging system based on:
- tumour size
- local invasion
- nodal disease
- metastases.

Unlike in differentiated thyroid cancer, age is not a factor in the staging of medullary thyroid cancer (see Table 19.3).

Table 19.1 AJCC TNM classification system for differentiated thyroid cancer

Primary tumour (T) classification

T1	Tumour diameter <2 cm
T2	Primary tumour diameter 2–4 cm
T3	Primary tumour diameter >4 cm limited to the thyroid or with minimal extrathyroid extension
T4a	Tumour of any size extending beyond the thyroid capsule to invade subcutaneous soft tissues, larynx, trachea, oesophagus, or recurrent laryngeal nerve
T4b	Tumour invades prevertebral fascia or encases carotid artery or mediastinal vessels
TX	Primary tumour size unknown but without extrathyroid invasion

Regional lymph nodes (N)

Nx	Nodes not assessed at surgery
N0	No regional lymph node metastases
N1a	Metastases to level VI (pretracheal, paratracheal, and prelaryngeal lymph nodes)
N1b	Metastases to unilateral, bilateral, contralateral cervical or superior mediastinal lymph nodes

Metastasis (M) classification

Mx	Unable to assess distant metastases
M0	No distant metastases
M1	Distant metastases

With permission from Edge SE, Byrd DR, Carducci MA, Compton CA, eds. AJCC Cancer Staging Manual, 7th ed. New York, NY: Springer, 2009.

Table 19.2 AJCC stage groupings for differentiated cancer of the thyroid

	Patient <45 years old	Patient ≥45 years old
Stage I	Any T, any N, M0	T1, N0, M0
Stage II	Any T, any N, M1	T2, N0, M0
Stage III		T3, N0, M0
		T1, N1a, M
		T2, N1a, M0
		T3, N1a, M0
Stage IV A		T4a, N0, M0
		T4a, N1a, M0
		T1, N1b, M0
		T2, N1b, M0
		T3, N1b, N0
		T4a, N1b, M0
Stage IV B		T4b, any N, M0
Stage IV C		Any T, any N, M1

With permission from Edge SE, Byrd DR, Carducci MA, Compton CA, eds. AJCC Cancer Staging Manual, 7th ed. New York, NY: Springer, 2009.

Table 19.3 Staging system for medullary carcinoma of the thyroid

Stage I	Primary tumour <1 cm with no evidence of disease outside the thyroid gland
Stage II	Primary tumour >1 cm or the presence of extrathyroidal invasion without nodal or distant metastases
Stage III	Local or regional nodal metastases
Stage IV	Distant metastases

Surgery for thyroid cancer

Differentiated (papillary) carcinomas

For the primary tumour (papillary, follicular)

- Surgery is the primary mode of treatment.
- The aim is to perform definitive surgery at the outset.
- At least, a total lobectomy must be performed on the side of the tumour with identification of the recurrent laryngeal nerve. Prognosis following incomplete surgery (e.g. removal of a suspicious nodule) and subsequent further surgery (e.g. completion thyroidectomy) may be less good than if a total thyroidectomy had been performed at the start.

Surgical options include:

Unilateral total lobectomy

- May be appropriate for selected low-risk patients, e.g. pT1 (<1 cm) N0 women <45 years old.

Total thyroidectomy

- The procedure of choice in most cases.
- Advantages include:
  - many papillary tumours are multicentric
  - up to 1 in 5 will recur after partial thyroidectomy
  - local recurrence is associated with a poor prognosis, with up to 40% risk of death from metastatic disease (others argue this can be treated with radioactive iodine)
  - small risk of progression to anaplastic carcinoma
  - subsequent monitoring for recurrence is easier (permits diagnostic/therapeutic radio-iodine scans)
  - up to 50% of completion thyroidectomies are tumour positive.

More extensive resection

- In pT4 tumours the options are:
  - extensive resection of all involved structures, e.g. larynx, oesophagus, with potential loss of organ function, or
  - conservative surgery with preservation of local structures but residual foci of disease followed by external beam radiotherapy.
- Rates of local control and disease-free survival are similar but quality of life appears better following the more conservative surgery.

Long-term data (30 years) from the Mayo Clinic show a 2% 30-year mortality irrespective of extent of surgery.

Those who argue for a total lobectomy (only) quote the increased risk of recurrent laryngeal nerve damage and hypocalcaemia after total thyroidectomy.

Frozen section is rarely used for the thyroid mass with good pre-operative fine needle cytology. However, there may be a role for intraoperative frozen section to investigate enlarged lymph nodes found at surgery.

Potential complications of thyroid surgery
- Hypoparathyroidism
- Recurrent laryngeal nerve injury → hoarse voice and 'bovine' cough (should be less than 1% in experienced hands)
- Superior laryngeal nerve injury → inability to reach higher registers with voice
- Follow-up with thyroglobulin (serum) measurement is standard for differentiated thyroid cancers.

Selective neck dissection

Extent of neck dissection should be dependent on:
- size of primary tumour, e.g. up to 80% of pT4 tumours will have regional nodal involvement at presentation
- clinical examination, e.g. presence of palpable nodes
- intra-operative findings, e.g. suspicious nodes at surgery ± histological examination of frozen section
- gross cervical metastatic disease should be treated with a modified radical neck dissection.

Recurrent or metastatic disease

- If there is metastatic disease at presentation, total thyroidectomy and ablation are usually still required because optimal management is based on the ability of most differentiated cancers to concentrate radioiodine.
- Re-excision can be considered for locally recurrent disease.
- Occasionally, resection may also be appropriate for a solitary metastatic deposit.
- Further surgery is usually followed by ^{131}I therapy ± external beam radiotherapy.

Anaplastic (undifferentiated) carcinomas

- Usually inoperable at presentation (50% have lung secondaries at presentation).
- If appears localized, surgery offers the best chance of a prolonged period of symptom-free survival. Total thyroidectomy may not produce any survival advantage over ipsilateral thyroid lobectomy with wide margins of adjacent soft tissue. This is rarely possible.

Medullary carcinoma

- Pre-operative screening for phaeochromocytoma (MEN type 2) and hyperparathyroidism with ↑Ca^{2+}(MEN type 2a).
- All patients should be treated by **total** thyroidectomy where possible because:
  - surgery is the only potentially curative intervention
  - 20% have intra-glandular lymphatic spread
  - 20% are *RET* oncogene positive even if the case is apparently 'sporadic'
  - hereditary background may not be known
  - radioactive iodine is not effective.

- Quality of lymph node dissection is paramount and appears to be the sole surgical factor that can improve prognosis. The size of the primary correlates with the chances of metastatic lymphatic spread:
  - <1 cm → 11–50%
  - >2 cm → 60%
  - Palpable tumour → 85%.
- Usually surgery involves total thyroidectomy, central and ipsilateral neck node dissection.
- In medullary thyroid cancer, involvement of central neck nodes is a strong pointer to involvement of ipsilateral lateral neck nodes (77%).
- Surgery with palliative intent can also produce long-term survivors, e.g. re-operation for local recurrence or even resection of solitary metastases.
- Screening for disseminated disease prior to further surgery should include laparoscopy to assess for liver metastases. Up to 20% of patients with no hepatic disease identified on conventional imaging will have liver secondaries seen at laparoscopy.
- All familial cases (frequently bilateral) must have total thyroidectomy.

There are a number of subgroups of well-differentiated thyroid cancer that are aggressive and require total thyroidectomy; these include tall-cell variant, columnar cell variant, insular carcinoma and Hurthle cell carcinoma.

Radioiodine treatment for thyroid cancer

^{131}I is used in the diagnosis and treatment of differentiated thyroid carcinoma for:
- ablation of residual thyroid tissue
- assessment of possible disease recurrence
- treatment of residual or recurrent disease.

Post-thyroidectomy there are typically up to 2 g of functioning thyroid remnant.

^{131}I is administered at doses sufficient to ablate residual thyroid tissue including microscopic foci of malignancy. This:
- reduces the risk of local recurrence by ~60% compared to thyroid suppression alone
- prolongs overall and disease-free survival
- is effective against microscopic disease only; it is not a treatment for macroscopic residual cancer
- increases the sensitivity and specificity of the subsequent screening programme to identify persistent or recurrent disease. Screening may be by:
  - monitoring changes in serum thyroglobulin (TG) levels (TG is secreted by normal and >90% of cancerous thyroid cells, so ablation of all active thyroid tissue should mean that TG is undetectable)
  - diagnostic ^{131}I scans.

Preparation for treatment with ^{131}I includes:
- total thyroidectomy approximately one month previously
- no thyroid hormone replacement, a low-iodine diet, and no iodine-containing medication, to maximize the chance of avid uptake of the iodine (NB beware the iodine load of CT contrast agents)
- confirm biochemically hypothyroid prior to administration (patient likely to be feeling unwell by this stage)
- explanation to the patient: they will be confined to a single room during their admission, interaction with nurses will be minimal, and visitors will be limited, etc.

Post-ablation diagnostic ^{131}I scans are performed to confirm the absence of residual active thyroid tissue. The serum TG level should become undetectable.

Potential acute toxicity of therapeutic ^{131}I treatment includes nausea, sialadenitis, radiation cystitis/gastritis. Very rarely it may precipitate haemorrhage into metastases.

Late effects include a persistent dry mouth, accelerated dental caries, and a very small risk of late second malignancies, particularly if repeated cycles of treatment have been necessary, e.g. leukaemias, salivary gland tumours.

Men should be offered sperm storage, particularly if repeated administrations are likely.

Replacement thyroid hormone therapy should be commenced following ablation of active glandular tissue.

The aim is for lifelong suppression of thyroid-stimulating hormone (TSH), i.e. the dose of exogenous hormone aims to maintain biochemical hyperthyroidism to avoid theoretical overstimulation of occult residual tissue.

Diagnostic ^{131}I scans can be repeated as part of post-treatment surveillance; >60% of differentiated thyroid cancers take up enough iodide to be detected by radioiodine imaging.

Treatment doses of ^{131}I can be repeated if:
- serum TG begins to rise
- further activity is observed on a diagnostic ^{131}I whole-body scan, indicating inoperable or metastatic disease, e.g. pulmonary metastases.

There is no role for ^{131}I treatment in medullary or anaplastic carcinoma – these tumours are not iodine avid.

External beam radiotherapy for thyroid cancer

Differentiated (papillary and follicular) carcinoma

Following complete resection

- Adjuvant external beam radiotherapy should be offered to selected patients whose tumours do not concentrate radioiodine.
- It should also be considered after surgery and ^{131}I therapy if:
  - the primary tumour is large (pT4)
  - there is extracapsular spread or lymph node involvement
  - there are other poor prognostic features (see 📖 p.371).
- A typical treatment regime would involve 60 Gy administered in 30 fractions. Treatment is usually in two phases, with lead shielding in the second phase to avoid exceeding spinal cord tolerance.
- Conformal techniques, CT planning and intensity-modulated radiation therapy (IMRT) allow reduction in the dosage to normal tissue.
- Potential acute side-effects include cutaneous erythema, desquamation, mucositis, and dysphagia. Late side-effects include skin pigmentation and formation of telangiectasia.

Palliation

- Role for external beam radiotherapy:
  - after incomplete resection – to improve local control of residual tumour. One trial comparing outcome in patients with incompletely resected disease treated with either surgery alone or post-operative radiotherapy found an iincrease in 5-year survival from 38% to 77%
  - for symptomatic metastatic disease, e.g. painful skeletal secondaries, when radioiodine is often less effective.

Anaplastic (undifferentiated) carcinoma

- Consider post-operative radiotherapy for the small number of patients whose tumours are completely resected.
- More frequently used with palliative intent for local control of inoperable tumours or for symptomatic metastatic disease. Up to 80% will have a partial response for a short period of time.
- Stridor or superior vena cava obstruction (SVCO) are urgent indications for radiotherapy.

Medullary carcinoma

- Post-operative external beam radiotherapy for macroscopic remnant to maximize local control.
- Alternatively, pre-operative radiotherapy may cause an inoperable tumour to become operable.
- Occasional avidity of uptake to meta-iodobenzylguanadine (MIBG) makes radioiodinated MIBG therapy a possibly useful therapeutic modality.

Chemotherapy for thyroid cancer

- Very limited role.
- Only if surgery, ^{131}I, or external beam radiotherapy no longer appropriate and patient remains fit.
- Few prospective randomized trials
- Response rates are poor (10–30%), incomplete, and of short duration
- No evidence for improvement in overall survival
- Standard first-line agent is doxorubicin.
- There are several trials supporting the use of dacarbazine-combination chemotherapy in medullary thyroid cancer.
- Other options are largely trial based.

Novel therapies for thyroid cancer

- The hypervascularity of many relapsed thyroid carcinomas (and the high levels of expression of vascular endothelial growth factor (VEGF)) has led to interest in novel therapies known to have antiantiogenic properties.
- For example, sorafenib:
  - multi-targeted small-molecule tyrosine kinase inhibitor (see 📖 Chapter 10, 'Biological and targeted therapies'), which inhibits multiple kinases and blocks the intracellulat domain of the VEGF receptor
  - a phase II trial of 30 patients with thyroid cancer treated with sorafenib reported disease stabilization in 16 patients and partial responses in seven.
- Studies of immunotherapy and approaches using gene therapy are in the very early stages.

Surveillance, follow-up, and prognosis for thyroid cancer

Surveillance and follow-up

Differentiated (papillary and follicular) carcinomas

- Most recurrences occur within 5 years.
- Regular physical examination particularly of the neck.
- Serum T4, TSH, and TG at each visit. TG in the presence of a suppressed serum TSH requires investigation.
- ~5% of recurrent disease is not associated with ↑TG.
- ± Chest X-ray (CXR), ultrasound scan of the neck, and diagnostic radioiodine imaging depending on risk factors.

Medullary carcinoma

- Clinical examination
- Serial serum calcitonin levels
- Screen for familial disease – all new cases of medullary carcinoma of the thyroid should be offered genetics referral.

Prognosis

Papillary

- Most patients with papillary carcinoma do not die of their disease.
- >90% 10-year survival.
- Prognosis for the follicular subtype is less good than for common-type papillary carcinoma, e.g. 92% versus 98% 10-year survival.
- Stage IV disease still has a 5-year survival of ~25%.
- Poor prognostic features include:
  - >45 years old
  - larger primary tumour, e.g. >7 cm
  - bilateral or mediastinal lymph node involvement, or distant metastases
  - lymphocytic infiltration
  - male sex
  - soft tissue or regional organ invasion, e.g. trachea, oesophagus, etc.
- The commonest site of initial relapse is local neck lymph nodes – treatment is usually further surgical resection followed by ^{131}I therapy.

Anaplastic (undifferentiated) carcinoma

- Aggressive cancer with very poor prognosis.
- Median time from first symptom to death is 3–7 months.
- 1-year survival 20–35% and 5-year survival only 5–14%.

Medullary carcinoma

- No effective treatment in advanced disease. However, patients may live for years despite a high metastatic load, e.g. median survival for stage III/IV disease is 3–5 years.
- Stage-for-stage there seems to be no difference in prognosis between sporadic and hereditary disease. However patients with MEN type 2b are more likely to have invasive disease at diagnosis and hence fall into a worse prognostic group.

Adrenal cancer

The adrenal gland is composed of:
- an outer cortex:
  - mainly controlled by the renin–angiotensin system that regulates the release of aldosterone
- an inner cortex:
  - mainly controlled by the corticotrophin-releasing hormone-corticotrophin (ACTH) system that regulates the release of cortisol and adrenal androgens
- a medulla:
  - which is part of the sympathetic nervous system.

Tumours arising in the cortex and the medulla are aetiologically and functionally different, reflecting their cells of origin.

Epidemiology and aetiology

Adrenocortical tumours
- Rare: incidence approximately 1.0 per 10^6 population
- Account for only 0.2% of cancer deaths
- Aetiology generally unknown: rare familial cases
- Carcinomas even more rare: bimodal age distribution. Peak incidence before 5 years of age and in the 4th–5th decades.

Medullary tumours
- Even rarer: incidence approximately 0.6 per 10^6 population
- ~10% currently identified as familial although this is likely to increase with improvements in genetic analysis
- Associated with MEN type II (germline mutation in *RET* proto-oncogene – see sections on 'Medullary carcinoma of the thyroid') and occasionally von Hippel–Lindau disease.

Pathology

Adrenocortical tumours
- Adenomas or adenocarcinomas of the adrenal cortex.
- If malignant, spread is via:
  - local invasion of lymph nodes and liver
  - distant dissemination.
- 60% of all adrenocortical tumours are non-functioning.
- 40% are functioning, secreting steroids that may include oestrogens, testosterone, and/or aldosterone.

Medullary tumours
- Commonest adrenomedullary tumour is a phaeochromocytoma: golden or tan-coloured appearance macroscopically.
- Majority are benign. Only ~10% are malignant.
- Tumoral hypersecretion of epinephrine, norepinephrine, and/or dopamine.
- 10% of phaeochromocytomas are extra-adrenal, i.e. arise elsewhere in the sympathetic chain. 10% are multiple.
- Hereditary phaeochromocytomas:
  - often occur in younger age groups
  - more likely to be bilateral and benign.

Presentation

Adrenocortical tumours (see Table 19.4)

- Incidental finding. The current National Institues of Health (NIH) position statement is that the incidentaloma less than 4 cm (non-functioning) can be monitored. Above 6 cm they should be excised laparoscopically because 30–80% will contain malignancy.
- 'Pressure symptoms', e.g. pain in the abdomen, symptoms from metastatic disease.
- In functioning tumours symptoms and signs will vary according to the predominant steroid hormone produced, e.g.:
  - virilization – commonest presentation of adrenocortical carcinoma in children
  - Cushing's syndrome – commonest presentation of adrenocortical carcinoma in adults
  - feminization – very rarely
  - hypertension.

Medullary tumours

- Incidental finding
- During screening for associated familial syndromes
- Intermittent, severe hypertension or essential hypertension
- Classical presentation with episodic:
  - headache
  - sweating
  - tachycardia/palpitations
  - ± pallor or tremor.

Investigations

- Careful family history
- Haemoglobin, electrolytes, urea, liver function tests
- Plasma catecholamines
- Plasma aldosterone-to-renin activity ratio
- Urinary vanillylmandelic acid (VMA) and urinary catecholamines
- Chromogranin assays
- Serum and urinary cortisols
- Blood oestrogen and testosterone
- CXR, ultrasound, CT, MRI abdomen to assess for potential metastatic disease
- Ultrasound of the thyroid gland (MEN)
- ^{123}I-MIBG, octreoscan: medullary tumour
- Selenocholesterol imaging: cortical tumour.

Surgery

- Surgery is the only treatment likely to achieve cure in benign disease or in the small group of patients with localized malignant disease without occult micrometastases.
- It may still be appropriate to resect the primary tumour in the presence of metastases if it is slow growing, or where there are a small number of metastases, in order to achieve local control.
- Radical resection (with adjacent nephrectomy if necessary) is essential for cure.

Table 19.4 Endocrine syndromes associated with adrenocortical tumours

Syndrome	Steroid
Cushing's syndrome (ACTH independent)	Cortisol
Conn's syndrome/primary hyperaldosteronism	Aldosterone
Virilization syndrome	Androgen
Feminization syndrome	Oestrogen
Precocious puberty syndrome/adrenogenital syndrome	Sex hormones
Non-functioning	None

- Special pre-operative considerations:
  - correction of electrolyte abnormalities
  - appropriate specialist blood pressure control.
- Surgery may be:
  - open – preferable for larger adenomas and carcinomas. Open surgery is still preferred for obvious carcinomas, although there are encouraging results for laparoscopic adrenalectomy with small cancers; some centres are performing laparoscopic resections for tumours over 6 cm
  - laparoscopic – longer operating time, less post-operative pain, shorter hospital stay post-operatively. Long learning curve
  - *en bloc* major resections of the tumour with adjacent organs are usually done with open surgery.

Non-surgical options

Adrenocortical tumours

- Mitotane:
  - orally administered adrenocorticolytic drug with some efficacy in patients with adrenal carcinoma
  - first-line treatment in patients with unresectable or metastatic tumours
  - common side-effects include nausea and anorexia. It may also cause cortisol and aldosterone deficiency necessitating replacement therapy
  - control of disease is usually transient with symptomatic or biochemical progression typically occurring after only 6–12 months.
- Metyrapone, aminoglutethimide, and ketoconazole:
  - potential second-line medical therapies that can also reduce excessive cortisol secretion.
- Chemotherapy:
  - limited benefit
  - no randomized clinical trials
  - most active drugs appear to be cisplatin and etoposide
  - patients should be referred for consideration of treatment within the context of randomized clinical trials wherever possible.

- Radiotherapy:
  - no established role in the management of adrenal carcinoma as it is rarely effective
  - occasionally used for the treatment of symptomatic metastases, usually in bone.

Medullary tumours

- Anti-hypertensive medication:
  - may be required for phaeochromocytomas with residual or unresectable disease to control the blood pressure.
- ^{131}I-MIBG:
  - if the tumour takes up the radionuclide MIBG a therapeutic dose may be administered
  - symptomatic, hormonal, and radiological improvements can be seen, although these are transient
  - treatment can be repeated.
- Radiotherapy:
  - appropriate for painful skeletal metastases.
- Chemotherapy:
  - may be considered for tumours that will not take up MIBG
  - a combination of dacarbazine, vincristine, and cyclophosphamide shows activity.

Prognosis

Adrenocortical tumours

- Almost all patients with benign disease are cured by surgery (usually laparoscopic).
- Prognosis is poor for patients with malignant disease. Untreated, the median survival is 3–9 months. Even if the carcinoma is small volume and apparently confined to the adrenal gland, survival following surgery may be as little as 14–36 months.
- Prognosis may be better in children.

Medullary tumours

- Surgical resection is not always curative even in benign disease. Long-term monitoring is therefore required. Subsequent recurrence may have malignant characteristics.
- 5-year survival for malignant phaeochromocytoma is <50%, although some patients live for many years without significant symptoms.

Neuroblastoma

- Commonest extracranial solid tumour in childhood.
- Incidence: peak age 1–3 years.
- Tumours arise in sympathetic nervous tissue:
  - 60% adrenal or elsewhere within the abdomen → pain, abdominal distension, general malaise
  - 15% intrathoracic → cough, pain, Horner's syndrome, incidental finding on CXR
  - ± bone or bone marrow metastases → non-specific limb, joint, or back pain often misdiagnosed as arthritis or an irritable hip. May also become pancytopenic from marrow involvement.
- Investigations:
  - abdominal ultrasound scan
  - CT/MRI chest and abdomen
  - MRI spine
  - urinary catecholamines
  - bloods including serum LDH (lactate dehydrogenase; elevation is a poor prognostic sign)
  - serum neurone-specific enolase (NSE)
  - ± techetium or ^{123}I-MIBG scan.
- Pathology:
  - ranges from an undifferentiated, small, round cell tumour (that may be difficult to distinguish from rhabdomyosarcoma, primitive neuroectodermal tumour (PNET) or non-Hodgkin's lymphoma (NHL)) to a highly differentiated ganglioneuroblastoma
  - biopsy can be done percutaneously, thorascopically, or with the laparoscope.

Management

- Depends on tumour stage and the presence of certain genetic features that may indicate a less good prognosis, e.g. amplification of the *n-myc* oncogene.
- 'Watch and wait' policy: an option for tumours of early stage with favourable biology. Spontaneous regression can be seen.
- **Surgical clearance:**
  - if possible
  - most thoracic, pelvic, and cervical primaries, and those abdominal tumours that do **not** cross the midline, are resectable
  - even subtotal resection in infants is beneficial
  - local recurrences can be usually managed surgically
  - many centres offer resection to patients with stage IV neuroblastoma, and if combined with systemic therapy, there is some evidence of benefit.
- **Neoadjuvant chemotherapy:**
  - may be used with the aim of making a localized but inoperable tumour resectable
  - chemotherapy is also used in disseminated, high-risk disease
  - occasionally high-dose chemotherapy followed by autologous haemopoietic stem cell rescue may be considered.

- **Radiotherapy:**
  - following incomplete resection or for tumours that remain unresectable after induction chemotherapy.

Prognosis

- Depends on stage of tumour (see Table 19.5), tumour genetics, and age at diagnosis.
- Children <1 year old have a good prognosis even in the presence of widely disseminated disease, e.g. 85% overall survival for stage 4S.
- This compares with an overall survival of <40% in children >5 years old with neuroblastoma of any stage.

Table 19.5 International staging system for neuroblastoma

Stage 1	Localized tumour with complete gross excision with, or without, microscopic residual disease; representative ipsilateral and contralateral lymph nodes negative for tumour microscopically (nodes attached to, and removed with, the primary tumour may be positive)
Stage 2a	Localized tumour with incomplete gross excision; representative ipsilateral and non-adherent lymph nodes negative for tumour microscopically
Stage 2b	Localized tumour with complete or incomplete gross excision; with ipsilateral non-adherent lymph nodes positive for tumour. Enlarged contralateral lymph nodes must be negative microscopically
Stage 3	Unresectable unilateral tumour infiltrating across the midine with, or without, regional lymph node involvement; or localized unilateral tumour with contralateral regional lymph node involvement; or midline tumour with bilateral extension by infiltration (unresectable) or by lymph node involvement
Stage 4	Any primary tumour with dissemination to distant lymph nodes, bone, bone, marrow, liver skin, and/or other organs (except as defined in stage 4S)
Stage 4S	Localized primary tumour (as defined for stage 1, 2a, or 2b) with dissemination limited to skin, liver, and/or bone marrow (limited to infants less than one year old)

Further reading

Bastian P, Fleischhack F, Zimmermann M, et al. (2004) The role of complete surgical resection in Stage IV neuroblastoma. World J Urol **22**, 257–60.

Baudin E, Schlumberger M (2007) New therapeutic approaches for metastatic thyroid carcinoma. Lancet Oncol **8**, 148.

Carling T, Ocal IT, Udelsman R (2007) Special variants of differentiated thyroid cancer: does it alter the extent of surgery versus well-differentiated thyroid cancer? World J Surg **31**, 916–23.

Eisenhofer G, Bornstein SR, Brouwers FM, et al. (2004) Malignant phaeochromocytoma: current status and initiatives for future progress. Endocr Relat Cancer **11**, 423–36.

Greenblatt DY, Woltman T, Harper J, et al. (2006) Fine needle aspiration optimizes surgical management in patients with thyroid cancer. Ann Surg Oncol **13**, 859–63.

Hero B, Simon T, Spitz R, et al. (2008) Localized infant neuroblastoma often shows spontaneous regression; results of the prospective trials NB95-S and NB97. J Clin Oncol **16**, 1504.

Libe R, Fratticci A, Bertherat J (2007) Adrenocortical cancer: pathophysiology and clinical management. Endocr Relat Cancer **14**, 13–28.

Machens A, Hauptmann S, Drake H (2008) Prediction of lateral lymph node metastases in medullary thyroid cancer. Br J Surg **95**, 586–91.

Maris JM, Hogarty MD, Bagatell R, et al. (2007) Neuroblastoma. Lancet **369**, 2106–20.

McIver B, Hay ID, Giuffrida DF, et al. (2001) Anaplastic thyroid carcinoma – a 50 year experience at a single institution. Surgery **130**, 1028–34.

Mureasan MM, Olivier P, Leclere J, et al. (2008) Bone metastases from differentiated thyroid carcinoma. Endocr Relat Cancer 15, 37.

Palazzo FF, Sebag F, Sierra M, et al. (2006) Long term outcome following laparoscopic adrenalectomy for large solid adrenal cortex tumours. World J Surg **32**, 893–8.

Patel KN, Shaha AR (2005) Locally advanced thyroid cancer. Curr Opin Otolaryngol Head Neck Surg **13**,112–16.

Quagle FJ, Moleey JF (2005) Medullary thyroid carcinoma: including MEN 2A and MEN 2B syndromes. J Surg Oncol **89**, 122–9.

Remy H, Borget I, Leboulleux S, et al. (2008) [131]I effective half-life and dosimetry in thyroid cancer patients. J Nucl Med **49**, 1445.

Genitourinary cancers

Renal cancer

Epidemiology and aetiology
- 2% of all cancers, 6000 cases annually in the UK.
- Increasing frequency with age, most >60 years.
- 1.5 times more common in men.
- Association with smoking (relative risk double).
- Other associations include urban dwellers, occupational exposure (e.g. asbestos, benzenes, cadmium, nitrosamines, aflatoxins), obesity, and chronic renal dialysis.

Genetics
The vast majority of adult renal cancers are sporadic, but an inherited predisposition causes 2%, and these may be multifocal/bilateral.
- von Hippel–Lindau syndrome (1/36 000 births):
  - *VHL* gene on chromosome 3 is a tumour suppressor gene
  - germline loss/mutation of this gene leads to a multiorgan syndrome including cerebral haemangioblastoma and risk of renal cell carcinoma.
- Hereditary clear-cell carcinoma (germline alteration in chromosome 3 without other features of VHL).
- Hereditary papillary renal carcinoma syndrome.
- Increased risk also in patients with autosomal dominant polycystic kidneys or tuberous sclerosis.

Pathology
Adenocarcinomas make up 85% of renal cancers and arise from the renal tubular epithelium. These renal cell carcinomas were previously known as 'hypernephroma' or 'Grawitz tumours' and demonstrate several histological types:
- clear cell (75%)
- papillary
- chromophobe
- spindle cell or sarcomatoid.

Renal cell carcinoma typically arises as a solitary mass in one pole of the kidney, and as it progresses may invade directly through the renal capsule, along the renal vein towards the inferior vena cava (IVC) or even right atrium, and via lymphatics to regional nodes (para-aortic). Systemic metastases are common; macroscopic spread is present in 25% at presentation, typically to lung or bone, but also liver, adrenal, brain, and skin.

Transitional cell carcinomas (TCCs) can arise within the urothelium of the renal pelvis and represent the majority of the remaining tumours. They vary from low-grade superficial papillary tumours to high-grade invasive TCC with propensity for direct invasion into perinephric tissues and lymphovascular spread.

Investigations

Many are picked up on ultrasound scan or intravenous urography (IVU), but computerized tomography (CT) is the preferred imaging modality. Contrast-enhanced CT scan of the abdomen characteristically shows an enhancing mass, at least partly solid. CT should also be used to image:

- chest, for lung and mediastinal lymph node metastases
- extrarenal direct tumour extension, e.g. into psoas muscle
- renal vein and IVC tumour thrombus
- regional para-aortic lymph nodes
- spread to other organs, e.g. liver, adrenals, bones, and contralateral kidney.

Biopsy is usually omitted prior to surgical treatment of renal cancer because of the risk of haemorrhage and tumour seeding along the biopsy tract. However lesions 1.5–3 cm diameter are not uncommonly benign, so biopsy under ultrasound or CT is often performed prior to surgery for these. Other required investigations include:

- full blood count (FBC), biochemical profile
- isotope bone scan, particularly in patients with bone pain or elevated alkaline phosphatase (note that renal bone metastases may be photopaenic or invisible on bone scan)
- CT brain if there is clinical evidence of central nervous system (CNS) spread
- occasionally magnetic resonance imaging (MRI) angiography or cavogram is required for locally advanced tumours to assess IVC extension
- isotope renogram to assess function of contralateral kidney if renal function impaired/small or scarred remaining kidney.

Staging

The Robson staging system is simple and commonly used (see Table 20.1).

Presenting symptoms and signs

Up to 30% are asymptomatic and are discovered coincidentally during abdominal imaging for other reasons. Symptoms may relate directly to the primary tumour, but paraneoplastic effects are not uncommon:

- haematuria (50%)
- loin pain (50%)
- palpable mass (30%)
- anaemia (40%)
- weight loss (35%)
- pyrexia (20%)
- hypertension (37%)
- hypercalcaemia (6%)
- polycythaemia (<5%).

Renal tumours may invade directly into adjacent psoas muscle or lumbar spine causing pain, or may present *de novo* with symptoms from metastatic disease in the lungs, lymph nodes, bone, brain, or skin.

Table 20.1 The Robson staging system

Stage	Description	% of cases	5-year survival
I	Confined to the kidney	20–40	50–60%
II	Extends into peri-renal fat but confined to Gerota's fascia	4–20	30–60%
III	Involvement of renal vein or IVC or lymph node involvement	10–40	20–50%
IV	Involvement of adjacent organs or metastatic disease	11–50	0–20%

Surgery

Resection of all the tumour is the only established curative treatment and should be offered to patients with operable disease without metastases, who are fit for surgery. Patients with metastatic disease but good performance status and resectable primary tumour may benefit from nephrectomy as a palliative procedure or to prevent development of local symptoms:

• to provide control of local symptoms
• nephrectomy followed by immunotherapy provides a modest survival benefit compared with immunotherapy alone
• although there are documented cases of regression of metastases following nephrectomy, this is extremely rare (<1%), and nephrectomy cannot be justified on this basis in patients who are frail or have extensive metastatic disease.

Surgical notes

• Radical nephrectomy includes removal of Gerota's fascia and its contents, including the kidney and the adrenal gland:
  • some surgeons believe that the adrenal gland can be left safely
  • laparoscopic nephrectomy is commonly performed to decrease the morbidity of the open procedure – survival seems equivalent to the open procedure.
• Partial nephrectomy (open or laparoscopic) is performed for small localized tumours or in patients without a second kidney, or in the rare case of bilateral renal cancer. Laparoscopic partial nephrectomy can be difficult, but with small tumours survival seems to be equivalent to the radical procedure, in selected cases.
• For patients who are frail or elderly, small tumours may not require resection, but can be successfully managed by percutaneous radiofrequency ablation.
• Surgery for solitary metastases (e.g. lung, brain) is indicated for isolated metastases particularly those that occur after a long (>1 year) disease-free interval, and can result in prolonged survival in up to 30%.

Although surgery is the cornerstone of management of localized disease, some patients are unfit for nephrectomy, or their tumour is unresectable. Tumour embolization (infarction) may provide some tumour control but can itself cause considerable morbidity. In some elderly asymptomatic patients, conservative management is appropriate, and tumour growth may be slow.

Spontaneous remissions

One of the most pervasive tales of 'oncological folklore' is the expectation of spontaneous remissions in renal cancer. Although these certainly occur, the true rate is less than 1%, and they tend to occur in metastases following resection of the primary tumour or after an episode associated with immune activation, such as following severe sepsis. Such regressions are not usually durable.

Adjuvant therapy

Adjuvant therapy has not been proven to offer a survival benefit when combined with nephrectomy. Cytotoxic chemotherapies, endocrine therapy, radiotherapy, and immunotherapy have been tested. Clinical trials using novel targeted agents are ongoing.

Radiotherapy

Renal cancer, in general, is radioresistant. Palliative radiotherapy is appropriate for:
- painful or bleeding primary tumour
- non-resectable metastatic disease, e.g. bone, brain, soft tissue.

Higher palliative doses and large doses per fraction compared with other malignancies may be appropriate to give durable control of disease, in particular with isolated non-resectable metastases after nephrectomy in good performance status patients.

Endocrine therapy

Progestins are widely prescribed for advanced renal cancer following the identification of progesterone receptors in some renal tumours and observation of anti-tumour activity in animal models. The objective response rate for systemic progestagen therapy is less than 10% and probably only 1–2% by modern response criteria. However, the anabolic effects of progesterone are often valuable in patients with advanced disease, whose quality of life may improve on this treatment. These agents increase the risk of venous thromboembolic disease, which is already high in this disease.

Chemotherapy

Cytotoxic drugs are of little value in renal carcinoma. The chemoresistance may, in part, be due to the high expression of a multidrug-resistance phenotype in both normal and malignant renal tissue. Response rates for single agents are generally under 10%. 5-Fluorouracil (5-FU) is one of the consistently active agents, and recent interest has focused on the combination of gemcitabine and 5-FU.

Biological therapy

The management of patients with unresectable and/or metastatic renal cancer is palliative. There is, however, good evidence that a small subset of patients, who have complete responses to biological therapy, may enjoy disease-free survival for several years.

Biological therapy has been extensively tested in renal cancer, partly because of its chemoresistance, but mainly because of the presumption that immunological mechanisms underlie:

- occasional spontaneous regression of metastases
- very late relapses in some patients
- increased incidence of renal cancers in immunosuppressed patients.

Interleukin-2 (IL-2)

- Most widely tested biological agent in advanced renal cancer.
- Induces responses in 10–25% of patients with advanced disease.
- Patients with a complete radiological response have a significant survival benefit, with remissions of several years in a few.
- Original studies of IL-2 employed high-dose intravenous IL-2, either alone or in combination with lymphokine-activated killer (LAK) cells.
- No evidence from randomized studies that LAK cells improve efficacy of IL-2.
- These regimens are associated with serious morbidity, in particular capillary leak syndrome, including hypotension and pulmonary oedema.
- Less toxic subcutaneous (s/c) IL-2 regimens are probably equally effective and can be combined with other agents, perhaps with greater anti-tumour effects.
- Other toxicities include flu-like symptoms and effects on bone marrow, hepatic, and renal function, CNS, and thyroid.

Interferon-α (IFN)

- Has been the preferred biological treatment for advanced renal cancer in the UK.
- As a single agent, s/c IFN provides a response rate of 8–15% but without prolonged remissions.
- A Medical Research Council (MRC) trial compared s/c IFN with medroxyprogesterone acetate in the treatment of metastatic renal cancer, and demonstrated a modest improvement in median survival with s/c IFN (8.5 versus 6 months).
- Toxicities of this drug are significant but not life threatening, in particular flu-like symptoms, lethargy, anorexia, and nausea.
- Other side-effects include deranged liver function tests (LFTs), and effects on bone marrow, renal function, and CNS.

Prognostic factors that predict higher response rates and prolonged survival time after biological therapy include:

- long disease-free interval
- previous nephrectomy
- good performance status (0–1)
- normal lactate dehydrogenase (LDH), haemoglobin, calcium
- pulmonary metastases as the sole site of disease.

Combined biological and chemotherapy

Although phase II studies have reported higher objective response rates with combinations of IL-2 and IFN, with or without chemotherapy, so far phase III studies have failed to demonstrate a significant benefit with any one combination regimen. The MRC RE04 study compared an IL-2/IFN/5-FU regimen developed by German investigators led by Atzpodien, with a reported response rate >30%, against single-agent IFN. Disappointingly, although the response rate was higher with the combination regimen (24% vs 16%), survival was equivalent in both arms (median survival 18 months).

Targeted therapy for renal cell carcinoma (see Table 20.2)

The systemic treatment of this disease has been transformed in the last few years with the advent of treatments targeted against vascular endothelial growth factor (VEGF). The majority of sporadic clear cell carcinomas of the kidney demonstrate inactivation of the tumour suppressor gene *VHL*, with resultant overexpression of VEGF. The pro-angiogenic effects of VEGF are mediated by its activation of the VEGF cell surface receptor, and this has proved a fruitful target for therapies:

Neutralizing antibody against VEGF

Bevacizumab is a recombinant human monoclonal antibody against VEGF:
- bevacizumab + interferon improves response rate and progression-free survival compared with interferon alone (responses in 25% vs 13%).

Small-molecule inhibitors of VEGFR pathway
- Sunitinib – oral tyrosine kinase inhibitor:
  - sunitinib versus interferon – response rate 39% vs 8%, with improved progression-free survival
- Sorafenib – oral tyrosine kinase inhibitor:
  - response rate relatively low (5%), but a large number of patients have prolonged stable disease
- Temsirolimus – inhibitor of mTOR, key component in intracellular control of angiogenesis and cell cycle:
  - temsirolimus versus interferon in poor-prognosis advanced renal cancer – 3.6m survival benefit

Despite these results, and approval for their use in this disease in Europe and the US, NHS patients are currently denied access to most of these on the grounds of cost efficacy. Indeed sunitinib was only approved by the National Institute for Health and Clinical Excellence (NICE) in 2009 for the treatment of renal cancer patients.

Management of transitional cell carcinoma

These tumours arise in the renal collecting system and may be associated with TCC in the ureter and bladder. Their biology, management, and prognosis are similar to those of TCC of the ureter.

Treatment outcomes

The prognosis for non-metastatic renal carcinoma is related to the pathological stage of disease post-nephrectomy, with 5-year survival rates between 60 and 20% as above.

Although the prognosis for metastatic renal cancer is poor, with median survival time <1 year, the outlook for good-prognosis patients as defined above is better, with a median survival >2 years.

Controversies in the treatment of renal cancer

Current areas of uncertainty in advanced disease include:
- optimum use of targeted therapies, sequence, or combination
- prediction of response to targeted therapies
- importance of nephrectomy as an adjunct to these therapies
- role of immunotherapy
- vaccine therapy.

Table 20.2 Targeted therapies for renal cell cancer

Drug	Dose regimen	Licensed indications	Side-effects
Sunitinib	50 mg oral daily for 4/52, then 14-day break	First-line therapy advanced disease in good-risk patients	Fatigue, nausea, stomatitis, diarrhoea, hypertension, bleeding/bruising, hypothyroidism, cardiac dysfunction, rarely gastrointestinal (GI) perforation
Sorafenib	400 mg oral bd	Second-line therapy after interferon	Skin rashes, diarrhoea, hypertension, hand–foot syndrome
Temsirolimus	25 mg IV weekly	First-line therapy in poor-risk patients	Lethargy, skin rash, hyperglycaemia, hyperlipidaemia
Bevacizumab	10 mg/kg IV every 2/52 in combination with interferon	Awaiting licence	Fatigue, hypertension, bleeding, rarely GI perforation

Wilms' tumour

Wilms' tumour (WT) is an embryonal neoplasm arising in the kidney, and is the commonest abdominal malignancy in childhood. Multidisciplinary management in specialist centres combined with international collaborative research over the last 30 years has resulted in cure rates rising from 50% to currently almost 90%.

Epidemiology

- Accounts for ~6% of childhood malignancies.
- Around 70 cases per annum in the UK.
- Male:female ratio ~1.
- Peak age at diagnosis 3–4 years.
- Rare after the age of 10 years, but occasionally present in adults.
- A number of conditions are associated with the development of WT:
  - congenital genitourinary abnormalities
  - hemihypertrophy
  - aniridia.

However, the majority of patients demonstrate none of these features.

Genetics

WT1 is a tumour suppressor gene, located on chromosome 11, constitutively deleted in patients with WAGR syndrome (Wilms' tumour Associated with Aniridia, Genitourinary abnormalities, and mental Retardation). This gene is also mutated or deleted in a number of sporadic cases of WT. Beckwith–Wiedemann syndrome (WT associated with overgrowth) is also linked with changes in chromosome 11, involving e.g. *IGF2*.

Presenting symptoms and signs

- Abdominal mass, smooth, rounded, or lobulated arising in the loin
- Pain
- Haematuria
- Fever, weight loss
- Hypertension.

Investigations

- Abdominal ultrasound to confirm organ of origin of mass, determine extent of spread within the abdomen, confirm patency of the inferior vena cava
- Chest X-ray (CXR) to detect pulmonary metastases
- FBC, biochemistry
- Clotting screen – may acquire von Willebrand disease
- Urinalysis
- Urinary catecholamines to exclude neuroblastoma
- Staging CT scan of chest and abdomen.

It is important to know that the contralateral kidney is functioning adequately before surgery, and IVU, dimercaptosuccinic acid (DMSA) scan, or excretion of contrast at the end of a CT scan of the chest/abdomen are useful in this role.

Pathology

Two broad groups of tumours may be recognized by their histological appearances.

Favourable histology (90%)

- Classical triphasic histology: epithelial, blastemal, and stromal elements are all present
- Rhabdomyoblastic differentiation
- Monomorphic epithelial variant

Unfavourable histology

- Anaplasia is an unfavourable feature occasionally observed in triphasic tumours.
- The major unfavourable histological types are probably distinct cancers, rather than true variants of Wilms' tumour:
  - bone-metastasizing renal tumour of childhood
  - malignant rhabdoid tumour.

Staging

The National Wims' Tumor Study Group (NWTS) staging system is commonly used:

- **stage I** – tumour confined within renal capsule and fully resected
- **stage II** – tumour beyond renal capsule but fully resected; pre-operative biopsy; ruptured; confined to the flank
- **stage III** – tumour outside capsule and incompletely resected; lymph node involvement at the hilum or para-aortic chain
- **stage IV** – haematogenous metastases, e.g. to lungs, liver, bone, or brain
- **stage V** – bilateral renal tumours.

Management

There is overwhelming evidence that WT must be treated only in paediatric oncology centres and there is no place for the casual therapist. Surgeons, radiotherapists, paediatricians, or nephrologists not working in a centre with paediatric oncological expertise who find themselves unexpectedly dealing with a child with WT should make an urgent referral to an appropriate unit.

Surgery

Surgical resection is, and almost certainly will remain, the cornerstone treatment for Wilms' tumour. There is debate about the timing of surgery, the place of percutaneous needle biopsy, and the use of pre-operative chemotherapy. US practice (NWTSG) remains steadfastly in favour of immediate surgery followed by adjuvant therapy dictated by the surgical stage. In contrast, the SIOP (International Society of Paediatric Oncology) group in Europe has conducted a series of trials based on the use of pre-operative therapy and, while it remains to be proven that the latter approach is superior, there is increasing recognition that pre-operative treatment may be of benefit in some circumstances. Only 5% are suitable for partial nephrectomy. Usually surgery is done by open technique (**not** laparoscopic) (best by a specialized paediatric surgeon) with wide excision taking care to avoid rupture or spillage of tumour. The latter is associated with peritoneal recurrence.

In bilateral tumours, one tumour is usually smaller and may be amenable to partial nephrectomy

Adjuvant therapy

The use of chemotherapy and radiotherapy as adjuvants to surgery is now an essential part of WT treatment. Major advances in treatment have come as a result of multicentre cooperative trials run by the US NWTS group (Table 20.3), SIOP, and the UK Children's Cancer Study Group (UKCCSG).

In general, treatment is tailored to the stage and pathology of the individual child, each successive study aiming to maximize the probability of cure, but minimize exposure to chemotherapy and radiotherapy. For example, radiotherapy can now be safely omitted in patients with stage I and stage II with favourable histology.

The initial studies of adjuvant chemotherapy used vincristine and dactinomycin, and these remain the mainstay of treatment for the majority of patients. Doxorubicin improves the outcome in stages III and IV, and other agents such as carboplatin, etoposide, and ifosfamide are active in poor-prognosis and relapsed disease.

Outcome of treatment

The favourable outcome of treatment for the majority is illustrated in Tables 20.4 and 20.5. Currently around 75% of children with WT can be successfully treated without doxorubicin or radiotherapy, minimizing the risk of late effects. Nonetheless, close follow-up including CXR and abdominal ultrasound scan is mandatory. Following relapse, 30–40% long-term survival may be achieved through salvage therapy.

Late effects may include impairment of:
• growth
• lung function
• cardiac function
• renal function
• hepatic function
• fertility
• second malignancy.

Table 20.3 Main findings in NWTS 1, 2, and 3

NWTS 1	
Group I	Patients under two years of age do not all need radiotherapy
Group II/III	AMD plus VCR is better than either alone
Group IV	Pre-operative vincristine is of no benefit
Other findings	Unfavourable histology and lymph-node involvement are adverse features
NWTS 2	
Stage I	No patients benefit from radiotherapy regardless of age 6 months of VCR and AMD is as good as 15 months
Stages II, III and IV	Addition of doxo to VCR and AMD improves survival
Other findings	Stages II and III have the same survival. Local spillage and invasion of the renal vein do not affect outcome
NWTS 3	
Stage I	10 weeks therapy with VCR/AMD is as effective as 6 months
Stage II	Intensive VCR/AMD is as effective as three drugs Addition of radiotherapy does not affect survival
Stage III	Intensive VCR/AMD is as effective as three drugs. 10 Gy flank irradiation is as effective as 20 Gy
Other findings	Addition of cyclophosphamide to VCR/AMD/doxo does not improve survival

Key: VCR = vincristine; AMD = actinomycin D; doxo = doxorubicin

Table 20.4 Outcome for patients in NWTS III

Stage	2-year relapse-free survival (%)	2-year overall survival (%)	Treatment
I	92	97	10 weeks vincristine + actinomycin D
II/III	87	91	15 months vincristine + actinomycin D + doxorubicin
III	78	86	10 Gy + vincristine + actinomycin D + doxorubicin
IV + UH	72	81	

UH = Unfavourable histology.

Table 20.5 Outcome for patients in UKWI

Stage	3-year event-free survival (%)	3-year overall survival (%)	6-year event-free survival (%)	6-year overall survival (%)
I	90	96	89	96
II	85	94	85	93
III	82	83	82	83
IV	58	65	50	65

Current treatment for Wilms' tumour

Stage	Treatment
I low risk	No adjuvant therapy
I intermediate risk	Adjuvant vincristine, actinomycin
I high risk	Adjuvant vincristine, actinomycin, doxorubicin
II low risk	Vincristine, actinomycin
II–III intermediate risk	Vincristine, actinomycin, +/– doxorubicin
II–III high risk	Cyclophosphamide, doxorubicin, etoposide, carboplatin, and radiotherapy
Metastatic	Neoadjuvant vincristine, actinomycin, doxorubicin, then surgery, then further chemotherapy +/– etoposide, carboplatin, and radiotherapy

Cancer of the bladder and ureter

Epidemiology
- 4th commonest male cancer
- Male: female ratio ~2:1
- 10 700 new cases in the UK each year
- Two-thirds occur aged >70 years.

Aetiology
- Cigarette smoking increases the risk by 2–6-fold.
- Occupational exposure to a number of carcinogens including aromatic amines is associated with increased risk with a latent interval of 20–30 years.
- Occupations at risk include:
  - aniline dye and the rubber industries
  - gas works
  - rodent care and other laboratory work
  - sewage treatment
  - textile printing
  - firelighter manufacturers.
- Chronic irritation of the bladder, e.g. infection, stones, long-term catheter, or schistosomiasis – associated with squamous cancer of the bladder.
- Previous pelvic radiotherapy, e.g. for gynaecological cancer.

Pathology
The majority (>90%) of urothelial tumours presenting in the UK are transitional cell carcinomas (TCCs). Less common pathologies include:
- squamous carcinomas associated with chronic irritation
- adenocarcinomas arising from urachal remnants in the bladder dome
- metaplasia in a transitional cell carcinoma may give rise to carcinomasarcoma or neuroendocrine carcinoma, both associated with poor outcome.

Typically the disease presents with superficial tumour involving only the bladder epithelium, but in 25% there is tumour invasion into the detrusor muscle of the bladder, and 5% present with metastatic disease to the regional lymph nodes, lung, liver, or bone. Pathological grading (I–III) correlates well with the natural history of the disease. Multifocal disease is not uncommon through exposure of the entire lining of the urinary tract to the relevant carcinogens, and a history of TCC of bladder carries an increased risk of TCC arising anywhere in the urothelium.

Genetics
No convincing evidence of a hereditary predisposition exists. Transitional carcinomas have a number of characteristic chromosomal abnormalities including, in particular, loss of chromosome 9. Other common abnormalities include a mutation of the $p53$ gene that appears more often in advanced cancers and has been associated with an increased risk of treatment failure.

Staging (see Table 20.6)

The management and prognosis of TCC of the bladder are largely determined by the stage of disease and its pathological grading. There is a strong association between well-differentiated tumours and early stage at presentation.

Seventy per cent of new patients present with superficial disease, of which at least half have Ta tumours. Although around 50% of these develop recurrent superficial bladder cancers, few progress to advanced disease. Carcinoma *in situ* has a worse outlook, with up to 60% progressing to invasive disease if recurrent disease is not eradicated.

There is a significant risk of metastatic disease with high-grade T1 disease, and this rises with increasing stage of muscle-invasive disease.

Table 20.6 Staging of TCC of the bladder

Stage	Description
Ta	Non-invasive papillary carcinoma
Tis	Carcinoma *in situ*, dysplasia confined to epithelium
T1	Invades subepithelial connective tissue
T2a	Invades superficial muscle
T2b	Invades deep muscle
T3a	Invades perivesical tissue microscopically
T3b	Invades perivesical tissue with a palpable mass
T4a	Invades prostate, uterus, or vagina
T4b	Invades pelvic wall or abdominal wall
N0	No regional lymph node metastasis
N1	Metastasis in one lymph node up to 2 cm
N2	Metastasis in one or more lymph nodes, none >5 cm
N3	Metastasis in one or more lymph nodes >5 cm
M0	No distant metastasis
M1	Distant metastasis present

Investigation

- FBC, biochemistry profile.
- Cystoscopy and transurethral resection of bladder tumour (TURBT):
  - provide pathological diagnosis and stage
  - should include resection through underlying detrusor muscle to confirm/refute muscle invasion
  - biopsy other areas of abnormal-looking epithelium (*in situ* carcinoma often appears as a red patch)
  - following cystoscopic resection, pelvic examination under anaesthetic should confirm the presence/absence of a residual pelvic mass (presence indicates at least T3 disease).
- For low-grade superficial tumours, no further imaging is required. High-grade superficial tumours do carry a significant risk of synchronous disease in the upper urinary tract, and should have IVU after diagnosis.

- For G3 pT1 and muscle-invasive disease, staging with CXR and either CT or MRI scan of the abdomen and pelvis is required, looking particularly at:
  - tumour extent in the bladder and extravesical extension of tumour into adjacent fat/organs
  - pelvic and para-aortic lymphadenopathy
  - ureteric obstruction
  - bone, liver and lung metastases.

Presentation
- 80–90 % have frank haematuria, usually painless.
- Irritative bladder symptoms, e.g. frequency and dysuria, may be associated with muscle-invasive disease or carcinoma *in situ*.
- Less often present with unexplained microscopic haematuria.
- Asymptomatic disease may be picked up at routine cystoscopy in patient with previous bladder cancer or upper tract TCC.

Management options
Superficial tumours (70% newly diagnosed cases)
- Ta and low-grade (G1–2) T1 tumours are resected cystoscopically.
- A single post-resection infusion of intravesical mitomycin reduces the risk of recurrence.
- Because of the risk of recurrent disease, regular cystoscopic follow-up is required.
- Recurrent disease managed by intravesical therapy with mitomycin, epirubicin, or bacillus Calmette–Guérin (BCG).
- Tis commonly responds to intravesical BCG but recurrences are common and may be multifocal.
- Refractory Tis often best managed by cystectomy.
- G3T1 tumour management is controversial:
  - >50% risk of recurrence, up to half of which may be invasive TCC
  - significant risk of regional and metastatic disease
  - initial treatment of solitary tumour often comprises TURBT followed by intravesical therapy
  - multifocal or recurrent disease require staging and management as for muscle-invasive disease
  - radiotherapy is not of benefit in preventing recurrence.

Muscle-invasive bladder cancer
Given the high rate of recurrence and metastatic spread after TURBT, all patients with invasive disease should be considered for further treatment. Options should be discussed both by the multidisciplinary team and with the patient including:
- radical cystectomy
- radiotherapy and bladder conservation
- neoadjuvant or adjuvant chemotherapy.

Radical surgery
The usual procedure is cystoprostatectomy in male patients, or anterior bladder exenteration in female patients, with dissection of local lymph nodes. Bladder resection is associated with urinary diversion, most commonly a non-refluxing ileal conduit and urinary bag. Complications include

loss of erectile function in the male and shortening of the vagina in the female. It is important for patients to have advice from a stoma therapist before surgery.

Increasingly, excellent results can be achieved in selected patients treated by radical cystectomy with continent diversion based on urinary tract reconstruction by ileocystoplasty. This can produce urinary continence and, in experienced centres, the surgical complication rates are less than 10% and operative mortality less than 2%.

The role of laparoscopic cystectomy and robotic surgery is currently unclear.

Radical radiotherapy

Many UK patients with invasive TCC of bladder, in particular elderly with significant co-morbidities, have been treated with radiotherapy.

- Radiotherapy is planned using a CT scan to define the target volume.
- Conventionally the entire bladder and prostatic urethra are treated using a 3- or 4-field plan.
- Common treatment regimens include 64 Gy/32 fractions or 52.4 Gy/20 fractions.
- Side-effects include cystitis and diarrhoea, and late reduction in bladder capacity.
- Cystoscopic follow-up is particularly important:
  - to diagnose and resect recurrent bladder tumour
  - to offer salvage cystectomy to selected patients with recurrent invasive disease who remain fit for surgery.
- Frail patients unfit for radical surgery or radiotherapy may benefit from short-course palliative radiotherapy to the bladder, ideally CT planned, e.g. 21 Gy/3 fractions/5 days.
- A number of studies have reported improved results when radical radiotherapy is combined with systemic chemotherapy either given prior to radiotherapy or concomitant with radiotherapy.
- For patients with unifocal bladder cancer, it may be unnecessary to irradiate the whole bladder, and clinical trials are under way exploring the benefits of partial bladder radiotherapy +/− chemotherapy.

Table 20.7 compares these two treatment modalities. Surgery remains the preferred option for many good performance status patients, particularly those with multifocal disease and/or irritative bladder symptoms.

Table 20.7 Surgery versus radiotherapy as curative treatment for invasive bladder cancer

	Radical surgery	**Radical radiotherapy**
In favour	Complete pathological staging Best local and loco-regional control rates Best survival rates	Bladder conservation Option for salvage cystectomy Feasible in patients with extravesical extension and significant co-morbidity
Against	Major pelvic surgery, not feasible in many patients because of co-morbidities and frailty Loss of normal bladder and sexual function	Poor results in multifocal disease and Tis Normal tissue damage, radiation cystitis, and enteritis May worsen urinary symptoms by reducing bladder capacity

Chemotherapy (see Table 20.8)

Combination chemotherapy has an established role in the palliation of patients with advanced bladder cancer. Cisplatin-based regimens such as MVAC (methotrexate, vinblastine, doxorubicin, cisplatin) were developed in the 1980s, and found to have high objective response rates (~50%), although few patients survive beyond 2 years. During this time the preferred regimen in the UK was CMV (cisplatin, methotrexate, vinblastine, no doxorubicin).

These regimens were found to be toxic, especially for patients with poor performance status and impaired renal function. Life-threatening toxicity, e.g. neutropenic sepsis, was common. The combination of gemcitabine and cisplatin has been shown to be as effective as MVAC with reduced toxicity, and has largely superseded the older regimen.

In view of the chemosensitivity of this disease, a number of trials have examined the benefits of neoadjuvant and adjuvant chemotherapy in combination with either surgery or radiotherapy. Meta-analysis of these trials has demonstrated that cisplatin-based chemotherapy given before cystectomy or radical radiotherapy affords a modest survival benefit, ~5% improvement at 5 years. Patient selection for this treatment is crucial, but fit patients with muscle-invasive disease should be considered for chemotherapy prior to local treatment.

Future treatments

• Other cytotoxics including the taxanes are active in this disease.
• Molecular-targeted therapies are being investigated.
• Molecular markers are being sought which may optimize selection of local treatment (surgery versus radiotherapy) for individual patients.

Table 20.8 Examples of chemotheraphy regimens for bladder cancer

MVAC		
Methotrexate	30 mg/m^2 d1, 8, 15	
Vinblastine	3 mg/m^2 d2, 8, 15	q4/52
Doxorubicin	30 mg/m^2 d2	
Cisplatin	70 mg/m^2 d2	
CMV		
Methotrexate	30 mg/m^2 d1&8	
Vinblastine	4 mg/m^2 d1&8	q3/52
Cisplatin	100 mg/m^2 d2	
Gemcitabine cisplatin		
Gemcitabine	1000 mg/m^2 d1, 8, 15	q4/52
Cisplatin	70 mg/m^2 d2	
or		
Gemcitabine	1250 mg/m^2 d1, 8	q3/52
Cisplatin	70 mg/m^2 d1	

Treatment outcomes

The prognosis for superficial disease is good, with 5-year survival rates in excess of 80%.

The outlook for invasive disease is less good, estimated 5-year survival rates after cystectomy:

- T2 50–70%
- T3 30–40%
- T4 20%.

There are no randomized studies comparing the results of bladder conservation using modern radiotherapy against primary treatment with radical cystectomy. Many patients treated with radiotherapy would not be candidates for radical surgery, but may still achieve successful bladder conservation. The best results with radical radiotherapy appear to follow TURBT for a solitary T2 tumour. Poor results are obtained with T4 disease, and squamous carcinomas.

For metastatic disease, treatment with chemotherapy is associated with a median survival time of around 1 year, but <10% survive 2 years.

Renal pelvis and ureteric TCC

These uncommon tumours range from superficial low-grade disease to aggressive muscle invasive cancer with a high propensity for distant spread. Presentation may be with ureteric obstruction, haematuria, or symptoms related to advanced disease. The tumour is commonly visible on IVU, and may be biopsied via a flexible ureteroscope. Staging requires CT or MRI scan of the abdomen and pelvis, as well as cystoscopy to look for synchronous bladder TCC.

Localized disease is usually treated by nephroureterectomy with removal of a cuff of bladder. Adjuvant therapy trials have not been conducted but advanced disease may be treated with chemotherapy and palliative radiotherapy as for TCC of bladder.

Prostate cancer

Cancer of the prostate gland is one of the most controversial malignancies with regard to its treatment. Despite its high incidence – now the commonest male cancer in Europe and the US – for many men with this diagnosis the optimum management is uncertain, with a spectrum of treatment options ranging from surveillance only to complex surgery or intensity-modulated radiation therapy.

Epidemiology

Prostate cancer has now overtaken lung cancer as the commonest male cancer in the UK.
- >30 000 new cases per annum and the incidence is continuing to rise.
- Lifetime risk 1 in 14 men.
- Rare in men <50 years.
- 85% of men are diagnosed at age 65 years or older.
- Autopsy studies have estimated that 70% of men >80 years have histological evidence of cancer in the prostate.
- Despite the rising incidence, only 9500 deaths per annum are caused by prostate cancer in the UK, and many men with this diagnosis die of other causes.

Aetiology

Its pathogenesis is clearly androgen dependent, and men who are castrated or develop hypopituitarism before 40 years rarely develop prostate cancer.
- Age is the most important risk factor.
- 5–10% of cases appear to be linked to inheritance of a susceptibility gene, particularly cases arising at a young age.
  - at present the only identified genes include *BRCA1* and *2*, but these do not account for the majority of cases with a family history
  - linkage analysis suggests that there is a hereditary prostate cancer locus on chromosome 1q 24–25.
- Race: 60% increased incidence in African-Americans often with poor prognosis compared with White Americans; uncommon in Asian men.
- Dietary factors may explain some racial differences.

Pathology

Ninety-five per cent are adenocarcinomas; rare pathologies include neuroendocrine and transitional cell carcinomas; 70% arise in the peripheral zone of the gland, and many are multifocal.

The natural history of the disease correlates well with its histological grade, assessed by Gleason score. Low-grade cancers (Gleason 6) are typically small and slow growing, confined to the prostate gland. High-grade cancers, Gleason 8–10, grow faster and frequently invade through the prostate capsule, can directly infiltrate adjacent organs (seminal vesicles, bladder, rectum), and commonly disseminate early to regional lymph nodes and by vascular invasion typically to bone, but also occasionally to lung and liver.

Screening for prostate cancer

Since the development of assays to measure serum prostate-specific antigen (PSA) to diagnose prostatic disease, this condition has been increasingly diagnosed at an earlier stage. In 1974, in the UK, more than 50% of patients presented with metastatic disease. Thirty-five years later, the majority of patients are diagnosed with organ-confined disease as a result of PSA testing, with few if any symptoms of prostatic disease. Although population screening is not recommended in the UK (the topic is again currently under political review), PSA testing is recommended in all men with lower urinary tract symptoms, and is also performed frequently as part of general health screening in primary care. As a result, increasing numbers of patients are now diagnosed with asymptomatic early-stage disease.

PSA

Measurement of serum PSA has limitations as a screening test for prostate cancer. Conventionally PSA >4 µg/l was viewed as an indication for prostatic biopsy. However:

- normal PSA range increases with age
- some centres have adopted these cut-off levels to guide selection of patients for prostate biopsy:
  - 6.5µg/l age >70 years
  - 4.5µg/l age 60–70 years
  - 3.5µg/l age 50–60 years
  - 2.5µg/l age 40–50 years
- PSA may be elevated in the absence of prostate cancer, e.g. benign prostatic hyperplasia, prostatitis
- 1 in 4 men with a PSA >4 µg/l will be found to have cancer on biopsy of the prostate
- but around one-third of prostate cancers will have a PSA <4 µg/l
- specificity but not sensitivity can be improved by measuring free or total PSA, or both
- digital rectal examination findings are important – 40% of men with palpable abnormality have tumour
- higher levels of PSA (> 20 µg/l) correlate well with tumour stage and grade.

PSA screening in the US

Currently, PSA testing is recommended for all US men aged 50–75 years, although the optimum frequency of testing is uncertain, every 2–4 years suggested. In the US, in 1995 with widespread use of PSA testing in asymptomatic men, nearly 400 000 patients were diagnosed with prostate cancer; in the same year approximately 38 000 patients died of prostate cancer. In Europe with largely no screening, 85 000 patients were diagnosed and around 20 000 died of prostate cancer. These figures suggest that too many cases of clinically insignificant disease were diagnosed in the US and treated without clear evidence of survival benefit. However, over the last 10 years the mortality rate from prostate cancer in the US has fallen, and advocates of PSA screening have claimed this as

evidence of success of the programme. Certainly a number of positive features are observed in screening detected prostate cancer:
- majority have low-grade early-stage disease
- treatment outcomes are excellent with most patients free of disease after 10 years' follow-up.

However this is at enormous cost to health resources, with significant morbidity in a number of patients, many of whom were destined never to have clinically significant prostate cancer. Interestingly, the number of patients receiving radical treatment for prostate cancer in the UK has quadrupled in the last 15 years, and it is anticipated that survival improvements similar to those in the US may be observed in UK prostate cancer deaths in the next decade.

Clinical trials of PSA screening
Conventionally, the establishment of population screening for a malignant disease requires that randomized studies have demonstrated that the screening process results in a reduction of mortality from the relevant cancer. Such trials have now been completed, in particular the American PLCO (Prostate, Lung, Colorectal, and Ovarian) Cancer Screening trial and the European Randomised Screening for Prostate Cancer trial. These should report in the next few years.

Staging
The TNM staging system is used (see Table 20.9).

Investigations
Patients with lower urinary tract symptoms should have digital rectal examination and PSA testing offered. All patients having PSA tested should be counselled:
- that the test may detect cancer in ~5% of men aged 50–65 years
- that the test will fail to detect up to 25% of cancers
- that biopsy and further treatment if cancer is found carries the risk of some morbidity with no guarantee of improved life expectancy.

Asymptomatic patients with elevated PSA should also be assessed by digital rectal examination (40% of palpable nodules are malignant). Transrectal ultrasound scan and prostatic biopsy is required for patients with PSA >4 µg/l or age-adjusted normal range, and patients with normal PSA but a palpable abnormality in the gland. Up to four biopsy cores are taken from each lobe, with antibiotic cover. The prostate volume is measured by ultrasound, relevant symptoms recorded e.g. by International Prognostic Scoring System (IPSS) questionnaire, and urinary flow rate may also be measured.

In patients with biopsy-proven cancer, further investigation depends on the stage, grade, and PSA, and planned treatment.

MRI scan of the prostate and pelvis provides the most accurate estimate of loco-regional tumour extent for patients being considered for surgery or radiotherapy.

Isotope bone scans are required only for T3–4 tumours, Gleason 8–10, PSA >15 µg/l, or patients with symptoms/signs/biochemical evidence of bone metastases.

Presenting symptoms and signs
- ~50% are asymptomatic with elevated PSA.
- Urinary symptoms, e.g. frequency, nocturia, poor stream, retention, haematuria:
  - these are commonly due to coincident benign prostatic hyperplasia
  - symptoms may be scored, e.g. using the IPSS.
- Locally advanced disease may cause:
  - impotence due to neurovascular bundle infiltration
  - haemospermia
  - ureteric obstruction and renal failure
  - rectal symptoms, e.g. tenesmus, bleeding
  - lymph node spread with lymphoedema in legs and genitals
  - bone metastases with pain, fracture, nerve root or spinal cord compression, or malignant hypercalcaemia
  - rarely liver, pleura, or lung metastases.

Table 20.9 TNM staging of prostate cancer

T0	No evidence of tumour
T1a	Tumour, incidental finding at TURP (<5% chippings)
T1b	Tumour, incidental finding at TURP (>5% chippings)
T1c	Impalpable tumour identified by raised PSA
T2a	Tumour involves half of a lobe or less
T2b	Tumour involves more than a half of a lobe but not both lobes
T2c	Tumour involves both lobes
T3a	Extracapsular extension (unilateral or bilateral)
T3b	Tumour involves seminal vesicle(s)
T4	Tumour invades bladder neck, rectum, pelvic side wall

TURP: transurethral resection of the prostate.

Management of prostate cancer

Metastatic disease

Although distant spread of prostate cancer is incurable, the majority of patients can have excellent palliation of their symptoms and a survival time of at least 2 years with appropriate hormone therapy. The growth of prostate cancer is androgen dependent, and a number of hormone treatment options are effective.

Surgical castration

- Achieves permanent reduction in circulating androgens
- Inexpensive
- Major toxicities include impotence and loss of libido, fatigue, mood disturbance, and muscle weakness
- In long-term survivors causes osteoporosis
- May not be acceptable to patient.

Medical castration

- Luteinizing hormone-releasing hormone (LHRH) agonist, e.g. goserelin, buserelin, leuprorelin
- Administered as depot subcutaneous injection (expensive)
- Causes initial flare with rise in testosterone followed by fall to castrate level
- Therefore requires anti-androgen cover for the first 2 weeks after the first injection (e.g. bicalutamide, flutamide, or cyproterone acetate)
- Similar toxicities to surgical castration, but also flushing and sweats, weight gain
- Reversible effects, but may take many months for testosterone level to recover after withdrawal of LHRH agonist.

Androgen blockade

- Non-steroidal agents, e.g. bicalutamide or flutamide:
  - anti-cancer effects are rather less, but may preserve libido and sexual potency because of incomplete androgen blockade
  - may cause gynaecomastia
- Steroidal – cyproterone acetate:
  - not recommended for long-term use because of toxicities (thromboembolic disease, hepatotoxicity).

Maximal androgen blockade

- Combination of surgical or medical castration plus androgen blockade
- No clear evidence of superior outcomes compared with castration alone.

Hormonal treatment options are summarized in Table 20.10.

Table 20.10 Hormonal treatment options for prostate cancer

1st line	2nd line	3rd line	4th line
Surgical castration	Add androgen antagonist		
LHRH agonist	Add androgen antagonist	Withdrawal of androgen antagonist	Adrenal suppression or Oestrogens
Androgen antagonist	Add LHRH agonist		

Hormone-refractory metastatic disease

After a median of 2 years' androgen deprivation, patients with metastatic prostate cancer demonstrate evidence of hormone-refractory disease, initially asymptomatic with rising PSA, then with symptomatic progression of disease, most commonly painful bone metastases. These patients may be treated with second-line hormone therapy.

- Introduction of androgen blocker, e.g. bicalutamide in combination with surgical or medical castration, leads to PSA response in ~20%, duration of response 2–6 months.
- Patients who respond to maximal androgen blockade and then have PSA rise may respond again following withdrawal of the oral anti-androgen.
- Inhibition of production of adrenal androgens by low-dose steroids or ketoconazole.
- Low-dose oestrogens (diethylstilbestrol 1 mg daily, often with aspirin thromboprophylaxis).
- Recent trials of abiraterone, an inhibitor of the enzyme CYP17A1, key to synthesis of testosterone, have shown promising results after failure of established second- and third-line treatments.

Radiotherapy and chemotherapy for metastatic disease

Palliative external beam radiotherapy has been used successfully for many years to alleviate symptoms from metastatic prostate cancer.

- Painful bone metastases may be treated with low-dose radiotherapy, e.g. 8 Gy/1 fraction.
- Spinal cord or nerve root compression may be treated with short-course radiotherapy, e.g. 20 Gy/5 fractions.
- Symptomatic soft-tissue disease, e.g. prostatic primary or lymph node metastasis, may be treated with similar doses.
- Radioactive strontium administered as a single IV injection (150 MBq) provides targeted irradiation to multiple bone metastases:
  - gives pain relief and delays need for further analgesia and radiotherapy
  - well tolerated but does cause significant myelosuppression.

Chemotherapy traditionally was viewed as ineffective and inappropriate for the majority of patients, due to the limited number of active agents, age, and frailty of these patients, and marrow compromise by both metastatic disease and radiotherapy. Radiological assessment of objective response to treatment can be difficult in patients with only sclerotic bone metastasis. However, chemotherapy can be of benefit:

- mitoxantrone, usually in combination with low-dose prednisolone, causes PSA response (>50% reduction in PSA) in around 1/3, with accompanying symptom relief
- docetaxel has been shown to cause more frequent PSA responses and improves the median survival time by about 2 months when compared with mitoxantrone.

Bisphosphonate therapy using monthly infusions of zoledronic acid has also been shown to delay symptomatic progression of bone metastases, but the optimum timing to commence bisphosphonates and duration of therapy remains to be defined.

Organ-confined prostate cancer

For patients diagnosed with early-stage prostate cancer, several treatment options may be considered. Selection of the most appropriate option depends on consideration of:

- the life expectancy of the patient, taking into account age and co-morbidities
- the predicted natural history of the prostate cancer, determined by stage, PSA, and Gleason score
- the patient's preferences, often with consideration of likely toxicities of treatment.

Risk stratification for localized prostate cancer

Commonly, disease is categorized as follows:

- Low risk   T1–2a and PSA <10 μg/l, and Gleason 6
- Intermediate risk   T2b–c, or PSA 10–20 μg/l, or Gleason 7
- High risk   T3–4, or PSA >20 μg/l, or Gleason 8–10.

Radical prostatectomy

For patients <70 years, without significant co-morbidities, and low- or intermediate-risk disease, radical surgery gives excellent disease-free survival rates. The approach may be retropubic or perineal, the former allowing pelvic lymph node sampling. Alternatively, initial lymph node sampling may be performed laparoscopically, avoiding major surgery in patients who have positive lymph nodes. Post-operative problems have been reduced with improvements in surgical technique but may include:

- urinary incontinence, rarely (~5%) persists beyond 6 months
- impotence, previously inevitable after prostatectomy, with nerve-sparing procedures may be prevented in 50%.

After prostatectomy, the PSA should fall promptly to <0.1 μg/l. Patients with positive resection margins with slowly rising PSA levels may benefit from post-operative radiotherapy to the prostate bed. The role of adjuvant hormonal therapy in such patients is being explored (MRC RADICALS (Radiotherapy and Androgen Deprivation in Combination After Local Surgery) trial).

- Increasingly, radical prostatectomy is being undertaken laparoscopically with excellent results. Laparoscopic radical prostatectomy in experienced hands (there is a definite learning curve) gives as good functional and oncological results as the open procedure, with more rapid recovery. The advantage for robotic prostate surgery is unclear, although a number of specialized centres have this expensive facility.

Radical radiotherapy

For patients with low-, intermediate-, or high-risk disease, where metastatic disease has been excluded by isotope bone scan and MRI or CT scan of the pelvic and retroperitoneal lymph nodes, radical radiotherapy offers an alternative curative treatment option. There are no randomized trials comparing surgery and radiotherapy for early prostate cancer, but stage-for-stage rates of disease-free survival after radiotherapy compare favourably with surgery. In addition, many patients treated by radiotherapy are unfit or have disease that is too extensive for surgery.

External beam radiotherapy

High doses of ionizing radiation are required to eradicate prostate cancer. Using CT-planned, conformal radiotherapy, doses of 74 Gy in 37 fractions can be safely delivered to the prostate, with acceptable normal tissue reactions and a high rate of disease-free survival. Prior treatment with 3–6 months' anti-androgen therapy reduces the prostatic volume by about 30%, and is recommended in intermediate- and high-risk disease. In high-risk disease there is now good evidence to support the continuation of adjuvant anti-androgen therapy (usually an LHRH agonist) for 2–3 years after radiotherapy, with improvement in survival at least in locally advanced disease. External beam radiotherapy fields can encompass tumour that is invading through the prostate capsule.

Common toxicities of radiotherapy to the prostate include:

- acute radiation cystitis/urethritis with urinary frequency, poor stream, and dysuria
- acute radiation proctitis with tenesmus, pain, and passage of mucus and blood
- late effects include impotence in ~50% (and all patients receiving anti-androgen therapy) and rectal bleeding from telangiectasia.

There is evidence that irradiation of the pelvic lymph nodes as well as the prostate gland reduces the risk of relapse in men with intermediate- or high-risk disease. Many centres are currently using intensity-modulated radiotherapy (IMRT) techniques to facilitate irradiation of the lymph nodes and prostate with reduced normal tissue damage, in particular bladder and rectum. Clinical trials are also under way to compare prolonged-course radiotherapy using 2 Gy fractions with shorter hypofractionated regimens using IMRT.

Brachytherapy

Permanent implantation of radioactive iodine seeds (^{125}I) under transrectal ultrasound control may be used to deliver a dose of ~140 Gy to the prostate, again with excellent results in organ-confined prostate cancer. This treatment is contraindicated in patients who have marked urinary outflow symptoms, very small or large prostate volumes, or previous TURP. It avoids the inconvenience of 7–8 weeks of external beam radiotherapy, and has similar toxicities:

- radiation urethritis, may require a urinary catheter for some days
- radiation proctitis
- impotence, probably less frequent than with external beam radiotherapy.

Neoadjuvant and adjuvant hormone therapy may be used with brachytherapy, as for external beam radiotherapy.

An alternative approach is to combine brachytherapy with external beam radiotherapy, the former commonly delivered using a single temporary insertion of a high-dose-rate (HDR) applicator.

Hormone therapy alone

Androgen deprivation has been used for many years to treat patients with localized prostate cancer if they are unfit for radical surgery or radiotherapy. However, such treatment has only temporary impact in terms of delay of tumour progression and, although normal PSA levels may be maintained for a number of years, hormone-refractory disease eventually develops if patients survive many years. There is controversy surrounding the timing of hormone therapy for non-metastatic prostate cancer, particularly when this is asymptomatic. For unfit elderly patients with high-risk disease for whom radical treatment is not appropriate or feasible, immediate treatment with androgen deprivation may be preferred to watchful waiting.

Active surveillance

Particularly for patients >70 years with low-risk cancers, a policy of expectant management is appropriate. The Scandinavian Prostate Cancer Group has recently published 10-year results of their randomized study of watchful waiting versus radical prostatectomy. This study clearly demonstrates benefits of radical treatment for prostate cancer, in terms of reduction in the risk of local recurrence, metastatic disease, need for hormone therapy, and death from prostate cancer. However, these benefits appear to be in patients who are <65 years, often with intermediate-risk disease. Patients who develop progressive disease (rising PSA, clinical evidence of disease progression, or worsening grade on repeat biopsy after two years) during active surveillance should be considered for radical treatment or androgen deprivation.

PSA failure

A rising PSA level after a radical prostatectomy or radical radiotherapy may herald the development of local recurrence or metastatic disease. Predictors of the latter are:
- a short interval from treatment to PSA rise
- PSA doubling time <6 months
- involved surgical margins, pelvic lymph nodes, or seminal vesicles at prostatectomy.

Patients with features suggesting local recurrence after surgery may be candidates for radiotherapy. Rising PSA after radiotherapy may be managed expectantly, or with androgen deprivation, or with salvage local therapy, e.g. prostate cryotherapy. There is controversy surrounding the benefits, morbidities, and timing of these interventions.

Treatment outcomes

The prognosis of early prostate cancer is excellent, with median survival times >10 years for patients treated by either radical prostatectomy or radiotherapy. Reassuringly, the number of deaths from prostate cancer in the US is falling. Although disease progression as measured by rising PSA occurs in around 40% of surgical patients and ~50% of patients treated by radiotherapy, the natural history of recurrent disease may be very slow. US data have shown that the median time from PSA rise post-prostatectomy to the development of metastatic disease may be as long as 8 years. The median time from PSA rise after radical radiotherapy until metastatic disease is shorter, around 5 years, almost certainly reflecting the more advanced stages of disease treated with this modality.

For metastatic disease, the median duration of response to hormone therapy is 18–24 months. The median survival time after development of hormone-refractory disease is 12–18 months.

Testicular cancer

The treatment of advanced testicular cancer represents one of the great successes of medical oncology in the last 30 years. This is one of the few solid tumours for which the majority of patients with metastatic disease can expect to be cured. Efforts are now focusing on minimizing the late effects of curative therapy as well as improving the outlook for poor-prognosis advanced disease.

Epidemiology and aetiology

Ninety-five per cent of testicular tumours are of germ cell origin. These are relatively uncommon malignancies, almost 2000 cases in the UK each year, the 14th most common cancer in men overall. They are, however, the commonest cancer in men aged 20–40 years, and their incidence has doubled over the last 30 years. The reason for this increase is not clear. The age distribution is dependent on pathology.

- Seminoma is the most frequent pathology (55%):
  - peak incidence age 30–40 years
  - occasionally 60–70 years.
- Non-seminoma (45%):
  - peak incidence age 20–30 years.

An increased risk of testicular cancer is observed in men with:

- history of undescended testis (relative risk 8×)
- previous testicular cancer (relative risk 25×)
- testicular carcinoma *in situ*
- family history of testicular cancer
- Klinefelter's syndrome
- atrophic testis and infertility
- *in utero* exposure to oestrogens.

It is believed that both environmental and genetic factors combine to give rise to testicular dysgenesis, manifested as either Leydig cell malfunction with failure of normal testicular descent, or impaired germ cell differentiation with poor sperm production and/or malignant change.

Screening

There is no evidence to support population screening for this disease.

Genetics

Testicular germ cell tumours are invariably aneuploid. Gain of the 12p chromosome arm, most commonly as an isochromosome, is highly consistent.

Pathology

Germ cell tumours arise from the germinal epithelium, and both seminomas and non-seminomatous germ cell tumours (NSGCTs) are thought to arise from pre-existing carcinoma *in situ*. The British classification has been replaced by the World Health Organization (WHO) system (see Table 20.11).

The natural histories of seminoma and NSGCT differ, and these differences dictate the variation in management between the two pathologies. The majority of seminomas (75%) present with disease confined to the testis. Spread tends to be predictable, to the para-aortic lymph nodes in the first instance and, subsequently, to the supradiaphragmatic lymph nodes and then to other metastatic sites. Tumour growth can be very slow, so that untreated microscopic metastatic disease may take up to 10 years to become clinically apparent.

In contrast only 50% of testicular NSGCTs present with localized disease. Blood-borne and lymphatic spread occurs earlier than with seminoma.

Tumour markers

NSGCT produces serum markers in the form of human chorionic gonadotrophin (HCG) and/or alpha fetoprotein (AFP) in 75% of cases. Seminomas on the other hand have no reliable tumour marker to monitor disease, although the HCG may be moderately elevated in about 25% of cases. The lactate dehydrogenase (LDH) may be raised in both tumours and is useful for defining a prognostic group, correlating with tumour bulk, but it is not a reliable marker for monitoring response to treatment or subsequent relapse.

Table 20.11 Pathological classification of testicular cancers

British	WHO	Relative frequency
Seminoma	Seminoma	55%
Teratoma	Non-seminomatous germ cell tumour	33%
Mixed seminoma teratoma	Mixed germ cell tumour	12%
Teratoma differentiated (TD)	Mature teratoma	
Malignant teratoma intermediate (MTI)	Embryonal carcinoma with teratoma (teratocarcinoma)	
Malignant teratoma undifferentiated (MTU)	Yolk sac tumour, embryonal carcinoma	
Malignant teratoma trophoblastic (MTT)	Yolk sac tumour; choriocarcinoma	

Presentation

Most commonly presents with a hard testicular lump, which may be painless, or may be mistaken for epididymo-orchitis. Patients with testicular symptoms that persist despite one course of antibiotics should be referred to a urology clinic for assessment including ultrasound examination of the testes.

Men with tumours producing high levels of HCG may develop gynaecomastia which resolves with treatment of the cancer.

Metastatic disease may present with:
- lumbar back pain associated with bulky (>5 cm) para-aortic lymphadenopathy
- cough and dyspnoea with multiple lung metastases
- superior vena cava obstruction (SVCO) with mediastinal lymphadenopathy
- CNS symptoms/signs with brain metastasis.

Many patients with relapsed disease are diagnosed with asymptomatic spread of disease picked up on routine monitoring of serum markers, CXR, or CT scan.

Investigation of testicular germ cell tumours

This initially includes:
- ultrasound scan of of both testes
- CXR
- tumour markers (AFP, HCG, LDH).

Where the patient has obvious and widespread metastases, immediate referral for chemotherapy may be necessary, but for the majority the initial management will be inguinal orchidectomy. A biopsy of the contralateral testis should be considered where there is a high risk of carcinoma *in situ*. Patients at risk include those with a history of maldescent, a small testis (less than 12 ml), and patients aged less than 30 years. Further staging investigations will usually be performed post-operatively.

Staging investigations and prognostic grouping

Staging investigations will include, in all patients, a CT scan of the thorax, abdomen, and pelvis. In patients with a greatly elevated HCG (>10 000 iu/l) or bulky mediastinal disease or symptoms/signs of CNS disease, a CT brain scan is advisable. Post-operative tumour markers should be serially checked, if raised, to assess whether or not they are falling with an appropriate half-life (4–6 days for AFP, 24 h for HCG). Other investigations such as a bone scan may be necessary if clinically indicated.

Until recently the Royal Marsden Hospital (RMH) staging (Table 20.12) has been used for both NSGCT and seminomas. The IGCCC (International Germ Cell Consensus Classification) prognostic grouping (see Table 20.14, 📖 p.417) is now applicable for all patients with stage >I disease.

Sperm storage

Sperm count and storage should be considered at an early stage where patients are likely to require further therapy. It should be remembered that up to 50% of patients with testicular germ cell tumour may be subfertile at presentation.

Table 20.12 RMH staging

I	No evidence of disease outside the testis
IM	As above but with persistently raised tumour markers
II	Infra-diaphragmatic nodal involvement
IIA	Maximum diameter <2 cm
IIB	Maximum diameter 2–5 cm
IIC	Maximum diameter 5–10 cm
IID[a]	Maximum diameter >10 cm
III	Supra- and infra-diaphragmatic node involvement
	Abdominal nodes a, b, c, as above
	Mediastinal nodes M+
	Neck nodes N+
IV	Extralymphatic metastases
	Abdominal nodes a, b, c, as above
	Mediastinal or neck nodes as for stage III
	Lungs:
	L1 <3 metastases
	L2 multiple metastases <2 cm in diameter
	L3 multiple metastases >2 cm in diameter
	Liver involvement H+
	Other sites specified

[a]The Stage IID category was formulated at the 1989 Seminoma Consensus Conference.

Management of testicular cancer

The management of seminoma and NSGCT depends on the stage of disease and involves all three major modalities for the treatment of cancer – surgery, radiotherapy, and chemotherapy.

Carcinoma *in situ*

Germ cell carcinoma *in situ* may progress to invasive cancer, either seminoma or NSGCT, with 50% producing invasive tumours 5 years from diagnosis. Once this diagnosis is made, treatment should be offered, although this may not need to be given immediately. Carcinoma *in situ* can be eradicated by low-dose radiotherapy to the testis (20 Gy in 10 fractions). The advantage of this treatment is that, in the majority of cases, it will avoid orchidectomy and not affect Leydig cell function, and long-term hormone therapy should not be necessary.

Stage I seminoma

Orchidectomy must be radical and the incision must be in the groin to avoid tumour seeding in the scrotal skin.

Despite a negative staging CT scan, 20% of these patients develop recurrent seminoma after orchidectomy; 90% of relapses are in para-aortic nodes, but some of these are late, up to 10 years after orchidectomy. Relapse is commoner after orchidectomy for testicular tumours >4 cm diameter, but is usually marker negative and only detectable on CT scan. The prognosis is excellent: almost all patients with relapsed disease are cured by salvage therapy (see below).

Currently there are three management options for patients with stage I seminoma:
- adjuvant radiotherapy to the para-aortic nodes, T11–L5 (20 Gy in 10 fractions):
  - reduces the relapse rate to 4%
  - well tolerated, but risk of radiation induced abdominal malignancy.
- surveillance including annual CT scan of abdomen and pelvis.
- adjuvant chemotherapy with one cycle of carboplatin chemotherapy:
  - recent results suggest similar reduction in relapse rate as with radiotherapy to retroperitoneal lymph nodes.

Stage IIA and IIB seminoma

These patients are best treated with radiotherapy to the para-aortic and ipsilateral iliac lymph nodes.
- IIA: 30 Gy in 15 fractions leads to 95% disease-free survival after 5 years.
- IIB: 36 Gy in 18 fractions leads to 90% disease-free survival after 5 years.

Stage I NSGCT

After orchidectomy alone, the relapse rate is around 30%, with the majority of relapses occurring in the first 2 years, and many detected by a rise in tumour markers with only low volume disease in the para-aortic nodes or lungs. As a result, the outcome of treatment for relapsed stage I disease is excellent, with cure rates >95%. The best predictor of relapse is the presence of vascular invasion in the tumour – 50% of these men develop metastatic disease if given no adjuvant therapy.

The treatment options are:
- surveillance including frequent clinic visits, CXR, tumour marker monitoring, and regular CT scans particularly in the first 2 years
- adjuvant chemotherapy particularly for tumours with vascular invasion:
  - 2 cycles of BEP (bleomycin, etoposide, cisplatin) chemotherapy
  - 97% disease-free survival
- nerve-sparing retroperitoneal lymph node dissection with adjuvant chemotherapy for node-positive disease:
  - not commonly used in UK.

Each of these results in >95% long-term disease-free survival.
- In the USA there is a more aggressive surgical approach to resection of retroperitoneal nodes for stage I NSGCTs.

Stage IIc–IV–seminoma and stage IM–IV NSGCT

Chemotherapy is the mainstay of treatment for all these stages of testicular cancer and has been the key to the improvement in prognosis for this disease over the last 20 years. For the vast majority of patients treatment is based on the BEP regimen. All patients should be assigned an IGCCC prognostic group to guide treatment (see Table 20.14).

Good-prognosis disease

Standard treatment comprises 3 cycles of BEP chemotherapy, monitoring tumour markers weekly, and restaging by CT scan at the end of chemotherapy. In patients in whom bleomycin is unsafe (older patients with poor lung function), an alternative regimen with equivalent results is four cycles of EP chemotherapy.

The toxicities of BEP chemotherapy include:
- nausea and vomiting (largely prevented with appropriate anti-emetics including $5-HT_3$ antagonist and dexamethasone)
- neutropenic sepsis:
  - dose delays and reductions should be avoided
  - granulocyte colony-stimulating factor (G-CSF) may be used as secondary prophylaxis after one episode of neutropenic sepsis
- neuropathy:
  - cisplatin causes sensory peripheral neuropathy and high-tone hearing loss
  - toxicity is reduced when cisplatin dose fractionated over 5 days
- nephropathy:
  - cisplatin causes a fall in glomerular filtration rate (GFR) and tubular damage, often associated with hypomagnesaemia;
  - best managed by prevention (pre-and post-hydration, diuretic, e.g. furosemide and mannitol, IV magnesium supplements)
- pulmonary fibrosis:
  - risk relates to the cumulative dose of bleomycin
  - this toxicity can be fatal.

Residual tumour masses post-chemotherapy

After completion of chemotherapy, CT scan may show persistent masses at the site of the original metastatic disease. For patients with seminoma, such masses are managed expectantly, and the majority are seen to slowly regress on serial scans. However, for patients with NSGCT in whom residual tumour is apparent, surgical resection should be performed. The majority of these will be in the retroperitoneum, and extensive and

difficult surgery is often necessary for a complete resection. The assistance of a vascular surgeon is required not infrequently. Morbidity can be up to 10% and mortality 0.5%. The residual masses may contain:
• necrotic tumour (50%)
• mature teratoma (35%); although histologically benign, excision is important as this tissue can give rise to malignancy if left *in situ*
• viable tumour (15%); may require additional chemotherapy.
Surgery should usually only be undertaken when markers have normalized. Residual pulmonary masses should also be resected where possible. The problems of surgical technique and anaesthetic risk, particularly as most patients will have been exposed to bleomycin, demand that patients are operated on in a centre experienced in this surgery.

Retroperitoneal node dissection can be performed laparoscopically in experienced centres.

Intermediate- and poor-prognosis disease
Although no chemotherapy regimen has yet been proven to be superior to four cycles of BEP chemotherapy for these groups of patients, the outcomes of treatment are significantly poorer, with 5-year survival:
• intermediate group 80%
• poor group 48%.
All such patients should be considered for clinical trials exploring novel or more intensive treatment options.

Follow-up

Following primary management of metastatic disease, regular follow-up is necessary as, in those patients who relapse, salvage therapy can be effective in ~25% of cases.

Non-germ cell testicular tumours

These represent a very small proportion of testicular tumours. Stromal tumours such as those arising from Leydig cells are generally benign, but metastases have been reported in approximately 10% of cases. Testicular lymphomas are the commonest testicular cancer in elderly men and should be treated along the same principles as lymphomas arising at other sites.

Table 20.13 Examples of chemotherapy regimens for testicular cancer

BEP			
Bleomycin	30 mg	d1, 8, 15	
Etoposide	100 mg/m²	d1–5	q 3/52
Cisplatin	20 mg/m²	d1–5	
EP			
Etoposide	100 mg/m²	d1–5	q3/52
Cisplatin	20 mg/m²	d1–5	
VIP			
Etoposide	75 mg/m²	d1–5	q3/52
Ifosfamide	1.2 g/m²	d1–5	
Cisplatin	20 mg/m²	d1–5	

Table 20.14 IGCCC prognostic grouping for metastatic germ-cell tumours

Teratoma (NSGCT)	Seminoma
Good prognosis with all of:	
Testis/retroperitoneal primary	Any primary site
No non-pulmonary visceral metastases	No non-pulmonary visceral metastases
AFP <1000 ng/ml	Normal AFP
HCG <5000 iu/ml	Any HCG
LDH 1.5 times upper limit of normal	Any LDH
56% of teratomas: 5-year survival 92%	90% of seminomas: 5-year survival 86%
Intermediate prognosis with any of:	
Testis/retroperitoneal primary	Any primary site
No non-pulmonary visceral metastases	Non-pulmonary visceral metastases
AFP >1000 and <10 000 ng/ml	Normal AFP
HCG >5000 and <50 000 iu/ml	Any HCG
LDH >1.5 times normal <10 times normal	Any LDH
28% of teratomas : 5-year survival 80%	10% of seminomas: 5-year survival 73%
Poor prognosis with any of:	
Mediastinal primary	No patients in this group
Non-pulmonary visceral metastases	
AFP >10 000 ng/ml	
HCG >50 000 iu/ml	
LDH >10 normal	
16% of teratomas: 5-year survival 48%	

Penile cancer

Epidemiology
This is an uncommon cancer, with around 350 new cases per annum in the UK. The majority occur in the over 70s, but up to 20% occur under the age of 40 years. The disease is relatively more common in Africa, India, and South America.

Aetiology
- Human papilloma virus (HPV 16 and 18) infection.
- Associated with poor hygiene and phimosis.
- Pre-malignant lesion—carcinoma *in situ*:
  - on the glans – erythroplasia of Queyrat
  - on the shaft – Bowen's disease
  - progresses to invasive carcinoma in ~10%.
- Increased risk with cigarette smoking and immunosuppression including HIV infection.
- Neonatal circumcision gives lifelong protection.

Pathology
The vast majority are squamous carcinomas, which may be exophytic or locally invasive and destructive, and can spread initially via lymphatics to inguinal and then pelvic lymph nodes. Locally advanced disease can spread to other organs including liver, lungs, bone, and skin.

Staging
The TNM system is commonly used (see Table 20.15).

Investigations
- Careful examination of the penis with cytological assessment or biopsy of any lesion.
- General examination including palpation of inguinal lymph nodes.
- >50% have inguinal lymphadenopathy, but less than half of these have metastatic disease within the nodes – reactive lymphadenopathy is more common.
- Fine needle aspiration (FNA) suspicious lymph nodes or review lymph nodes after treatment of the primary carcinoma.
- Further staging, e.g. cross-sectional imaging of the abdomen and pelvis, is only required if inguinal nodes involved or clinical suspicion of metastatic disease.

Presentation
At least 50% arise on the glans, appearing as an area of erythema, warty tumour, or ulceration; 20% involve the foreskin only. In advanced disease there may be considerable destruction of the penis. Patients not uncommonly conceal the diagnosis until there is advanced loco-regional disease with considerable secondary infection. Patients may present with metastatic disease, e.g. inguinal and pelvic lymphadenopathy.

Table 20.15 TNM staging for penile cancer

Tis	Carcinoma *in situ*
Ta	Non-invasive verrucous carcinoma
T1	Tumour invades subepithelial connective tissue
T2	Tumour invades corpus spongiosum or cavernosum
T3	Tumour invades urethra or prostate
T4	Tumour invades other adjacent structures
N0	No regional lymph node metastases
N1	Single superficial inguinal lymph node metastases
N2	Multiple or bilateral superficial inguinal lymph node metastases
N3	Deep inguinal or pelvic lymph node metastases

Management

Primary tumour

Early-stage disease may be successfully managed with organ conservation:

- Tis – topical 5-FU, laser therapy, cryotherapy, local excision
- T1 – excision or radiotherapy.

More advanced disease or local recurrence often requires at least partial amputation of the penis. Patients with inoperable disease may be treated with chemotherapy and radiotherapy.

Regional lymph nodes

Inguinal lymph nodes may be managed by surveillance if impalpable after completion of local treatment to the primary. However, with high-grade T2 and more advanced cancers, the incidence of positive regional lymph nodes is 60% or higher, and elective bilateral inguinal lymphadenectomy should be considered in the absence of clinical involvement of lymph nodes. Patients with persistent lymphadenopathy after clearance of the primary tumour and any infection should be considered for bilateral inguinal lymphadenectomy. Patients who are unfit for surgery or have inoperable disease may benefit from chemotherapy and radiotherapy. The role of sentinel node biopsy is unclear and it is not in widespread use.

The disease is moderately chemosensitive, and active regimens include methotrexate, bleomycin, and cisplatin (MBP). Chemotherapy is recommended both for advanced disease and as adjuvant therapy for node-positive disease.

Outcomes

Overall, 50% survive disease-free beyond 5-years, with better results in node-negative (60%) compared with node-positive (30%). The majority of relapses occur in the first 2 years, and close follow-up is recommended at least during this time.

Further reading

Advanced Bladder Cancer Meta-analysis Collaboration (2003) Neoadjuvant chemotherapy in invasive bladder cancer: a systematic review and meta-analysis. *Lancet* **361**, 1927–34.

American Society of Clinical Oncology (2007) Update of a practice guideline: initial hormonal management of androgen-sensitive metastatic, recurrent, or progressive prostate cancer. *Clin Oncol* **25**, 1596–605.

Atzpodien J, Kirchner H, Jonas U, et al. (2004) Interleukin-2- and interferon alfa-2a-based immunochemotherapy in advanced renal cell carcinoma: a prospectively randomized trial of the German Cooperative Renal Carcinoma Chemoimmunotherapy Group (DGCIN). *J Clin Oncol* **22**, 1188–94.

Barry MJ (2008) Screening for prostate cancer among men 75 years of age or older. *N Eng J Med* **359**, 2515–16

Chistoph F, Weikert S, Miller K, et al. (2005) New guidelines for clinical Stage I testicular seminoma. *Oncology* **69**, 455–62

Cookson MS, Herr HW, Zhang ZF, et al. (1997) The treated natural history of high risk superficial bladder cancer: 15 year outcome. *J Urol* **158**, 62–7.

Damber JE, Aus G (2008) Prostate cancer. *Lancet* **371**, 1710–21.

Dehn T (2008) Management of renal cell carcinoma. *Ann R Coll Surg Engl* **90**, 278–81.

Frankel S, Smith GD, Donovan J, Neal D (2003) Screening for prostate cancer. *Lancet* **361**, 1122–8.

Graham J, Baker M, Macbeth F, et al. (2008) Diagnosis and treatment of prostate cancer. Summary of NICE Guidance. *BMJ* **336**, 610–12.

Horikawa Y, Kamazawa T, Narita S, et al. (2007) Lymphatic invasion is a prognostic factor for bladder cancer treated with radical cystectomy. *Int J Clin Oncol* **12**, 131–6.

Hungerhuber E, Schlenker B, Frimberger D (2006) Lymphoscintigraphy in penile cancer: limited value of sentinel node biopsy in patients with clinically suspicious nodes. *World J Urol* **24**, 319–24.

Jani AB, Hellman S (2003) Early prostate cancer: clinical decision-making. *Lancet* **361**, 1045–53.

MRC Renal Cancer Collaborators (1999) Interferon-α and survival in metastatic renal carcinoma: early results of a randomized controlled trial. *Lancet* **353**, 14–17.

National Institute for Health and Clinical Excellence (NICE) (2008) *Clinical Guideline. Prostate Cancer – diagnosis and treatment.* London: NICE.

Ogan, K., Cadeddu, J.A., and Stifelman, M.D. (2003). Laparoscopic radical nephrectomy—stop oncologic efficacy. *Urol Clin North Am* **30**, 543–50.

Raghavan D, Shipley WU, Garnick MB, Russell PJ, Richie JP (1990) Biology and management of bladder cancer. *N Engl J Med* **322**, 1129–38.

Rini BI, Small EJ (2005) Biology and clinical development of vascular endothelial growth factor targeted therapy in renal cell carcinoma. *J Clin Oncol* **23**, 1028–43.

Scottish Intercollegiate Guidelines Network (SIGN) (1998) *Management of Adult Testicular Germ Cell Tumours: a national clinical guideline.* Guideline 28. Edinburgh: SIGN. http://www.sign.ac.uk/pdf/sign28.pdf (accessed 29 June 2009).

Scottish Intercollegiate Guidelines Network (2005) *Management of Transitional Cell Carcinoma of the Bladder: a national clinical guideline.* Guideline 85. Edinburgh: SIGN. http://www.sign.ac.uk/pdf/sign85.pdf (accessed 29 June 2009).

Tomita Y (2006) Early renal cell cancer. *Int J Clin Oncol* **11**, 22–7.

Volpe A, Panzarella T, Rendon RA (2004) The natural history of incidentally detected small renal masses. *Cancer* **100**, 738–45.

Gynaecological cancer

Ovarian cancer

- Fifth commonest cancer in women with over 6000 cases diagnosed and over 4000 women dying of the disease each year in UK. Incidence slowly rising.
- Majority of cases occur over the age of 55 years with the peak in the 65–75-year age group.

Aetiology

- Risk of ovarian cancer relates to the number of ovulatory cycles in a woman's lifetime and multiple pregnancies.
- Use of the oral contraceptive pill now shown to offer protection; infertility or its treatment may increase the risk.
- About 5% are clearly hereditary – associated with *BRCA1* or *BRCA2* or Lynch families (see 📖 Chapter 15, 'Breast cancer').

Pathology

- 80% of ovarian malignancies are epithelial. Serous and endometrioid are the commonest forms but about 5% are mucinous or clear cell. Clear-cell cancers account for up to 20% in the Far East.
- The rest comprise germ cell, sex cord/stromal tumours, sarcomas, and neuro-endocrine cancers.

CA125

Eighty per cent of women with advanced ovarian cancer have elevated serum CA125 and this marker is valuable in monitoring response to therapy and in the detection of early relapse. However, it is not specific for ovarian cancer and is elevated in association with other peritoneal pathologies. A ratio of CA125 and carcinoembryonic antigen (CEA) that is higher than 25 may help to support the diagnosis of epithelial ovarian cancer (EOC).

Presentation and staging

- Majority of women present with disease that has spread beyond the ovary to involve the peritoneum and other abdomino-pelvic organs.
- Most common symptoms are of abdominal discomfort and swelling, bloating, and change in bowel habit.
- Gastrointestinal and urinary symptoms also occur.

The two main prognostic factors in ovarian cancer are stage (see Table 21.1) and the amount of residual disease after surgery. Five-year survival rates according to stage are as follows:

- stage I, 80%; but over 90% for stage IA
- stage II, 45%
- stage III, 20%
- stage IV, less than 10%.

Table 21.1 A simplified staging of ovarian cancer

Stage	Description
Ia	Tumour confined to one ovary
Ib	Tumour confined to both ovaries
Ic	Tumour stage I but with capsule ruptured or malignant ascites
II	Tumour with pelvic extension only
III	Tumour with peritoneal implantation outwith the pelvis or involved small bowel; retroperitoneal or inguinal nodes
IV	Distant metastases eg intra hepatic, pleura or lung

Treatment of epithelial ovarian cancer

- The primary treatment remains surgery, with the aim to achieve complete surgical removal or maximal debulking effort.
- This should also include thorough staging with removal of the omentum, peritoneal washings, inspection of the subdiaphragmatic areas, and, more controversially, lymphadenectomy.
- The amount of residual disease correlates with worse prognosis.
- Majority of patients present with advanced disease (stage II–IV), with a correspondingly poor prognosis.
- Patients who have greater than 2 cm disease after their initial surgery have a poor prognosis, with only 20% of patients surviving 3 years.
- Median survival times for patients with suboptimally debulked disease (greater than 1 cm) range from 16 to 29 months and from 26 to 96 months for patients with optimally debulked disease.

Surgery

Patients must undergo full surgical staging. A surgical staging procedure consists of:
- a midline incision
- total abdominal hysterectomy
- bilateral salpingo-oophorectomy (BSO)
- omentectomy
- multiple peritoneal biopsies and washings
- lymph node sampling of the para-aortic and pelvic regions
- careful assessment of the subdiaphragmatic areas.

The case should be discussed at the local tumour board or multidisciplinary team meeting (MDT). There is good evidence to support referral for surgery to a specialized gynaecological oncology surgeon.

Radical surgery plays an important role in the treatment of ovarian cancer.

A randomized trial has shown that, for patients who cannot be optimally debulked at initial laparotomy, interval debulking surgery after three cycles of chemotherapy confers a significant survival benefit. However, this is only applicable when the original surgery was performed by a non-specialist gynaecological oncology surgeon.

For patients who are not fit or who have supra-omental stage III disease and some stage IV patients with positive pleural effusions only, and where optimal debulking cannot be achieved, neo-adjuvant chemotherapy (NACT) and delayed primary surgery (DPS) may be considered as an alternative.

Laparoscopic surgery is becoming established and is especially helpful for lymph node dissection of the pelvic side wall. Over the past decade, in specialized referral centres, laparoscopic ovarian radical surgery is being assessed with less morbidity, faster recovery, and equal oncological results to open surgery. The procedure is technically difficult; often specialists work in pairs.

First-line chemotherapy

Chemotherapy is usually offered to all patients except possibly stage Ia G1. Platinum and a taxane are usually standard but there is a body of opinion which recommends carboplatin alone based on the ICON 3 (International Collaborative Ovarian Neoplasm) trial reserving taxanes for relapse.

- Platinum-based therapy is usual – carboplatin is equivalent to cisplatin but with less toxicity.
- Taxanes are usually given in combination in most centres.
- In older or unfit patients, single-agent carboplatin is used.
- To date, the addition of a third drug or alternating doublets has failed to improve survival.
- Maintenance treatments have also failed to show survival benefit as yet.
- Intra-peritoneal chemotherapy in optimally debulked patients has been shown to improve survival in four randomized trials but has been slow to be adopted universally because of toxicity and inconvenience.
- Currently there are many trials investigating the addition of targeted anti-cancer treatments but their exact role remains to be defined until these trials are complete; at the time of writing the vascular endothelial growth factor (VEGF) receptor antagonists seem to offer greatest potential.

Treatment at relapse

- Patients who relapse after first-line therapy are incurable.
- The majority of patients relapse within 15–24 months and the length of the treatment-free interval before relapse is an important factor in predicting response to second-line therapy.
- Patients who relapse on treatment are termed platinum refractory and should be entered into clinical trials of new agents, or treated with new drugs or non-platinum-containing regimes such as pegylated liposomal doxorubicin or topotecan
- Patients who relapse within 6 months are termed platinum resistant, and retreating with platinum produces response rates less than 10% so should be treated as above
- Patients with a treatment-free interval of greater than 12 months are generally termed platinum sensitive and should be re-challenged with a platinum-containing regimen. Other indicators of response are the bulk of disease, serous pathology, previous response to treatment, and the number of disease sites.

- A number of new agents including topotecan, liposomal doxorubicin, etoposide, gemcitabine, epothilones, new taxane analogues, and trabectedin have response rates of 15–25% in this setting.
- Dose-dense and dose-intense regimes are active in these settings and following initial reports of cisplatin and etoposide, weekly carboplatin and paclitaxel are becoming established alternatives; 40–50% response rates are reported.

Follow-up

Clinical dilemmas arise after first-line therapy – what follow-up protocol is appropriate and when should second-line therapy be instituted? All patients usually have serial CA125 estimations but, as soon as the marker rises, much anxiety is caused and many patients expect treatment. The OV05 trial may help to answer whether early-intervention treatment with a rising CA125 improves outcome. Data are expected in 2009.

Treatment of rare ovarian cancers

- Special consideration should be given to mucinous tumours which respond less well to carboplatin and paclitaxel. Investigation of regimes being used to treat gastrointestinal tumours is being undertaken.
- Similarly, clear-cell tumours have a worse prognosis and Japanese experience suggests novel regimes should be tested.
- Primary ovarian sarcomas are believed to behave more aggressively, although recent experience suggest carboplatin and paclitaxel with or without an anthracycline should be considered.
- Small-cell cancers are often lethal and may be associated with hypercalcaemia. They tend to be more common in younger age groups. Aggressive treatments programmes are offered but even so only 20–30% survive 2 years.
- Germ-cell tumours usually carry an excellent prognosis, and fertility-sparing surgery is advised with use of BEP (bleomycin, etoposide, cisplatin) chemotherapy in stage Ic and above. Early disease is treated more conservatively.
- Sexcord and stromal tumours may behave variably, sometimes with delayed relapse.
- All of these rare and uncommon cancers are best managed by centralized teams.

Cancer of the uterine corpus

- Carcinoma of the endometrium accounts for over 90% of tumours.
- Less common are the uterine sarcomas. Carcinosarcomas are almost certainly poor prognostic carcinomas but endometrial stromal sarcomas and smooth muscle tumours (leiomyosarcomas) may account for 3–8%.

Endometrial adenocarcinoma

Epidemiology and aetiology

- Occurs principally in post-menopausal women and the incidence rises with age.
- Aetiology has not been fully determined; however, obesity and unopposed oestrogen as hormone replacement therapy are thought to increase the risk.
- Women with breast cancer taking tamoxifen, which exerts oestrogenic agonist effects on the endometrium, have an increased risk of polyps, hyperplasia, and sometimes carcinoma.
- Commoner in obese women in whom oestrogen is peripherally produced in fat.
- Lynch syndrome leads to 40–60% additional risk of endometrial cancer.

Pathology

- Two types of endometrial cancer are usually recognized, type 1 and type 2.
- Type 1 is usually endometrioid and occurs in younger women with obesity and excess oestrogen exposure and generally carries a better prognosis.
- Type 2 occurs in older women with serous, clear-cell or other variants, and has a more aggressive pattern. Carcinosarcomas may be associated with this type. The prognosis is usually much worse.
- The major prognostic factors are the depth of invasion of the myometrium (if more than 50%) and grade of tumour (G3), and this is reflected in the International Federation of Gynecology and Obstetrics (FIGO) staging classification (see Table 21.2). This is due to be revised in 2009.
- Surgery should include total hysterectomy, and BSO, and washings. While many gynaecological oncologists argue for pelvic lymphadenectomy, two randomized trial have not shown any survival advantage but there may be prognostic value from staging and help in planning adjuvant therapies.
- The ovaries are also removed because they are frequently the site of secondary deposits or synchronous tumours.
- If the cervix is known to be involved pre-operatively, an extended or radical hysterectomy should be performed.

Table 21.2 Carcinoma of the corpus uteri (FIGO 2008)

Stage I*	**Tumour confined to the corpus uteri.**
IA*	No or less than half myometrial invasion.
IB*	More than half myometrial invasion.
Stage II*	**Tumour invades cervical stroma, but does not extend beyond the uterus.****
Stage III*	**Local and/or regional spread of the tumour.**
IIIA*	Tumour invades the serosa of the corpus uteri and/or adnexae#.
IIIB*	Vaginal and/or parametrial involvement#.
IIIC*	Metastases to pelvic and/or para-aortic lymph nodes#.
IIIC$_1$*	• Positive pelvic nodes
IIIC$_2$*	• Positive paraortic lymphnodes with or without positive pelvic lymphnodes.
Stage IV*	**Tumour invades bladder and/or bowel mucosa, and/or distant metastases.**
IVA*	Tumour invasion of bladder and/or bowel mucosa.
IVB*	Distant metastases, including intra-abdominal metastases and/or inguinal lymph nodes.

* Either G1, G2 or G3.
** Endocervical glandular involvement only should be considered as Stage I and no more as Stage II.
# Positive cytology has to be reported separately without changing the stage.

Management

Mainstay of treatment for stage I disease is total hysterectomy, BSO, peritoneal washings. While not recommended routinely, pelvic (and para-aortic) lymphadenectomy should be considered in high-risk cases such as clear-cell, serous carcinomas and carcinosarcomas.

The laparoscopic-assisted procedure is now being evaluated in a number of centres. The role of routine pelvic nodal dissection has not been supported in recent clinical trials (Hockel and Dornhofer, 2009).

Radiotherapy

• Adjuvant radiation post-operatively reduces the risk of local relapse. However none of the radiotherapy studies has shown any survival benefit in low or intermediate risk disease. The place of adjuvant radiotherapy is undergoing re-evaluation and should probably be reserved for cases with stage 1C and grade 3, doses given are usually between 45 and 52 Gy in 25–28 fractions. Vaginal brachytherapy only may be considered as an option for intermediate risk stage 1 patients. Brachytherapy is usually advised when there is cervical extension. Increasing evidence supports the use of sequential chemotherapy and radiation in high risk stage 1 and 2 cancers.

- In stage 3 cancers chemotherapy and tailored radiation are advised, discuss at tumour board/MDT
- A recent trial has demonstrated that neo-adjuvant chemotherapy and delayed primary surgery should be considered in selected cases
- Less commonly radiation may be required as primary treatment for women unfit to undergo surgery, usually through a combination of co-morbidity and marked obesity. Cure rates are only about 50–60%.

Chemotherapy

Recent studies have shown that combined chemotherapy and radiation in high-risk stage I cancers can reduce risk of local recurrence and improve overall survival. While traditionally Adriamycin® (doxorubicin) and cisplatin were used, this is being replaced as the community standard by carboplatin and paclitaxel.

Prognosis

- Best survival rate of the gynaecological cancers
- 70–75% overall 5-year survival
- Low-risk stage I disease carries a 15-year survival in excess of 90%
- High-risk stage I disease nearer 50%
- In stage II, III, and IV disease the 5-year survival falls to 50%, 30%, and 10%, respectively.

Sarcomas

The classification of sarcomas has recently been reviewed. Most experts now consider carcinosarcomas (previously known as MMMT – malignant mixed mesodermal tumours) as poorly differentiated carcinomas. Molecular markers support this. Uterine sarcomas are now divided into high grade and low grade, but many clinicians still refer to stromal sarcomas and leiomyosarcomas. They have different patterns of behaviour and spread. Nodal metastases are commoner with carcinosarcomas and stromal sarcomas, but leiomyosarcomas tend to spread haematogenously so lung and liver metastases are common and CT scanning is advised for staging.

Successful treatment depends very much on surgery for localized disease. Debulking is helpful for extensive disease. Residual disease or tumours with nodal or distant metastases are usually incurable. Hysterectomy and BSO should be performed, together with pelvic lymphadenectomy to stage the disease. Residual disease can be treated with radiation. Adjuvant radiation may improve pelvic control but does not confer a survival benefit and thus is not routinely recommended. As for endometrial carcinomas, adjuvant chemotherapy is increasingly used. Chemotherapy (e.g. doxorubicin, cisplatin and ifosfamide, or carboplatin and paclitaxel) can be prescribed for metastatic stromal disease, especially outside the pelvis, but long-term survival is very poor under these circumstances. However, leiomyosarcomas have different chemosensitivities, and Adriamycin® (doxorubicin) with or without ifosfamide remains standard. Docetaxel and gemcitabine maybe used for relapsed disease.

The future

Endometrial cancer will probably continue to increase in incidence as more women live longer. Long-term tamoxifen treatment for breast cancer may merit endometrial screening to identify early change, but screening on a population basis is not currently regarded as an effective strategy.

Cancer of the cervix

Aetiology
- Unprotected sexual intercourse
- Human papillomavirus (HPV)
- HPV types 16, 18 – USA and Europe
- Vaccination programme started in Europe in 2008
- Highly variable incidence rates in different countries
- Globally second commonest cancer in females

Epidemiology
The epidemiology of this disease has been extensively studied and strong associations demonstrated with:
- social deprivation
- multiparity
- cigarette smoking
- early onset of sexual intercourse (before 17 years)
- non-barrier forms of contraception
- reduced incidence and mortality in those countries with population screening.

More recent studies have focused attention specifically on papillomavirus transmission and the increased susceptibility of the cervical epithelium of the sexually active teenage female.

Pathology
When the disease is confined to the cervix, patient management depends on the cytology and/or histology specimens. These can reveal a spectrum of changes in the epithelium of the cervix:
- slight dysplastic changes to the cell architecture
- viral cytoplasmic changes
- intra-epithelial neoplasia (CIN 1, 2, or 3)
- micro-invasive carcinoma
- frank invasive carcinoma.

These early changes may first be identified by examination of a smear of cells, collected by a special wooden (Ayers) spatula or a brush, from the vaginal surface of the cervix. The specimen is a sample of the cells that are being shed from the ectocervix along, sometimes, with cells that are being shed from the endocervix and the endometrium. They are examined on a slide after staining with Papanicolou stain, and an impression of the health of the epithelium can be formed.

To accurately map changes in the cervical epithelium, patients require colposcopy, where the cervix is examined by binocular microscopy at 10× normal magnification.

Viral changes, dysplasia, CIN 1, and 2 are common in the sexually active adult female, particularly among those in their 20s when multiple partners and non-barrier contraception are involved. They can all revert to normal without treatment and are monitored by regular smears. CIN 3 changes are more commonly part of a process that can progress over months or years to invasive carcinoma.

Table 21.3 FIGO staging system for cervical cancer

Stage	Definition
Ia	Micro-invasive disease (max depth 5 mm, max width 7 mm)
Ib	Clinical disease confined to the cervix
IIa	Disease involves upper 1/3 vagina but not parametrium
IIb	Disease involves parametrium but does not extend to pelvic wall
III	Disease involves lower 2/3 vagina and/or pelvic wall
IV	Involvement of bladder, rectum, or distant organs

Staging
The FIGO staging system (Table 21.3) is based predominantly on the extent of the primary tumour. Metastatic spread is normally by the lymphatic system.

Presentation
- CIN and micro-invasive carcinoma usually have no symptoms.
- The earliest symptoms of invasive carcinoma are:
  - vaginal discharge
  - postcoital bleeding
  - intermenstrual or post-menopausal bleeding
  - back ache from hydronephrosis and nodal spread.

Investigation
Asymptomatic patients with CIN 1, 2, or 3, or micro-invasive carcinoma do not require any further investigation prior to treatment. Symptomatic patients should have an examination under anaesthetic to complete FIGO staging, cystoscopy, or sigmoidoscopy if these adjacent organs appear to be involved. CT or MRI scanning of the pelvis and abdomen define more fully the size of the primary tumour and any lymphadenopathy. Positron emission tomography (PET) CT is increasingly used as it is more likely to show occult metastases and change treatment plan. Intravenous urography (IVU) now considered obsolete.

Management
Surgery
- CIN 3 disease localized to ectocervix – colposcopy and loop diathermy, cryoprobe, or laser:
  - laser produces less distortion and more-rapid healing. Diathermy is inexpensive and easy to learn.
- CIN 3 disease extending into endocervical canal or microinvasion – cone biopsy.
- Complete excision still requires follow-up or, if patient wants no more children, hysterectomy and surveillance for vaginal vault.
- Invasive carcinoma (less than 4 cm, confined to cervix) – Wertheim's hysterectomy removes parametrium and pelvic nodes. A recent

study with 30-month survival data has shown Stage Ibi cervical cancer has an equally good oncological outcome with laparoscopic radical hysterectomy and pelvic lymphadenectomy.

Radiotherapy

- Radiotherapy if:
  - incomplete excision of tumour
  - poor tumour differentiation
  - vascular invasion
  - node involvement
  - all other stages/medically unfit
- External-beam irradiation followed by ICT
- 45–52 Gy – pelvis over 5 weeks
- Sterilizes pre-menopausal patients
- ICT gamma sources (^{137}Cs or ^{192}Ir) in uterus/upper vagina
- Inserted for minutes (HDR); multiple fractions
  - Inserted for ~24 h for MDR
- ICT – dose to central pelvic structures:
  - target dose 75–85 Gy to tumour volume 'A' point
  - dose to bladder and rectum below 70 Gy
  - moving towards customized planning with CT/MR
- Pelvic radiotherapy for advanced cancer:
  - minor side-effects are common, e.g. 10–20%
  - up to 5% serious late morbidity (bowel and urinary tract)
  - bleeding from proctitis or cystitis
  - stricture or ulceration
  - fistula
  - vaginal shortening/dryness.

Chemotherapy

Patients with recurrent pelvic or systemic metastatic disease may benefit from palliative chemotherapy. The principal active agents are:

- cisplatin
- mitomycin C
- ifosfamide
- methotrexate
- 5-fluorouracil (5-FU)
- bleomycin
- paclitaxel
- topotecan.

Concomitant chemo-irradiation

The National Cancer Institute (NCI) consensus statement of 1999 of clinical trials of chemo-irradiation for cervical carcinoma concluded that there was significant improvement in overall survival, local control, and risk of metastatic disease compared with radiotherapy alone, with greatest evidence of benefit in stage IB–II disease. All trials demonstrate increased toxicity with combined modality treatment, so that patient selection is important. A recent update has confirmed this benefit and again shown maximal benefit in earlier-stage disease.

Results

Survival at 5 years is typically as follows: stage Ia, 100%; stage Ib, 70–90%; stage II, 50–70%; stage III, 25–60%; stage IV, 10–20%. The wide ranges reflect the large variation in disease volume seen within the present staging system, which is based on tissue involvement rather than volume of disease. Relapse after 5 years is unusual.

Concomitant chemoirradiation

The NCI Consensus statement of 1999 of clinical trials of chemo-irradiation for cervical carcinoma concluded that there was significant improvement in overall survival, local control, and risk of metastatic disease compared with radiotherapy alone, with greatest evidence of benefit in stage IB–II disease. All trials demonstrate increased toxicity with combined modality treatment, so that patient selection is important. A recent update has confirmed this benefit and again shown maximal benefit in earlier stage disease. There is some limited evidence to support maintenance chemotherapy but this needs validation.

Vaginal and vulval cancer

Vaginal cancer
- Most vaginal malignancies are metastatic, from primaries in the cervix, vulva, endometrium, or trophoblast (choriocarcinoma).
- Most common histological types of primary cancer are squamous (80%) and adenocarcinoma (10%).

Aetiology
- Recognized association with squamous intra-epithelial and invasive neoplasia at other anogenital mucosal and cutaneous sites such as the cervix, vulva, and anus.
- Oncogenic HPV likely to be important in this tumour's biology.
- Smoking is almost certainly a co-factor as in cervix cancer and long-term survivors of cervix cancer who continue to smoke are most at risk.

Symptoms and signs
Symptoms
- Abnormal vaginal bleeding
- Vaginal discharge
- Bladder, rectal symptoms.

Signs
- Vaginal examination: best method of detection
- Soft tissue mass – speculum examination
- Most lesions in upper third and are exophytic
- Submucosal lesions may indicate metastatic spread from endometrium or bowel.

Staging and investigations
- MRI is the preferred investigation for evaluating local spread, particularly if body or transvaginal coils are used.
- Negative predictive values of CT and MRI for regional nodal involvement remain unsatisfactory.

Management
- Radical radiotherapy with a combination of pelvic external-beam and utero-vaginal intracavitary brachytherapy is the treatment of choice, especially in stage II.
- Overall 5-year survival is 40%, and salvage after first relapse is uncommon.
- Bad prognostic features are primary adenocarcinoma, large tumour bulk, tumour site (lower vaginal lesions fare worse), and posterior vaginal wall involvement.
- One in five long-term survivors will suffer from serious radiotherapy-related complications.
- Surgery has a limited role – early tumours of upper posterior vaginal wall need a radical hysterectomy and partial vaginectomy.
- Some USA centres use surgery alone for stage II disease.

Vulval cancer
- Primary invasive vulval cancer; occurs as commonly as cervical cancer in women over 60 years.
- One in four tumours occur in women under the age of 65 years.
- Majority (85%) are squamous carcinoma.
- Other types include basal carcinoma (10%) and malignant melanoma (4%).

Aetiology
- Associations with oncogenic HPV DNA
- Pre-existing abnormal vulval skin conditions such as a thickened epidermis (squamous hyperplasia)
- Lichen sclerosis
- Intra-epithelial atypia.

Symptoms and signs
- Tumours are preceded by chronic vulval skin symptoms such as pruritus and irritation.
- Sensation of a painful lump.
- Abnormal genital tract bleeding or haematuria may occur.
- Examination of the external genitalia will identify the majority of tumours.

Staging and investigations
- Combination of surgical and histopathological investigations.
- Incidence of nodal metastases rises from less than 1% for tumours with less than 1 mm depth of invasion to over 10% for tumours over 3 mm in depth.
- Routine node dissection and pathology assessment.
- Sentinel lymph node biopsy may be useful in early disease to spare the sequelae of a full lymphadenectomy.

Management
- Surgical excision with clear margins and removal of groin nodes (infection and wound seroma occur in 15% of cases). The role of sentinel node biopsy is not yet established.
- Extensive disease may require complex reconstruction involving anus, rectum, urethra after radical vulvectomy, and block dissection of inguinal nodes (morbidity is considerable).
- Chemo-irradiation for advanced disease: 5-FU and mitomycin C or cisplatin and 5-FU combined with radiotherapy give encouraging results.
- For very advanced inoperable disease, neo-adjuvant chemotherapy may downsize tumours and render them respectable.
- 5-year survival: 85% if node negative.
- Bad prognosis if:
  - >3 regional nodes involved
  - stage III, IV disease
  - large tumour bulk
  - node metastases
  - poor performance status
  - specific tumour type (melanoma).

Trophoblastic tumours

Introduction
Gestational trophoblastic disease (GTD) includes a spectrum of disorders:
- complete hydatidiform mole (CHM)
- partial hydatidiform mole (PHM).
- malignant invasive mole, gestational choriocarcinoma.
- highly malignant placental-site trophoblastic tumour (PSTT).
- both CHM and PHM can develop into invasive moles.

Difficulty in diagnosis occurs most frequently with choriocarcinomas and PSTT, which can arise after any type of pregnancy and may not present until many years later, with widespread metastases.

These rare tumours are best managed in specialist centres.

What is trophoblast?
Within a few days following conception, a ball of cells is formed called the blastocyst and the outer layer of this ball differentiates into trophoblast. This consists of an inner layer of cytotrophoblast cells that migrate outwards and fuse to form large multinucleate syncytiotrophoblast cells. The latter produce the pregnancy-associated hormone, human chorionic gonadotrophin (HCG), and invade the myometrium, triggering the formation of new maternal blood vessels that are leaky and supply nutrition to the growing fetus. Trophoblast tissue frequently invades these blood vessels, in both normal and molar pregnancies, and circulates in the blood.

Hydatidiform moles
Epidemiology
- 1/1000 pregnancies in UK
- Two-fold increase in frequency in South-East Asia
- More common after pregnancy when aged <16 years or >40 years.

Pathology
- Ovum lacking maternal nucleus DNA fertilized by one or two sperm – duplicate its chromosomes
- Conceptus is androgenetic
- Proliferate to give abnormal trophoblastic tissue
- Partial mole – arises when two sperm fertilize an ovum that has retained nuclear DNA:
  - triploid conceptus proliferation, to give abnormal trophoblast and variable fetal tissue
  - abnormal trophoblast forms hydropic villi that resemble grapes.

Histology
- Dilated villi of hyperplastic syncytiotrophoblast and cytotrophoblast
- Later, cisterns form
- Large arteriovenous (AV) shunts form – facilitates spread.

Presentation and staging
- Bleeding in early pregnancy.
- Anaemia.

- Toxaemia, hyperemesis, hyperthyroidism.
- About 15–20% of complete moles and 0.5% of partial moles will require chemotherapy. Staging of the disease involves ultrasound of the pelvis, serum HCG, and chest X-ray (CXR). In most instances the CXR will be normal but metastatic disease can present with:
  - cannonball secondaries
  - pleural effusions
  - wedge infarcts
  - oligaemic areas
  - cavitating lesions
  - miliary appearance.

If there are chest lesions then a CT or preferably MRI brain scan is indicated prior to lumbar puncture for HCG analysis of the cerebrospinal fluid (CSF) (an HCG ratio of >1:60 (CSF: blood) indicates central nervous system (CNS) involvement).

Diagnosis
- Ultrasound: large uterus for dates
  - CHM – snow-storm appearances, no fetal parts
  - PHM – abnormal placenta, fetal parts seen
- HCG level high
- Ductal carcinoma *in situ* (DCIS) in 2%
- Trophoblastic embolism.

Management
- Gentle suction curettage.
- Spontaneous abortion.
- Hysterotomy, Caesarean section increases the risks two-fold of chemotherapy required to eradicate persistent trophoblastic disease.

The information from the staging investigations is used in the scoring system (Table 21.4) to determine the risk of developing drug resistance to methotrexate. Patients who score <5 will be cured with methotrexate alone in at least 75% of cases, while only 30% are cured who score 5–8. Nevertheless, the latter patients are also offered methotrexate therapy to start with since this treatment carries no risk of long-term sequelae. Methotrexate may cause bleeding through rapid involution of metastases. Patients scoring >9 receive 'high-risk' intravenous combination chemotherapy comprising etoposide, methotrexate, and actinomycin D (EMA), alternating weekly with cyclophosphamide and vincristine (CO). Treatment with either methotrexate or EMA/CO regimens continues until the HCG has been normal for 6 weeks.

Registration
Three specialist centres in the UK register and oversee therapy of this rare tumour: Charing Cross (London), Dundee, Sheffield.

Follow-up
- Regular HCG measurement.
- Subsequent pregnancies increase risk of further molar pregnancy.
- Rise in HCG means persistent gestational trophoblastic disease or invasive mole or choriocarcinoma has developed.

If the HCG plateaus or starts to rise, this indicates that the patient has persisting molar disease or has developed an invasive mole (progression to choriocarcinoma and PSTT is rare). If a repeat ultrasound shows evidence of trophoblastic proliferation within the uterus, suction curettage may be performed. However, performing more than two dilation and curettages (D&Cs) is not usually beneficial and will not prevent the subsequent need for chemotherapy. Uterine perforation is more likely if the HCG is >20 000 iu/l, when a second D&C is contraindicated.

Other factors that increase the risk of needing subsequent chemotherapy include age >50 years and use of the oral contraceptive pill while HCG is still elevated. Accordingly, all patients are advised to use a barrier method of contraception following evacuation of a mole.

Table 21.4 Scoring system for gestational trophoblastic tumours

Prognostic factor	Score[a]			
	0	1	2	6
Age (years)	<39	>39		
Antecedent pregnancy (AP)	Mole	Abortion or unknown	Term	
Interval (end of AP to chemotherapy in months)	<4	4–7	7–12	>12
HCG iu/l	10^3–10^4	<10^3	10^4–10^5	>10^5
ABO blood group (female × male)		A × 0, 0 × A 0 or A × unknown	B × A or 0 AB × A or 0	
No of metastases	Nil	1–4	4–8	>8
Site of metastases	Not detected Lungs Vagina	Spleen Kidney	GI tract	Brain Liver
Largest tumour mass	<3.0	3–5 cm	>5 cm	
Prior chemotherapy			Single drug	2 or more drugs

[a]The total score for a patient is obtained by adding the individual scores for each prognostic factor. Lower risk, 0–5; medium risk, 6–8; high risk, >9.

Choriocarcinoma

Epidemiology
- Follows any type of pregnancy
- Incidence 1/50 000
- 3% of CHM develop into choriocarcinoma
- No geographical trends.

Pathology
- Highly malignant
- Soft, purple, haemorrhagic mass
- Histology:
  - mimics early blastocyst
  - cores of mononuclear cytotrophoblast
  - rim of multinucleated syncytiotrophoblast
  - no chorionic villi
  - surrounding necrosis, bleeding
  - tumour in venous sinuses.

Presentation
- Presents within 1 year of pregnancy
- Vaginal bleeding
- Abdominal pain
- Pelvic mass
- One-third present with metastases to liver, brain, or lung.

Management
- In most instances the patient will be transferred to the specialist centre.
- In addition to the staging investigations previously outlined, patients may undergo further tests including:
  - measurement of other tumour markers
  - whole-body CT/MRI
  - PET scanning
  - anti-HCG antibody scanning.

Where it can be safely achieved, excision biopsy of a metastasis should be considered. This not only enables histological confirmation of the diagnosis but also permits genetic analysis to prove the gestational nature of the tumour. If there are only maternal genes and no paternal genes present, then the patient has a non-gestational tumour (an ovarian choriocarcinoma or, more rarely, an epithelial tumour that has differentiated into choriocarcinoma). Frequently, however, biopsy is not possible and the diagnosis is made on the clinical history and other investigation findings. The patients are then scored and treated as described for molar disease.

The indications for chemotherapy are:
- evidence of metastases in brain, liver, or GI tract or radiological opacities >2 cm on CXR
- histological evidence of choriocarcinoma
- heavy vaginal bleeding or evidence of GI or intraperitoneal haemorrhage
- pulmonary, vulval, or vaginal metastases unless HCG falling
- rising HCG after evacuation

- serum HCG = 20 000 iu/l more than 4 weeks after evacuation, because of the risk of uterine perforation
- raised HCG 6 months after evacuation even if still falling.

Any of these are indications to treat following the diagnosis of GTD.

Placental-site trophoblastic tumour

PSTT can develop following a term delivery, non-molar abortion, or CHM. There are currently about 100 recorded cases of PSTT in the literature, and so estimates of its true incidence may well be inaccurate. Nevertheless, PSTT is thought to constitute about 1% of all trophoblastic tumours (choriocarcinoma, invasive mole, and PSTT).

PSTTs are slow-growing, malignant tumours composed mainly of cytotrophoblast with very little syncytiotrophoblast, so producing little HCG. However, they often stain strongly for human placental lactogen (HPL), which helps to distinguish this tumour from carcinomas, sarcomas, exaggerated placental-site reaction, and placental nodule. The raised HPL may cause hyperprolactinaemia that can result in amenorrhoea and/or galactorrhoea. In most cases spread occurs by local infiltration with distant metastases occurring late via the lymphatics and blood.

The behaviour of PSTT is thus quite different from other forms of GTD and it is relatively chemoresistant. The best management is hysterectomy when the disease is localized to the uterus. When metastatic disease is present, patients can respond and be apparently cured by multi-agent chemotherapy either alone or in combination with surgery.

Patient follow-up and prognosis

On completion of their chemotherapy, patients are advised to avoid pregnancy for 1 year and remain on HCG follow-up for life to confirm that their disease is in remission. About 2% of low-risk and 4% of high-risk patients will relapse. All low- to middle-risk patients are salvaged with further chemotherapy (EMA/CO or alternative regimens) and the cure rate is almost 100% in this group. The high-risk group has 90% survival rate beyond 10 years. With the addition of platinum and other new agents, salvage rates for patients relapsing following EMA/CO therapy can be in excess of 70%. Neither methotrexate nor EMA/CO therapy reduce fertility or cause abnormalities. Thus, women treated for GTD can expect to have healthy children.

Further reading

Advanced Ovarian Cancer Triallist Group (1998) Chemotherapy in ovarian cancer: four systematic meta-analyses of individual patient data from 37 randomized trials. *Br J Cancer* **78**, 1479–87.

Amant F, Moerman P, Nevin P, *et al.* (2005) Endometrial cancer. *Lancet* **366**, 491–505.

Cannistra S (2004) Cancer of the ovary. *N Eng J Med* **351**, 2519–30.

Green JA, Kirwan JM, Tierney JF, *et al.* (2001) Survival and recurrence after concomitant chemotherapy and radiotherapy for cancer of the uterine cervix: a systematic review and meta-analysis. *Lancet* **358**, 781–6.

Hockel M, Dornhofer N (2009) Treatment of early endometrial carcinoma: is less more? *Lancet* **373**, 97–8.

Kim JJ (2008) Human papilloma virus vaccination in the UK. *BMJ* **337**, 303–304.

Onda T, Yoshikawa M, Mizutani K, *et al.* (1997) Treatment of node positive endometrial cancer with complete node dissection, chemotherapy and radiation therapy. *Br J Cancer* **75**, 1836–41.

Papadopoulos AJ, Foskett M, Seckl MJ, *et al.* (2002) Twenty-five years clinical experience with placental site trophoblastic tumours. *J Reproduct Med* **47**, 460–4.

Pellegrino A, Vizza E, Fruscio R, *et al.* (2009) Total laparoscopic radical hysterectomy and pelvic lymphadenectomy in patients with 1BI stage cervical cancer – analysis of surgical and oncological outcome. *Eur J Surg Oncol* **35**, 98–103.

Rose PG, Bundy BN, Watkins EB, *et al.* (1999) Concurrent cisplatin based chemotherapy and radiotherapy for locally advanced cervical cancer. *N Engl J Med* **340**, 1144–53.

Head and neck cancers

Introduction

- Head and neck cancer encompasses a range of neoplasms arising from different anatomical sites (see Fig. 22.1):
  - **the larynx**: including the supraglottic, glottic, and subglottic regions
  - **the oral cavity**: including the lips, gums, anterior tongue, floor of the mouth, hard palate, and buccal mucosa
  - **the pharynx**: including the nasopharynx, oropharynx, and hypopharynx
  - **the nasal cavity and paranasal sinuses**: maxillary, frontal, ethmoid, and sphenoid
  - **the salivary glands**.
- Malignancy of the head and neck cancer is the fifth most common cancer worldwide and the most common in central Asia.
- In the UK:
  - incidence of cancer at each separate anatomical site is relatively low
  - >8000 new diagnoses per year.
  - 85% of cases arise in patients >50 years old.
  - 'tends to be a disease of deprivation, with the risk of developing disease four times greater for men living in the most deprived areas' (Scottish Intercollegiate Guidelines Network)
  - increasing incidence amongst young people of both sexes.
- The term 'head and neck cancer' includes many different diseases. However, most of the skills required to assess and manage these patients are broadly similar.

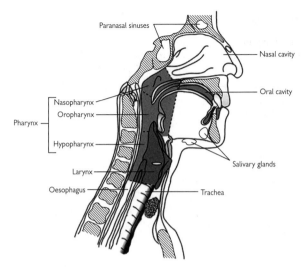

Fig. 22.1 Anatomy of the head and neck.

Aetiology

Smoking and alcohol

- Major modifiable risk factors in the Western world.
- Together are believed to account for >75% of cases of head and neck cancer.
- Effect on the risk of malignancy is synergistic (multiplicative).
- Cigarette smoking is associated with >10 times greater risk of all head and neck cancers.
- Heavy smoking combined with excess alcohol consumption results in >35 times the risk of oral cancer of a person who does neither.
- Chewing tobacco and pipe smoking are particularly associated with oral cancer.
- These carcinogens do not have a significant role in the development of cancers of the nasal cavity, paranasal sinuses, or salivary glands.

Diet

- Low risk associated with well-balanced diet rich in vegetables and fruit.
- Increased risk with a poor diet, particularly deficient in vitamins A and C.
- Nitrosamines in salted fish implicated in Chinese diet.

Infections

Virally induced cancers may have a better prognosis than those attributable to smoking and alcohol use.

Human papillomavirus (HPV) infection

- Risk factor for cancer of the larynx, pharynx, and oral cavity.

Herpes simplex viruses 1 (HSV-1) and 2 (HSV-2)

- Associated with oral cancer.

Epstein–Barr virus infection (EBV)

- Associated with the undifferentiated form of nasopharyngeal cancer:
  - analyses of tissue from these tumours confirm all are EBV positive, with monoclonal viral copies identified within malignant cells
  - precise role of EBV in malignant transformation remains to be established.
- Also implicated in some salivary gland tumours.

Chronic syphilis infection

- Implicated in cancer of the oral cavity, in particular the tongue.

Genetic susceptibility

- There is a believed to be a genetic susceptibility to some of the head and neck cancers:
  - germline mutations in *p53* have been associated with oral cancer
  - certain major histocompatibility complex profiles are associated with nasopharyngeal cancer.

Other environmental agents
- Formaldehyde: cancers of the pharynx and oral cavity
- Hard wood dust: adenocarcinoma of the ethmoids – woodworkers have a 70 times greater relative risk
- Soft wood dust: squamous cell carcinoma of the nasal cavity and paranasal sinuses
- Radiation exposure: salivary gland tumours.

Epidemiology

Laryngeal cancer
- Second most common of the head and neck cancers, although it comprises <2% of all carcinomas in men.
- Annual incidence is 3–10 per 100 000.
- Predominantly male disease, as are most head and neck cancers.
- Typically age 40–80 years.
- Higher incidence in urban than rural areas.

Cancer of the oral cavity
- Worldwide, oral cancer has the highest incidence of the head and neck cancers.
- Relatively uncommon in the UK.
- Patients of South Asian origin are at increased risk.
- More common in men than in women.
- 10–30% of patients with cancer of the oral cavity subsequently develop a second head and neck primary.
- The incidence of lung and bladder tumours is also increased in this population.

Cancer of the pharynx
- Rare in the UK, where the most common site is the tonsil; 400 cases per annum in England.
- Nasopharyngeal cancer rare in the UK but more frequent in those of southern Chinese and South East Asian origin, reflecting a combination of differing genetic, dietary, and viral aetiological factors.

Cancer of the nasal cavity and paranasal sinuses
- Sinonasal malignancy is rare, <3% of head and neck cancer.
- Global figures suggest an incidence of <1/100 000 people per year in most countries.
- Occupational factors produce regional differences.
- Male to female ratio is approximately 2:1.
- Majority present between 50 and 70 years.

Cancer of the salivary glands
- 3–6% of all head and neck neoplasms.
- Incidence of 1–3 per 100 000/year.
- Cancerous tumours present at a mean age of 60 years; benign disease is more common in a younger age group.

Screening and prevention

- Currently there is no national screening programme for this group of cancers.
- In the UK the emphasis is on public health education to:
  - tackle the major modifiable risk factors of tobacco and alcohol use
  - raise awareness of these cancers and their presenting symptoms
  - reduce the number of patients presenting with advanced-stage disease.

Pathology

Squamous cell carcinoma

- Account for >90% of cancers of the head and neck particularly those involving the larynx and oral cavity.
- Categorized as well, moderately, or poorly differentiated depending on the degree of keratinization.
- Typically they invade adjacent structures depending on the site of origin, and spread via lymphatics to regional lymph nodes in the cervical chain, in preference to blood-borne spread.
- Distant metastases are usually associated with advanced or recurrent primary tumour and may include mediastinal lymph nodes, lung, liver, and bone spread.
- There is an association between squamous cell malignancy of the head and neck and several pathological diagnoses believed to represent pre-malignant conditions:
  - **leukoplakia**: hyperparakeratosis ± underlying epithelial hyperplasia. If this is an isolated abnormality there is believed to be ≤5% chance of subsequent malignant change
  - **erythroplakia**: superficial red patches adjacent to normal mucosa. Frequently associated with epithelial dysplasia. Associated with carcinoma *in situ* or invasive disease in up to 40% of cases
  - **dysplasia**: or carcinoma *in situ* (if it involves the full mucosal thickness). Progression to invasive disease is believed to occur in 15–30% of cases.
- A verrucous tumour (also named Ackerman's tumour):
  - variant of well-differentiated squamous cell carcinoma
  - presents as a whitish, cauliflower-like growth.
  - histology confirms a pushing margin with a marked surrounding inflammatory cell response
  - lymphatic spread is rare.
- Spindle cell carcinomas behave as squamous cell carcinomas.

Other pathologies

Histology

- Adenocarcinomas arising from salivary tissue, e.g. in the oral cavity
- Melanoma
- Sarcoma, e.g. rhabdomyosarcoma

Timing

Patients with head and neck squamous cancer are more likely to develop second primary cancers than any other group of patients with malignancies. These may be:

- synchronous:
  - occurring at or near the same time as the original tumour
- metachronous:
  - occurring >6 months later.
- Approximately 15% of 'cured' patients with previously treated head and neck cancer present with further primaries (at a rate of 3–5% per year).

- Mucosa adjacent to the carcinoma frequently contains areas of dysplastic changes, *in situ* carcinoma, or occult invasive carcinoma.
- High risk of multiple primaries reflects the carcinogenic effects of prolonged exposure to tobacco and alcohol over the whole of the aerodigestive tract and urothelium ('field effect').
- Second tumours are often clonally distinct and therefore are not felt to represent loco-regional recurrence or metastatic spread from the original primary.

Tumours of the salivary glands

- Represent a very different spectrum of diseases compared to the more common head and neck tumours.
- Most common location of a salivary gland tumour is the parotid gland (70–85%).
- Most parotid tumours are benign (>75%).
- Tumours of the minor salivary glands represent only 5–8% of salivary gland disease but >80% of these are cancerous.
- Most frequent salivary gland tumour is the pleomorphic adenoma (also known as the mixed parotid tumour):
  - a benign epithelial tumour that only rarely undergoes malignant transformation
  - local recurrence following enucleation is common
  - treatment is most commonly with formal parotidectomy.
- Malignant tumours that occur in the salivary glands include:
  - mucoepidermoid carcinoma
  - adenocarcinoma
  - squamous carcinoma
  - adenoid cystic carcinoma
  - undifferentiated carcinoma
  - metastasis from other primary sites, e.g. breast or lung cancer
  - lymphoma.

Presentation

- Characteristic local symptoms depend on the site and size of the primary lesion.
- Malignancy of the head and neck may not uncommonly present with painless cervical lymphadenopathy.

Laryngeal cancer

- A hoarse voice is typical if the cancer is affecting the glottis (most common site of laryngeal cancer in UK and USA).
- A persistent irritating cough and dysphagia or odynophagia (painful swallowing) are characteristic of supraglottic carcinoma, which typically presents with advanced disease often including a palpable neck mass.
- Dyspnoea/stridor can be caused by subglottic cancers that grow circumferentially. These are rare (<5%).
- ±Referred pain in the ear.
- ±Haemoptysis.

Cancer of the oral cavity

- Persistent mouth ulcers, painful ulcerative lesion on lip, or exophytic growth
- White or red patches on tongue, gums, or lining of mouth
- Dental problems, e.g. loose teeth, dentures no longer fitting
- Dysphagia/odynophagia
- Referred pain in the ear
- Dysarthria if there is involvement of the tongue
- Lymphadenopathy
- Weight loss

Tumours commonly extend to involve >1 region within the oral cavity:

- tongue, 60%
- floor of mouth, 15%
- alveolar ridge/retromolar trigone, 10%
- buccal mucosa, 10%
- hard palate, 5%.

Cancer of the pharynx

Pattern of symptoms tends to differ according to the primary site of disease.

Nasopharyngeal cancer

- Cervical lymphadenopathy (up to 90% of patients)
- Nasal symptoms: bleeding, obstruction, or discharge
- Unilateral hearing loss ± serous otitis media (2° to Eustachian tube blockage) ± tinnitus
- Headache
- Cranial nerve palsies due to base of skull invasion

Oropharyngeal cancer

- Sore throat or lump in the throat
- Pain referred to ear

Hypopharyngeal cancer
- Dysphagia and lump in the throat
- Odynophagia
- Pain referred to ear
- Hoarse voice

Cancer of the nasal cavity and paranasal sinuses
- Epistaxis
- Unilateral nasal obstruction ± serosanguinous or purulent discharge
- Pain and paraesthesia
- Ulceration
- Proptosis, diplopia, chemosis ± visual loss if there is involvement of the orbit with displacement of the globe

Tumours of the salivary glands
- Painless lump within the substance of a salivary gland, as opposed to enlargement of the whole gland.
- Differentiation between an enlarged gland and a lump in the gland is often difficult.
- Benign and malignant salivary gland tumours may be indistinguishable clinically.
- Features highly suggestive of malignancy include:
  - infiltration of surrounding structures
  - facial nerve palsy.

Investigations

The aims of investigations include:
- identifying the primary tumour site and extent: including cytological or histological confirmation of the diagnosis
- detecting any other synchronous primaries: not uncommon in this group of patients
- staging the disease
- assessing the general fitness of the patients: significant co-morbidities such as ischaemic heart disease and obstructive airways disease are common in patients with head and neck cancer, primarily because these conditions share aetiological risk factors.

Physical examination

This should include:
- inspection of the region including mirror examination. This has largely been superseded by flexible fibreoptic endoscopy – to allow visualization of nasopharynx, hypopharynx, base of tongue, larynx, and vocal cord mobility
- bimanual examination of the oral cavity
- palpation of regional lymph nodes: cervical lymph node spread is an important determinant of prognosis. However, clinical examination should be combined with appropriate imaging due to the high false-negative rate (15–30% for cervical lymph nodes) and false-positive rate (30–40% for cervical nodes) from clinical examination alone
- general physical examination: as a clinical assessment of potential metastatic disease (which is commonly asymptomatic)
- ±examination and biopsy under anaesthesia.

Bloods

- Full blood count (FBC) and urea and electrolytes (U&Es)
- Liver function tests and coagulation screen: commonly abnormal because of concomitant alcohol excess

Imaging

- The extent of imaging will depend on the site and size of the primary tumour, e.g. early laryngeal cancer has a very low risk of distant spread and requires only loco-regional cross-sectional imaging.
- Computerized tomography (CT) scan:
  - to determine:
  - the extent of local tumour infiltration, particularly invasion of bone/cartilage (T4 disease)
  - radiological evidence of regional nodal involvement
  - the presence of distant metastases
  - the most common sites of dissemination are lungs, then liver, then bones.
- Magnetic resonance imaging (MRI) of head and neck:
  - may provide better soft tissue definition.

- Skeletal scintigraphy:
  - if bone metastases suspected but not identified on CT
  - for example, in nasopharyngeal cancer 725% of patients with low cervical or supraclavicular nodes who have a positive bone scan will have secondaries.
- Positron emission tomography (PET):
  - increasing role, particularly in patients where tumour staging is unclear despite CT/MRI
  - at least as sensitive and specific as CT and MRI for detecting primary tumours, e.g. metastatic squamous carcinoma in cervical lymph nodes but no visible ear, nose, and throat (ENT) primary.
  - superior to MRI and CT for detecting second primaries, regional and distant metastases
  - not used in isolation as provides inadequate anatomical detail.

Histology

- Biopsy: if the primary tumour is identified and accessible. The exception are salivary gland tumours when fine needle aspiration (FNA) is preferred to biopsy to minimize the risk of tumour seeding.
- FNA: of a metastatic lymph node mass; non-diagnostic in up to 15% of cases although this figure improves with the use of ultrasound guidance.

TNM staging

- Staging systems for head and neck cancers are based on the 'TNM system' and are broadly similar for each of the anatomical sites of origin.
- Details that differ between the staging systems typically take into account if involvement of particular local structures will affect whether radical treatment is appropriate and hence the effect on overall prognosis.
- **T** – extent of primary tumour:
  - generally reflects the size of the tumour ± involvement of bone or cartilage (T4)
  - for some sites T4 tumours are further divided into potentially resectable (T4a) or unresectable (T4b)
- **N** – involvement of regional lymph nodes
- **M** – absence (0) or presence (1) of distant metastases or inability to assess for their presence (X).

The American Joint Committee on Cancer (AJCC) staging system for laryngeal cancer, updated in 2002, is given as an example (see Tables 22.1 and 22.2).

Table 22.1 AJCC TNM classification for cancer of the larynx

Primary tumour (T) classification	
Tx	Primary tumour cannot be assessed
T0	No evidence of primary tumour
Tis	Carcinoma *in situ*
Supraglottis	
T1	Limited to one subsite of supraglottis, normal cord mobility
T2	Invades mucosa of >1 adjacent subsite of supraglottis, glottis, or region outside the supraglottis, e.g. mucosa of base of tongue, without fixation of the larynx
T3	Limited to larynx with vocal cord fixation and/or invades any of the following: post-cricoid area, pre-epiglottic tissues, paraglottic space, and/or minor thyroid cartilage erosion
T4a	Invades through the thyroid cartilage and/or invades tissues beyond the larynx, e.g. trachea, soft tissues of the neck including strap muscles, oesophagus, etc.
T4b	Invades prevertebral space, encases carotid artery, or invades mediastinal structures
T1a	Limited to one vocal cord with normal mobility
T1b	Involves both vocal cords with normal mobility

Table 22.1 (Cont'd)

Glottis	
T2	Extends to supraglottic and/or subglottis and/or with impaired cord mobility
T3	Limited to the larynx with vocal cord fixation and/or invades paraglottic space and/or minor thyroid cartilage erosion
T4a	Invades through the thyroid cartilage and/or invades tissues beyond the larynx, e.g. trachea, soft tissues of the neck including strap muscles, oesophagus, etc.
T4b	Invades prevertebral space, encases carotid artery, or invades mediastinal structures

Subglottis	
T1	Limited to the subglottis
T2	Extends to vocal cord(s) with normal or impaired cord mobility
T3	Limited to the larynx with vocal cord fixation
T4a	Invades cricoid or thyroid cartilage and/or invades tissues beyond the larynx, e.g. trachea, soft tissues of the neck including strap muscles, oesophagus, etc.
T4b	Invades prevertebral space, encases carotid artery, or invades mediastinal structures

Regional lymph nodes (N) in head and neck cancer (excluding nasopharyngeal cancer)	
Nx	Regional lymph nodes cannot be assessed
N0	No regional lymph node metastases
N1	Metastasis in a single ipsilateral lymph nodes ≤3 cm max diameter
N2	Single ipsilateral nodal metastasis >3 cm but ≤6 cm max diameter
N2a	Single ipsilateral nodal metastasis >3 cm but ≤6 cm max diameter
N2b	Mutiple ipsilateral nodal metastasis >3 cm but ≤6 cm max diameter
N2c	Bilateral/contralateral nodal metastases, all ≤6 cm max diameter
N3	Metastasis in a lymph node >6 cm in max diameter

U = metastasis above the lower border of the cricoid, i.e. nodal metastases in the lower neck.

L = metastasis below the lower border of the cricoid, i.e. nodal metastases in the lower neck.

(continued)

Table 22.1 (Cont'd)

Metastasis (M) classification

Mx	Unable to assess distant metastases
M0	No distant metastases
M1	Distant metastases

With permission from Edge SE, Byrd DR, Carducci MA, Compton CA, eds. AJCC Cancer Staging Manual, 7th ed. New York, NY: Springer, 2009.

Table 22.2 AJCC stage grouping for cancer of the larynx, oro-pharynx, hypopharynx, lip and oral cavity, and maxillary sinus

Stage 0	Tis N0 M0
Stage I	T1 N0 M0
Stage II	T2 N0 M0
Stage III	T3 N0 M0
	T1–3 N1 M0
Stage IVA	T4a N0/1 M0
	T1–4a N2 M0
Stage IVB	T4b any N M0
	any T N3 M0
Stage IVC	Any T any N M1

With permission from Edge SE, Byrd DR, Carducci MA, Compton CA, eds. AJCC Cancer Staging Manual, 7th ed. New York, NY: Springer, 2009.

Management

Pre-malignant lesions

- Pre-malignant lesions require specialist management because:
  - they may subsequently develop into frank carcinoma
  - patients with pre-malignant lesions are at high risk of other primary malignant neoplasms especially within the upper aerodigestive tract and lungs.
- Treatment is usually by excision followed by examination by an experienced pathologist.
- Classification should be based on grade of dysplasia as this has a bearing on prognosis.
- Radiotherapy may be appropriate for frequently recurring or diffuse lesions, e.g. on the vocal cords.

Malignant lesions

- Investigation and management should be co-ordinated by a multidisciplinary team with expertise in the complex medical, psychological, and functional issues that affect patients with head and neck cancers.
- Co-existing socio-economic deprivation can complicate management, and compliance may be problematic.
- The aim of treatment is to combine optimal rates of cure with the best functional results.
- Where cure is not feasible, every attempt should be made to provide loco-regional disease control.
- Before beginning treatment it is important to:
  - establish nutritional status – including baseline weight and risk of malnutrition during therapy (elective insertion of a nasogastric or enterostomy feeding tube, may be appropriate). A specialist dietician should be involved wherever possible
  - refer for dental assessment – including completion of any necessary dental treatment. Ongoing mouth care advice will be needed during and after treatment
  - correct anaemia – haemoglobin (Hb) must be maintained at ≥12 g/dl throughout treatment for optimal results from radiotherapy
  - undertake a speech and language assessment.
- There are few randomized trials comparing treatment modalities – the evidence is mainly at level III (i.e. based largely on retrospective case series). This is partly due to the relative rarity of tumours arising from each anatomical site.
- Most head and neck cancers are treated with surgery, radiotherapy, or a combination of the two:
  - generally T1–2, N0, M0 disease can be treated with single-modality treatment and retrospective data suggest the results achieved by surgery or radiotherapy alone are equivalent
  - In more advanced disease, combined-modality regimens are frequently adopted, depending on the primary site.

Management of early-stage disease
- 30–40% of patients with head and neck cancer present with stage I or II disease, with an overall prognosis of 60–98% depending on the site of primary, etc.

Surgery alone
- Potential advantages of surgery alone include:
  - provides complete pathological staging of the disease
  - quick local clearance of disease
  - newer surgical techniques, e.g. for early laryngeal cancer, may conserve the voice
  - treatment of metachronous head and neck tumours is not compromised
  - avoids the toxicity of radiotherapy, including the risk of radiotherapy-induced second malignancies
  - for salivary gland tumours, pre-operative open biopsy may be avoided (risk of tumour seeding). However, fine needle biopsy with an experienced head and neck cytopathologist is safe. Primary excision can be used as a simultaneous diagnostic and therapeutic procedure.

Radiotherapy alone
- A typical radiotherapy regime might comprise 60–70 Gy administered to the primary site over 6–7 weeks.
- Treatment may be with external photon beams alone or with photons followed by an electron boost, or by interstitial therapy, e.g. using iridium wire.
- Advantages of primary radiotherapy include:
  - avoidance of operative mortality in patients who have significant co-morbidities
  - surgical clearance may be difficult or impossible
  - organ conservation is more likely, including preservation of the voice and swallowing
  - option of elective radiotherapy treatment of clinically occult regional lymph node disease with relatively little extra morbidity (compared with elective neck dissection)
  - surgery remains an option as salvage therapy in the event of treatment failure. However, subsequent surgery is likely to be associated with greater morbidity, e.g. total laryngectomy is usually required after failure of primary radiotherapy for laryngeal cancer
  - allows the treatment of multiple synchronous primaries.
- Toxicity of radiotherapy includes:
  - mucositis and a dry mouth – may persist depending on the amount of salivary tissue spared from irradiation
  - chronic ulceration of the mucosa and osteonecrosis – particularly with locally advanced tumours involving the mandible
  - dry eye/cataract, pituitary dysfunction, and central nervous system (CNS) necrosis – radiation dose to the eyes, brain, and spinal cord must be kept within tolerance. Conformal techniques and CT planning allow reduction in the dosage to normal tissue.

Surgery versus radiotherapy?
- Cure rates with primary radiotherapy are generally believed to be equivalent to those for surgery for early-stage disease of many head and neck tumours.
- In certain clinical situations, radiotherapy is clearly the first-line treatment of choice, e.g. in nasopharyngeal carcinoma when the use of surgery is limited to staging and the elective dissection of neck nodes that have not regressed 3 months after radiotherapy.
- In other clinical situations surgery is the first choice if at all possible, e.g. tumours of the nasal cavity and paranasal sinuses.

Combined surgery and radiotherapy
- Combination therapy is generally the best choice for bulky tumours. The aim of using both modalities is to minimize the risk of loco-regional disease recurrence.
- The most important risk factors for prediction of recurrence and the need for post-operative radiotherapy are:
  - positive resection margins
  - extra-capsular lymph node spread
  - T3–4 primary tumour
  - perineural or vascular invasion
  - poorly differentiated tumour
  - ≥N2 disease.

Management of involved neck nodes
Options include the following:
- therapeutic radiotherapy:
  - appropriate for N1 disease particularly if radiotherapy is also being used to treat the primary
  - 60–65 Gy administered over 6 weeks will control 90% of N1 nodes
- therapeutic neck dissection:
  - should be considered for patients with more advanced nodal disease (N2–3) and an operable primary
  - there are no prospective trials to support subsequent adjuvant radiotherapy but retrospective series suggest it has a role if there is a high risk of local relapse
- radical neck dissection:
  - removes the superficial and deep cervical fascia with the enclosed lymph nodes (level I to V) along with sternomastoid muscle, omohyoid muscle, internal and external jugular veins, accessory nerve, and submandibular gland
- a modified neck dissection:
  - preserves vital structures such as the accessory nerve (functional dissection)

Complications after neck dissection include:
- haematoma
- seroma
- lymphoedema
- infection
- damage to VII, X, XI, XII cranial nerves
- carotid rupture.

Post-irradiation neck dissection
- May be planned electively after radiotherapy (e.g. 50 Gy) for advanced nodal disease
- More commonly used to salvage regional relapse after radiotherapy

The role of sentinel node biopsy and the management of micrometastases are uncertain. In some centres (but not all), sentinel node biopsy is being established.

Post-operative chemo-radiotherapy
- Results published in 2004 from two large randomized trials support the use of post-operative chemo-radiotherapy in selected high-risk, fit patients with resected squamous cell head and neck cancers.
- Radiotherapy with concurrent administration of cisplatin:
  - has been associated with fewer loco-regional relapses and improvements in disease-free survival
  - an improvement in overall survival has not been consistently demonstrated
  - the incidence of significant toxicity in the patients receiving both cisplatin and radiotherapy was over double the incidence in patients receiving radiotherapy alone.

Treatment of locally advanced unresectable disease

Chemo-radiotherapy
- >60% of squamous cell head and neck cancers have advanced loco-regional disease at presentation (stage III/IV M0).
- In some cases surgery remains an option and can result in 5-year survival rates of 20–50% if combined with radiotherapy.
- In many cases surgery is either technically not possible or would be associated with unacceptable morbidity, e.g. base of tongue cancer requiring glossectomy and consequent loss of normal voice and swallow.
- Significant co-morbidity may mean that operative risk is deemed too great.
- Primary radiotherapy for unresectable stage III or IV head and neck cancer is associated with a 5-year survival of only 10–30%.
- Combined modality therapy:
  - the use of radiotherapy with concurrent chemotherapy in such cases has been demonstrated to be associated with a modest survival advantage over treatment with radiotherapy alone (4–8% increase in 5-year survival)
  - the most commonly studied chemotherapy regime so far has been single-agent cisplatin, although combination regimes have also been used and may be associated with further improvements in outcome
  - associated with increased toxicity, in particular mucositis
  - most appropriate in patients with good performance status and relatively few co-morbidities.

Biological therapies

Cetuximab (Erbitux®):

- an intravenously administered human/mouse chimeric immunoglobulin G monoclonal antibody
- competitively binds to the epidermal growth factor receptor preventing tyrosine kinase activation (see 📖 Chapter 10, Biological and targeted therapies'). This receptor is overexpressed in many head and neck cancers
- a randomized trial compared radiotherapy alone versus the combination of radiotherapy and concurrent weekly cetuximab in >400 patients with locally advanced squamous cell carcinoma of the head and neck. The use of cetuximab was associated with significant improvements:
  - longer duration of loco-regional control (24.4 vs 14.9 months)
  - greater median overall survival (49 vs 29.3 months)
  - no increase in mucositis although significant skin toxicity was more frequent in the group receiving combined-modality treatment
- cetuximab was given National Institute for Health and Clinical Excellence (NICE) approval in 2008 for the treatment of fit patients (Karnowsky score ≥90%) with locally advanced head and neck cancer receiving radiotherapy for whom all platinum-based chemotherapy is inappropriate.

Management of metastatic disease

Chemotherapy

Advanced squamous cell carcinoma:

- Certain chemotherapy agents have been shown to be active, e.g. cisplatin, the taxanes (docetaxel and paclitaxel), 5-fluorouracil (5-FU), methotrexate, and pemetrexed.
- Cetuximab (Erbitux®) is also active in advanced disease.
- Single agent therapy:
  - median survival with treatment is only around 6 months
  - e.g. methotrexate, cisplatin or cetuximab (approved for use in the USA for platinum-refractory disease).
- Combination regimes:
  - appear to achieve the highest response rates (15–30%)
  - a survival advantage over single-agent treatment has not consistently been demonstrated
  - can only be considered in patients of good performance status.
  - e.g. a platinum agent with either 5-FU ± cetuximab (Erbitux®), or alternatively with a taxane.
- Nasopharyngeal carcinomas seem particularly chemosensitive, with response rates of up to 70% reported in advanced disease.

Disseminated or unresectable salivary tumours:

- Typically chemosensitive.
- Response rates of up to 50% are reported.
- Duration of response is usually only a few months.
- The regime chosen can be tailored to the histology of the disease.

Prognosis and follow-up

Follow-up is important in patients treated with curative intent for head and neck cancer. The aims of surveillance include:
- early detection of loco-regional recurrence:
  - occurs in 20–50% of patients
  - the major contributor to head and neck cancer-related deaths
  - early detection will improve the chances of successful salvage therapy
- detection of new primaries:
  - the incidence of new primary cancers is 3–5% per year (10–15% overall)
- management of the late effects of treatment.

The role of routine PET-CT scanning in follow-up is unclear. It may help to diagnose early relapse e.g. when CT shows equivocal abnormalities.

Laryngeal cancer
- 90% of recurrences occur within 3 years.
- High risk of second primary malignancies (12–20%).
- Patients with supraglottic laryngeal cancer are at particular risk of subsequent primary lung cancer – chest X-ray (CXR) and even bronchoscopy may be considered in regular follow-up. Spiral CT may also have a role.

Cancer of the oral cavity
- >80% 5-year survival for those presenting with early-stage, localized disease
- >40% 5-year survival for patients with loco-regional nodal involvement
- <20% 5-year survival for those with distant metastases

Cancer of the pharynx
- Reported 5-year survival rates for nasopharyngeal carcinoma range from >80% for stage I disease to <30% for patients presenting with advanced tumours.
- Follow-up after treatment for early-stage disease should be most intensive in the first 3 years, when the majority of recurrences occur.
- Prognosis is less good for localized oropharyngeal cancers, with a 5-year survival of ~50% for those presenting with stage I disease, although survival with advanced disease is similar to that with metastatic nasopharyngeal cancer.
- Tonsillar cancer in general has better prognosis, with survival of >80% at 5 years, even for stage III disease.

Cancer of the nasal cavity and paranasal sinuses
- Presentation is most commonly with locally advanced tumours that remain potentially curable with radical surgery and radiotherapy.
- Regional metastases are infrequent – occurring in <20% of patients at presentation.

Cancer of the salivary glands

- 5-year survival is 75–85% for those presenting with early-stage, localized (stage I) malignant disease of the salivary glands but falls to ~30% for patients presenting with disseminated disease (stage IV).
- More than one-fifth of recurrences occur over 5 years following treatment for the primary disease.

Rehabilitation

- The treatment of many head and neck cancers has significant associated long-term morbidity.
- Patients may have to adjust to huge changes in both appearance and function.
- A high level of specialist support from many different disciplines in the months and years following their treatment can significantly improve quality of life.

Specific difficulties that require ongoing input include:

Speech

- The greatest handicap for patients after a total laryngectomy is the loss of voice.
- Options include:
  - oesophageal speech – ~40% of patients acquire socially useful speech using this method
  - artificial larynx device – used successfully by some patients
  - fistula operations with insertion of speech valvulas – increasingly performed and well tolerated
  - specialist speech and language therapists – should be involved throughout the patient's care
  - support groups or web-based information sites helpful, e.g. www. larynxlink.com.

Airway management

- Patients may have to adjust to breathing through a stoma.
- If the airway has been separated from the gullet they will have to learn to manage their airway secretions.
- Heat and moisture exchangers are commonly used to lower the risk of respiratory problems and can be positioned in front of the stoma.

Dentistry

- Specialist dentists should be involved in follow-up due to the specific problems that occur following, e.g. radiotherapy to the mouth. These include:
  - frequent dental caries
  - poor healing after tooth extraction
  - potential for late osteonecrosis.

Nutrition

- Late effects from radiotherapy and surgery may affect nutritional intake in the long-term.
- Factors that need addressing include any alterations in:
  - normal swallow mechanism
  - salivary production
  - taste.
- Input from a dietician with expertise in patients treated for head and neck cancers is vital.

Coping with disfigurement and altered body image
- The adjustment to changes in appearance can be problematic for patients of both sexes and all ages as well as their relatives.
- Professional psychological input, patient support groups, and self-help literature each have a role in helping patients and their relatives to cope.

Ongoing alcohol and tobacco dependency
- Strenuous efforts must be made to encourage patients to stop smoking and to cut back on their alcohol intake.
- Currently there is little evidence to support formal smoking cessation programmes, e.g. in a trial of newly diagnosed patients with head and neck cancer, randomized to either 'usual care' or a formal smoking cessation programme, the rate of ongoing smoking after 1 year fell by the same amount (88% → 70%).

Intra-ocular tumours

Melanoma
- See 📖 Intra-ocular melanoma, p.518.

Retinoblastoma
- Rare intra-ocular tumour arising in young children, usually in the first 2 years of life, incidence 1 in 20 000.
- The disease is hereditary (autosomal dominant) and often bilateral.
- Patients should be managed in combined clinics by ophthalmologists experienced in management of retinoblastoma.
- Biopsy should not be performed.

Management
- Small tumours not adjacent to the macula or optic disc: photocoagulation.
- Small/moderate tumours: radioactive plaques (iodine, ruthenium plaques – 40 Gy).
- Large or multiple tumours: external radiotherapy.
- May need to irradiate whole eye (40 Gy, 20 fractions over 4 weeks); try to maintain vision.
- Occasionally enucleation is required: if tumour fills the whole globe.
- Tumour is also chemosensitive:
  - platinum
  - etoposide
  - vincristine
  - doxorubicin
  - cyclophosphamide.
- Chemotherapy is useful if tumour has a bad prognosis or in neoadjuvant setting.
- Prognosis: 90% survival; 80% of patients can have eye preserved.

Metastatic disease
- Metastatic disease involving the eye is usually associated with choroidal metastases.
- Commonest tumours implicated are lung and breast.
- An oncological emergency if vision threatened.
- Usually treatment with radiotherapy.

Further reading

Andry G, Hamoir M, Leemans CR (2005) The evolving role of surgery in the management of head and neck tumours. *Curr Opin Oncol* **17**, 241–8.

Argiris A, Karamouzis MV, Raben D, et al. (2008) Head and neck cancer. *Lancet* **371**, 1695–709.

Bradley P, McClelland L, Mehta D (2007) Paediatric salivary gland epithelial neoplasms. *ORL J Otorhinolaryngol Relat Spec* **69**, 137–45.

Culliney B, Birhan A, Young AV, et al. (2008) Management of locally advanced or unresectable head and neck cancer. *Oncology (Williston Park)* **22**, 1152–66.

Goudakos JK, Mankou K, Nikolaou A, et al. (2009) Management of the clinically negative neck (NO) of supraglottic laryngeal carcinoma – a systemic review. *Eur J Surg Oncol* **35**, 223–9.

Greenspan D, Jordan RCK (2004) The white lesion that kills. *N Eng J Med* **350**, 1382–5.

Haddad R, Shin DM (2008) Recent advances in head and neck cancer. *N Eng J Med* **359**, 1143–54.

Jeannon JP, Calman F, Gleeson M, et al. (2008) Management of advanced parotid cancer. A systematic review. *Eur J Surg Oncol* **Nov 20** epub ahead of print.

Lefebvre JL (2006) Laryngeal preservation in head and neck cancer – multidisciplinary approach. *Lancet Oncol* **7**, 747–755

Le QT, Raben D (2009) Integrating biologically targeted therapy in head and neck squamous cell carcinoma. *Semin Radiat Oncol* **19**, 53–62.

Misra S, Chaturvedi A, Misra NC (2008) Management of gingivobuccal complex cancer. *Ann R Coll Surg Engl* **90**, 546–53,

NICE (2004) *Guidance on Cancer Services: improving outcomes in head and neck cancers*. London: NICE.

NICE (2008) *Cetuximab for the Treatment of Head and Neck Cancer*. London: NICE.

Patetsios P, Gable DR, Garrett WV, et al. (2002) Management of carotid body paragangliomas and review of a 30 year experience. *Ann Vasc Surg* **16**, 331–8.

Scott AM, Gunawardana DH, Bartholomeusz D, et al. (2008) PET changes management and improves prognostic stratification in patients with head and neck cancer – results of a multicentre prospective study. *J Nucl Med* **49**, 1593–600.

Tumours of the central nervous system

Primary CNS tumours

Epidemiology

The incidence worldwide is very uniform with a few exceptions such as a higher incidence of pineal tumours in Japan and central nervous system (CNS) lymphoma in AIDS populations. Recent reports suggest that the incidence of glioma and (non-AIDS) lymphoma is increasing in developed countries. In the UK:

- approximately 6500 primary tumours of the CNS were recorded annually between 1995–2000 in England and Wales
- primary CNS tumours account for 2% of all malignancies
- almost half of intracranial tumours may not be registered so current statistics may significantly underestimate the true number
- peak incidence 70–80 years
- as the proportion of elderly in the population rises the incidence is expected to rise
- primary brain tumours show a bimodal age distribution:
  - in children they are the most common solid malignancies, predominantly arising in the posterior fossa;
  - second peak in (late) middle age with largely supratentorial tumours.

Aetiology

- Majority of primary CNS tumours are sporadic.
- The main risk factors are increasing age, female sex and higher socioeconomic status.
- Gliomas and meningiomas may be induced by radiation.
- There is an association between primary CNS lymphoma and immunosuppression, including HIV infection.
- A number of rare familial syndromes are associated with CNS tumours (see Table 23.1).
- Other candidate aetiological agents remain controversial and unproven, e.g. industrial and agricultural chemicals, electromagnetic fields, viruses, and trauma.

Pathology

Primary CNS tumour pathology is extremely varied reflecting diverse histogenesis.

The terms benign and malignant are not useful because:

- even small, slow-growing tumours may cause severe and detrimental symptoms because the brain is contained within a rigid structure
- surgery may be difficult due to infiltration of surrounding structures and/or close proximity to critical structures
- most tumours rarely metastasize outside the CNS
- slow-growing tumours may transform into a more aggressive type.

Table 23.1 Hereditary syndromes associated with primary CNS tumours

Syndrome	Gene	Chromosome	Associated tumours
Neurofibromatosis type 1	NF1	17q11	Neurofibroma, optic nerve glioma, astrocytoma, malignant nerve sheath tumour
Neurofibromatosis type 2	NF2	18q22	Astrocytoma, multiple meningioma, bilateral acoustic schwannoma, glial hamartoma
Li–Fraumeni syndrome	p53	17p13	Astrocytoma, primitive neuroectodermal tumour
Von Hippel–Lindau syndrome	VHL	3p25	Cerebellar haemangioblastoma
Gorlin's syndrome	PTCH	9q22	Medulloblastoma
Tuberose sclerosis	TSC1 TSC2	9q34 16p13	Subependymal giant cell astrocytoma
Turcots's syndrome	APC HMLP1 HPSM2	5q21 3p21 7p22	Medulloblastoma, glioblastoma
Cowden's disease	PTEN	10q23	Dysplastic gangliocytoma of the cerebellum

The most widely used classification system is the World Health Organization (WHO) 2000 scheme (see Table 23.4). This classifies CNS tumours into the basic types of tumours of neuroepithelial tissues, germ-cell tumours, tumours of the peripheral nerves, tumours of the meninges, lymphomas and haematopoeitic tumours, tumours of the sellar region, and metastatic tumours. Each type has further subdivisions.

The WHO classification also describes tumours by their histopathological grade: low grade (slow growing, type I and II) and high grade (rapidly growing and aggressive, type III and type IV).

Primary CNS tumours can be divided into primary intracranial tumours and spinal cord tumours, which account for 90% and 10% respectively. The frequency of intracranial pathologies is shown in Table 23.2. Spinal cord tumours can be described by their relation to the spinal cord and dura. The pathologies occurring at these sites are shown in Table 23.3. The commonest primary spinal tumour is schwannoma, followed by meningioma and ependymoma.

By far the most common primary CNS tumour is the glioma (approximately two-thirds of new cases) – behaviour and prognosis are strongly linked to histological grade:
- grade I – slow growing and may be cured by surgical excision
- grade II – slow growing but infiltrative, recurring after surgery

- grades III and IV – show typical features of malignancy with mitotic activity, invasion of adjacent normal brain, and occasionally distant spread
- overall, 50% of gliomas are grade IV glioblastoma multiforme (GBM) – typically areas of prominent abnormal vascularity, haemorrhage and necrosis.

Although imaging may be diagnostic of some primary CNS tumours, in most cases it offers only a differential diagnosis. Precise histological diagnosis is desirable to direct appropriate management. However, for many patients this is not possible either due to hazardous tumour location (e.g. brainstem) or poor performance status. In these cases a presumptive diagnosis is made on clinical and radiological findings.

Table 23.2 Frequency of primary intracranial tumours

Tumour type	Frequency (%)
Glioma	45
Meningioma	27
Pituitary	10
Nerve sheath	7
Lymphoma	4
Medulloblastoma and other primitive neuroectodermal tumours (PNETs)	2
All neurone and neurone/glial tumours	1
Germ-cell tumours	<1
Craniopharyngioma	1
Choroid plexus	<1
Other	3

Table 23.3 Classification of spinal cord tumours by their relation to the spinal cord and dura

Location	Tumour type
Extradural	Metastatic (carcinoma, lymphoma, melanoma, sarcoma)
	Chordoma
Intradural	
Intramedullary	Astrocytoma, ependymoma
Extramedullary	Schwannoma, meningioma

Table 23.4 Abbreviated WHO (2000) classification of CNS tumours

Tissue of origin	Tumour group	Pathological diagnosis
Neuroepithelial tumours	Glial tumours	Pilocytic astrocytoma
	Astrocytic tumours	Diffuse astrocytoma
	Oligodendroglial tumours	Anaplastic astrocytoma
		Glioblastoma
	Mixed gliomas	Oligodendroglioma
		Anaplastic oligodendroglioma
	Ependymal tumours	Oligoastrocytoma
		Anaplastic oligogastrocytoma
	Neuroepithelial tumours of uncertain origin	Myxopapillary ependymoma
		Subependymoma
		Ependymoma
		Anaplastic ependymoma
	Neuronal and mixed neuronal-glial tumours	Astroblastoma
		Gliomatosis cerebri
	Non-glial tumours	Gangliocytoma
	Embryonal tumours	Ganglioblastoma
		Ependymoblastoma
		Medulloblastoma
	Choroid plexus tumours	Choroid plexus papilloma
	Pineal parenchymal tumours	Pineoblastoma
		Pineocytoma
Meningeal tumours		Meningioma
		Haemangiopericytoma
Germ-cell tumours		Germinoma
		Embryonal carcinoma
		Yolk-sac tumour
		Choriocarcinoma
		Teratoma
		Mixed germ-cell tumour

(continued)

Table 23.4 (Cont'd)

Tissue of origin	Tumour group	Pathological diagnosis
Tumours of the sellar region		Pituitary adenoma
		Pituitary carcinoma
		Craniopharyngioma
Tumours of uncertain histogenesis		Capillary haemangioblastoma
Primary CNS lymphoma		
Tumours of peripheral nerves that affect the CNS		Schwannoma
Metastatic tumours		

Clinical presentation

Tumours of the CNS can present with a wide range of physical, cognitive, and psychological symptoms.

Intracranial tumours tend to present either with neurological dysfunction or with symptoms and signs of raised intracranial pressure, depending on their location within the brain. Presentation with epilepsy or with slow onset of symptoms carries a relatively favourable prognosis. The frequency of symptoms in patients with intracranial glioma is shown in Table 23.5. High-grade gliomas are typically associated with considerable oedema in the surrounding normal brain, and this contributes significantly to pressure symptoms. Symptom relief may be obtained through reduction of cerebral oedema by the introduction of steroids, e.g.dexamethasone 8–16 mg daily with proton pumpinhibitor (PPI) gastroprotection, prior to biopsy or craniotomy. Maintenance of symptom control can often be achieved with a reduced dexamethasone dose (2–4 mg daily), with reduced toxicity.

Pituitary tumours may present with a visual field defect due to the close proximity of the pituitary gland to the optic chiasm. The clinical features of pituitary tumours also correlate with the amount and type of hormone secreted.

Spinal cord tumours are likely to present with focal neurological symptoms related to compression or invasion of nerve roots or the cord itself. A common presenting symptom is pain along a nerve root. As the commonest primary cord tumours are slow growing, onset of symptoms may be insidious.

Skull base tumours may cause specific symptoms such as cranial nerve palsies, difficulty with balance or hearing. Of note, the most commonly occurring tumour at this site is schwannoma.

Table 23.5 Presenting symptom in patients with intracranial glioma

Symptom	Frequency as principal presenting symptom (%)	Overall frequency at presentation (%)
Epilepsy	30	53
Headache	25	71
Cognitive distance	12	52
Motor disturbance	8	43
Speech disturbance	5	27
Clouding of consciousness	4	25
Visual disturbance	4	25
Sensory change	2	14
Miscellaneous	10	

Investigations and staging

Investigation and management of all patients with a suspected primary CNS tumour should be co-ordinated by a neuro-oncology multidisciplinary team.

Investigation is dominated by CNS imaging:

- computerized tomography (CT) – contrast-enhanced CT of brain is readily available and frequently adequate to demonstrate CNS tumours. However, CT may miss early tumours especially in the temporal lobes and posterior fossa
- magnetic resonance imaging (MRI) – full-sequence scanning with gadolinium enhancement provides maximal tumour resolution in structural imaging
- functional imaging with single photon emission CT (SPECT), positron emission tomography (PET), and MR are gaining importance in both diagnosis and assessment of response to treatment:
  - imaging agents thallium-201 and ^{123}I-tyrosine in SPECT scanning
  - ^{18}FDG (fluorodeoxyglucose) in PET can give important insights into the functional activity of the tumour, albeit hindered by high background activity in grey matter
  - can aid differentiation between high- or low-grade neoplasms and treatment-induced necrosis
- tumours that spread via cerebrospinal fluid (CSF) pathways require whole neuraxis MRI (e.g. medulloblastoma, ependymoma).

Histological confirmation of the diagnosis should ideally be obtained in all cases. Methods of biopsy include:

- stereotactic biopsy
- neuroradiologically guided needle biopsy
- craniotomy and excision or debulking of tumour
- endoscopic biopsy (minimally invasive technique allowing direct visualization of intraventricular tumours)
- electrophysiologically guided resection (performed under local anaesthetic, this allows sparing of brain tissue involved in critical functions, thereby minimizing disability following surgery).

Other investigations are guided by initial findings:

- angiography (for surgical planning of spinal tumours)
- lumbar puncture and CSF cytology (medulloblastoma, ependymoma, germ-cell tumour)
- HIV status (primary CNS lymphoma)
- ophthalmology review (primary CNS lymphoma)
- assessment of pituitary function (pituitary tumour)
- serum/CSF tumour markers (germ-cell tumour)
- molecular genetics, for example: 1p,19q deletion and MGMT. (O^6-methylguanine-DNA methyl transferase expression (glioma).

The dominant prognostic factors for brain tumours are a combination of histological type and clinical features such as age and performance status. Spread to regional lymph nodes and blood-borne spread to distant sites are rare in the majority of pathologies. Therefore, staging systems that are commonly used for other tumour types are rarely used for brain tumours.

Treatment of primary CNS tumours

Multidisciplinary management

Patients with CNS tumours suffer a wide variety of related physical, cognitive, and emotional problems. Prominent are:

- movement disorders
- tumour-associated epilepsy
- pain (headache)
- speech disorders
- intellectual decline
- personality changes.

These are best managed jointly between primary care and a hospital neuro-oncology multidisciplinary team, including a neurosurgeon, neuro-oncologist, neurologist, nurse specialist, and rehabilitation team, whose goals are to maximize the quality of life as well as to improve survival. Early involvement of the specialist palliative care team can be valuable in patients with high-grade glioma.

Low-grade glioma (WHO grades I and II)

- Histological diagnosis is preferred where possible, as up to 40% of radiologically diagnosed low-grade gliomas have high-grade features histopathologically.
- Initial management is usually immediate surgery or watchful waiting.
- Immediate surgery is indicated if there is a large mass and/or extensive neurological symptoms, in patients in whom resection is technically feasible.
- Watchful waiting may be appropriate for small, minimally symptomatic tumours:
  - low-grade astrocytoma presenting with epilepsy alone with no mass effect on imaging may be managed for years with anticonvulsants, with only regular review and repeat scanning required
  - intervention (surgery or radiotherapy), may be indicated if new neurological symptoms develop or radiological evidence of mass effect, tumour growth, or transformation to high-grade tumour.
- European Organisation for Research and Treatment of Cancer (EORTC) criteria can help identify patients with poor prognostic features, who may benefit from early intervention. These are:
  - age >40 years
  - largest tumour diameter >6 cm
  - tumour crossing the midline
  - astrocytoma histology
  - presence of neurological deficit.
- Radiotherapy is used for:
  - persistent neurological symptoms and significant residual tumour after surgery
  - tumour regrowth after surgery
  - evidence of tumour progression to high grade
  - symptomatic unresectable tumour.
- Radiotherapy improves survival whether it is given initially or for progressive disease. Early post-operative radiotherapy may, however,

provide an improvement in disease-free survival in patients with good performance status.
- Role of chemotherapy as first-line treatment is unclear.
- Chemotherapy does have benefit in the treatment of relapsed or progressive disease post-radiotherapy.

High-grade glioma (WHO grades III and IV)
- Includes glioblastoma multiforme, anaplastic astrocytoma, anaplastic olidodendroglioma, and anaplastic ependymoma.
- Age and performance status are strong determinants of survival.
- Main aims of treatment are to maximize patient's quality of life and improve survival where possible.
- Role of surgery:
  - surgery alone is not curative
  - for rapid relief of pressure symptoms (emergency decompression or shunt insertion for hydrocephalus)
  - elective surgery for fit patients for biopsy and tumour debulking
  - maximal tumour debulking improves survival and provides tissue for histology
  - re-operation is occasionally appropriate for relapsed disease, although the indications for this are not firmly established (may be more appropriate e.g. for frontal lobe tumours with pressure symptoms)
  - advances in surgery, which include MRI-guided neuro-navigation, intra-operative MRI, functional MRI, intra-operative mapping and fluorescence-guided surgery, have improved the extent and safety of resection
  - patients with diffuse brainstem tumours are **not** amenable to surgery, but if the lesion is local, resection (if possible) is the treatment of choice, usually via a posterior fossa approach. Surgical morbidity can be high.
- The mainstay of treatment is radiotherapy:
  - radical radiotherapy should be restricted to younger patients (commonly maximum 60–70 years) with good performance status (WHO 0–1)
  - palliative radiotherapy may be appropriate for younger patients of performance status 2–3, or older patients of performance status 0.
- Concurrent radical radiotherapy and temozolomide chemotherapy followed by adjuvant temozolomide chemotherapy has been shown to improve 2-year survival to 26%, compared to 10% in those who did not receive chemotherapy.
- Chemotherapy also of benefit in the treatment of relapsed disease.
- Regardless of age, patients of poor performance status may not benefit from any treatment and should be offered supportive care.

Ependymoma
- Arise from ependymal cells lining ventricular system and central canal of spinal cord to filum terminale.
- Safe resection of all tumour is the optimal primary treatment.
- Residual tumour carries poor prognosis.
- Low-grade tumours treated by surgery and local radiotherapy.
- Anaplastic tumours require additional craniospinal irradiation (CSI).

Pineal tumours

- Hydrocephalus due to blockage of third ventricle is common, requiring shunt insertion/surgical decompression prior to surgical excision, or debulking. At least a biopsy is essential for optimum management. Stereotactic biopsy or an open microsurgical procedure requires careful discussion at a multidisciplinary meeting. The former gives rise to fewer complications but the latter removes maximal tumour burden and may improve prognosis.
- Pineocytoma is treated by surgery and radiotherapy. Stereotactic radiotherapy may be used for low-grade tumours.
- Pineoblastoma requires CSI.

Meningioma

- Management depends on signs, symptoms, patient fitness and size and site of tumour.
- Watchful waiting may be appropriate (small incidental tumour in asymptomatic patient).
- Surgery is the mainstay of treatment although complete excision may be difficult as some are very vascular and/or may be in inaccessible areas. Total excision (Simpson grade I) is ideal but probably unusual in practice. Total excision for meningiomas involving the cavernous sinus, petroclival region, posterior aspect of superior sagittal sinus, and optic nerve sheath is not possible without major neuropathic morbidity. Most convexity and spinal meningiomas can be excised with minimal morbidity.
- Indications for radiotherapy:
  - radical primary treatment
  - tumour at inoperable location (cavernous sinus, optic nerve).
- Radical post-operative treatment:
  - invasion by tumour of adjacent critical structure
  - WHO grade II/III tumour
  - unresectable recurrence.
- Stereotactic radiotherapy and radiosurgery may be useful in selected cases.

Germ-cell tumours

Germinoma

- Standard treatment is radical radiotherapy.
- Role of chemotherapy is unclear.
- Urgent radiotherapy may be necessary to prevent blindness due to predilection of germinoma for optic chiasm and suprasellar cistern.

Non-germinoma

- Chemotherapy first line
- Surgery if residual tumour in selected cases
- Radiotherapy to primary site

Pituitary tumours

Pituitary adenoma
- Macroprolactinoma:
  - bromocriptine first line
  - surgery
  - post-operative radiotherapy to residual tumour.
- Microprolactinoma:
  - treat only if symptomatic
  - surgery
  - post-operative radiotherapy if high pre-operative prolactin fails to normalize post-operatively, or locally invasive tumour
- Functionless tumour:
  - surgery
  - post-operative radiotherapy to reduce local recurrence
- Acromegaly/gigantism
  - surgery
  - post-operative radiotherapy to reduce local recurrence
  - bromocriptine if high growth hormone post-operatively, or surgery not possible
  - octreotide for refractory growth-hormone-secreting adenoma.

Craniopharyngioma
- Surgical resection
- Post-operative radiotherapy if subtotal resection.

Surgery for pituitary tumours is via the trans-sphenoidal route. Most microadenomas and many macroadenomas can be resected via the trans-sphenoidal route. Endoscopic trans-sphenoidal approaches are increasingly used in specialized centres.

Primary CNS lymphoma
- Chemotherapy is mainstay of treatment:
  - adjuvant radiotherapy if partial response to chemotherapy
  - role of radiotherapy after complete response unclear.
- In AIDS patients antiretroviral therapy and cranial radiotherapy may modestly improve an otherwise dismal prognosis.

Acoustic neuroma (vestibular schwannoma)
- Often associated with neurofibromatosis: patients may have other tumours therefore management may be complex.
- Treatment required only if disease progression.
- Treatment options are surgery or radiotherapy.

Surgery
- Should be curative if complete excision with microsurgical techniques.
- Hearing loss was previously inevitable but selected patients may preserve hearing with a partial labyrinthectomy.
- After failure of primary radiotherapy.
- Surgical risks include:
  - CSF leaks
  - meningitis

- headache
- hearing loss
- facial nerve paralysis.

Radiotherapy
- Single fraction stereotactic radiosurgery (SRS)
- Fractionated stereotactic radiotherapy (FSRT)

Medulloblastoma

- Is predominantly a tumour of childhood and is very rare in adults.
- Usually occurs in the posterior fossa presenting with cerebellar symptoms and raised intracranial pressure, and commonly spreads through craniospinal axis.
- Management and prognosis is guided by staging using modified Chang criteria based on extent of disease. See Table 23.6:
  - Standard-risk disease is T1–3a, M0, and no residual disease after surgery
  - high-risk disease is T3b-4, any M+, or post-operative residual disease.
- Combined modality treatment, including maximal surgical resection, tumour bed and craniospinal irradiation, and chemotherapy is the standard of care
  - standard-risk disease is treated with CSI with boost to tumour bed
  - high-risk disease is treated with chemotherapy prior to radiotherapy, with maintenance chemotherapy if M1–M3 disease.
- As clinical experience in adults is limited, treatment should be patterned after that in children.

Table 23.6 Modified Chang system for staging of medulloblastoma

Extent of tumour	Metastatic spread
T1: <3 cm diameter	M0: no evidence of metastases
T2: >3 cm diameter	M1: microscopic tumour cells in CSF
T3a: >3 cm diameter with extension into aqueduct of Sylvius and/or foreamen of Luschka	M2: macroscopic tumour seeding in cerebellar/cerebral subarachnoid space or in third or lateral ventricles
T3b: >3cm diameter with extension into the brainstem	M3: macroscopic tumour seeding in spinal subarachnoid space
T4: >3 cm diameter with extension above the aqueduct of Sylvius and/or below the foreamen magnum	M4: metastases outside the cerebrospinal axis

Spinal cord tumours

Schwannomas and meningiomas
- Usually amenable to complete resection with high rates of local control.
- Inoperable/recurrent disease treated with radical radiotherapy.

- High grade tumours usually treated with post-operative radical radiotherapy.

Ependymoma
- Gross total resection improves survival.
- Post-operative radiotherapy given if subtotal resection or anaplastic pathology.

Glioma
- Standard treatment is resection followed by post-operative radiotherapy for low- and high-grade tumours.
- No survival benefit for gross total resection over subtotal resection.
- Higher radiotherapy dose for high-grade tumours.

Radiotherapy for primary CNS tumours

Radical radiotherapy

Treatment should be 3D conformal, and the principles of treatment are the same regardless of tumour type:

Patient position
- Depends on tumour location
- Supine has advantage of patient comfort
- Prone for posterior lesions

Patient immobilization
- Perspex or thermoplastic shell immobilization allows accurate reproducibility, essential for radical treatment planning, given close proximity of critical normal structures (e.g. lens, optic chiasma, brainstem, spinal cord)

Volume localization
- CT planning scan
- Co-registered with pre-operative CT or MRI if possible
- Gross tumour volume (GTV) defined on each slice with margin to create clinical target volume (CTV), and planning target volume (PTV), dependent on tumour type (see Table 23.7), edited to avoid organs at risk
- Organs at risk (OAR) outlined

Dose fractionation (see Table 23.7)
- Fraction size 1.8–2.0 Gy to minimize late radiation damage
- Attention to dose tolerances of OAR (see Table 23.8)
- Tumour dose reflects balance of probability of tumour control against risk of late radiation damage

Palliative radiotherapy

Palliative radiotherapy is appropriate for young glioma patients of performance status 2–3, or older patients of performance status 0. In these patients palliative radiotherapy may help symptom control. However, life expectancy is short regardless, therefore treatment duration and toxicity should be kept to a minimum. Examples of radiotherapy schedules include 30 Gy/6 fractions/2 weeks and 40 Gy/15 fractions/3 weeks.

Craniospinal irradiation (CSI)

CSI is a complex technique which should only be attempted in radiotherapy centres with clinicians, physics, and radiographer staff experienced in its delivery.

- Traditionally in most centres patients have been treated in the prone postion but supine positioning is now increasingly used, to improve patient comfort and stability.
- Immobilization is crucial, a perspex or thermoplastic shell for the head/neck, and body immobilization may also be used e.g. vac-bag and foot stocks. The CTV is the intracranial and spinal meninges preferably outlined on a planning CT scan of head and spine.

- The field arrangement is usually lateral opposed cranial fields with usually two posterior fields in adults carefully matched to the lower border of the cranial fields.
- To avoid the risk of overdosing or underdosing at the spinal field junctions, moving junctions are used.

Table 23.7 Details of radiotherapy planning for primary CNS tumours

Tumour type	GTV to CTV margin (GTV is primary tumour prior to any intervention) (cm)	Dose/fractionation (Gy/fractions)
Glioma		
High-grade	2.5	60/30
Low-grade	1.5	54/30
Medulloblastoma	2.5	55/33 (+CSI 35/21)
Ependymoma	1.5–2.5	50–54/30–33 (+CSI 35/21 if anaplastic)
Pineocytoma	0.5	45–50/25
Meningioma		
High-grade	1.5–2.5	50–55/30–33
Low-grade	0.0–0.5	50–55/30–33
Germinoma	1.0–2.0	40/24 (+CSI 25/15)
Pituitary		
Adenoma	0.5	45/25
Craniopharyngioma	0.5	50/30
Primary CNS lymphoma	2.5	45/25

NB: CTV to PTV margin using a Perspex or thermoplastic head shell is usually ~0.5 cm.

Table 23.8 Normal CNS tissue tolerance doses

Structure	Tolerance dose, Gy (2 Gy/fraction)
Brain parenchyma	54–60
Brainstem	48
Optic nerves and chiasm	50–55
Pituitary gland/hypothalamus	40–60
Middle/inner ear	60
Lacrimal gland	20
Lens	6–10
Retina	50

Stereotactic radiotherapy

Stereotactic radiosurgery (SRS) is a highly specialized technique available in a limited number of cancer centres. It focuses high doses of radiation to a tumour in a single fraction, sparing normal tissues by limiting its use to small tumours and treating with minimal margins around the GTV. This technique is most widely used for acoustic neuroma.

Fractionated stereotactic radiotherapy (FSRT) is planned in a similar way to radical radiotherapy. The difference is that high-precision immobilization in a relocatable stereotactic frame means that no CTV to PTV margin is required. The margin to PTV with stereotactic immobilization should be in the region of 0.2–0.3 mm. This allows sparing of nearby critical normal structures. This technique is most commonly used for treatment of acoustic neuroma treating to a dose of 50–54 Gy/30 fractions. It has also been used in management of skull base meningioma and solitary intracranial metastases.

The advantage of theses techniques for treatment of acoustic neuroma is hearing preservation compared to surgery. FSRT has slightly better reported hearing preservation rates compared to SRS, of 85% and 75% respectively.

CNS radiotherapy side-effects

The common side-effects of CNS radiotherapy are shown in Table 23.9.

Table 23.9 Side-effects of brain and spinal irradiation

Radiotherapy site	Acute toxicity	Late toxicity
Brain	Alopecia	Pituitary hypofunction
	Skin reaction	Optic chiasm damage
	Fatigue	Risk of second malignancies (brain)
	Nausea and vomiting	Neurocognitive impairment
		Memory loss
Spine	Sore throat	Risk of second malignancy (chest/abdomen/pelvis)
	Nausea and vomiting	Ovarian failure
	Diarrhoea	Spinal cord damage
	Myelosuppression	

Chemotherapy for primary CNS tumours

Most CNS tumours are traditionally considered poor targets for chemotherapy:

- many, e.g. gliomas, demonstrate intrinsic chemoresistance to many conventional cytotoxics
- the blood–brain barrier normally provides an obstacle to drugs except lipophilic agents
- however, the blood–brain barrier is disrupted in many primary CNS tumours (as demonstrated by contrast uptake on axial imaging) allowing penetration of chemotherapy.

The current indications for chemotherapy in primary CNS tumours include:

- in selected fit patients with GBM, concomitant radical radiotherapy and oral temozolomide chemotherapy (75 mg/m^2 daily) followed by 6 cycles of post-radiation therapy oral temozolomide (200 mg/m^2 for 5 days of a 28-day cycle)
- for relapsed glioma (low grade and high grade), examples of chemotherapy regimes are:
  - oral temozolomide (200 mg/m^2 for 5 days of a 28-day cycle until tumour progression)
  - PCV (1-(20chloroethyl)-3-cyclohexyl-1-nitrosurea (CCNU) 110 mg/m^2 oral day 1 q 6/52, procarbazine 60 mg/m^2 oral day 8–21, vincristine 1.4 mg/m^2 (max 2 mg) IV days 8 and 22)
  - single-agent CCNU 200–240 mg oral day 1, 6 weekly
- intra-operative carmustine implants are licensed for the treatment of patients with newly diagnosed high-grade glioma in whom more than 90% of tumour has been resected
- the agents used in the management of medulloblastoma include cisplatin, vincristine, and cyclophosphamide
- the agents used in the management of non-germinoma are bleomycin, etoposide, and cisplatin.

Prognosis for primary CNS tumours

Prognosis varies widely dependent on tumour type. See Table 23.10. The overall survival of patients with high-grade glioma remains fairly dismal. However, some tumours, for example pituitary adenomas, may not affect long-term survival at all. Overall, the 5-year survival of malignant brain tumours is approximately 17%.

Table 23.10 Prognosis of primary CNS tumours

Tumour type	Prognosis
High-grade glioma	
Anaplastic astrocytoma	Surgery only: MS 1 year Surgery +RT: MS 3 years
Glioblastoma	Surgery only: MS 3/12 Surgery + RT: MS 10/12 Surgery + chemoRT: 14.6/12
Low-grade glioma	MS >5 years
Medulloblastoma	
Standard-risk disease	5YS 70%
High-risk disease	5YS 20–50%
Ependymoma	
Low grade	5YS 30–50%
High grade	5YS 0%
Pineocytoma	5YS 85%
Meningioma	
Grade I	RR: 7–20%
Grade II	RR 29–40%
Grade III	RR 50–78%
Germ-cell tumours	
Geminoma	5YS >90%
Non-germinoma	5YS 60%
Pituitary tumours	
Adenoma	5YS >95%
Craniopharyngioma	10YS 85%
Primary CNS lymphoma	5YS 30%
Acoustic neuroma	SRS: 5YLCR 92% FSRT: 5YLCR 98%

RT: radiotherapy; 5YS: 5-year survival; 10YS: 10-year survival; MS: median survival; 5YLCR: 5-year local control rate; RR: recurrence rate.

Predictors of outcome for patients with glioma include:
- tumour grade
  - most important predictor
  - low-grade gliomas have a relatively good prognosis
  - results of treatment of high-grade gliomas remain poor
- extent of surgical excision
- age (worse survival >50 years)
- performance status at presentation
- presence of fits confers a better prognosis
- low score correlates with poor prognosis
- Mini-mental score. See Table 23.11.

Table 23.11 Mini-mental test

Maximum score	Patient's score	Questions
5		What is the date? day, month, year?
5		Where are we now?
3		Examiner names three unrelated objects and asks the patient to repeat these
5		Subtract serial 7s from 100
3		Ask patient to recall the same three objects
2		Ask patient to name two simple objects, e.g. watch and pen
1		Ask patient to repeat 'no ifs, ands, or buts'
3		Give patient a piece of paper and ask him/her to take the paper in their right hand, fold it in half, and put it on the floor
1		Give patient written instruction, e.g. 'close your eyes'
1		Ask patient to make up and write one sentence
1		Ask patient to copy a picture
30		Total

Impairment: score 10–20 moderate; 0–10, severe.

Recent advances and future treatments for primary CNS tumours

- Surgical neuronavigation:
  - recently acquired images of the patient's brain are projected intra-operatively on to the operating field.
  - facilitates accurate laser or ultrasound resection of tumour.
- Radiotherapy: improved accuracy and dose escalation is feasible with stereotactic localization, although results so far disappointing in high-grade glioma. Intensity-modulated radiotherapy (IMRT) can undoubtedly facilitate dose escalation and sparing of normal tissues, but has yet to prove any survival benefit.
- Novel therapies under evaluation include
  - tyrosine kinase inhibitors
  - farnesyl transferase inhibitors
  - epidermal growth factor receptor inhibitors
  - vascular endothelial growth factor inhibitors and other anti-angiogenesis inhibitors.
- Gene therapy:
  - much attention has focused on the HSVtk/aciclovir suicide gene system
  - other therapeutic strategies are possible but the lack of effective vectors currently limits the applicability of this approach
  - using adenovirus or herpes simplex virus might overcome the limitations inherent in the current retroviral approaches.

Brain metastases

Epidemiology
Metastases to the brain from an extracranial primary are common – at least 10× more common than primary CNS tumours:
- symptomatic metastases have an incidence of around 6 per 100 000
- autopsy studies have revealed an overall occurrence in 24% of patients with known cancer
- found in 40% of patients with systemic cancer at postmortem
- slight male preponderance and incidence increases with age.

The incidence of brain metastases is rising, in part due to improvements in and availability of brain imaging, but also due to better control of extracerebral malignancy as a result of improved local and systemic therapy:
- breast cancer especially lung metastases and/or HER2 +ve (trastuzumab does not cross blood–brain barrier)
- colorectal cancer – prolonged survival with advanced disease through effective systemic treatment
- non-small cell lung cancer – improved loco-regional therapy and axial imaging.

While brain metastases may arise from any primary site, the most common are from:
- lung cancer (50%)
- breast cancer (15%)
- melanoma (10%)
- renal cancer
- gastrointestinal (GI) cancer
- unknown primary (10%).

Some cancers that commonly metastasize to other organs rarely involve the brain, e.g. prostate, bladder, cervix, and ovary. The reason for this is not clear. Rare tumours that have a predilection for the brain include choriocarcinoma and malignant germ-cell tumours with trophoblast elements.
Carcinomatous meningitis is less common but may occur in:
- lung cancer
- breast cancer
- leukaemia and lymphoma.

Pathology
The histology reflects the original primary tumour. Vascular proliferation and tumour necrosis are common features. There is often demarcation from adjacent brain:
- 30% single
- 80% cerebral hemispheres, 15% posterior fossa, 5% brainstem
- different tumours have predilection for metastases to different areas of brain:
  - pelvic and GI tumours more commonly metastasize to posterior fossa
  - small-cell lung cancer equally distributed in all areas of brain
- commonly considerable cerebral oedema adds to the mass effect of metastases.

Presentation

The presentation of brain metastases is similar to that of primary brain tumours:
- headache
- focal neurological deficit, e.g. loss of power, dysphasia, visual field defect
- confusion or personality change
- seizures – focal or generalized
- ataxia
- with the additional features of systemic malignancy if other organs involved.

Investigation

Imaging is most commonly with contrast-enhanced CT of brain because of its availability. However, the most sensitive investigation is high-resolution contrast-enhanced MR scan:
- metastases most frequently appear as multiple, discrete, well-demarcated lesions
- hypointense on T_1
- hyperintense on T_2
- marked gadolinium enhancement
- often considerable associated vasogenic oedema
- up to 20% of lesions revealed on MRI are not seen on CT.

In patients who present with brain metastases with no previous diagnosis of cancer, a detailed history and examination can identify the primary in ~30%. Subsequent investigations may include chest X-ray, CT chest/abdomen/pelvis, PET-CT, and biopsy; 60% will have a primary lung cancer or concomitant pulmonary metastases. Other frequent unknown primary cancers include melanoma, breast, and colorectal, with the primary unidentified in 25–30%.

Management

Management includes:
- symptom control
- specific treatment directed again the brain metastases
- systemic treatment.

Appropriate management is guided by an assessment of prognosis. Several studies have assessed prognostic features in patients with brain metastases (see Table 23.12). Patients of intermediate prognosis fall into the favourable- or poor-prognostic group, depending on likelihood of controlling systemic disease. For the third group, appropriate management comprises steroids and symptom control.

Table 23.12 Predicting prognosis in brain metastasis

Prognosis	Characteristics
1 Favourable	KPS >70
	Age <65 years
	Controlled primary
	No extracranial metastases
2 Intermediate	KPS >70
	With 1+ of: age>65 years; uncontrolled primary; extracranial metastases
3 Poor	KPS <70

KPS, Karnofsky Performance Status score.

Symptom control

Control of symptoms similar to primary brain tumours:
- dexamethasone in the majority of patients
- frequently produces a reversal of symptoms and neurological deficit
- starting dose of 8–16 mg daily along with proton pump inhibitor (PPI) gastroprotection.
- improvement can often be maintained with doses of 2–4 mg.

Treatment directed against brain metastases

For patients with multiple brain metastases, with favourable prognostic characteristics at presentation, or patients improved following dexamethasone, treatment with palliative radiotherapy can be offered with the following aims:
- temporary tumour control
- modest improvement in survival time
- allows reduction in the steroid dose without deterioration in symptoms (reducing problems of candidiasis, proximal myopathy, Cushingoid appearance).

Typically the whole brain is irradiated. A dose of 20 Gy in 5 fractions has been shown to be as effective as any of the more protracted fractionation schemes. For patients presenting with solitary or small number of brain metastases:
- defined as metastatic disease within the brain in the absence of demonstrable malignancy elsewhere in the body
- biopsy may be required especially when there is no history of previous cancer.
- In patients with favourable prognostic features:
  - surgical excision should be considered
  - post-operative whole-brain radiotherapy is given (20 Gy in 5 fractions or 30 Gy in 10 fractions) with or without a local boost
  - an alternative to surgery is stereotactic radiosurgery (20 Gy in a single fraction), followed by whole-brain irradiation.

Systemic treatment
While many cytotoxics do not cross the blood–brain barrier, this barrier is disrupted in many patients with CNS metastases. Chemotherapy may be useful in chemosensitive tumours:
- germ-cell tumours
- small-cell lung cancer
- breast cancer.

Targeted therapies under investigation
- Lapatinib
- Bevacuzimab

Outcome
Overall, the prognosis is poor for patients with brain metastases from the common cancers. For patients with poor prognostic features, the median survival is 6–8 weeks, irrespective of treatment. Patients with 'favourable-prognosis' solitary metastases that are treated with surgery and radiotherapy have a median survival of ~10 months.

Further reading

Akay KA, Izci Y, Baysefer A (2004) Surgical outcomes of cerebellar tumours in children. *Pediatr Neurosurg* **40**, 220–5.

Bhagavathi S, Wilson J (2008) Primary central nervous system lymphoma. *Arch Pathol Lab Med* **132**, 1830–4.

Bruce JN, Ogden AT (2004) Surgical strategies for treating patients with pineal region tumours. *J Neurooncol* **69**, 221–36.

Davies E, Hopkins A, ed. (1997) *Improving Care for Patients with Malignant Glioma*. London: Royal College of Physicians.

Henry RG, Berman JI, Nagarajan SS, *et al.* (2004) Subcortical pathways serving cortical language sites: initial experience with diffusion tensor imaging fiber tracking combined with intraoperative language mapping. *NeuroImage* **21**, 616–22.

Recinos PF, Sciubba DM, Jallo GI (2007) Brainstem tumours – where are we today? *Pediatric Neurosurg* **43**, 192–201.

Wen PY, Kesari SL (2008) Malignant gliomas in adults. *New Engl J Med* **359**, 492–507.

Whittle IR, Smith C, Navoo P, Collie E (2004) Meningiomas. *Lancet* **363**, 1535–43.

Skin cancers

Introduction

- Skin cancers constitute the most common group of cancers in the UK (20% of all cancer registrations).
- The registered incidence of 60 000 cases in England and Wales each year is felt to under-represent the true incidence, due to differing practices for registering cases – National Institute for Health and Clinical Excellence.
- Management of this group of cancers may be co-ordinated in the community, at the local hospital or in a specialist centre, depending on the diagnosis and stage. However, it is recommended that any health professional involved in the treatment of any type of skin cancer should be a member of the appropriate multidisciplinary team.

Malignant melanoma

Primary cutaneous malignant melanoma arises from the melanocytes found in the basal layer of skin, which produce melanin pigment and are responsible for the tanning response after ultraviolet (UV) radiation exposure.

Epidemiology and aetiology

- Incidence rates are rising faster than for any other cancer worldwide:
  - lifetime risk is currently estimated at >1:80 for Caucasians, but as low as 1:1200 amongst those with pigmented skin.
  - rates in Australia are the highest in the world and continue to double each decade.
  - incidence in women is at least comparable to the incidence in men, although death from melanoma is more common in men.
- Sunlight:
  - main environmental cause of melanoma
  - excess exposure to UV radiation, particularly in early life, is strongly associated with subsequent risk of developing melanoma
  - a history of severe sunburn or intense intermittent exposure may be particularly relevant
  - artificial exposure to UV (sun-beds) radiation has also contributed to the increased incidence of melanoma over the past decade.
- Genetic risk:
  - ~10% of cases will have a strong family history of melanoma
  - a melanoma susceptibility gene *CDKN2A* on chromosome 9 has been identified as a tumour suppressor gene
  - germline mutations are implicated in up to 40% of patients with familial melanoma and may have a role in sporadic cases.
- Benign pigmented naevi (Figs. 24.1 and 24.2):
  - some may be precursor lesions to malignant disease
  - more frequently these are markers of a more general increased risk within the individual.
- Immunosuppression:
  - e.g. following organ transplantation
  - appears to be associated with an increased risk of developing melanoma
  - conversely there is currently no evidence that melanoma is more prevalent in the HIV-positive population.

Screening and prevention

- Strenuous efforts must be made to minimize the occurrence of melanoma and to maximize the chances of early diagnosis while curative treatment remains possible.
- Exposure to sunlight has been identified as the major modifiable risk factor. This has led to public health drives to promote sun avoidance, including:
  - the successful Australian 'Slip (on a shirt), Slap (on a hat), Slop (on sun-screen)' campaign
  - the promotion of artificial tanning products as an acceptable cosmetic alternative to UV exposure
  - the introduction of sun hats as part of the uniform in some schools.

- Screening may be an appropriate option for patients deemed at particular risk of the disease, e.g. those with a strong family history of melanoma or with a personal history of any skin cancer or of blistering sunburn in early life.
- Serial photographs can be useful in patients with a high mole burden, as can inspection via a magnifying dermatoscope.

Malignant melanoma: clinical presentation

Typically present with:
- alteration in a pre-existing pigmented mole on the skin
- a new pigmented lesion – this is particularly relevant if aged ≥40 years, when the acquisition of new moles is uncommon
- irregular brown/black pigmentation of a lesion
- irregular border or new asymmetry of a lesion
- ±oozing, crusting, itching, or bleeding
- differential diagnosis:
  - benign melanocytic naevi
  - seborrhoeic keratoses (older ages).

Less commonly:
- palpable regional lymphadenopathy
- metastatic disease to viscera (1° lesion may not be identified).

Investigations

- Full clinical examination including skin, regional and distant lymph node assessment, palpation of the abdomen, and neurological examination if indicated.
- Excision biopsy required for any pigmented lesion of concern (see Figs. 24.3 and 24.4 for examples of cutaneous malignant melanoma). Complete excision with normal skin margins is optimal. Initial biopsy should be with a miminum lateral clearance of 2 mm and a cuff of subcutaneous deep fat to allow the pathologist to diagnose the lesion and give depth of invasion (Breslow).
- Incision biopsy is only acceptable for large lesions in cosmetically sensitive areas (face). Punch biopsy should **not** be done, because of inadequate depth to allow histological staging.
- Shave biopsy should be avoided if possible, to minimize the risk of incomplete excision and to allow appropriate staging which requires depth measurement.
- Chest X-ray (CXR) and serum biochemistry, including lactate dehydrogenase (LDH), once the diagnosis of melanoma has been confirmed.
- Further imaging, e.g. computerized tomography (CT) chest/abdomen, should probably be restricted to those patients with confirmed regional metastatic disease or clinical symptoms/signs suggestive of dissemination. This is because of the high false-positive rate following speculative imaging.

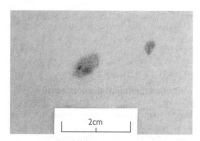

Fig. 24.1 Benign pigmented lesion. (See Plate 1 for a full colour version.)

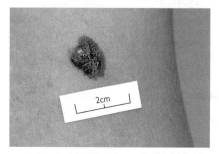

Fig. 24.2 Benign naevus close-up. (See Plate 2 for a full colour version.)

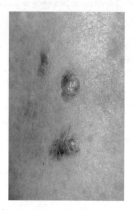

Fig. 24.3 Malignant melanoma close-up. (See Plate 3 for a full colour version.)

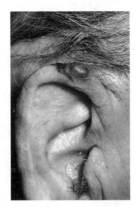

Fig. 24.4 Malignant melanoma close-up. (See Plate 4 for a full colour version.)

Pathology

- Confirms neoplastic melanocytic cells invading beneath the basement membrane into the underlying dermis.
- Histological subtype, e.g. superficial spreading melanoma, nodular or acral lentiginous melanoma.
- Tumour thickness (Breslow depth) in millimetres from the epidermal granular layer to the base of the tumour at its thickest point.
- Any invasion of dermal blood vessels and lymphatics.
- Presence or absence of ulceration.
- Margins: whether involved or width of normal tissue surrounding melanoma. Identifies microsatellites of melanoma.

Staging

The American Joint Committee on Cancer (AJCC) Staging 2002 has produced a revised validated staging system based on tumour thickness, the presence of ulceration, and the identification of metastases to provide guidance for management decisions and likely prognosis (see Tables 24.1 and 24.2).

Table 24.1 AJCC TNM classification for melanoma

Tumor (T) classification		
Tx	Primary melanoma cannot be assessed	
Tis	Melanoma *in situ*	
T1	≤1 mm	a: Without ulceration b: With ulceration
T2	1.01–2.0 mm	a: Without ulceration b: With ulceration
T3	2.01–4.0 mm	a: Without ulceration b: With ulceration
T4	>4.0 mm	a: Without ulceration b: With ulceration
Node (N) classification		
N1	1 lymph node (LN)	a: Micrometastasis b: Macrometastasis
N2	2–3LNs	a: Micrometastasis b: Macrometastasis c: In-transit/satellite disease without LNs
N3	>4 LNs or in-transit disease with metastatic nodes	
Metastasis (M) classification		
M1a	Distant skin or LNs	Normal LDH
M1b	Pulmonary metastases	Normal LDH
M1c	All other visceral metastases	Normal LDH
	Any metastatic disease	Elevated LDH

With permission from Edge SE, Byrd DR, Carducci MA, Compton CA, eds. AJCC Cancer Staging Manual, 7th ed. New York, NY: Springer, 2009.

Table 24.2 AJCC stage groupings for cutaneous melanoma

Stage	Clinical stage grouping			Pathological stage grouping		
0	Tis	N0	M0	pTis	N0	M0
IA	T1a	N0	M0	pTa	N0	M0
IB	T1b	N0	M0	pT1b	N0	M0
	T2a	N0	M0	pT2a	N0	M0
IIA	T2b	N0	M0	pT2b	N0	M0
	T3a	N0	M0	pT3a	N0	M0
IIB	T3b	N0	M0	pT3b	N0	M0
	T4a	N0	M0	pT4a	N0	M0
IIC	T4b	N0	M0	pT4b	N0	M0
III	any T	N1–3	M0			M0
IIIA				pT1–4a	N1a	M0
IIIB				pT1–4b	N2a	M0
				pT1–4b	N1a	M0
				pT1–4b	N2a	M0
				pT1–4a	N2b	M0
				pT1–4a	N2b	M0
				pT1–4a/b	N2c	M0
IIIC				pT1–4b	N1b	M0
				pT1–4b	N2b	M0
				any T	N3	M0
IV	any T	any N	any M	any T	any N	any M

With permission from Edge SE, Byrd DR, Carducci MA, Compton CA, eds. AJCC Cancer Staging Manual, 7th ed. New York, NY: Springer, 2009.

Management of malignant melanoma

Surgical management

Surgery at the primary site

- The treatment for primary malignant melanoma is complete excision of the lesion.
- The recommended margin of excision of normal skin varies according to the thickness of the tumour:
  - *In situ* disease only: 0.5 cm
  - <2 mm thick: at least 1 cm
  - ≥2 mm but <4 mm thick: at least 2 cm
  - ≥4 mm: 3 cm margin recommended although superiority of this over more conservative excision not yet proven.
- Excision must be adequate in depth as well as laterally.
- Unusual sites of disease, e.g. foot sole, nail bed, require tailored surgical techniques.
- Most patients with primary melanoma have the defect closed directly. A small number may require either a flap or a graft to achieve closure.

Surgery for the regional lymph nodes

- One in five patients who are clinically node negative will have metastatic deposits.
- False-positive nodal assessment is probably equally as common.
- **Regional lymph node dissection** in patients with clinical evidence of lymph node involvement:
  - therapeutic lymphadenectomy of palpable or histologically proven metastatic lymph nodes may be curative, e.g. 10-year disease-free survival of ~25% for all node-positive patients treated surgically
  - lymph node dissection also minimizes the risk of local ulceration or fungation
  - complications following surgery are common and include infection and seroma formation in the short-term and lymphoedema in the longer-term.
- **Elective lymph node dissection** in patients without definite evidence of regional nodal involvement:
  - more complex
  - has not been shown to improve survival in patients with tumours that are <1 mm or ≥4 mm thick. There is some suggestion of a survival benefit in younger patients with tumours of intermediate depth
  - main benefit of establishing the status of regional lymph nodes is for accurate staging, provided this will not affect options for subsequent adjuvant therapy.
- Sentinel lymph node biopsy:
  - using either blue dye or a radiolabelled tracer
  - identifies patients with a definite lymph node metastasis who can then proceed to formal regional nodal dissection. If the sentinel node is negative for tumour deposit then formal nodal dissection is not performed, avoiding the associated morbidity

- a staging investigation rather than a therapeutic intervention
- early studies have suggested that the sentinel node can be identified in up to 90% of cases and the false-negative rate may be as low as 2%. In 30–50% of patients, the sentinel node is the only positive node identified
- risk of detecting malignant deposits in the sentinel node increases with primary tumour thickness (see Table 24.3). The results of several large-scale trials that should help clarify whether this approach compromises long-term survival are awaited
- in the UK, use is limited to centres with established expertise, ideally within the context of a clinical trial, of which a number are ongoing.

Table 24.3 Risk of identifying a metastatic deposit in a sentinel lymph node according to primary tumour thickness

	Risk of metastatic deposit in sentinel node (%)
Breslow depth <0.75 mm	1
≥0.75 Breslow depth <1.5 mm	8
≥1.50 Breslow depth <4.0 mm	23
Breslow depth ≥4.0 mm	36

Prognosis and risk of relapse
- Most patients present with stage I to IIA disease, when appropriate surgery is curative in the majority of cases, e.g. Stage IB – 90% cured by surgery, falling to 78% for those with Stage IIA disease.
- Relapse rates following resection escalate rapidly with advancing stage:
  - stage IIB disease – risk of recurrence of 40% following local excision
  - stage III disease (which includes regional node involvement) associated with relapse rates of >80%.
- Median survival with stage IV disease is typically <9 months, and with leptomeningeal involvement is 5–16 weeks.

Chemotherapy, immunotherapy, and radiotherapy
Surveillance
- In the UK, the current standard management following resection of a primary melanoma ± regional lymph node dissection is a surveillance regime, often shared between:
  - the patient,
  - their general practitioner (GP)
  - a plastic surgeon
  - possibly an oncologist.

Adjuvant therapy
- Aims to minimize the risk of relapse particularly in patients with stage III disease (resected node-positive disease).

- In the UK there is currently no standard adjuvant treatment in patients at intermediate and high risk of disease relapse. Entry to clinical trials should be offered wherever possible.
- Multiple trials have examined using several modes of therapy.
- High-dose intravenous (IV) interferon-α (HDI):
  - most encouraging adjuvant regime
  - typically involves 4 weeks of daily HDI (e.g. 20 Mu/m²) often followed by a lower dose for a further 1–4 years
  - there is agreement that HDI affects the natural history of the disease in some way
  - several large trials have produced conflicting results, and comparison of the outcomes is complex
  - all trials of HDI in intermediate- and high-risk patients have demonstrated that treatment with HDI is associated with modest improvements in relapse-free survival (~11–25%)
  - any effect on overall survival is unknown. Comparison between trials is complex and results have been inconsistent. A meta-analysis of 14 trials comparing interferon-α treatment to a control showed no impact on overall survival
  - side-effects include 'flu-like' symptoms, myelosuppression, fatigue, hepatotoxicity, and depression ± mania
  - no consensus as to the optimal regime
  - any additional benefit of ongoing subcutaneous low-dose interferon-α (IFN-α) remains to be established
  - mechanism of action is unknown, although suggestions include:
  - immune modulation
  - direct cytotoxic action (at high doses)
  - anti-angiogenic role.
  - treatment with HDI in the UK remains limited to the context of clinical trials.
- Low- and intermediate-dose interferon:
  - alternative regimes using lower doses of IFN-α have been studied, occasionally in combination with interleukin-2 (IL-2; see 📖 Chapter 10, 'Biological and targeted therapies')
  - aimed to establish whether equivalent benefit can be achieved with fewer side-effects
  - no trial evaluating lower doses has shown equivalent benefit to HDI.
- Vaccines:
  - there is no randomized phase III trial to support the use of any vaccine as adjuvant treatment following resection of node-positive melanoma
  - strategies have included attempts to enhance cellular immunity, or alternatively to induce humoral immunity
  - clinical trials of a number of different types of vaccine are ongoing
  - tumour heterogeneity, tumour-reinforced tolerance, and poor immunogenicity of relevant antigens have all probably contributed to disappointing results to date.

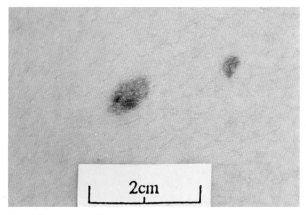

Plate 1 Benign pigmented lesion.

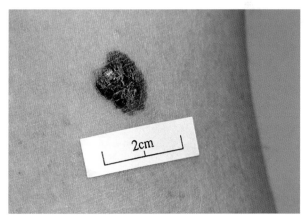

Plate 2 Benign naevus close-up.

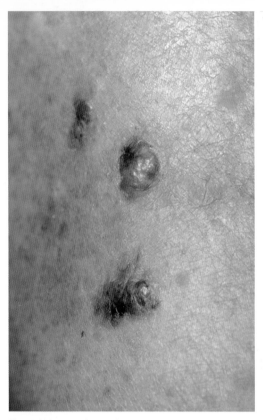

Plate 3 Malignant melanoma close-up.

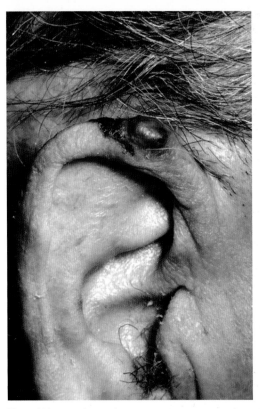

Plate 4 Malignant melanoma close-up.

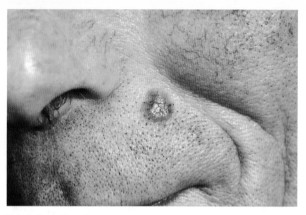

Plate 5 Basal cell carcinoma.

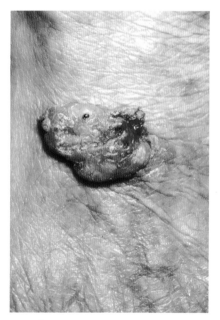

Plate 6 Squamous cell carcinoma.

Loco-regionally advanced disease
- Includes:
  - recurrence at the site of the resected primary disease
  - in-transit and satellite metastases
  - regional lymph node metastases.
- If there is no evidence of disseminated disease, further resection should be considered as this approach can sometimes produce long-term survivors.
- Alternative approaches for local control of unresectable disease include hyperthermic isolated limb perfusion ± melphalan infusion and occasionally radiotherapy.

Management of metastatic disease

- No curative treatment for patients with stage IV disease.
- Aim of treatment is to palliate symptoms and maximize quality of life.

Surgery
- Procedures to debulk the tumour and optimize local control are occasionally appropriate.

Chemotherapy
- The lack of efficacious agents for use in metastatic disease is also concerning, and referral for entry into a phase I trial remains a reasonable option for patients of a good performance status in this group.
- Dacarbazine (DTIC):
  - response rates of 7–20% are documented in the literature, with a median duration of response of 4–6 months
  - treatment is generally well tolerated
  - randomized data demonstrating an associated survival advantage are still lacking
  - combining DTIC with either tamoxifen or IFN-α has produced no compelling evidence of benefit.
- Temozolomide:
  - an oral analogue of DTIC
  - phase III data to support its equivalent activity in metastatic melanoma
  - potential advantage of greater central nervous system (CNS) penetration (crosses the blood–brain barrier)
  - ongoing clinical trials to establish the optimal regime and whether concurrent use of other therapies, e.g. radiotherapy, novel enzyme inhibitors, may improve efficacy
  - use is restricted to the context of clinical trials (UK and USA). Further National Institute for Health and Cllinical Excellence (NICE) guidance expected 2010.
- Combination regimes, e.g. with cisplatin, vinblastine, and DTIC:
  - consistent evidence to support superiority over single-agent DTIC is lacking, and toxicity is significantly greater.

Biological therapy
- IFN-α:
  - self-administered subcutaneously, typically three times per week on an uninterrupted schedule
  - response rates of 10–20% are reported
  - median duration of response is only 4 months, although occasional durable responses can be seen and treatment is usually well tolerated
  - appears most appropriate for those with small-volume, non-visceral metastatic disease
  - combination with dacarbazine or temozolomide has demonstrated no increase in survival.

- High-dose IL-2:
  - response rates of up to 20% are documented although trials have generally been non-randomized to date
  - multi-organ toxicity including arrhythmias, hypotension, and capillary leak syndrome limit this approach
  - remains within the context of clinical trials.
- Other:
  - novel therapies targeting specific molecular abnormalities identified in melanoma are under investigation
  - examples include oblimersen, an antisense oligonucleotide which suppresses expression of Bcl-2 (see 📖 Correction of mutant oncogenes, Chapter 39, p.730), and sorafenib, which inhibits many targets including BRAF and tyrosine kinases involved in the vascular endothelial growth factor (VEGF) pathway (see 📖 Chapter 10, 'Biological and targeted therapies').

Radiotherapy
- Melanoma in general is not responsive to radiotherapy.
- Skeletal metastases: can achieve good palliation in the case of pain.
- Cerebral metastases: relatively common in long-term survivors from melanoma. If asymptomatic there is controversy as to whether or not they should be treated. If cerebral metastases are symptomatic then corticosteroid therapy should be commenced and cranial irradiation considered.

Intra-ocular melanoma

- A rare malignancy affecting the uveal tract, most frequently involving the choroid.
- **Risk factors** appear to include UV exposure, light iris colour, inability to tan, and previous personal or family history of melanoma.
- **Presentation** is often an incidental finding at a routine visit to the optician in an asymptomatic individual. Alternatively, patients may present with visual loss.
- **Investigation**: biopsies should not be performed. Diagnosis should be made by an ophthalmologist with experience in this field.
- **Management** is ideally carried out in a combined ophthalmic–oncology clinic. Options include observation, brachytherapy with radioactive eye plaques (e.g. ruthenium-106 or iodine-125), charged particle irradiation, local resection, or enucleation.
- **Prognosis** is generally poor, with death from metastatic disease in >50% of affected patients. Dissemination is purely haematogenous, with hepatic involvement in 90% of those with metastatic disease.

Non-melanoma skin cancer

- The two main forms of primary skin cancer in this group are:
  - basal cell carcinoma (BCC, see Fig. 24.5), i.e. keratinocyte skin cancers
  - squamous cell carcinoma (SCC, see Fig. 24.6).
- Malignant skin lesions may also represent metastases, e.g. from breast, lung, or gastrointestinal (GI) primaries.
- There are also several uncommon skin cancers beyond the scope of this chapter, e.g. Kaposi's sarcoma (see 📖 Chapter 29, 'AIDS-related malignancies'), and cutaneous angiosarcoma.

Epidemiology and aetiology

- These cancers are the commonest malignancies in Western populations, occurring particularly in fair-skinned Caucasians.
- Risk factors for development include:
  - UV radiation: sunlight remains the principal environmental cause of the keratinocyte skin cancers
  - ionizing radiation
  - chronic inflammation
  - human papilloma virus (HPV)
  - immunosuppression, e.g. post organ-transplant
  - hereditary conditions, e.g. 0.5% of BCCs occur in patients with the autosomal dominant basal cell naevus syndrome.

Presentation

Squamous cell carcinomas

- Represent ~20% of non-melanoma skin cancers.
- Arise on sun-exposed sites or at sites of chronic inflammation.
- Rapidly growing, red papule or non-healing skin lesion.
- ±Background of actinic keratosis.
- Ulceration and bleeding may occur.
- 5–10% metastasize, initially to regional lymph nodes.
- Risk factors for metastasis include:
  - recurrent disease
  - large size
  - deep invasion
  - disease associated with chronic scars, sinus tracts, and certain anatomical sites, e.g. lip.
- Loco-regionally, metastatic disease is associated with a 5-year survival of ≤65%. Disseminated disease has a very poor prognosis.

Basal cell carcinomas

- Represent ~75% of non-melanoma skin cancers.
- Lesions arising on sun-exposed areas, e.g. face, ears, scalp.
- Normally confined to hair-bearing skin.
- Slow-growing, pink papule with telangiectasia.
- Typically indolent although can be locally invasive causing significant disfigurement.
- Metastases are rare (0.1%).

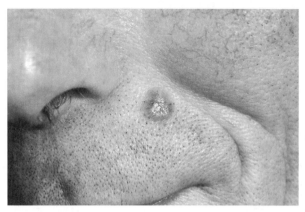

Fig. 24.5 Basal cell carcinoma. (See Plate 5 for a full colour version.)

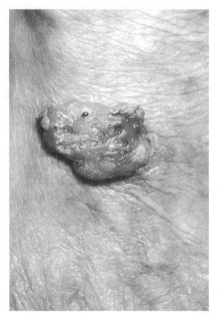

Fig. 24.6 Squamous cell carcinoma. (See Plate 6 for a full colour version.)

Management

Basal cell carcinomas (BCC)

- Usually curable (≥90% for 1° disease). Certain factors predict a higher risk of local recurrence, including:
  - a sclerosing, micronodular, or mixed growth pattern
  - perineural invasion
  - baso-squamous differentiation.
- Despite their low metastatic potential, early definitive treatment is important as local invasion can be associated with significant morbidity.
- Surgical excision:
  - allows assessment of histological features and adequacy of resection margin.
- Mohs' surgery:
  - specialized surgical technique
  - micrographic surgery in which the tumour is excised at an oblique angle in a series of stages and examined microscopically
  - oblique angle of surgery maximizes examination of the peripheral margin
  - further excision continues until all margins are negative
  - advocated for tumours in which it is essential to obtain a clear margin whilst preserving the maximum amount of normal surrounding tissues, e.g. recurrent BCCs or tumours on the face
  - in the UK, the requirement for specialist training and equipment means there is currently limited availability of this technique
  - a recent trial (December 2008) has clarified the use of traditional excisional surgery versus Mohs' procedure. The latter is preferable for facial recurrent BCC (fewer recurrences) , but for a primary BCC on the face, surgical excision is sufficient in most cases.
- Cryotherapy or electrosurgery:
  - used for the treatment of low- and intermediate-risk lesions
  - 5-year recurrence rate for primary BCCs ~8–13%.
- Radiotherapy:
  - appropriate for both 1° and recurrent disease, particularly in elderly patients
  - generally avoided in those <50 years old due to the long-term risk of secondary cutaneous malignancies within the radiation field
  - 5-year cure rates of >90% for previously untreated lesions
  - especially useful around the eyelids, nose, and lips, when the cosmetic result is likely to be superior to surgical techniques
  - contraindicated in patients with the hereditary basal cell naevus syndrome.
- Photodynamic therapy:
  - uses light and a topical photosensitizing agent to produce tumour destruction, with response rates of 82–100% reported
  - advantages: good cosmetic results, well tolerated
  - disadvantages: lengthy treatment, long-term recurrence rates unknown.
- Chemotherapy:
  - may achieve cure rates of >90% in selected patients with low-risk BCCs, e.g. with topical 5-fluorouracil (5-FU).

- Ongoing surveillance:
  - 80% of recurrences will occur within the first 5 years
  - ~40% of patients will develop a new 1° BCC within the same period, and patients are also at risk of other cutaneous malignancies.

Squamous cell carcinomas (SCC)
- Surgical excision:
  - resection of the primary ± loco-regional lymph node dissection of any clinically evident lymph node metastases
  - the most common treatment for cutaneous SCC
  - allows histological assessment of the adequacy of the margin of excision
  - 5-year cure rate of >90% is reported for excision of localized 1° disease
  - a potential role for sentinel lymph node biopsy awaits further study.
- Cryotherapy (e.g. using pressurized liquid nitrogen) or electrosurgery:
  - can be used for *in situ* disease or small, low-risk lesions
  - disadvantage of these techniques is they prevent confirmation of clear margins.
- Radiotherapy:
  - most useful for small, well-localized lesions
  - reported 5-year cure rate is ~90%
  - can also be used as adjuvant treatment following incomplete surgical excision or in patients with nodal involvement.
- Chemotherapy:
  - has been used for disseminated disease, e.g. with cisplatin.
- Ongoing surveillance:
  - 95% of relapses will occur within 5 years
  - ~50% of patients will also develop a new non-melanoma skin cancer also within 5 years.

Prevention and future directions
- Any patient with a non-melanoma skin cancer should be advised about the importance of sun avoidance to minimize future risk.
- New research on non-invasive treatments for BCCs and SCCs is ongoing and includes trials of cyclo-oxygenase-2 (COX-2) inhibitors and biological response-modifying agents. Results are awaited.

Merkel cell carcinoma

- Rare malignant skin tumours, most commonly arising in the head and neck area or on the limbs.
- Propensity for local recurrence and regional and distant spread.
- Pathologically these tumours have neuroendocrine features.
- Clinical presentation is typically with a red or purple nodule with shiny overlying epithelium.
- Staging requires at a minimum CXR and assessment of regional lymph nodes, commonly by CT or MRI scan.
- Sentinel node biospy may have a role in this tumour.
- At presentation:
  - 40% localized
  - 50% regional spread
  - <10% metastatic disease.
- The optimum management of these tumours remains controversial.
- Although they are sensitive to both radiotherapy and chemotherapy, the role of the adjuvant treatment of localized disease is uncertain.
- Patients with operable disease are best managed by surgery, but adjuvant radiotherapy and chemotherapy (e.g. platinum and etoposide) may be considered for patients with regional spread.
- Treatment outcome is dependent on stage at presentation:
  - localized node-negative disease – >90% 5-year survival
  - positive lymph nodes – 50–60% 5-year survival
  - metastatic disease – 9 months' median survival.

Further reading

Chakrabarty A, Geisse JK (2004) Medical therapies for non-melanoma skin cancer. *Clin Dermatol* **22**, 183–8.

Chung ES, Sabel MS, Sondak VK (2004) Current state of treatment for primary cutaneous melanoma. *Clin Exp Med* **4**, 65–77.

Fang L, Lansdorf AS, Hwang SJ (2008) Immunotherapy for advanced melanoma. *J Invest Dermatol* **123**, 2596–605.

Hauschild A, Gogas H, Tarhini A, *et al.* (2008) Practical guidelines for the management of interferon-alpha-2b side effects in patients receiving adjuvant treatment for melanoma. Expert opinion. *Cancer* **112**, 982–94.

Mosterd K, Krekels GAM, Nieman FHM, *et al.* (2008). Surgical excision versus Mohs' micrographic surgery for primary and recurrent basal cell carcinoma of the face – a prospective randomised controlled trial with 5 years' follow-up. *Lancet Oncol* **9**, 1149–56.

Rigel DS (2008) Cutaneous ultraviolet exposure and its relationship to the development of skin cancer *J Am Acad Dermatol* **58(5 Suppl 2)**, S129–32.

Tadiparthi S, Panchani S, Iqbal A (2008) Biopsy for malignant melanoma – are we following the guidelines? *Ann R Coll Surg Engl* **90**, 322–5.

Thirlwell C, Nathan P (2008) Melanoma – Part 2 Management clinical review. *BMJ* **337**, 1345–8.

Thompson JF, Scolyer RA, Kefford RF (2005) Cutaneous melanoma. *Lancet* **365**, 687–701.

Haematological malignancies

Acute leukaemia

Epidemiology

The incidence of acute leukaemia is 4–7 cases per 100 000. The peak incidence of acute lymphoblastic leukaemia (ALL) is 2–4 years and of acute myeloid leukaemia (AML) is over 60 years.

Aetiology

The cause of most cases is unknown. Some congenital and inherited diseases carry an increased risk:

- Down syndrome
- Fanconi anaemia
- Bloom syndrome
- Klinefelter syndrome
- neurofibromatosis
- ataxia telangiectasia.

There is a 3–5 times increased risk in identical twins.

Environmental factors implicated in leukaemogenesis include ionizing radiation, including *in utero* for childhood ALL, chemical carcinogens especially benzene and including cigarette smoking (2-fold increase), chemotherapeutic drugs, and infectious agents (e.g. T-cell leukaemia virus 1 in the Caribbean or Japan, causing adult T-cell leukaemia/lymphoma). It seems that in at least some cases of childhood ALL, a genetic predisposition is acquired *in utero* in that markers of the leukaemic clone. e.g. a single copy of the t(12;21) translocation producing the *TEL-AML1* fusion gene or a clonal *IgH* gene rearrangement are identifiable on testing Guthrie card blood spots or umbilical blood samples. Subsequent additional genetic mutations, e.g. deletion of the second *TEL* gene occurring after birth, perhaps following exposure of naive immune systems to infections, then lead to childhood ALL.

Pathology

Acute leukaemias arise from the malignant transformation of haemopoietic stem cells or early lineage-committed progenitor cells. The leukaemic progeny proliferate but fail to differentiate properly, leading to the accumulation of poorly differentiated leukaemic blast cells in the marrow, and bone marrow failure.

Clinical presentation

Acute leukaemia presents with features of bone marrow failure:

- anaemia
- thrombocytopenic bleeding
- infection, mainly bacterial or fungal.

There may also be features of extramedullary leukaemic infiltration, more commonly in ALL or monocytic forms of AML:

- hepatosplenomegaly
- lymphadenopathy
- leukaemic meningitis
- testicular infiltration
- skin nodules.

Patients with acute promyelocytic leukaemia (APL) can present with excessive bleeding as a result of primary fibrinolysis and disseminated intravascular coagulation (DIC).

Diagnosis and classification

Peripheral blood pancytopenia is the commonest finding, but a minority has an elevated white blood cell count (WCC).

A marrow examination using morphology, immunophenotyping, cytogenetics, and increasingly molecular genetics, is the basis of diagnosis. This will allow classification into myeloid or lymphoid leukaemia and give important prognostic information. Acute leukaemia is diagnosed when the bone marrow blast count is >20% of nucleated cells. The present World Health Organization (WHO) classification of acute leukaemia is shown in Table 25.1. Central nervous system (CNS) infiltration can be a feature of ALL and requires a diagnostic lumbar puncture.

Table 25.1 WHO classification of acute leukaemias

WHO classification of acute lymphoblastic leukaemias (ALL)
B lymphoblastic leukaemia/lymphoma, not otherwise specified
B lymphoblastic leukaemia/lymphoma with recurrent genetic abnormalities
T lymphoblastic leukaemia/lymphoma

WHO classification of acute myeloid leukaemias (AML)
AML with recurrent genetic abnormalities
AML with myelodysplasia-related changes
Therapy-related AML
AML not otherwise specified
Myeloid sarcoma
Myeloid proliferations related to Down syndrome
Acute leukaemia of ambiguous lineage

Reproduced with kind permission of the World Health Organization (WHO).
www.who.int.

Acute lymphoblastic leukaemia (ALL)

ALL is the commonest cancer in children (23% of cancer diagnoses in children under 15 years), with modern treatment producing an ~80% leukaemia-free survival at 5 years. Most of these will be cured. Adult disease responds less well, with only 30–50% long-term survivors. This relates to an excess of poor-prognostic features in adults, with some 30% having one or more of a high white cell count, older age, poor genetics such as t(9;22), t(4;11), or t(1;19), or delayed disease clearance (>4 weeks) with induction chemotherapy.

Management of ALL

It is important that children and adults with ALL are treated in expert centres. Increasingly, it is recognized that adolescents benefit from treatment in an environment that deals with patients of the same age and provides the type of support needed by teenagers. Recently, it has been accepted that patients up to the age of early 20s have better outcomes when treated on childhood protocols.

Children with ALL are now treated according to risk groups, and increasingly this approach will apply to adults. Clinical and laboratory features of prognostic significance in children include the following:

- age at diagnosis – infants <1 year poor prognosis; children 1–9 years do better than children 10–18 years
- WCC at diagnosis – <50 × 10⁹/l better prognosis than higher WCCs
- presence or absence of CNS disease at presentation
- gender – girls have slightly better prognosis than boys
- hypodiploidy (<45 chromosomes) of ALL cells on karyotyping carries a poorer prognosis than normal numbers or hyperdiploidy
- specific acquired genetic abnormalities, including the Philadelphia chromsome t(9; 22) and rearrangement of the *MLL* (mixed lineage leukaemia) gene on chromosome 11q23, carry a worse prognosis. *MLL* rearrangements are common in infantile ALL
- response to treatment – children who clear their bone marrow of blasts within 7–14 days of induction have a better prognosis than those who do not. Early clearance of blasts in the blood with steroids is also favourable
- The level of minimal residual disease (MRD) by molecular or flow cytometric technology post-induction is important, with negative MRD being favourable.

Chemotherapy
Patients with B-ALL (Burkitt leukaemia) are generally treated as Burkitt lymphoma with short intensive courses of chemotherapy (see below).

Philadelphia-positive cases are treated on experimental protocols based around stem cell transplantation and imatinib mesilate. All others are treated on ALL protocols adapted to the risk group of the patient. Treatment is in three stages: induction of remission, intensification (consolidation), and maintenance.

Induction of remission
This is routinely achieved by combining vincristine, steroids (prednisolone or dexamethasone), and L-asparaginase. Additional anthracycline is used in adults and poor-risk children. Remission rates are 90–95% in children and a little less in adults.

Intensification
This is a crucial phase during which exposure to new drugs (e.g. cyclophosphamide, cytarabine) is a key strategy, as is clearance of the CNS as a sanctuary site. This may be achieved by CNS irradiation or methotrexate intrathecally or by intermediate- or high-dose intravenously (IV).

In high-risk cases there remains a 10% risk of CNS relapse and there are concerns about the long-term effects of different treatment modalities.

Maintenance
For about 2 years patients in remission continue on a cyclical schedule of methotrexate, mercaptapurine, vincristine, steroids, and intrathecal prophylaxis if cranial irradiation has not been given.

Management of high-risk disease
Various approaches are in use for high-risk disease. Intensification in consolidation with cyclophosphamide or methotrexate in higher dosage has brought some success, and allogeneic stem cell transplantation has been vigorously pursued for its graft versus leukaemia effect in reducing relapse risk. Recent data in adults from the Medical Research Council (MRC) UKALL XII, HOVON study group and others have helped clarify the role of transplantation. Using a biological randomization and intention-to-treat analysis based on whether a patient has a sibling donor or not, there is clearly a 5-year disease-free survival (DFS) advantage (~60% vs ~40%) for having a donor, the majority of whom receive an allogeneic stem cell transplant in first remission. For those without a donor UKALL XII demonstrated that standard maintenance therapy was better than receiving an autologous transplant.

When treatment fails, outcome depends on age and length of first remission. In children with long remissions, further chemotherapy may achieve salvage; for others allogeneic stem cell transplant is indicated including from matched unrelated donors.

Philadelphia chromosome-positive ALL carries a very poor prognosis when treated with chemotherapy alone. Recent results with the addition of the BCR-ABL inhibitor imatinib mesilate and planned allogeneic stem cell transplant from a matched donor of any source have been encouraging, with remission rates of >90% and 3-year DFS approaching 50%.

Acute myeloid leukaemia (AML)

At diagnosis with AML, the patient's age, performance status, and whether or not the subtype is of APL determine the initial clinical approach.

* APL must be identified at diagnosis to ensure that all-*trans* retinoic acid (ATRA) is included promptly in the treatment schedule.
* It is now usual that patients under 60 years who are relatively fit are offered intensive treatment with curative intent that may include allogeneic stem cell transplantation.
* Older patients constitute the majority, and often are not considered suitable for intensive treatment. The outcome for this age group has not improved during the last 20 years, and therapy is centred on palliation with blood product-based supportive care and trials of novel therapeutic agents.
* A major contributor to better survival over the last 30 years has been improved supportive care. This includes appropriate use of blood product support, including platelets, and the succesful management of neutropenic sepsis with antibiotics and an increasing range of effective anti-fungal drugs.

Chemotherapy
Anthracycline and cytarabine, given over 7–10 days, has been the backbone of treatment for 30 years. The addition of a third drug (thioguanine or etoposide) is widely used, but there is little evidence that one or other is superior. Recent data from MRC AML 15 has shown that the addition of targeted chemotherapy in the form of anti-CD33-bound calicheomycin (gemtuzumab ozogamycin – GO) to daunorubicin and cytarabine leads to

better DFS for good- and possibly standard-risk patients, but not poorer-risk patients.

Successful induction is defined as achieving first remission (normal blood counts and bone marrow blasts <5%), and depends on patient age (90% in children, 75% 50–60 years, 65% 60–70 years); 70–80% of all patients achieve complete remission with the first course. Between two and four further intensive courses incorporating other drugs (e.g. amsacrine, etoposide, idarubicin, mitoxantrone, and cytarabine at higher doses) are usually given. It is not at present clear how many courses of consolidation are optimum. Older patients seldom tolerate more than two, and there seems little benefit for more than four courses of intensive chemotherapy in total in younger patients.

Non-intensive treatments

The standard therapy for older and frailer patients has been low-dose subcutaneous cytarabine. This produces a remission rate of ~20% and is superior to oral hydroxycarbamide. Present approaches for this difficult group of patients include randomizing novel agents such as FLT3 inhibitors, clofarabine, arsenic trioxide (ATO) and GO against low-dose cytarabine. The 'pick a winner' approach identifies such agents with promising clinical efficacy in phase II studies and carries them promptly on to phase III while discarding ineffective therapies. Histone deacetylase inhibitors, hypomethylating agents, and mTOR inhibitors are all classes of drugs that may be identified as beneficial through this approach.

Prognostic factors

A number of characteristics can identify different risks of relapse and therefore survival. Most powerful of these are cytogenetics (favourable, intermediate, poor), patient age (young better than elderly), and initial response of marrow blasts to treatment (remission with first course or not). Other factors associated with poor prognosis include:

- high WCC on presentation
- molecular markers such as *FLT3* internal tandem duplication (*FLT3 ITD*) – present in 30% of cases and predictive of relapse
- less cellular differentiation – undifferentiated leukaemia
- leukaemia secondary to prior chemotherapy (t-AML)
- leukaemia secondary to myelodysplasia (s-AML)
- the length of first remission – <6–12 months very poor.

Favourable cytogenetics are t(8;21), t(15;17), inv(16), which comprise about 25% of patients less than 60 years. Poor-risk cytogenetics are abnormalities of chromosomes 5 or 7, del(3q), or complex (multiple) abnormalities that tend to be more frequent in older patients and are associated with t-AML and s-AML. Intermediate-risk cytogenetics includes normal karyotype and abnormalities not defined by the other risk groups. The identification of molecular abnormalities within the normal cytogenetic group is helping improve predictions of treatment outcomes in this difficult group e.g. *FLT3* ITD+ poor risk, nucleophosmin (*NPM1*) mutation+ without *FLT3* ITD good risk, *CEPBA* mutation+ good risk. A chemoresistance phenotype of P-glycoprotein overexpression occurs particularly in the elderly and is associated with a lower rate of remission and higher relapse risk.

Stem cell transplantation

Allogeneic stem cell transplantation reduces the relapse risk in AML through the graft versus leukaemia effect (GVL).This benefit is offset by the toxicity of the transplant procedure and hence an overall survival advantage has been difficult to demonstrate. However, recent analyses of the large MRC dataset using a more sophisticated measure of risk than just cytogenetics and response clearly shows a survival benefit (33% vs 18%) for those defined as poor risk, even though only 30% of eligible patients received a transplant. No clear benefit has been shown in donor vs no donor analyses in standard/intermediate-risk patients however defined, though younger patients actually receiving a transplant probably do have a survival advantage and many centres adopt this strategy for younger standard-risk patients with a suitable donor. There is no benefit for good-risk patients transplanted in first remission. Overall, if the patient is relatively young (<60 years) and has a human leucocyte-associated antigen (HLA)-matched donor, allogeneic transplantation of blood or bone marrow stem cells will be considered in poor- and standard-risk in first remission. The development of less toxic reduced-intensity conditioning (RIC) regimens based on immunosuppression without myeloablation improve the risk–benefit analysis and allow transplantation of older, frailer patients. Maturing results with RIC allografts in AML appear to be as good as those achieved with myeloablative regimens in younger patients with ~60% 3-year overall survival (OS) for patients <60 years. At present, therefore, patients less than 40 years will generally be offered a conventional myeloablative allograft while older patients will be offered a RIC allograft. The encouraging data with RIC allografts may promote their use in increasingly younger patients.

Acute promyelocytic leukaemia (APL)

This is a separate entity, having FAB-M3 morphology (malignant promyelocytes) and the t(15:17) rearrangement creating the *PML-RARA* fusion gene. ATRA used alone can induce remission by differentiation without hypoplasia but is not curative. Additional chemotherapy, either given with, or subsequent to, ATRA, remains essential to eliminate the leukaemic clone and APL is very sensitive to anthracyclines. ATRA reduces the risk of early death through haemorrhage. The WCC at diagnosis is of key importance. Low count patients (<10 × 10^9/l) given ATRA and anthracycline will have >80% survival. The 25% of patients who present with higher WCC have a high risk of early death or relapse and only 60% survival. Italian and Spanish groups have developed less toxic regimens based on ATRA and idarubicin induction and consolidation followed with ATRA-based maintenance chemotherapy. In a randomized comparison with four cycles of traditional intensive AML therapy and ATRA, the remission and survival rates are as good with less toxicity and better compliance. However, the role of maintenance has not been proven. Patients with a higher WCC may benefit from the addition of cytarabine. The *PML-RARA* fusion transcript is detectable by sensitive reverse transcription polymerase chain reaction (RT-PCR) and allows monitoring of molecular minimal residual disease. It is now clear that achieving molecular negativity is associated with prolonged survival, whereas persistent or relapsed positivity in bone marrow invariably predicts for haematological relapse. Therefore, patients in remission are monitored for molecular relapse and offered treatment before full haematological relapse, with the differentiating agent ATO followed, where appropriate, by transplantation. Indeed, recent data suggest that low-risk patients can be treated at presentation with a non-chemotherapy regimen of ATRA and ATO with careful molecular monitoring, and only given chemotherapy for molecular positivity.

Treatment outcome in AML

Remission is achieved in 80% of patients under 60 years and 60–65% of patients over 60 years. Survival is age related and will depend on the prognostic factors outlined above. At present some 50% of patients under 60 years will be long-term survivors, while only 10–15% of older patients survive beyond 3 years. Therefore, most patients will relapse. If first remission is short (<6–12 months) and cytogenetics are not favourable, the outlook is grave.

Future prospects

AML is a heterogeneous disease and the increasing characterization of biological and clinical features associated with disease outcome will allow better risk-directed therapy. There will be ongoing refinements in the techniques of stem cell transplantation allowing harnessing of GVL independently of graft versus host disease. The disease in the elderly remains a major challenge. Standard chemotherapy approaches have not improved the outcome in this age group, and 5-year survival is of the order of 10%. It must be established which elderly patients, if any, benefit from an intensive approach. Improved, more targeted, non-intensive treatment is needed for the majority, and to this end the 'pick a winner' approach discussed may allow the timely identification of efficacious novel agents.

Chronic myeloid leukaemia (CML)

Epidemiology
Chronic myeloid leukaemia (CML) can occur in either sex and in any age group. The disease most commonly presents between the ages of 40 and 60 years. There is an association with exposure to radiation – for example, atomic bomb survivors.

Pathology
CML is a malignancy arising from a mutated haemopoietic pluripotential stem cell. In CML, a clone of cells replaces the normal bone marrow with enhanced proliferative capacity, but, unlike in acute leukaemia, the cells retain their ability to differentiate during the chronic phase of the disease. In 97.5% of cases there is a reciprocal translocation between chromosomes 9 and 22, which in most cases can be recognized in standard karyotypes as a Philadelphia chromosome (small chromosome 22). This t(9;22) results in a new fusion gene called BCR-ABL1. The protein product of this gene behaves as an abnormal tyrosine kinase and is the cause of the leukaemia. Knowledge from the pathogenesis has been utilized to develop novel therapeutic agents.

The disease runs a chronic phase for a number of years. Eventually the leukaemia loses its ability to differentiate normally and enters 'blast crisis', resembling an acute leukaemia of myeloid or, less frequently, lymphoid origin, which is fatal. Modern therapy has been incredibly successful in preventing or delaying this transformation and prolonging survival.

Clinical features
In the chronic phase, the presenting symptoms are anaemia, weight loss, and splenomegaly. Patients can develop gout.

Rarely, altered consciousness, blurred vision, and cardiorespiratory failure can occur from hyperviscosity with a very high WCC.

Investigations
• Full blood count (FBC)
• Blood film
• Bone marrow
• Cytogenetics
• Molecular genetics.

Leucocytosis is a uniform feature, and WCC can be in excess of $300 \times 10^9/l$. A normochromic anaemia is usually present whilst platelets are commonly increased (sometimes over $1000 \times 10^9/l$). The blood film resembles a bone marrow aspirate with all stages of myeloid differentiation present. The bone marrow is hypercellular with predominant granulocytopoiesis. In blast crisis, increased numbers of blast cells become evident in blood and bone marrow. Correspondingly, anaemia and thrombocytopenia are more marked. Approximately 95% of patients have the Philadelphia chromosome on routine G-banding, and a further 2.5% will have an occult t(9;22) translocation identified by a positive PCR for the BCR-ABL1 transcript. Approximately 2.5% are negative for the t(9;22) translocation (by G-banding and PCR) and are termed atypical chronic myeloid leukaemia, BCR-ABL1 negative.

Management

Chronic phase

Initial treatment may involve leukapharesis if the WCC is very high and there are signs and symptoms of hyperviscosity. If there is no ready access to tyrosine kinase inhibitors (TKIs), hydroxycarbamide is used to reduce the white cell count. Patients with high WCC and hyperviscosity should not be transfused red cells until this is corrected.

Imatinib mesilate

Imatinib mesilate (Glivec®) at a dose of 400 mg per day is now considered standard initial therapy in all adult patients. This drug binds to the ATP binding site of BCR-ABL1 and inhibits the function of the tyrosine kinase protein. Complete haematological responses are achieved in 95% of patients. At a median follow-up of 5 years, the IRIS randomized study of imatinib vs interferon-α with cytarabine demonstrated complete cytogenetic responses of 69% by 12 months and 87% by 60 months for imatinib. OS of patients who received imatinib as initial therapy was 89% at 60 months. However, 30% of patients were no longer taking imatinib, for a variety of reasons including resistance, intolerance, and withdrawal of consent. Complete cytogenic response and a maximum molecular response (3-log reduction in BCR-ABL1 transcripts) was associated with a 100% freedom from progression at 60 months, though most patients still have detectable BCR-ABL1 transcripts. Interestingly, the rate of progression on imatinib falls off year by year beyond 3 years. This is a landmark targeted therapy that has revolutionized the outlook for this disease. The term 'operational cure' has been suggested for long term non-progressors on imatinib with residual small detectable quantities of BCR-ABL1. Only time will tell if this is the case.

However, as discussed, one-third of patients stop taking imatinib over the longer term. The European LeukaemiaNet has recently defined criteria for imatinib failure or suboptimal response at various time points on therapy. Prospectively, these criteria predict for poor outcome. The options for such patients are higher doses of imatinib, second-generation TKIs nilotinib and dasatinib, or allogeneic stem cell transplantation.

Allogeneic stem cell transplantation

Allogeneic stem cell/bone marrow transplantation offers the potential of cure for CML. The precise role of allogeneic transplantation following the introduction of TKI therapy has been controversial. However, it is predominantly now seen as a second-line therapy for appropriate patients defined as failing imatinib therapy. It might be considered in children or adolescents as first line if an appropriate donor is available. The best results are achieved in young (less than 30 years) fit patients with a suitable fully matched donor. The transplant-related mortality ranges from 15% to 40%. The relapse rates are usually less than 20%. Cured patients have no detectable BCR-ABL1 by PCR, which is the benchmark for alternative therapies.

Second-generation tyrosine kinase inhibitors: nilotinib and dasatinib

Nilotinib is a more potent inhibitor of BCR-ABL1 and dasatinib is more potent and inhibits a wider spectrum of kinases including src. Both are now used for patients who are defined as imatinib failures. Responses in imatinib-resistant patients are at least as good as using higher doses of imatinib (600 mg or 800 mg) except for the kinase domain mutation *T315I* which is resistant to both second-line TKIs and high-dose imatinib. Dasatinib produces complete cytogenetic responses in 40% of imatinib-resistant patients and 70% of imatinib-intolerant patients with a progression-free survival of 90% at a median follow-up of 15 months.

Accelerated phase and blast phase

Patients who progress from chronic phase still fare poorly. Imatinib, often used at the higher doses, and second-generation TKIs produce responses in advanced disease but the benefits are relatively short lived. Combination chemotherapy may return the patient to chronic phase, especially from lymphoid blast crisis. Allogeneic or autologous transplantation may prolong the second chronic phase.

Myelodysplastic syndromes (MDS)

MDS are a group of neoplastic disorders of the bone marrow, characterized by dysplastic haemopoiesis and peripheral blood cytopenias. As part of the family of myeloid neoplasms, there is a tendency for the disease to progress to AML.

Epidemiology

The incidence of MDS is about 4 per 100 000 per year, with a peak incidence of >20 per 100 000 in the over 80s. The median age is in excess of 70 years. Risk factors for developing MDS include exposure to previous chemotherapy, especially alkylating agents, radiation, and benzene.

Pathology

The hallmarks of these diseases are hypercellular bone marrow with dysplastic cell morphology and paradoxical peripheral blood cytopenias. The paradox may result from apoptosis of dysplastic bone marrow progenitor cells, in turn leading to ineffective production of differentiated cells for release into the blood, especially in early stages of disease. The disease subtypes are classified according to WHO criteria, based on the number of lineages involved, the presence of ring sideroblasts, the blast count, and the presence of specific cytogenetic abnormalities (see Tables 25.2 and 25.3).

Clinical features

Symptomatic anaemia is the most common presentation, but patients may also present with bleeding from thrombocytopenia or with recurrent infections owing to neutropenia. Patients with chronic myelomonocytic leukaemia (CMML) may have hepatosplenomegaly or other evidence of tissue infiltration by leukaemic cells. Patients die from the effects of bone marrow failure or progression to AML, which occurs in about one-third of cases.

Investigations

- FBC
- Blood film
- Bone marrow
- Cytogenetics

A macrocytic anaemia is usual, and neutropenia, thrombocytopenia, and monocytosis may also be evident. The peripheral blood film shows evidence of dysplasia including misshapen red cells, agranular neutrophils, and circulating blast cells.

The bone marrow is usually hypercellular, with dysplasia in at least 10% of the cells in one or more cell lines. Typical dysplastic features in the marrow are megaloblastoid change, binucleated erythroblasts, megakaryocytes with multiple separate nuclei, micro-megakaryocytes, and increased blast cells of 5–20%. Ring sideroblasts may be present and are >15% of erythroblasts in sideroblastic subtypes. Bone marrow cytogenetics often demonstrates a clonal cytogenetic abnormality of prognostic importance.

Table 25.2 WHO classification of myelodysplastic syndromes

Refractory cytopenia with unilineage dysplasia
Refractory anaemia with ring sideroblasts (RARS)

Refractory cytopenia with multilineage dysplasia with or without ring sideroblasts (RCMD)

Refractory anaemia with excess blasts-1 (RAEB-1; 5–9% blasts)
Refractory anaemia with excess blasts-2 (RAEB-2; 10–19% blasts)

Myelodysplastic syndrome unclassified (MDS-U)
MDS associated with isolated del(5q)

Reproduced with kind permission of the World Health Organization (WHO). www.who.int.

Table 25.3 WHO classification of myelodysplastic/myeloproliferative syndromes

Chronic myelomonocytic leukaemia (CMML)

Myelodysplastic/myeloproliferative neoplasm: unclassifiable

Juvenile myelomonocytic leukaemia (JMML)

Reproduced with kind permission of the World Health Organization (WHO). www.who.int.

Management

Blood and platelet transfusion

The mainstay of management is supportive care with blood and platelet transfusions as required. Iron chelation therapy for patients with MDS remains controversial. It might be considered appropriate and may improve survival for patients with excessive iron loading (ferritin >1000 µg/l) with repeated transfusions (>15–20 units) and with a good prognosis (IPSS (International Prognostic Scoring System) low and intermediate-1). The oral iron chelator deferasirox is available for patients who cannot tolerate subcutaneous desferrioxamine.

Erythropoietic stimulating agents (ESAs) and colony-stimulating factors

Treatment with the growth factors erythropoietin (EPO), darbopoietin and granulocyte colony-stimulating factor (G-CSF) can improve the anaemia in a proportion of patients and the neutrophil count in the majority, which may help through the transient use of G-CSF at the time of infections. Patients are predicted to be more likely to respond to ESAs if they have a mild anaemia, no or minimal transfusion requirements (<2 units per month), and a low endogenous EPO level. Seventy per cent of such patients will respond. Patients with ring sideroblasts are more likely to respond to the combination of EPO and G-CSF than EPO alone. Recent retrospective data have suggested that responders to EPO may have a survival advantage.

Chemotherapy

Selected patients with increased blast cells may achieve temporary remission with AML-type chemotherapy. This is most useful in patients with normal cytogenetics and as a way of achieving remission prior to allogeneic transplantation. Patients with MDS seldom tolerate more than one or two courses of combination chemotherapy.

Allogeneic stem cell transplantation

This is currently the only treatment with curative potential and is considered for appropriately fit patients with IPSS score intermediate-2 and high. Conventional myeloablative stem cell transplants are reserved for younger, fitter patients, but recent use of RIC allografts in older patients up to 65 years is encouraging. Patients with increased blasts or a clonal cytogenetic abnormality probably benefit from one or two cycles of remission-induction chemotherapy prior to transplantation.

Hypomethylating agents

There is excess methylation of gene promoter regions in MDS. This may lead to inhibition of tumour suppressor genes. Two prospective randomized trials of the hypomethylating agent azacitidine have demonstrated a survival advantage in MDS patients compared to patients receiving supportive care, low-dose chemotherapy or remission-induction chemotherapy. The European AZA-001 phase III study randomized 179 patients to azacitidine and 179 to best supportive care, low-dose, or conventional chemotherapy. OS at a median of 21 months was 24.4 months vs 15 months in favour of azacitidine. This is the first time a therapy other than allogeneic stem cell transplantation has clearly offered an improved overall survival in MDS. Azacitidine is licensed for all subtypes of MDS in the USA, but the European licence will be restricted to patients with IPSS Intermediate-2 and high, CMML with 10-29% blasts and AML with 20-30% blasts. A second hypomethylating agent decitabine is also available. Hypomethylating agents are likely to become the standard of care in high-risk MDS.

Lenalidomide

The karyotypic abnormality deletion (5q) is the commonest abnormality identified in MDS. Recently the gene encoding the ribosomal protein RPS14 has been identified as the likely crucial gene lost from the critically deleted area leading to haplo-insufficiency. The immune modulator drug lenalidomide (Revlimid®) has recently been shown to alleviate anaemia and produce transfusion independence in 67% of MDS patients with del(5q). Cytogentic responses and thrombocytopenia on treatment predict for transfusion independence, suggesting lenalidomide suppresses the MDS clone carrying del(5q). Lenalidomide is licensed in the USA. However, a license has not been granted in Europe because of the limitations of the present phase II data and a controversial concern that lenalidomide might promote progression to AML. Lenalidomide is a very expensive drug and regulatory bodies in the UK such as The Scottish Medicines Committee (SMC) have not supported its licensed indication for multiple myeloma.

Anti-lymphocyte globulin (ALG)

ALG produces impressive responses in some patients with low-risk MDS including those with a hypocellular marrow akin to responses in aplastic anaemia.

Prognosis

The International Prognostic Scoring System (IPSS) predicts prognosis based on the number of cytopenias (anaemia, neutropenia, and thrombocytopenia), the blast cell percentage, and the cytogenetic abnormalities (good risk, intermediate risk or poor risk) (Table 25.4) and ranges from a few months (patients with excess blasts) to several years (refractory anaemia with ring sideroblasts). Patients die from either transformation to AML or the effects of bone marrow failure and its treatment.

Table 25.4 IPSS for myelodysplastic syndromes

Score value	0	0.5	1.0	1.5
Marrow blast %	<5	5–10	11–20	
Karyotype	Good	Intermediate	Poor	
Cytopenias	0/1	2/3		

The scores for each of the above are totalled to produce the prognostic score and predicted survival as follows:

Scores	Survival in years for age (years)		
	<60	>60	>70
Low (0)	11.8	4.8	3.9
Intermediate-1 (0.5–1.0)	5.2	2.7	2.4
Intermediate-2 (1.5–2.0)	1.8	1.1	1.2
High (>2.5)	0.3	0.5	0.4

Chronic lymphoid leukaemias

These are a heterogeneous group of conditions associated with accumulation of lymphoid cells in the peripheral blood. They are classified by morphology, surface immunophenotype, cytogenetics, and molecular biology. Some lymphomas may present with lymphoid cells in the blood and bone marrow infiltration-leukaemic phase. The present WHO classification of mature lymphoid leukaemias is shown in Table 25.5).

B-cell chronic lymphocytic leukaemia (B-CLL)

Epidemiology

This is the commonest leukaemia in the Western world. It occurs predominantly in late middle age and old age, with accumulation of small, mature-looking B lymphocytes in the peripheral blood, bone marrow, and lymphatic tissues.

CLL accounts for 30–40% of all leukaemias diagnosed in adults in Europe and North America. Annual incidence, 2.5 per 100 000; male to female ratio 2:1; median age at diagnosis 65–70 years; 79% of patients over 60 years of age at diagnosis. There are no well-defined environmental risk factors. Genetic factors may have a role – compare, for example, the low incidence of CLL in Japanese people both in Japan and after emigration. Familial cases are well described.

Pathology

Lymphocyte clonal expansion is the result of prolonged survival of CLL cells through failure to respond to apoptotic signals. CLL cells constitutively express high levels of BCL-2 protein, inhibiting apoptosis.

Gradual accumulation of small lymphocytes in the lymph nodes, spleen, bone marrow, and blood causes slowly progressive enlargement of the lymph nodes and infiltration of spleen and bone marrow. Recent data have distinguished two related subtypes of B-CLL. Both arise from B-cells that have rearranged their immunoglobulin genes. However, in one subtype the leukaemic cells have acquired additional somatic mutations in their immunoglobulin heavy chain variable region genes (*IgVH*), in keeping with antigen affinity maturation (mutated), and in the other subtype this has not occurred (unmutated). Other pathological features include:

- a positive direct Coombs' test in some 15% with clinical autoimmune haemolytic anaemia in a smaller percentage; CLL cells seem adept at presenting Rhesus antigens and promoting an immune response to the antigens on red cells
- idiopathic thrombocytopenic purpura (ITP)
- hypogammaglobulinaemia
- disorders of T-lymphocyte function.

Table 25.5 Mature lymphoid leukaemias as classified by WHO

B-cell

B-cell chronic lymphocytic leukaemia/small lymphocytic lymphoma (B-CLL/SLL)

B-cell prolymphocytic leukaemia (B-PLL)

Hairy-cell leukaemia and variants

Splenic marginal zone lymphoma/leukaemia

Leukaemic phase of mantle cell lymphoma

Leukaemic phase of follicle centre cell lymphoma

Leukaemic phase of lymphoplasmacytoid lymphoma

T-cell

T-cell prolymphocytic leukaemia (T-PLL)

T-cell large granular lymphocytic leukaemia (T-LGL)

Chronic lymphoproliferative disorders of NK cells

Aggressive NK cell leukaemia

Adult T-cell leukaemia/lymphoma

Leukaemic phase of mycosis fungoides/Sézary syndrome

Reproduced with kind permission of the World Health Organization (WHO).
www.who.int.

Clinical presentation

Presentation is variable, but CLL generally runs an indolent clinical course. It is now frequently diagnosed early, often after routine blood count for an unrelated reason. Presentation is with painless lymphadenopathy, anaemia, or infection, e.g. shingles. Constitutional symptoms are restricted to patients with advanced disease including fatigue, drenching night sweats, and weight loss. In advanced disease there is bone marrow failure with variable degrees of anaemia, thrombocytopenia, and neutropenia.

Lymphadenopathy is symmetrical, often generalized. Splenomegaly at presentation is present in 66%; hepatomegaly is much less frequent at presentation but common in advanced disease; involvement of other organs is infrequent at diagnosis. The diagnosis of CLL requires a peripheral blood lymphocytosis $>5 \times 10^9/l$. Occasional patients present with lymphadenopathy without the leukaemic phase; small-cell lymphocytic lymphoma (CLL/SCLL).

Diagnosis

Updated National Cancer Institute (NCI) Working Group guidelines (2008) recommend the following diagnostic tests:

• FBC and differential

• blood film

• bone marrow aspirate and trephine biopsy

• lymphocyte immunophenotyping

• cytogenetics by fluorescence in situ hybridization (FISH) targeted at recognized abnormalities of prognostic significance

• abdominal ultrasound.

There are NCI working group criteria for the diagnosis of CLL (see Table 25.6). The lymphocyte count is raised and the blood film shows small lymphocytes with many disrupted 'smear cells'. Surface antigen immunophenotyping is essential to exclude reactive causes (usually T-lymphocytosis) and lymphocytosis due to other lymphoid neoplasms. CLL cells are typically identified as positive for CD19, CD20, CD5, CD23, and demonstrate weak expression of surface immunoglobulin M (IgM). Cytogenetic abnormalities of prognostic significance include del(11q) and del(17p).

Monoclonal B-lymphocytosis (MBL)

Recently, the group of Hillmen *et al.* in Leeds has identified circulating clonal lymphocytes in approximately 3% of people with normal lymphocyte counts (<5 × 10^9/l); this has also been confirmed by others. The majority of these have the phenotype of CLL cells and a minority of non-Hodgkin lymphoma (NHL) cells. This finding is more common in the elderly and relatives of those with known CLL. The spectrum of genetic abnormalities is similar to good-prognosis CLL, with the majority carrying mutated *IgVH* genes. The rate of progression to CLL is documented at ~1% per year.

Management

Patients are staged by the Binet system in Europe and the Rai staging in USA. There is no evidence that treatment prolongs survival of patients with lymphocytosis or uncomplicated lymphadenopathy (early-stage CLL, Binet stage A). Systemic therapy is indicated for symptomatic and advanced disease (progressive Binet stage A or stages B and C).

British Committee for Standards in Haematology (BCSH) CLL Working Party guidelines (2004) for initiating treatment are as follows:

- constitutional symptoms referable to CLL (weight loss >10% in 6 months, fatigue, or performance score 2 or worse, fever without overt infection, night sweats)
- symptomatic lymphadenopathy; symptomatic hepatosplenomegaly
- progressive anaemia with haemoglobin <10 g/dl
- progressive thrombocytopenia with platelets <100 × 10^9/l
- progressive lymphocytosis >300 × 10^9/l or rapid rate of increase (short WCC doubling time)
- autoimmune disease refractory to prednisolone
- repeated infections with, or without, hypogammaglobulinaemia.

Table 25.6 NCI Working Group revised criteria for diagnosis of CLL

Peripheral blood lymphocytosis

1. Absolute lymphocyte count >5 × 10^9/l
2. Morphologically mature-appearing cells

Characteristic phenotype

1. Expansion of CD19 +, CD20 + B-cells, CD19 and CD5 + and CD23 + co-expressing B-cells
2. Light chain restriction i.e. monoclonal-γ or λ expression
3. Low-density surface immunoglobulin (sIgM) expression

Bone marrow examination

>30% lymphocytes in bone marrow if peripheral blood lymphocytosis is relatively low, i.e. close to 5 × 10^9/l

First-line therapy

The alkylating agent chlorambucil or the nucleoside analogue fludarabine have historically been most commonly used as first-line therapies. Both can be given orally. Generally they produce a partial response: reduction in peripheral blood lymphocytosis and improvement in haemoglobin and platelet count, shrinking of lymphadenopathy and splenomegaly, and improvement in constitutional symptoms. The UK CLL4 trial and the German CLL4 trial have shown better overall and complete response rates for fludarabine and cyclophosphamide (FC) compared with either chlorambucil or fludarabine used alone, though with higher rates of infective complications and no overall survival advantage. The combination of fludarabine, cyclophosphamide and rituximab (FCR) has produced very high response rates in the single-centre phase II setting and the recent German CLL8 trial has provisionally reported that FCR is better than FC for overall response (OR) 95% vs 88% and complete remission (CR) 52% vs 27%, but again there is no difference in overall survival (OS) at 2 years. In most Western practice FC or FCR has become first-line therapy for the majority of patients who are deemed fit enough to receive combination chemotherapy.

Fludarabine-based therapy is usually given for 4–6 courses. Fludarabine is profoundly immunosuppressive, especially for the CD4 subset of lymphocytes, and patients are at risk of opportunistic infections such as herpes viruses and *Pneumocysti jivori* for many months following treatment; patients are given prophylaxis with septrin and aciclovir for 6–12 months. Alkylating agents or fludarabine-based therapy can trigger autoimmune haemolysis and they should be used with care in direct antiglobulin (DAT)-positive patients. In the recent UK CLL4 trial, 10% of DAT-positive patients developed haemolysis, and DAT positivity predicted for the triggering of haemolysis by treatment. Patients treated with chlorambucil or fludarabine were twice as likely to develop haemolysis as those treated with FC combination, and four haemolytic deaths occurred on fludarabine alone. FC, therefore, may protect against haemolysis. FC and FCR are heavily myelosuppressive, and prolonged cytopenias and morphological bone marrow dysplasia are well recognized, requiring careful monitoring of multiple course therapy, especially in the elderly.

Corticosteroids

Single-agent prednisolone (1 mg/kg/day) produces reduction in lymphocytic infiltration of bone marrow and can result in significant improvement in cytopenias and symptoms. This is useful initial treatment (1–2 weeks) for patients with advanced disease and pancytopenia at diagnosis prior to chemotherapy. Also given for autoimmune haemolysis or thrombocytopenia.

Second-line and subsequent therapy

Elderly patients relapsing after an initial response to oral chlorambucil can be treated again if the first remission is long. Patients refractory to low-dose chlorambucil or with short/poor initial responses should be treated with fludarabine-based therapy. Combination chemotherapy such as cyclophosphamide, vincristine, and prednisolone (CVP) or cyclophosphamide, doxorubicin, vincristine, and prednisolone (CHOP) are alternative treatments for patients that are unsuitable for fludarabine. Patients who develop progressive disease more than 1 year after receiving fludarabine-based therapy and whose CLL responded to fludarabine initially may be treated again with fludarabine alone or as FC or FCR, providing there is care to observe the blood counts. A multicentre phase III trial randomized relapsed or refractory patients to FCR or FC. Patients could not have received these combinations before. The median progression-free survival was better for FCR (30.6 months vs 20.6 months).

Patients who develop progressive disease within 1 year of previous fludarabine-based therapy may be treated with FC or FCR, but second responses are not as good.

Patients who are refractory or become resistant to fludarabine currently have a poor prognosis.

Alemtuzumab

Alemtuzumab is a chimeric anti-CD52 antibody expressed on a wide range of lymphocytes including CLL cells. Several hundred patients refractory to fludarabine have been treated with alemtuzumab producing an overall response rate (ORR) of ~40% (10% complete remission (CR) and 30% partial remission (PR)), with a prolonged median survival compared with historical data on fludarabine-resistant patients. Alemtuzumab is licensed for the treatment of fludarabine-failed CLL and is the treatment of choice for patients with a known p53 deletion who respond poorly to other currently available therapies and have a poor prognosis. A randomized trial of first-line therapy with alemtuzumab vs chlorambucil showed a better progression-free survival (PFS), with time to alternative treatment of 23.3 vs 14.7 months. Alemtuzumab is given for up to 12 weeks and seems more effective at clearing disease in the blood and marrow than bulky lymph nodes. Small numbers of patients have been treated with alemtuzumab maintenance. There is an improved PFS but at the cost of significant infection rates, which led to the halting of a randomised phase III trial. Alemtuzumab is profoundly immunosuppressive and is associated with an increased risk of viral infections including reactivation of cytomegalovirus (CMV), which should be monitored.

Stem cell transplantation

Conventional allogeneic transplantation has rarely been carried out in CLL and is associated with a very high transplant-related mortality (40–70%), predominantly relating to the age of the patients and the co-morbidity associated with previous multiple courses of chemotherapy. However, there does seem to be a graft vs leukaemia effect for CLL, and use of RIC allografts shows promising early results. Autologous stem cell transplantation can produce very good quality responses including molecular negativity; however there is an association with a high rate of treatment-related MDS.

Radiotherapy

Radiotherapy is effective local treatment for lymph nodes compromising vital organ function. Splenic irradiation is effective for painful spleno-megaly, though splenectomy is better for massive splenomegaly if the patient is fit for surgery.

Splenectomy

This is effective for massive splenomegaly, anaemia, or thrombocytopenia owing to hypersplenism, and for autoimmune haemolytic anaemia refrac-tory to prednisolone and cytotoxic therapy.

While laparoscopic splenectomy is increasingly used in small or moderate splenectomy, in those cases of massive splenomegaly, open surgery is still sometimes favoured because of the difficulty of access to the pedicle and risk of massive blood loss. Careful pre-operative counselling is required regarding the risk of infection post-operatively.

Prior to splenectomy the patient requires pneumococcal, meningococcal and haemophilus vaccination. Following splenectomy lifelong penicillin prophylaxis must be given to avoid infection, especially overwhelming post-splenectomy infection (OPSI).

Most spleens can be removed laparoscopically with little morbidity, but huge spleens may still require open surgery.

Prognosis

Patients with CLL containing mutated *IgVH* genes have a long median sur-vival of the order of 25 years. Patients with CLL containing unmutated *IgVH* genes have a shorter median survival of the order of 8 years. The expression of certain antigens including CD38 and ZAP-70 is associ-ated with a poorer prognosis, and ZAP-70 expression correlates with *IgVH* gene mutation status. Genetic abnormalities including del(11q) and del(17p) (p53 deletion) and resistance to fludarabine are associated with poor prognosis. Small percentages of patients undergo a transformation to large B-NHL (Richter transformation) which carries a poor prognosis.

Future directions

It is increasingly recognized that the quality of the response in CLL corre-lates with the length of remission. Data from treatment with high-dose che-motherapy or alemtuzumab have emphasized the importance of achieving a complete response using sensitive techniques to detect minimal residual

disease, such as 4-colour flow cytometry. Further attempts to reduce minimal residual disease burden and affect a cure will involve:
• combinations of high-dose therapy with alemtuzumab
• combinations of antibodies, e.g. alemtuzumab and rituximab
• maintenance antibody/chemotherapy
• allogeneic transplantation with newer conditioning regimens
• therapies that overcome the acquired blocks in apoptosis, e.g. flavopiridol.

Hodgkin lymphoma (HL)

Epidemiology and aetiology

HL is a rare malignancy, with an annual UK incidence of 3 per 100 000. The age distribution in the West shows a large peak in the 20–30-year age group, and a smaller peak in old age. In developing countries there is a higher frequency of childhood cases. There have been associations described with higher socio-economic class, Caucasian race, and previous clinical/severe glandular fever. The cause is unknown, and may differ between the various histological subtypes. An association between infection with Epstein–Barr virus (EBV) and HL is well documented. It occurs in about 30% of cases, particularly classical mixed cellularity HL and lymphocyte-depleted HL in older patients.

Pathology

Classical HL

The characteristic diagnostic feature is the binucleate Reed–Sternberg (RS) cell, seen in a variable cellular background of small lymphocytes, eosinophils, neutrophils, histiocytes, plasma cells, and fibrosis. The infiltrating lymphocytes are T-regulatory cells, which favour an anergic-type immune response within the nodal environment, perhaps contributing to the survival of the malignant cells. The RS cell is the malignant cell in HL, and molecular studies have confirmed its B-cell lineage in 97% of cases.

Nodular lymphocyte-predominant HL (NLPHL)

NLPHL is a distinct entity, characterized by 'L&H Hodgkin cells' also known as 'popcorn cells', which are of B-cell lineage and express CD20. Approximately 10% of NLPHL develop into diffuse large B-cell NHL. This subtype has a favourable prognosis, though it may run a chronically relapsing and remitting course over many years, akin to low-grade NHL. The WHO classification of HL is summarized in Table 25.7.

Table 25.7 The WHO classification of HL

Classical Hodgkin's lymphoma
Nodular sclerosis classical HL (NSCHL) (~50%)
Mixed cellularity classical HL (MCHL) (30–40%)
Lymphocyte rich classical HL (LRCHL)
Lymphocyte depleted classical HL (LDHL) – rare

Presentation

- Painless rubbery lymphadenopathy (cervical nodes especially)
- May be generalized lymphadenopathy
- Later spread to liver, lungs, marrow
- 'B' symptoms:
  - fever
  - night sweats
  - weight loss >10% over 6 months

- Other systemic symptoms:
  - itch
  - alcohol-induced pain in lymph nodes (rare).

Diagnosis

The mainstay of diagnosis is a good-sized lymph node or involved tissue biopsy, which is analysed by expert haematopathologists using routine morphology and immunohistochemistry. Fine needle aspirates may suggest HL but should not be used alone for diagnosis.

Staging

Spread of HL is typically to contiguous lymph node groups. As a result, anatomical staging using the Ann Arbor system (see Table 25.8) has been the basis of treatment decisions in HL. The staging procedure now involves a CT scan of the neck, chest, abdomen, and pelvis rather than laparotomy. Bone marrow involvement is rare at presentation but more likely with disease below the diaphragm when a marrow trephine should be included in the staging process. The identification of prognostic factors other than anatomical staging has refined treatment decisions, which are now rarely made on the basis of anatomical stage only.

Table 25.8 Ann Arbor staging system

Stage	Feature
I	Disease in a single lymph node region
II	Disease in two or more regions on the same side of the diaphragm
III	Disease in two or more regions on both sides of the diaphragm
IV	Diffuse or disseminated disease in extra-lymphatic sites including liver and bone marrow
Various suffixes are added to each anatomical stage:	
	A No systemic symptoms
	B Systemic symptoms present
	E Extranodal disease

Prognostic factors

Recent studies have identified various presenting factors that may influence outcome in HL. For patients with early-stage (I and II) disease, several studies have identified prognostic groups based on histological subtype, age, sex, symptom status, number of nodal regions involved, and the presence of bulky mediastinal disease (see Table 25.9).

For patients with advanced (stage IIB to IVB) disease, seven prognostic factors have been identified in an analysis of over 5000 patients treated conventionally (Table 25.10).

Table 25.9 EORTC prognostic groups in early-stage HL

Group	Prognostic factors
Very favourable	Stage I and age <40 years or 'A' + ESR <50 mm/h or female and MT ratio[a] <0.35
Favourable	All other patients
Unfavourable	Age ≥40 years, or 'A' and ESR ≥50 mm/h, or 'B' and ESR ≥30, or stage II$_{4/5,}$ or MT ratio ≥ 0.35

EORTC: European Organisation for Research and Treatment of Cancer.

ESR: erythropcyte sedimentation rate.

* MT ratio = size of mediastinal mass compared with transverse diameter of the chest on chest X-ray.

Table 25.10 The adverse factors of the Hasenclever International Prognostic Index for advanced HL

Albumin <40 g/dl
Haemoglobin <10.5 g/l
Male gender
Lymphocytes <0.8 × 10⁹/l
WCC >15 × 10⁹/l
Lymphocytes less than 15% of total WCC
Stage IV

In the absence of any adverse factors, the 5-year failure-free survival (FFS) rate is 84%. The presence of each of these factors reduces the expected 5-year FFS by about 7%. Having three or more factors is generally considered a poor prognostic group.

The Role of ^{18}FDG-positron emission tomography (PET) scanning in HL

PET scanning is rapidly becoming an integral part of HL management, especially within clinical trials. HL tissue is PET avid and takes up radio-labelled-flurodeoxyglucose (^{18}FDG) producing an intense positron signal in involved tissue compared with background. Patients staged with PET are upstaged in approximately 16% of cases but this leads to a change in therapy in a minority, so staging with PET is not accepted as routine practice. However, assessment of early response to treatment or end-of-treatment response has significant prognostic bearing. Negative predictive values are high (~80–90%) and positive predictive values are ~60–70%. Such use of PET scanning may allow patient-adapted therapy such as the avoidance of mediastinal radiotherapy in young women with early-stage disease who are PET negative post-therapy, or the intensification of treatment in patients with advanced disease who remain PET positive after one or two courses of standard chemotherapy. The less reliable positive predictive value results from a number of causes of false positivity, including inflammation post-radiotherapy, infection etc. Therefore, long-term monitoring of remission by PET scanning is not recommended.

Management

Since HL predominantly affects young adults, potential long-term toxicities of therapy become of major importance now high cure rates are achieved. A recent analysis of the late effects after HL shows that at 30 years of follow-up, twice as many patients have died from second cancers as from relapsed HL. The recognition of the long-term toxicity of radiation therapy, particularly to the mediastinum (second malignancies, including lung and breast cancer, pulmonary fibrosis, coronary artery disease), has led to a major re-evaluation of the use of extensive radiotherapy. The use of mantle radiotherapy in women aged less than 20 years has been associated with breast cancer rates of up to 1 in 3 by age 50 years, and such therapy is rarely if ever used now. Alkylating agent-based chemotherapy is associated with t-MDS, t-AML and NHL, and infertility and these issues are also taken in to account when planning treatment. The aim is to maintain high cure rates but reduce long-term toxicity, especially in early-stage disease.

Early-stage (IA and IIA) disease

The majority of patients with early-stage HL present with supradiaphragmatic disease. For these patients, treatment should be determined by prognostic factors that predict the likelihood of occult subdiaphragmatic disease not detected by routine clinical staging techniques.

Patients with very favourable stage IA NLPHL or NSCHL involving the high cervical region and a low ESR are at very low risk of occult sub-diaphragmatic disease and may be treated with involved field radiotherapy (IFR) alone. However, most patients with good-prognosis early-stage HL treated outside a clinical trial would be offered 2–4 courses of standard ABVD (Adriamycin®, bleomycin, vinblastine, dacarbazine) chemotherapy, followed by involved field radiotherapy (IFR). In early-stage patients without adverse risk factors, such limited-course (2–4 cycles) ABVD or 'ABVD-like' chemotherapy combined with IFR is superior to nodal radiotherapy alone. Using this approach, German and French HL study groups have produced 5-year PFS and OS rates of >85% and >90% respectively. The big question in early-stage HL, therefore, is whether the same cure rates can be maintained with chemotherapy alone so removing the long-term complications of radiotherapy. The Eastern Co-operative Oncology group (ECOG) study of ABVD vs ABVD + RT or RT alone showed a small PFS advantage for using radiotherapy without any OS benefit. Therefore, significant numbers of patients may be cured by chemotherapy alone. PET scanning at the end of standard therapy has been shown to have a high negative (>90%) predictive value for relapse of early-stage disease and may allow selection of PET-negative patients for omission of radiotherapy without increasing the risk of relapse The current National Cancer Research Network (NCRN) RAPID trial is assessing this. Early-stage supradiaphragmatic patients receive 3 cycles of ABVD. Those who are then shown to be PET negative are randomized to no further therapy or IFR. PET-positive patients all receive a fourth cycle of ABVD and IFR. To date, 79% of 331 patients are PET negative post-three cycles ABVD. After a median follow-up of 13 months post-randomization, 245 of 255 (96%) patients are alive and progression free, confirming the very high negative predictive value of PET in the first year. The trial continues with no data on the randomization outcome as yet. Patients with early-stage disease but including poor prognostic features would be treated like those with advanced disease in many centres.

Advanced-stage disease (IIB–IV)

The major trial by the Cancer and Leukemia Group B (CALGB) compared doxorubicin-based chemotherapy as ABVD alone with MOPP (mustine, vincristine, procarbazine, and prednisolone) and MOPP alternating with ABVD. The respective 5-year freedom from salvage (FFS) rates were 61%, 50%, and 65%, demonstrating that ABVD and MOPP/ABVD were equivalent and both superior to MOPP alone. Therefore, in advanced-stage HL the gold standard therapy has become 6–8 cycles of ABVD producing PFS rates of 63–87%. It is important that ABVD is delivered optimally. This has been shown to consist of full dose being delivered every two weeks without dose reduction or delay for neutropenia, and without the need for growth factor support. The German HD9 study showed superior 5-year freedom from treatment failure rates of 87% with more intensive dose-escalated BEACOPP (bleomycin, etoposide, doxorubicin, cyclophosphamide, vincristine, procarbazine, prednisolone) chemotherapy compared with baseline BEACOPP (76%) and alternating COPP/ABVD (69%), though with considerable acute and chronic toxicity including an increase in t-MDS and more infertility. OS at 5 years was superior for escalated BEACOPP vs COPP/ABVD (91% vs 83%, $P = 0.002$). A mixture of four courses of baseline BEACOPP and four courses of escalated BEACOPP seems to maintain the very high response rates and reduce the rate of t-MDS. In contrast, the UK NCRI study of ABVD vs 12-week intensive Stanford V regimen has shown no difference in EFS or OS between the therapies. There was extensive use of radiotherapy in both arms of this study. The big question in advanced-stage HL, therefore, is whether patients can be stratified into those likely to be cured by gold standard ABVD from those who need intensification of therapy. The Hasenclever prognostic index identifies poor risk patients with a score of 3 or more. However, recent prospective data from a Danish and Italian study have shown that 50% of patients with poor-risk Hasenclever scores are cured by ABVD, and in the German studies the benefit from escalated BEACOPP requires all Hasenclever risk groups to be treated. Using this approach, significant numbers of patients will still be exposed to the complications of treatment intensification who can be cured by ABVD. Therefore, as an alternative approach, the Danish and Italian study explored the use of the PET scan as a dynamic prognostic marker. An early interim PET scan was completed after two cycles of ABVD. Patients who were PET negative had a 2-year PFS of 95% irrespective of Hasenclever score. Patients who were PET positive had a 2-year PFS of only 13% irrespective of Hasenclever score. Hence the early interim PET scan may distinguish good-risk advanced-stage patients who should continue treatment with ABVD and may even be able to undergo dose reduction from poor-risk advanced stage patients who may benefit from dose intensification. This is being tested prospectively in the NCRI RATHL (randomized phase III Trial to assess Response-Adapted therapy using FDG-PET imaging in patients with newly diagnosed advanced Hodgkin Lymphoma) trial.

The role of radiotherapy in advanced HL

A total of 333 stage III and IV patients treated with MOPP/ABV who achieved CR were randomised to 24 Gy IFR or not. There was no difference in PFS or OS, leading to the standard practice of not offering IFR to advanced-stage patients who achieve CR with chemotherapy. However, recent analysis of the UK Lymphoma Group (UKLG) LY09 trial in which patients were randomized to ABVD, alternating ChlVPP/PABLOE (chlorambucil, vinblastine, procarbazine, prednisolone, doxorubicin, bleomycin, vincristine etoposide) or hybrid ChlVPP/EVA (etoposide, vincristine, doxorubicin) challenges this approach. IFR was recommended only for incomplete response or bulk disease. The allocated chemotherapy had no influence on response rate, PFS, or OS at median follow-up of 6.5 years. EFS at 5 years post-chemotherapy was better for those given radiotherapy (86% vs 71%) and, of most concern, 5-year OS was also superior for receiving radiotherapy (93% vs 87%). The PET scan may in the future help clarify which advanced patients will benefit from the addition of radiotherapy, and this is being studied prospectively.

Salvage therapy

The prognosis for the majority of patients with HL of all stages is now very good. However, 30–40% will relapse from CR or demonstrate primary resistant/refractory disease. Patients relapsing after more than 12 months in first CR show better responses to salvage chemotherapy than those with shorter first CR. Commonly used salvage regimens include IVE (ifosfamide, etoposide, epirubicin), DHAP (cisplatin, ara-C, dexamethasone) or ESHAP (cisplatin, cytarabine, etoposide, methylprednisolone). Patients treated with salvage chemotherapy alone have a long-term DFS of only 20–25%, whereas the addition of high-dose chemotherapy and autologous stem cell transplantation (ASCT) produces long-term DFS of 40–50% if patients have chemosensitive disease going into the transplant. Results of ASCT are poorer for chemorefractory disease and, as recently recognized for patients not in functional CR defined by positive PET scan after salvage. Salvage therapy and ASCT is presently the standard of care for the majority of relapsed patients. Recent data with RIC allografts are encouraging for patients who relapse after ASCT. A UK study compared 38 patients receiving a RIC allograft after failed ASCT with a carefully selected historical control who survived for 12 months post-ASCT and would have nowadays been considered for a RIC allograft. The RIC group had a 5-year survival from the autograft of 65% compared to a 5-year survival from the autograft of only 15% for the historical control. Because of the apparent graft vs HL effect, RIC allografting may be a more appropriate therapy for chemorefractory or PET-positive patients after salvage than ASCT, though as yet RIC allografting remains experimental in this situation.

Future directions

- Removal of radiotherapy for early-stage disease
- Antibodies against CD30 antigen on R–S cell; some responses in phase II trials
- Anti-CD20 and radiolabelled anti-CD20 for treatment of NLPHL
- Anti-CD25 to target the TReg infiltrating cells and promote better immune clearance of malignant R–S cells.

Non-Hodgkin lymphomas (NHL)

Definition and aetiology

NHL is a group of malignant diseases arising from lymphocytes and their precursors. The spectrum of NHL ranges from indolent low-grade lymphomas that are incurable yet compatible with a number of years of survival, to aggressive high-grade lymphomas that, left untreated, are rapidly fatal, but which modern treatment can cure in a significant proportion of patients.

NHL is increasing in frequency, and in the USA this increase has been 3–4% per annum since the early 1970s, with a current incidence of approximately 15 per 100 000. The pathogenesis of the majority of NHL is unknown, but identified aetiological factors include the following:

- longevity
- prolonged immunosuppression, e.g. congenital immunodeficiencies, HIV-associated NHL, and post-transplant lymphoproliferative disease (PTLD)
- Epstein–Barr virus (EBV) infection in Burkitt lymphoma, HIV- and PTLD (immunosuppression related), and human T-cell lymphocytotrophic virus (HTLV-1) infection in adult T-cell leukaemia/lymphoma (ATLL)
- *Helicobacter* infection in gastric lymphoma and coeliac disease in small bowel lymphoma
- Chlamydia infections in ocular marginal zone lymphomas
- hepatitis C in some marginal zone lymphomas
- regular use of pre-1980 hair dyes.

Classification of NHL

Immunological identification of lymphocytes and molecular analysis of immunoglobulin and T-cell receptor gene rearrangements have allowed improved classification of NHL based on the biology of the cells rather than just morphological description. The majority of cases of NHL are B-cell type.

The pathological classification currently employed is the WHO classification (see Table 25.11). This is based on whether lymphoma cells are B-lymphocytes or T-lymphocytes, the perceived original cell of origin of the lymphoma, and whether or not a group of expert pathologists agree that the lymphoma can be reproducibly identified as a distinct entity.

In day-to-day practice, the clinical behaviour of NHL is a useful parameter, and treatment strategies are still based on classification systems that divide NHL into indolent (low-grade) and aggressive (high-grade) diseases. The general differences between low- and high-grade NHL are summarized in Table 25.12.

Table 25.11 WHO classification of NHL

B-cell lymphoma

Precursor B-cell neoplasms
Precursor B-lymphoblastic leukaemia/lymphoma

Mature B-NHL

Small lymphocytic lymphoma (lymphomatous manifestation of chronic
   lymphocytic leukaemia)
Lymphoplasmacytic lymphoma
Splenic marginal zone lymphoma
Extranodal marginal zone lymphoma of mucosa-associated lymphoid tissue
   (MALT-lymphoma)
Nodal marginal zone lymphoma
Follicular lymphoma
Mantle cell lymphoma
Diffuse large B-cell lymphoma (DLBL)
Mediastinal (thymic) large B-cell lymphoma
Intravascular large B-cell lymphoma
Primary effusion lymphoma
Burkitt lymphoma/leukaemia
B-cell lymphoma, unclassifiable with features intermediate between DLBL and
Burkitt lymphoma, or between DLBL and classical HL.

T-cell and NK-cell lymphoma

Precursor T-cell neoplasm
Precursor T-lymphoblastic lymphoma/leukaemia

Mature T-cell and NK-cell neoplasm

Cutaneous
Mycosis fungoides
Sézary syndrome
Primary cutaneous anaplastic large cell lymphoma
Lymphomatoid papulosis

Extranodal
Extranodal NK/T-cell lymphoma, nasal type
Enteropathy-associated T-cell lymphoma
Hepatosplenic T-cell lymphoma
Subcutaneous panniculitis-like T-cell lymphoma

Nodal
Angioimmunoblastic T-cell lymphoma
Anaplastic large T-cell lymphoma (ALK positive or negative)
Peripheral T-cell lymphoma, unspecified

Leukaemic
T-cell prolymphocytic leukaemia
T-cell large granular lymphocytic leukaemia
Aggressive NK cell leukaemia
Adult T-cell leukaemia/lymphoma

Table 25.12 Differences between low-grade and high-grade NHL

Low-grade NHL

Indolent clinical course with relatively long survival

Incurable with present therapy – relapsing and remitting course

Non-destructive growth patterns

CNS involvement rare

High-grade lymphoma

Aggressive clinical course and rapidly fatal without treatment

Curable in a significant proportion of patients

Destructive growth pattern

CNS and extranodal involvement common

Clinical features and staging of NHL

The majority of adult patients (60–70%) present with nodal disease, whereas the majority of children present with extranodal disease. One or more areas of lymph nodes are painlessly enlarged and may remain unchanged or slowly increase in size in low-grade NHL, or rapidly increase in size in high-grade lymphomas. Hepatosplenomegaly is common and extranodal sites are protean and include the gut, testes, thyroid gland, bone, muscle, lung, CNS, facial sinuses, and skin. Systemic symptoms include drenching night sweats, loss of weight, and culture-negative fever.

Medical emergencies associated with NHL include mediastinal obstruction, obstructive nephropathy, spinal cord compression, hypercalcaemia, and metabolic derangement. Ascites and pleural effusions (sometimes chylous) are common end-stage features, especially in high-grade NHL. Patients may develop bone marrow failure from lymphomatous involvement, and low-grade NHL can cause immune-mediated haemolysis or thrombocytopenia.

Diagnosis requires a lymph node biopsy or, in the absence of lymphadenopathy, biopsy of an involved extranodal site. Immunohistochemistry and cytogenetic and molecular techniques aid morphological diagnosis. Once again expert haematopathology diagnosis and multidisciplinary team review (MDT) is mandatory.

The extent or stage of the disease should be determined by clinical rather than pathological (surgical) staging. This involves:

- chest X-ray (CXR)
- computerized tomography (CT) scanning of the chest, abdomen, and pelvis to define areas of nodal and extranodal involvement
- blood count and blood film for leukaemic involvement
- bone marrow aspiration and trephine biopsy for morphology, immunophenotyping, and cytogenetic analysis
- renal biochemistry, liver function, calcium, and uric acid
- markers of tumour burden: serum lactate dehydrogenase (LDH) and beta2-microglobulin
- others, depending on circumstances, e.g. CT brain scan, magnetic resonance imaging (MRI) of spine, lumbar puncture, bone scan.

Clinical staging is based on a modification of the Ann Arbor classification of Hodgkin lymphoma (see Table 25.8). The PET scan is increasingly being used in the staging and response assessment of NHL, particularly in high-grade disease. However, the roles of PET scanning in NHL are less well defined than in HL.

Low-grade NHL

The low-grade lymphomas comprise 20–45% of NHL. They tend to be disseminated at the time of presentation, with widespread lymphadenopathy, hepatosplenomegaly, and, often, blood and marrow involvement.

Follicular lymphoma (FL)

This is the archetypal low-grade B-cell NHL and the most common subtype of indolent NHL (30% of cases). It typically presents at an older age, though it is also seen in young people. Rarely, it presents as an apparent true stage I, when it may be cured by IFR. More commonly, it presents as stage III or IV, when it remains incurable in the majority with current treatments, but runs a relapsing and remitting course with an improving median survival of 10–12 years. This lymphoma can transform to high-grade NHL in 30–60% of cases, which carries a high mortality. High-grade transformation seems to be very rare in patients surviving beyond 15 years or so.

The lymphoma cells contain a reciprocal chromosomal translocation – t(14;18) (q32;q21). This leads to the oncogene *BCL-2*, from chromosome 18, coming under the regulation of the immunoglobulin heavy chain gene (*IgH*) on chromosome 14. The increased production of *BCL-2* protects the lymphoma cell from apoptosis (programmed cell death) and, as such, follicular lymphoma represents a relentless accumulation of malignant cells.

Management strategies: presentation
- IFR for the small number of patients who are apparently stage I. This can be curative though most patients will prove to have occult systemic disease and relapse.
- For advanced disease (>stage I), avoid chemotherapy-based treatment until significant symptoms. This so-called 'watch and wait' approach remains valid, though needs to be re-tested with each new development in primary therapy. There are some registry data suggesting 'watch and wait' might be associated with an increase risk of high-grade transformation.
- Consider patients with asymptomatic advanced disease for the present NCRI UK trial of 'watch and wait' versus rituximab to see if rituximab can delay the need for chemotherapy.

For symptomatic patients (bulky lymphadenopathy, systemic symptoms, cytopenias, organ dysfunction), recent randomized data, confirmed by a meta-analysis, have demonstrated a higher response rate (RR), longer time to disease progression (PFS) and now OS for first-line treatment with rituximab (R-) based immunochemotherapy. Rituximab is a chimeric anti-CD20 monoclonal antibody. The optimal chemotherapy to combine with rituximab remains unclear, and rituximab is now licensed for use with a range of first-line chemotherapies. The recently completed randomized

PRIMA (a multicentre phase III, open-label, randomized study in patients with advanced follicular lymphoma evaluating the benefit of maintenance therapy with rituximab (monoclonal antibody therapy) after induction of response with chemotherapy plus rituximab in comparison with no maintenance therapy) study may help define the benefit of a particular chemotherapy regimen. At present R-CVP rather than CVP (cyclophosphamide, vincristine, prednisolone) (at median 53 months: OS 83% vs 77%, time to treatment failure (TTF) 34 months vs 15 months), R-CHOP rather than CHOP (cyclophosphamide, doxorubicin, vincristine, prednisolone) (at median 18 months: OS 95% vs 90%, TTF not reached vs 29 months) and R-MCP rather than MCP (mitoxantrone, chlorambucil, prednisolone) (at median 47 months: OS 87% vs 74%, TTF not reached vs 26 months) are the mainstays of initial therapy. Very elderly or infirm patients are still appropriately treated with the oral alkylating agent chlorambucil or R-chlorambucil. There may be further benefit for prolonged rituximab maintenance therapy in first remission. At present, rituximab maintenance is not licensed in first remission and the results of the randomized maintenance component of PRIMA are awaited.

Treatments at time of progression from first response
As at presentation, there is no rush to treat asymptomatic patients at first or subsequent relapses, and watch and wait remains appropriate. Available therapies are similar to first-line with some additional options and include:
• CHOP or CVP or alkylating agents (chlorambucil) with or without rituximab
• purine analogues: fludarabine, and 2-CDA, with or without rituximab
• single-agent rituximab
• radiolabelled monoclonal antibody (radioimmunoconjugate), ^{131}I-anti-B1 (tositumomab) and ^{90}Y-anti CD20 (ibritumomab tiuxetan, Zevalin®, not licensed in the UK)
• patients relapsing from non-rituximab-based first-line therapy show a survival benefit for R-CHOP as second-line therapy followed by rituximab maintenance every 3 months for two years or until relapse. Rituximab has a licence for such maintenance therapy in second remission and is approved as such by the SMC in the UK. Whether or not patients receiving R-chemotherapy as first line (almost universal now) show the same benefit at relapse is unclear.

The role of stem cell transplantation
• Phase III randomized data for the use of high-dose chemotherapy and ASCT in first remission has demonstrated prolonged PFS vs interferon-α maintenance in the GLSG trial, but not in the GELF94 study and with no OS advantage to date. ASCT is associated with higher rates of morbidity, including second cancers. Therefore, ASCT is reserved for second and subsequent responses outside of clinical trials.
• The European Group for Blood and Marrow (EBMT)-sponsored CUP (conventional chemotherapy, unpurged, purged autograft) study suggests a PFS and OS advantage for randomization to ASCT in relapsed FL (4-year OS 46% vs 71% vs 77% for chemotherapy alone vs unpurged ASCT vs purged ASCT). However, this study suffered from

slow accrual and closed early with only 140 of a planned 250 recruited and only 89 randomizations.
- There is clearly an allogeneic graft vs lymphoma effect for FL and increasing interest in RIC allografting for relapsed patients. The EBMT has recently completed a retrospective comparison of 1394 patients receiving an ASCT and 110 patients receiving an RIC allograft for relapsed FL. The RIC patients, not surprisingly, had received more prior lines of therapy, took longer to get to transplant, and were more likely to have refractory disease at the time of transplant. The cumulative 100-day and 1-year transplant-related mortality (TRM) was 5% and 15% for RIC allograft and 2% and 3% for ASCT. However, there were no relapses beyond 30 months for RIC allografts, with the 3-year and 5-year PFS being 62% for RIC allografts vs 58% and 48% for ASCT. The usual story for allografting of higher TRM but reduced relapse risk clearly holds true for relapsed FL with the potential for long-term remission/cure via the graft vs lymphoma effect.
- Patients suffering from high-grade transformation of FL who respond to salvage chemotherapy and are fit enough may benefit from ASCT or RIC allografting, and these approaches are commonly pursued in this situation.

In summary it is clear that patients with FL should be treated with rituximab-based immunochemotherapy as first line and be considered for either rituximab maintenance or stem cell transplantation in second response. The best order of all other palliative therapies is unclear. Given that no therapy is clearly curative, most patients end up receiving all available therapies in a typical relapsing and remitting natural history over several years. Since the quality of the response (negative or low-level minimal residual disease) correlates with the length of response, intensive therapies like ASCT and RIC allografts are able to produce long remissions.

Prognosis
- Follicular lymphoma prognostic index (FLIPI) identifies three risk groups based on five clinical parameters – age, stage, haemoglobin combination, LDH, and number of nodal sites. Three prognostic groups are produced with 10-year survivals of approximately 76%, 52%, and 24%.
- Gene expression profiling is providing prognostic information. Interestingly, the gene expression signatures of the infiltrating T-cells and monocytes within the FL node have been shown to predict for survival.

Marginal-zone lymphomas (MZL)
After FL and CLL/SCLL the group of diseases known as MZL are the next most frequent low-grade lymphomas. There are three subtypes recognized:
- **extra-nodal MZL** (commonest presentation) involving the stomach, small bowel, salivary glands, thyroid, adnexa of the eye, lung, and other rarer sites. These lymphomas arise in acquired mucosa-associated lymphoid tissue (MALT) resulting from chronic inflammatory stimuli, either infective or autoimmune. Examples include *Helicobacter pylori*

in the stomach, *Chlamydia* in the eye, and Sjogren's syndrome with parotid MZL
- **splenic MZL** presenting as splenomegaly with bone marrow involvement, circulating villous lymphocytes, and a possible association with hepatitis C infection
- **nodal MZL** (rare).

Management

The archetypal gastric MZL without t(11;18) translocation has a high response rate to *H. pylori* eradication. Patients who fail this treatment respond well to IFR. MZL in general are very sensitive to radiotherapy and the treatment of choice for stage I disease at most sites is relatively low dose (up to 30 Gy) IFR. Ongoing trials include tetracycline for *Chlamydia* eradication for eye MZL, and the International Extranodal Lymphoma Study Group (IELSG)-19 trial for advanced extranodal MZL or failed local therapy, which randomizes to chlorambucil, rituximab or both.

Splenic MZL are often successfully treated with splenectomy, and nodal MZL are treated similarly to FL in many centres.

Mantle-cell lymphoma (MCL)

MCL accounts for ~6% of NHL. Whilst histologically low grade it carries the poorest prognosis of all NHL with a median survival of ~3 years. The disease presents predominantly as nodal, though a relatively benign leukaemic form is recognized most commonly in older men. A rarer high-grade blastoid variant is also recognized. Bowel involvement in the form of multiple lymphomomatous polyps is well recognized. The tumour, like CLL/SCLL, is CD5 positive, but carries the hallmark cytogenetic rearrangement t(11;14) leading to overexpression of cyclin D1 used for diagnosis.

Management

CHOP produces poor CR rates of ~30%. A meta-analysis has suggested a benefit in response rates for the addition of rituximab to front-line chemotherapy, and a recent update of the German Low-Grade Lymphoma Study Group has shown an advantage in overall response rate (92% vs 75%), response duration (29 months vs 18 months) and time to treatment failure (28 months vs 14 months), but no OS benefit for R-CHOP vs CHOP. An ongoing UK NCRI phase III trial is comparing FCR (fludarabine, cyclophosphamide, rituximab) with FC (fludarabine, cyclophosphamide).

There are high response rates for regimens using high-dose therapy in younger, fitter, patients. HyperC-VAD/methotrexate followed by ASCT or with rituximab and no ASCT has produced OR of 90–100% and CR 58–100%. Recently, the Nordic Lymphoma Group has treated 160 consecutive patients with alternating R-maxi CHOP/R-high-dose cytarabine followed by ASCT. The results are very encouraging, with OS ~70% and no relapses beyond 3 years. High-dose cytarabine-based regimens followed by ASCT are becoming the accepted standard of care for younger patients.

High-grade NHLs

High-grade NHLs can be considered as those with a strong tendency to involve the CNS – lymphoblastic, Burkitt, adult T-cell leukaemia/lymphoma (ATLL), primary CNS lymphoma (PCL), and those others with a lesser tendency to do so. However, these latter histological types (predominantly diffuse large B-NHL-DLBL) have an increased risk of CNS disease in certain situations: If they involve the testes or breasts, if they involve multiple extranodal sites, para-spinal sites, or, controversially, if they have a raised LDH. Such patients require CNS examination and prophylaxis. Most centres will not give CNS prophylaxis for a raised LDH alone, as this would account for 50% or so of patients, but only if it is associated with other risk factors.

Burkitt lymphoma

Burkitt lymphoma (BL) is a highly aggressive B-cell malignancy characterized by a rearrangement of the *cMYC* oncogene on chromosome 8 via t(8;14) or a variant translocation. cMYC deregulation leads to a cell cycle fraction approaching 100%, which is commonly used in the diagnostic process along with cytogenetics and a follicle centre phenotype. The disease sometimes presents as mature B-ALL (Burkitt leukaemia) with distribution in the blood and marrow rather than lymph nodes and solid organs. Some diffuse large B-cell non-Hodgkin lymphoma (DLBL) have very high cell cycle fractions (>90%) without *cMYC* rearrangements, and are commonly termed Burkitt-like lymphoma (BLL). Two epidemiological subtypes of BL are recognized:

- **endemic**:
  - endemic in equatorial Africa
  - 90% associated with EBV infection
  - young adults/children, present with head/neck tumours
- **sporadic**
  - associated with EBV in ~20%
  - abdominal disease more common
  - occurs as non-HIV related or HIV related.

Management

Rapidly cycling, high-intensity multi-agent chemotherapy with a backbone of methotrexate, cyclophosphamide, and ifosfamide including CNS prophylaxis is frequently curative in non-HIV BL. Aggressive management of tumour lysis risk is important, with IV fluids, rasburicase, and regular electrolyte monitoring. The regimen developed by Magrath of CODOX-M (cyclophosphamide, vincristine, doxorubicin, methotrexate, IT cytarabine) alone for low-risk disease (early-stage and normal LDH) or CODOX-M alternating with IVAC (ifosfamide, etoposide, cytarabine, IT methotrexate) for poor-risk disease is one frequently used example. Recent UK data from the LY10 trial using dose-modified CODOX-M/IVAC to limit toxicity produced 2-year PFS of 64% for non-HIV BL and 55% for BLL. Low-risk patients' 2-year PFS rose to 85%. Given the B-cell phenotype, recent attempts to improve outcome have included the addition of rituximab. Twenty-four patients (8 HIV related) received R-CODOX-M/R-IVAC producing EFS and OS of 67% and 75% at median 19 months. HIV-related BL has a poorer prognosis than non-HIV-related BL. Immunocompromised patients are less able to tolerate the regimen toxicity. However, increasing success is seen with the type of regimens described when used concurrently with highly active antiretroviral therapy (HAART).

Lymphoblastic lymphoma

Presents with or without leukaemia, is more common in children than adults, and is most often T-cell type, typically featuring a mediastinal mass and pleural effusion. Treatment includes emergency management of mediastinal obstruction and prevention of the tumour lysis syndrome as above. Intensive combination chemotherapy schedules similar to those used in ALL and including CNS-directed therapy have improved the outlook in children, but results in adults remain less good.

Poor prognostic features include bone marrow and/or CNS involvement, LDH >300 iu/l, age >30 years, and delayed achievement of CR. Allogeneic and autologous progenitor cell transplantation may improve survival in these cases.

Diffuse large B-cell NHL (DLBL)

This is the commonest high-grade NHL and accounts for ~40% of all NHL. It presents as nodal disease alone (60%) or as extranodal disease (primary extranodal DLBL) or with combined nodal and extranodal disease.

First-line therapy

Short course (3–4) CHOP-like chemotherapy (most commonly R-CHOP now) followed by involved field radiotherapy can cure ~90% of non-bulky stage IA disease.

For all other stages, 6–8 courses of R-CHOP has become the gold standard chemotherapy. This follows the landmark Groupe d'Étude des Lymphomes des Adultes (GELA) trial that showed an event-free and overall survival advantage at 5 years for patients over the age of 60 years treated with 8 courses of R-CHOP (EFS 47%, OS 58%) compared with CHOP (EFS 29%, OS 45%). Similar results have been produced for younger patients. In a German study, CHOP given every 14 days with G-CSF support produced a better complete remission rate (77% vs 63.2%) and longer time to treatment failure than CHOP given every 21 days. A UK National Cancer research Institute (NCRI) trial has just closed, with over 1000 patients randomized to R-CHOP-14 or R-CHOP-21.

While R-CHOP is a milestone development in the first-line management of DLBL, there remain significant issues in patients with advanced poor-prognostic disease, who fare less well with R-CHOP and in all patients who relapse after R-CHOP who from preliminary data may be less salvageable than relapses from CHOP. Attempts are being made to intensify first-line therapy for poor-risk patients (International Prognostic Index (IPI) ≥3). One example is the UK NCRI trial of modified R-CODOX-M/R-IVAC in such patients. A meta-analysis has failed to demonstrate a benefit for high-dose chemotherapy and ASCT in first remission.

Relapsed DLBL

Historically, patients relapsing after CHOP chemotherapy who respond to salvage chemotherapy have been shown to have a survival benefit with high-dose chemotherapy and ASCT, which is the accepted standard of care for patients who are fit. There are a number of widely used salvage therapies and no one is clearly superior. The addition of rituximab is beneficial in patients who did not receive rituximab in first line. In the GELA study, patients relapsing from the CHOP arm survived longer with R-salvage than salvage alone ($P = 0.00043$) but the benefit was not significant for

R-salvage in those relapsing from the R-CHOP arm (*P* = 0.073), with very small numbers. Taking all patients there was a benefit for R-salvage and this has become the standard of care. Commonly used regimens are R-ICE (ifosfamide, carboplatin, etoposide), R-DHAP (dexamethasone, high-dose cytarabine, cisplatin) and R-IVE (ifosfamide, etoposide, epirubicin), followed where possible by ASCT for chemoresponsive disease. There are data suggesting no benefit for trying more than one type of salvage therapy if there is chemoresistance, though this is often a difficult decision for physicians and patients to make. The recently completed CORAL trial has compared R-ICE vs R-DHAP followed by ASCT and randomization to maintenance rituximab or not. Hopefully, it will help clarify some of the uncertain issues in this difficult group of patients. The role of RIC allografting is less clear in DLBL than in HL or FL.

Prognosis of DLBL

- The IPI identifies prognostic groups based on a score of 1 for each of: age, stage, number of extranodal sites, LDH, and performance status. Score 0/1 is low risk, score 2 low-intermediate risk, score 3 high-intermediate risk, and score 4/5 high risk. The IPI remains prognostic in the era of R-CHOP with 4-year probability of OS being 95% for IPI 0, 90% for IPI 1, 70% for IPI 2, 55% for IPI 3, and 28% for IPI 4.
- Recent gene expression profiling has had a significant impact on identifying biological subgroups of DLBL with prognostic importance. A germinal centre signature is associated with a good prognosis, whereas an activated B-cell signature is associated with a poor prognosis.

Myeloma

Epidemiology and aetiology

Myeloma (multiple myeloma, myelomatosis) is due to the unregulated proliferation of monoclonal plasma cells in the bone marrow. Their accumulation leads to anaemia and eventually marrow failure and, indirectly, to bone resorption resulting in lytic lesions, generalized osteoporosis, and pathological fractures. The cell of origin has not been conclusively identified but may be a memory B-lymphocyte. The cause is unknown.

The overall incidence of the disease is 4 per 100 000 in the UK, but over 30 per 100 000 in subjects over 80 years of age. It is higher amongst African-Americans and much lower in Chinese- and Japanese-Asian populations. It is rare under the age of 40 years.

Pathology

Plasma cell dyscrasias can present in a number of ways:

- monoclonal gammopathy of uncertain significance (MGUS) – paraprotein in serum <30 g/l, marrow clonal plasma cells <10% with no features of myeloma end-organ damage or lymphoma or amyloidosis
- solitary plasmacytoma – either of bone or extramedullary
- asymptomatic myeloma – paraprotein in serum >30 g/l and/or marrow clonal plasma cells >10% but no features of myeloma-related end-organ damage (anaemia, hypercalcaemia, bone lesions, kidney impairment)
- systemic amyloidosis
- multiple myeloma – paraprotein in serum and/or urine, bone marrow clonal plasma cells and myeloma-related end-organ damage.

Some lymphomas can present with a paraprotein, most commonly lymphoplasmacytic NHL (Waldenstrom's macroglobulinaemia) but also CLL, MZL, and, less frequently, FL.

The clonal plasma cells in myeloma synthesize, and usually secrete, a monoclonal protein (M protein, paraprotein). This is most commonly intact immunoglobulin, but may be immunoglobulin together with free light chain, or free light chain only. IgG is secreted in 60% of cases, IgA in 20%, and free light chain in 20%. Light chains can pass through the glomerular filter, saturate the reabsorption mechanism, and appear in the urine as Bence–Jones protein. In rare cases there is synthesis of monoclonal IgD, IgE, or IgM, or of two clonal proteins. Also uncommon are non-secretory and non-synthesizing variants of the disease. However, more sensitive methods of detecting free light chain in the serum have recently suggested that many cases of non-secretory myeloma are in fact low-level light chain secretors.

Clinical features

The accumulation of plasma cells in bone marrow, induction of bone resorption, and paraprotein synthesis explains the clinical findings.

Marrow infiltration

Malignant plasma cells accumulate in the red marrow of the axial skeleton and flat bones. Anaemia is common, and frequently present at diagnosis. It results from the combination of the anaemia of chronic disease, renal impairment, and bone marrow suppression if the plasma cell burden is high. Overt bone marrow failure is more commonly a feature of end-stage disease.

Bone resorption

There is abnormal bone remodelling with increased bone resorption and inhibition of osteoblastic bone formation. This leads to lytic destruction of the skeleton and hypercalcaemia, usually with a normal alkaline phosphatase. The pathogenesis of the osteoclast bone resorption is understood to result from abnormal cytokine signalling between malignant plasma cells, osteoclasts, osteoblasts and marrow stromal cells. In particular, increased levels of receptor activator of NF-κB (RANK)-ligand produced by myeloma cells and marrow stromal cells coupled with a suppression of soluble osteopetegrin (OPG) favour osteoclast bone resorption. Other cytokines such as interleukin 6 further support excess osteoclast activity.

Bone pain is the most common presenting complaint, especially severe back pain. There may be fractures of proximal long bones, ribs, sternum, and vertebral crush fractures. The increased bone resorption also leads to hypercalcaemia and associated symptoms of thirst, polyuria, nausea, constipation, drowsiness, and even coma. Plain X-ray examination typically reveals osteoporosis and typical lytic lesions that are often visualized on skull films.

Secretion of paraprotein

Accumulation of M protein in the plasma may result in hyperviscosity with lethargy and confusion, progressing to fits and coma. There is a characteristic retinopathy in hyperviscosity syndrome, with distension of retinal veins and irregular vessel constrictions; haemorrhages and papilloedema may be present. IgA and IgM (almost exclusively lymphoma associated) paraproteins are especially likely to induce hyperviscosity, though IgG also if in high level or of IgG3 subclass. Bence–Jones protein is deposited in the renal tubules and leads to renal failure (cast nephropathy). Other factors contributing to renal failure are:

• hypercalcaemia and dehydration
• amyloid deposition
• infection.

Paraproteinaemia is typically accompanied by immuneparesis, which contributes to the infection risk. In non-secretory myeloma the only immunological abnormality may be immuneparesis, giving rise to diagnostic confusion.

Other features

Plasmacytomas may be palpable and also cause pressure effects. Spinal cord compression is most frequent and constitutes a medical emergency with the need for urgent assessment and local radiotherapy and/or decompressive surgery. Amyloidosis may present as macroglossia, renal failure, peripheral neuropathy, and cardiac failure. A syndrome of high-output cardiac failure is an occasional feature, unrelated to cardiac amyloid.

Very occasionally, the bone lesions appear sclerotic, and this variant of the disease is often accompanied by severe progressive peripheral neuropathy. This combination of sclerotic lesions and neuropathy may also occur as part of the 'POEMS' syndrome, where plasma cell dyscrasia is accompanied by:

- sensorimotor polyneuropathy
- organomegaly (principally hepatomegaly)
- endocrinopathy (diabetes mellitus, amenorrhoea, gynaecomastia)
- M protein
- skin changes (predominantly pigmentation).

Diagnosis

- FBC
- ESR/plasma viscosity
- Urea and electrolytes (U&Es) and serum calcium and albumin
- Electrophoresis and immunofixation of serum and urine for paraprotein
- Quantification of intact paraprotein in serum or free light chain in serum for light chain or non-secretory myeloma. This is expressed as a serum free light chain ratio (SFLCR)
- β_2 microglobulin quantification
- Bone marrow aspirate and trephine biopsy
- Skeletal survey

The classic diagnostic triad consists of bone marrow infiltration with monoclonal plasma cells, osteolytic lesions on skeletal X-rays, and para-proteinaemia/Bence–Jones' proteinuria. For diagnostic purposes the bone marrow clonal plasma cell count and the paraprotein do not have to be at any given level, providing there is evidence of myeloma-related organ or tissue impairment, including bone lesions. The distribution of plasma cells is notoriously patchy but is often over 30%, usually with morphologically abnormal forms.

Cytogenetic abnormalities, most commonly on chromosomes 13 and 14, and aneuploidy are usually present when analysed by FISH, although their demonstration is not necessary for diagnostic purposes. The myeloma cells tend to be positive for CD38 and syndecan-1 (CD138). Additional common features are:

- raised ESR and rouleaux on a blood film
- normocytic anaemia
- pancytopenia
- renal impairment.

In approximately 30%, hypercalcaemia is present at diagnosis and, typically, the serum alkaline phosphatase concentration is normal and the isotope bone scan negative (due to suppressed osteoblastic activity). The serum albumin may be low.

- The main differential diagnosis is '**monoclonal gammopathy of uncertain significance**' (MGUS). Its prevalence is around 20 times higher than that of multiple myeloma and it is age related – 1% of the population, rising to 3% of subjects over 80 years of age, have detectable paraprotein. There is a progression rate to multiple myeloma of 1% per year.
- Asymptomatic myeloma is associated with an initially stable course and relatively long survival.

- In plasma cell leukaemia there are greater than 20% plasma cells in peripheral blood. It may be a presenting feature or develop late in the disease course and is typically poorly responsive to therapy.
- Solitary plasmacytoma of bone (SBP) presents as a single bone lesion with normal bone marrow, and 60% have a paraprotein, often of low titre. The common sites are the axial skeleton, especially the vertebrae, and include the skull base. Despite normal marrow morphology, recent MRI data have shown that 25% of patients have an abnormal marrow signal at presentation and MRI of the spine should be performed before delivering radical radiotherapy to SBP. The tumour is radiosensitive, but myeloma subsequently develops in two-thirds of cases.
- Extramedullary plasmacytoma (SEP) is a rare soft-tissue plasma-cell tumour occurring most commonly in the upper airways of the head and neck especially the nasopharanx, sinuses, and tonsils. Again the bone marrow is normal and there is no paraprotein in the majority of cases. The tumour is radiosensitive. Multiple myeloma develops less commonly than in SBP, in up to 30% of cases.

Management

Myeloma remains an incurable malignancy. However, significant developments during the last decade have led to longer survival and better quality of life. The disease now runs a relapsing and remitting course over several years somewhat akin to low-grade lymphoma. Untreated, death usually occurs within months, especially from infection and renal failure, and is often preceded by intractable bone pain. Initial therapy should include:

- adequate analgesia, often necessitating the use of opiates, with radiotherapy to areas of persisting local bone pains
- rehydration and vigorous management of hypercalcaemia using intravenous bisphosphonate. Dialysis is occasionally necessary for management of renal impairment, and plasma exchange for rapid correction of hyperviscosity syndrome. A trial, 'MERIT', is currently looking at the benefit of early plasma exchange in patients with renal failure.

First-line therapy

- Trial-based therapy remains the best approach where possible. Recent large trials have led to a fundamental switch in approach to thalidomide-based therapy. In 1800 patients recruited to the two age groups of the MRC Myeloma IX study, the addition of thalidomide in the form of CTD (cyclophosphamide, thalidomide, dexamethasone) improved response rates compared to CVAD (cyclophosphamide, vincristine, daunorubicin, dexamethasone) or MP (melphalan, prednisolone). Older patients (>65 years) and patients not considered for high-dose chemotherapy are in the majority treated in the UK with dose-adjusted CTD or MPT (melphalan, prednisolone, thalidomide). The pivotal trial compared MPT (125 patients) with MP (196 patients) in patients aged 65–75 years. With a median follow-up of 51 months, OS was 51.6 months vs 33.2 months in favour of MPT, and subsequently MPT has been approved by the SMC. Treatment is given until maximum response assessed by intact paraprotein levels or SFLCR – known as plateau. The thalidomide side-effects of somnolence, constipation, peripheral neuropathy, and risk of venous thromboembolism (VTE) are important and limit the dose escalation (100–200 mg/day), and indeed any use in some patients.

- The proteosome inhibitor bortezomib is also approved for first-line use in the USA but not in the UK. In the VISTA trial BMP (bortezomib, melphalan, prednisolone) (344 patients) was compared to MP(338 patients) and the median time to progression was 24 months compared to 16.6 months in favour of BMP which converted into a reduction in the risk of death of 39% at 16 months' follow-up.

- Younger patients in the UK are commonly treated with non-dose adjusted CTD until maximum response/plateau, usually 4–6 courses, with a view to proceeding in first response to high-dose melphalan (200 mg/m^2) and ASCT. Randomized data from the last 15 years have shown increased CR rates and survival benefit for ASCT of about 18 months, pushing median survivals to 5 years and leading to its adoption as standard of care. However, recent analyses suggest the benefit may apply only to those who are not in CR following initial therapy. The move to more effective first-line therapies based on thalidomide and increasingly bortezomib and lenalidomide might allow the delay of ASCT until relapse for those who get a CR (no detectable paraprotein and plasma cells <5%) with initial treatment.

- All patients are treated with bisphosphonates as bone protection for up to one year from the achievement of CR, or lifelong in non-remitters (the majority). Commonly used drugs are oral sodium clodronate or intravenous pamidronate and zoledronic acid. The results of the randomized comparison of clodronate vs zoledronic acid in UK Myeloma IX are awaited.

- Important issues during the delivery of care include:
  - presribing thalidomide via a risk management programme to prevent exposure of unborn babies (e.g. Thalidomide Pharmion Pregnancy Prevention Programme)
  - prescribing thromboprophylaxis to patients on thalidomide, especially early on when the disease bulk is high and the risk of VTE is of the order of 6%
  - obtaining a dental check prior to giving bisphosphonates and stopping bisphosphonates prior to dental work to minimize the risk of osteonecrosis of the jaw.

- The role of thalidomide maintenance in first plateau has been investigated. In the UK Myeloma IX trial PFS was improved with maintenance thalidomide in all treatment groups but with no OS benefit. Patients not achieving at least a very good PR after ASCT might benefit from 6 months of maintenance thalidomide but it is not generally recommended for any other groups. It may be detrimental to patients with the cytogenetic abnormality del(17p).

- Interferon-α, administered as maintenance therapy, appears to extend the duration of the plateau phase according to a meta-analysis. However, this is probably not a meaningful survival, being of the order of 3 months, especially given that the therapy is associated with significant side-effects and impinges on quality of life.

- Allografting in myeloma remains controversial. Conventional allografting carries an unacceptably high TRM. Recent data with RIC allografting, including some randomized data, are more encouraging, and studies looking at RIC allografts in younger patients at a time of MRD post-ASCT are ongoing.

Treatment of relapse/progressive disease

New agents have offered significant benefit in the palliation of progressive disease. The proteosome inhibitor bortezomib (Velcade®) produces responses in one-third of pre-treated patients. An open-label randomized study of 669 patients with progressive myeloma after 1–3 prior therapies has shown a benefit for bortezomib over high-dose dexamethasone. The median TTP was 189 days vs 106 days with OS, at a median of 22 months of follow-up 29.8 months vs 23.7 months. Bortezomib is approved for second-line therapy in the UK in patients who have received or are unsuitable for ASCT.

The second-generation immunomodulatory drug (IMID), lenalidomide, when combined with dexamethasone produced better TTP (11.3 months vs 4.7 months) and OS (35 months vs 31 months) compared to placebo and dexamethasone in previously treated patients. It produces responses in patients who have failed thalidomide. Lenalidomide with dexamethasone has a licence for use in first relapse of myeloma in the UK.

These new agents in myeloma have highlighted the difficulty in funding effective yet expensive drugs within the UK healthcare system. Bortezomib is approved by the SMC for third-line use. NICE originally rejected bortezomib for use in myeloma but later approved it for second-line use in conjunction with a drug company-funded re-imbursement scheme for non-responders. Lenalidomide has been rejected for use in Scotland by the SMC on cost-effectiveness grounds.

Patients progressing after ASCT may benefit from a second high-dose therapy and ASCT. Tandem transplants in close succession probably offer little benefit over repeat ASCT at progression. The physical and psychological morbidity of two ASCTs needs to be taken into account.

Older therapies including weekly cyclophosphamide and single-agent dexamethasone remain useful palliative treatments for some in the advanced multiply treated setting.

Additional therapies

- Pain control is very important. Analgesics, oral when possible, should be given as appropriate for the level of pain. These range from regular paracetamol to high doses of long-acting morphine identified through the titration of short-acting morphine. Non-steroidal anti-inflammatory drugs (NSAIDs) should be avoided because of their potential renal toxicity.
- Involved field radiotherapy is given for intractable bone pain and pressure effects such as cord compression. Long bone fractures should be surgically stabilized and then treated with involved field radiotherapy. Very precarious lytic lesions within long bones may benefit from prophylactic surgical pinning.

- A recent promising surgical development is kyphoplasty, which allows re-expansion of collapsed vertebrae with a balloon, followed by support of the collapsed vertebrae with injectable cement.
- Erythropoietin (EPO) can be used to reduce transfusion requirements with responses of the order of 70%, especially in patients with renal failure. The cost has limited its use within the UK and recent concerns over the use of EPO in solid tumours have led to added caution.

Prognosis

A number of prognostic factors have been identified to predict survival in myeloma. A system based on β_2 microglobulin levels and albumin has been accepted as the international staging system for predicting prognosis (see Table 25.13).

Table 25.13 New international staging system for myeloma

Criteria	Median survival (months)
I. Serum β_2 microglobulin <3.5 mg/l (296 nmol/l) and serum albumin >3.5 g/dl (532 μmol/l)	62
II. Neither I or III[a]	45
III. Serum β_2 microglobulin >5.5 mg/l (465 nmol/l)	29

[a]There are two subcategories: serum β_2 microglobulin <3.5 mg/l, but serum albumin <3.5 g/dl, or serum β_2 microglobulin 3.5–5.5 mg/l irrespective of the serum albumin level.

Further reading

Harrosseau J-L (2007) Multiple myeloma – ESMO clinical recommendations for diagnosis, treatment and follow-up. *Ann Oncol* **18(Suppl 2)**, 44–6.

Hoffbrand AV, Catovsky Daniel, Tuddenham EGD, eds. (2005) *Postgraduate Haematology*, 5th edn. Oxford: Blackwell Publishing.

Jost L (2007) Hodgkin's Disease: ESMO Clinical recommendations for diagnosis, treatment and follow-up. *Ann Oncol* **18(Suppl 2)**, 53–4.

Ludwig H, Strasser-Weippl K, Schreder M, Zojer N (2007) Advances in the treatment of hematological malignancies – current treatment approaches in multiple myeloma. *Ann Oncol*, **18(Suppl 2)**, 64–70.

Pui C-H, Robison LL, Look AT (2008) Acute lymphoblastic leukaemia. *Lancet*, **371**, 1030–43.

Swerlow SH, Campo E, Harris NL, *et al.*, eds. (2008) *WHO Classification of Tumours of haematopoietic and Lymphoid Tissues.* Lyon: IARC Press.

Wiernick PH, Goldman JM, Dutcher JP, Kyle RA, eds. (2003) *Neoplastic Diseases of the Blood*, 4th edn. Cambridge: Cambridge University Press.

Bone and soft-tissue malignancies

Osteosarcoma

Epidemiology and aetiology

Malignant bone tumours are rare, <550 new cases per annum in the UK. They account for only 0.2% of all new cancers but 5% of childhood cancers. Osteosarcoma is the commonest primary bone tumour, accounting for 20%.

- Bimodal distribution: 75% under 20 years, second peak >60 years.
- Occurs predominantly in adolescence with a peak incidence coinciding with the growth spurt.
- Cases occurring over the age of 40 years are usually associated with a recognized predisposing lesion:
  - Paget's disease
  - irradiated bone
  - multiple hereditary exostoses
  - polyostotic fibrous dysplasia.
- Male:female 1.6:1.
- Usually arise in the metaphysis of long bones.
- 60% arise around the knee.

Pathology

- Composed of malignant spindle cells and osteoblasts that produce osteoid or immature bone.
- 'Classic' subtype is a central medullary tumour.
- Rarer types with a better prognosis include parosteal, periosteal, and low-grade intra-osseous osteosarcoma.
- Local invasion into the medulla and through the bony cortex.
- Soft tissue extension, less often joint space invasion.
- Vascular invasion is common.
- Typical sites for metastatic disease are lung and bone.
- 75% have occult or overt metastatic disease at presentation.

Genetics

Occasionally associated with Li–Fraumeni syndrome (germline mutation of *p53*) or hereditary retinoblastoma.

Presenting symptoms and signs

- Most present with pain at the tumour site.
- May have associated bone or soft tissue swelling.
- Overlying erythema and tenderness.
- Pathological fracture infrequently.

Investigations

Plain X-rays of the affected area are often sufficient to suggest the diagnosis of osteosarcoma. The classic radiological features of osteosarcoma:

- poorly delineated or absent margins around the bone lesion
- periosteal reaction, usually non-continuous and thin, with multiple laminations
- new bone formation with calcification of the matrix
- bone destruction.

There are no specific tumour markers, but serum alkaline phosphatase is elevated in 50% of cases.

> **Note**: Histological confirmation of the radiological diagnosis of a primary bone tumour must be deferred until the patient is assessed by a surgeon with expertise in the management of bone malignancies.

Staging investigations

- Magnetic resonance imaging (MRI) scan to assess local extent of tumour, intramedullary tumour, and skip metastases along the bone, soft tissue extension
- Computerized tomography (CT) chest for lung metastasis
- Isotope bone scan

Several staging systems for bone tumours exist, the most commonly used being that described by Enneking (see Table 26.1). The stage is derived from a combination of the histological grade of the tumour, the presence or absence of distant metastases, and the extent of local spread of disease.

Management of patients with osteosarcoma

Surgical resection (usually amputation of a limb) alone was used to treat osteosarcomas until the 1970s. Overall survival was only 15–20%, largely because of pulmonary metastatic disease. Subsequent use of chemotherapy in the adjuvant (post-operative) or neo-adjuvant (pre- and post-operative) setting has improved the 5-year survival rate to 55–70%. Surgical management has also improved in the past 20 years, with amputation being replaced in the majority of patients by limb-sparing surgery, usually with endoprosthetic replacement of the resected bone.

Pre-operative assessment

- Biopsy of suspected osteosarcoma must be performed by an orthopaedic specialist with experience of this technique. In 1990, only 20% of patients referred to MD Anderson Cancer Centre had correctly placed biopsy sites. Today, most patients have the biopsy performed by a specialist.
- Ideally the biopsy should be performed by the surgeon who will undertake the definitive resection.
- Trephine or core biopsy is recommended.
- Potential tumour contamination of all tissue planes and compartments traversed by the biopsy needle, so biopsy tract will have to be removed *en bloc* during definitive resection.
- Incorrectly sited biopsy may necessitate amputation instead of limb-sparing surgery.
- Angiography may be necessary when limb-sparing procedure is planned to determine individual vascular pattern before resection, especially proximal tibial lesions.

Table 26.1 Enneking staging of bone tumours

Stage	Grade	Site[a]	Metastasis
1A	Low	Intracompartmental	Absent
1B	Low	Extracompartmental	
2A	High	Intracompartmental	Absent
2B	High	Extracompartmental	
3	Low or high	Intracompartmental or extracompartmental	Present

[a]Extracompartmental disease breaches fascial planes.

Chemotherapy

The outcome for patients with osteosarcomas has been markedly improved with the addition of chemotherapy to surgery. The most active agents are:

- doxorubicin
- cisplatin
- high-dose methotrexate
- ifosfamide.

Chemotherapy is commonly given pre- and post-operatively. This has several potential benefits:

- treatment starts without delay (production of a customized endoprosthesis takes several weeks)
- tumour volume may be reduced by chemotherapy, making surgery easier
- allows the pathological assessment of response to chemotherapy in the resected tumour, with possibility of introducing alternative cytotoxics post-operatively.

Typically 2–3 cycles of chemotherapy are delivered, followed by surgery, followed by a further 3–4 cycles of chemotherapy.

Surgery

Sarcomas grow radially and produce a pseudocapsule. Osteosarcoma invariably spreads through the capsule and expert surgery is necessary to ensure *en bloc* resection with wide clear margins to remove all viable tumour. While previously amputation was almost always necessary for limb osteosarcomas, approximately 95% of osteosarcomas at these sites are now treated successfully with limb-sparing techniques. A wide variety of endo-prosthetic devices are available, including extendable prostheses for growing children and, again, success, both eradication of all local tumour and achievement of a functional limb, is dependent on the expertise of the surgeon.

Limb-sparing resection requires:

- no involvement of major neurovascular bundle
- wide resection of affected bone
- *en bloc* removal of previous biopsy sites
- resection of bone 4 cm beyond CT, MRI, bone scan uptake
- resection of adjacent joint
- adequate muscle reconstruction with transfers.

This is only done in designated specialized centres and the diseased bone is replaced by a custom-made endoprosthesis or nodular segmental prostheses. While vascular reconstruction is possible, having to sacrifice mixed nerves is a limiting step in functioning preservation of the limb. Relative contraindications to limb-sparing surgery include major neurovascular involvement, pathological fractures (tumour cells spread via the haematoma), infection, and extensive muscle involvement.

Previously, a tumour thought to be benign and which turned out to be malignant, after inappropriate surgery, would require amputation, but more recently limb salvage in selected cases may be possible.

Radiotherapy

Osteosarcomas are relatively radioresistant. Radiotherapy is rarely used in the primary treatment of this disease. Its use is limited to:

- high-dose palliative treatment for patients who refuse surgery or for axial osteosarcomas that are not respectable
- adjuvant therapy after surgery and chemotherapy when excision has been marginal
- palliative treatment of bone metastases.

Metastatic osteosarcoma

Around 15% of new cases have metastatic disease at presentation. With combination chemotherapy, followed by resection of the primary and, when feasible, resection of metastatic disease, long-term survival can be achieved in 20–30%.

Careful follow-up of patients with localized disease is essential.

- Most patients who relapse have pulmonary metastases.
- Up to 30% of relapsing patients may be salvaged by surgical resection of the metastases.
- Metastasectomy may be considered for multiple and bilateral lung deposits and on more than one occasion.
- Local recurrences are managed by surgical resection (usually amputation) or palliative irradiation.
- The role of chemotherapy after surgery for relapsed disease is uncertain.
- The outcome of palliative treatment with second-line chemotherapy for unresectable tumours is poor.

Treatment outcomes and prognostic factors

- Operable localized disease 60–70% 5-year survival:
  - limb conservation does not compromise survival compared with amputation.
- Metastatic disease 10–30% 5-year survival.
- Better prognosis with limb versus axial primary.
- Response to chemotherapy:
  - good response >95% cell kill in resected specimen conveys 80% 5-year survival and is seen in ~60% of patients with current regimens
  - poor response to chemotherapy conveys 40–50% 5-year survival.

Recent developments

A worldwide co-operative study is currently examining the benefits of maintenance interferon after MAP (high-dose methotrexate, doxorubicin, cisplatin) chemotherapy and of chemotherapy intensification with addition of ifosfamide and etoposide in poorly responding tumours after surgery – the EURAMOS-1 (European and American Osteosarcoma Study Group) trial.

Ewing's sarcoma

First described by James Ewing, New York pathologist, in 1926. This is another rare but highly malignant primary bone tumour. Until the introduction of combination chemotherapy in the 1970s, 90% of patients with this diagnosis died, usually from metastatic disease.

Epidemiology and aetiology

- Annual incidence 0.6 per million
- 6–10% of all primary bone tumours
- Less common in non-Caucasians
- Peak age 10–20 years
- Aetiology is unknown
- Not associated with cancer family syndromes
- May affect any bone; 55% arise in the axial skeleton
- May also arise in soft tissue.

Pathology

The Ewing's sarcoma family of tumours includes:

- Ewing's tumour of bone
- peripheral primitive neuroectodermal tumour (PNET)
- Askin tumour (arising on chest wall).

They are believed to arise from neural crest cells. Microscopy shows small round blue cells with rosette formation and positive staining for:

- MIC2 (CD99)
- neural markers (NSE, S100)
- glycogen (PAS).

Typically they arise in the diaphysis of long bones or in flat bones, e.g. pelvis, invade through the medulla, but also extend through cortex to form a significant soft tissue extra-osseous mass in at least 50%. Blood-borne spread to lung and bone is common, and 20–25% have overt metastases at presentation. Microscopic systemic disease is present in the majority of patients with radiologically localized disease.

Genetics

More than 95% have rearrangement of chromosome 22, usually an 11;22 translocation, to produce an oncogenic transcription factor.

Presenting symptoms and signs

- Painful bony swelling.
- Overlying tissues warm and red.
- Axial lesions may cause pain with compression of abdominal organs, urinary tract, or nerve.
- 10% have fever and a hot swollen limb mimicking osteomyelitis.

Investigations

- Plain X-ray typically shows a destructive, osteolytic lesion, with periosteal elevation, although 25% have a sclerotic component.
- MRI scan demonstrates both osseous and extra-osseous disease extent.

- May have anaemia, elevated erythrocyte sedimentation rate (ESR)/ C-reactive protein (CRP), and high LDH.
- Patients with suspected bone malignancy must be referred to an orthopaedic oncologist for biopsy – inappropriate biopsy siting can result in tumour spillage and unnecessary requirement for limb amputation.
- Core biopsy, with material sent fresh to the laboratory to allow cytogenetics.

Staging

- CT chest and abdomen
- Isotope bone scan
- MRI of primary lesion and any hot spots identified on bone scan, with estimate of primary tumour volume.
- Bone marrow aspirate (×2) and trephine from sites distant from known disease

Prior to therapy, tests of normal organ function should include:

- full blood count (FBC) and biochemistry
- renal function (EDTA (ethylenediaminetetra-acetic acid) clearance)
- electrocardiogram (ECG) and left ventricular ejection fraction (mutigated acquisition test (MUGA) or echocardiogram)
- pulmonary function tests
- viral titres.

Management of Ewing's tumours

All patients should be managed in a cancer centre with appropriate multidisciplinary expertise and experience. They should wherever possible be treated within multi-institutional trials, currently in Europe the Euro-Ewing 99 study.

Broadly, management consists of:

- initial chemotherapy, e.g. 6 cycles VIDE – vincristine, ifosfamide, doxorubicin, etoposide
- local therapy to the primary tumour, e.g. surgery, radiotherapy, or both (chemotherapy continues concomitant with radiotherapy)
- further chemotherapy (up to another 8 cycles of conventional chemotherapy or high-dose therapy with peripheral blood stem cell support).

Chemotherapy

Over the last 20 years dose intensification and incorporation of new cyto-toxics have led to significant improvement in the outcome of treatment, but at the cost of significant toxicities.

- Venous access requires Hickman line, portacath, or portable intensive care (PIC) line.
- Profound myelosuppression occurs in all patients during chemotherapy.
- Risk of neutropenic sepsis is reduced by prophylactic use of granulocyte colony-stimulating factor (G-CSF) and antibiotics.
- *Pneumocystis carinii* prophylaxis is required.
- Febrile neutropenia must be treated promptly with broad-spectrum antibiotics.

- Close attention to hydration, anti-emetics, and mouth care.
- Careful monitoring of renal, hepatic, and cardiac function.
- Risk of graft versus host reaction; blood products must be irradiated before use and leucocyte filters used for transfusion.
- These young patients require considerable psychosocial and educational support.

Local therapy of the primary tumour

Surgery should be considered in all cases and, if it is possible to remove the entire tumour without undue mutilation, then it is the local treatment of choice. Surgical developments mean that there are few bones in the body that are not amenable to surgery, including the pelvis. Overall randomized trials have shown that survival from Ewing's is better with surgery plus radiotherapy compared with radiotherapy alone. Limb salvage is increasingly used with a goal of 'wide' clear surgical margins.

Following surgery, radiotherapy is given if excision margins are close or positive (44–54 Gy in 1.8 Gy fractions), and inoperable tumours are treated with radiotherapy only (54–64 Gy). The volume irradiated includes the original tumour with 2–5 cm margins, often shrinking the volume after 44 Gy.

Management of metastatic disease

Patients presenting with metastatic disease are managed initially as above with induction chemotherapy followed by local therapy to the primary tumour.

- Patients with lung metastases may then be treated with conventional chemotherapy and whole-lung irradiation (18 Gy in 10 fractions) or high-dose chemotherapy, e.g. busulphan and melphalan with peripheral blood stem cell support.
- Patients with bone or marrow metastases have a poorer prognosis and high-dose chemotherapy may be considered for many of these.

Treatment outcomes and prognostic factors

- 5-year survival:
  - localized disease, 55–65%
  - metastatic disease, 10–20%
  - lung only metastases, 30%.

The major prognostic factors are:

- metastases at presentation
- site and volume of the primary:
  - tumour <100 ml in a long bone, 80% 5-year survival
  - pelvic tumour, 30% 5-year survival
- pathological response to chemotherapy
- local therapy (surgery better than radiotherapy).

Late effects

- Cardiomyopathy (anthracyclines)
- Nephrotoxicity (ifosfamide)
- Infertility
- Second malignancy (leukaemia, osteosarcoma).

Further reading

Burchill SA (2003) Ewing's sarcoma: diagnostic, prognostic and therapeutic implications of molecular abnormalities. *J Clin Pathol* **56**, 96–102.

Fuchs B, Ossendorf C, Leerapun T, Sim FH (2008) Intercalary segmental reconstruction after bone tumour resection. *Eur J Surg Oncol* **34**, 1271–6.

Gobel V, Jurgens H, Etspuler G, *et al.* (1987) Prognostic significance of tumour volume in localised Ewing's sarcoma of bone in children and adolescents. *J Cancer Res Clin Oncol* **113**, 187–91.

Iwamoto Y (2007) Diagnosis and treatment of Ewing's Sarcoma. *Jpn J Clin Oncol* **37**, 79–89.

Kelley SP, Ashford RU, Rao AS, *et al.* (2007) Primary bone tumours of the spine: a 42 year survey from the Leeds Regional Bone Tumour Registry. *Eur Spine J* **16**, 405–409.

Paulussen M, Bielack S, Jurgens H, Jost L (2008) Ewing's sarcoma of the bone – ESMO clinical recommendations for diagnosis, treatment and follow-up. *Ann Oncol* **19(Suppl)**, 97–8.

Schuck A, Ahrens S, Paulussen M, *et al.* (2003) Local therapy in localized Ewing tumours. Results of 1058 patients treated in the CESS 81, CESS 86, and EICESS 92 trials. *Int J Radiat Oncol Biol Phys* **55**, 168–77.

Scully SP, Temple HT, O'Keefe RJ, *et al.* (1995) Role of surgical resection in pelvic Ewing's sarcoma. *J Clin Oncol* **13**, 2336–41.

Skubitz KM, D'Adamo DR (2007) Sarcoma. *Mayo Clin Proc* **82(11)**, 1409–32.

Other primary bone tumours

Primary malignant spindle cell sarcoma of bone

Most often malignant fibrous histiocytoma, but other pathologies include liposarcoma, angiosarcoma, leiomyosarcoma, haemangiopericytoma.

- All are rare, <1% of all bone tumours.
- Arise in any bone (usually the metaphysis of a long bone).
- Occur mainly in middle age.
- Can occur after a previous insult to the bone, e.g. ionizing radiation, bone infarct, or fibrous dysplasia.

The treatment is surgical removal of all disease but, as with osteosarcoma, limb-sparing surgery and insertion of a customized endoprosthesis may be feasible. The role of adjuvant chemotherapy has been explored using agents including doxorubicin and cisplatin, or ifosfamide in pre-operative therapy, with promising results. Greater than 90% necrosis in the resected bone is reported after chemotherapy in ~40%.

Metastatic disease may require:
- lung resection for solitary metastasis
- palliative chemotherapy using the above agents.

Chondrosarcoma

- Cartilage-forming malignancy.
- Tumours of middle to late age.
- Second most common primary bone tumour (~20%).
- Typically presents with painful enlarging mass in the pelvis, proximal femur, humerus, or ribs; unusual in distal bones.
- Grade is a good guide to behaviour, although about 10% of low-grade tumours transform to a higher grade.
- Treatment is surgical resection with limb conservation if possible – for cure, surgical excision is essential – usually wide excision (tumour is often low grade) and limb-sparing surgery is possible.
- No proven role for adjuvant chemotherapy.
- Radiotherapy after incomplete resection or palliation of advanced disease.
- Grade 1, 90%, grade 3, 40% 5-year survival.
- Metastatic disease managed similarly to malignant fibrous histiocytoma (MFH) (see 📖 Soft tissue sarcomas, p.590), although palliative chemotherapy may not be appropriate for older patients. Some of these tumours are oestrogen receptor positive, and may respond to anti-oestrogen therapy.

Chordoma

- Slow-growing tumour that arises from notochord remnants.
- Accounts for 2–4% primary bone tumours.
- Sited in the sacrum/coccyx (50%), skull base/clivus (35%), or upper cervical vertebrae.
- Presents in middle age with persistent pain.
- Often only discovered on CT or MRI after 'normal' plain X-rays of the bone.
- Metastases are rare (lung or bone).

- Survival determined by the success or failure of local control.
- Surgery is the treatment of choice but may not be feasible or may cause significant morbidity because of the tumour site. Surgery with wide excision is the only chance of cure – removing the sacral bone one level higher than the tumour.
- Radiotherapy (55–60 Gy) after incomplete resection or as palliation.
- Particle therapy with protons has shown some promise.
- 30–50% survive 5 years but late recurrences are possible.

Solitary plasmacytoma

- Isolated painful lytic bone lesion rich in plasma cells.
- Age 50–60 years, males > females 2:1.
- Diagnosis depends on the exclusion of myeloma (no other skeletal lesions, no hypercalcaemia, no suppression of other immunoglobulins, and bone marrow contains <5% plasma cells).
- Paraproteinaemia is common.
- Treatment is with radiotherapy (40–45 Gy).
- Prognosis is good; median survival 10 years.
- Follow-up important as 50% developed multiple myeloma.

Primary bone lymphoma

- 3% of primary bone tumours; 2% of all non-Hodgkin's lymphoma (NHL) cases.
- Age 50–70 years.
- Painful lytic or mixed lytic sclerotic bone lesion.
- Core biopsy shows malignant, small, round, dark cell tumours of bone (differentiate from, e.g., Ewing's, metastatic neuroblastoma).
- Staging with CT, bone scan, and bone marrow examination is required to exclude systemic lymphoma.
- Localized high-grade NHL is treated with initial chemotherapy (e.g. CHOP (cyclophosphamide, hydroxodoxorubicin, vincristine, prednisolone)).
- Followed by either radiotherapy or surgical excision and endoprosthesis (latter is preferred for long, weight-bearing bones, where there is otherwise a high risk of fracture).
- 60% 5-year survival.

Soft-tissue sarcomas

Epidemiology
- Rare; ~1200 cases per annum in the UK.
- 1% of adult cancers, 6% childhood cancers.
- 15% occur in children; 4th commonest childhood cancer.
- Age distribution depends on pathology:
  - rhabdomyosarcoma in children/young adults
  - synovial sarcoma in young adults
  - MFH and liposarcoma in older adults.

Aetiology
- Genetic associations:
  - neurofibromatosis NF1 predisposes to malignant peripheral nerve sheath tumour
  - hereditary retinoblastoma;
  - Li–Fraumeni syndrome (germline mutation of p53).
- Radiation exposure, usually therapeutic many years previously, e.g. angiosarcoma following breast irradiation.
- Rarely, chemical exposure (vinyl chloride, herbicides, dioxins).

Pathology
Although the histological classification is complex, staging and management are similar for most. Histological grading is crucial. Low-grade sarcomas rarely metastasize, grow slowly with development of a pseudocapsule, and may be dealt with successfully by surgery alone. High-grade sarcomas are locally invasive, may recur after surgery, and metastasize typically to lung by blood-borne spread. High-grade tumours account for 50% of sarcomas, and of these 50% die of metastatic disease. Lymphatic spread is less common, but may occur in epithelioid or synovial sarcoma or rhabdomyosarcoma. Fresh tissue for cytogenetic analysis may assist in the classification of soft tissue sarcomas (see Table 26.2).

Presenting symptoms and signs
- Most present with a painless soft tissue mass.
- 45% lower limb, 15% upper limb, 10% head and neck, 15% retroperitoneal.
- Any enlarging mass, deep to deep fascia, should be regarded as a potential sarcoma.
- However, up to 30% of soft-tissue sarcomas are subcutaneous.

Investigations
- Imaging with MRI to assess local extent of the tumour mass and its relationship to adjacent structures including blood vessels and nerves.
- Chest X-ray and CT chest looking for lung metastases.
- Core biopsy and imaging should be performed before an attempt is made to excise any potentially malignant soft tissue tumour. The only exception to this rule may be retroperitoneal and pelvic sarcomas, where core biopsy may carry the risk of tumour spillage and spread.

- Multidisciplinary planning of individual patients' management is crucial, involving pathologist, radiologist, site specialist surgeons, clinical and medical oncologist.

Pathological classification of soft-tissue sarcomas

- Alveolar soft part sarcoma (ASPS)
- Angiosarcoma
- Clear cell sarcoma
- Dermatofibrosarcoma protuberans (DFSP)
- Desmoplastic small round-cell tumour
- Epitheliod sarcoma
- Extra-osseous Ewing's tumor
- Extraskeletal chondrosarcoma
- Extraskeletal osteosarcoma
- Fibrosarcoma
- Gastrointestinal stromal tumour (GIST)
- Kaposi's sarcoma
- Leiomyosarcoma
- Liposarcoma
- Malignant fibrous histiocytoma (MFH)
- Malignant giant cell tumor of tendon sheath
- Malignant hemangiopericytoma
- Malignant peripheral nerve sheath tumour (MPNST)
- Malignant solitary fibrous tumour
- Rhabdomyosarcoma (RMS)
- Synovial sarcoma.

Table 26.2 Cytogenetic abnormalities in sarcomas and the genes involved

Sarcoma	Translocation	Genes involved
Ewing's tumours	11;22	EWS-Fli1
Liposarcoma (myxoid and round cell)	12;16	TLS (FUS)-CHOP
Synovial sarcoma	x;18	SYT-SSX1 and 2
Rhabdomyosarcoma (alveolar)	2;13	PAX3-FKHR
Clear-cell sarcoma	12;22	EWS-ATF1

Staging system

- Combination of grading, tumour size, and evidence of metastatic spread (see Table 26.3).
- Primary tumour is staged by size:
  - T1 <5 cm
  - T2 >5 cm.

Table 26.3 Staging of soft tissue sarcomas

Stage groupings	Tumour grade	Primary tumour	Lymph node status	Metastasis
I	G1	T1–2	N0	M0
II	G2	T1–2	N0	M0
III	G3	T1–2	N0	M0
IVA	Any	Any	N1	M0
IVB	Any	Any	N0	M1

Management of soft-tissue sarcomas

Surgery

Ideally, localized sarcomas are managed by complete excision with clear margins and en bloc removal of any biopsy tract. For limb tumours surgery is classified according to its extent:

- **intralesional or intracapsular** – excision passes through the tumour with involved margins and the risk of local recurrence approaches 100%; most commonly such procedures are performed without a pre-operative diagnosis of sarcoma, and without pre-operative imaging. The outcome for patients managed this way is significantly poorer than with appropriately planned radical excision. They require urgent referral to an orthopaedic oncologist usually for staging and imaging of local residual disease and more radical surgery
- **marginal** – tumour shelled out through the pseudocapsule, recurrence rate 20–70% depending on tumour pathology
- **wide excision** – wide margin of local tissue removed along with tumour, adequate for low-grade sarcoma but up to 30% recurrence rate with high-grade disease, usually due to unsuspected non-contiguous tumour extension beyond the surgical field
- **radical excision** – en bloc dissection of tumour and muscular compartment; low risk of local recurrence, but may lead to unacceptable loss of function. Resection limits of 2 cm of uninvolved tissue is now adequate (previously attempts were made to excise full muscle from origin to insertion). Skin and bony involvement are unusual
- **limb amputation** is infrequently indicated, if disease cannot be completely excised with conservation of a functional limb. Amputation rate was 50% in the 1960s and is now 5%. Current data at 10 years show that, while local recurrence is higher with limb-salvage surgery, there is no difference in disease-free survival.

For the majority of soft-tissue sarcomas arising at other sites, surgery is the mainstay of local treatment. Locally advanced disease not amenable to primary surgery may be treated with pre-operative radiotherapy or chemotherapy in order to facilitate resection. Surgery may also be appropriate for local recurrence and for metastatic disease, in particular solitary pulmonary metastasis.

Chemotherapy

The majority of adult soft tissue sarcomas are only moderately chemo-sensitive. The most active agents are doxorubicin and ifosfamide, with response rates of 10–30% to these agents either singly or in combination in advanced disease. The role of adjuvant chemotherapy remains controversial, with little evidence to support its use in an effort to improve cure rates. For some specific pathologies (e.g. extra-osseous Ewing's/PNET), chemotherapy has a major impact on survival; the benefits of chemotherapy in other adult sarcomas are less clear. A meta-analysis has examined data from 14 trials involving >1500 patients. Although adjuvant chemotherapy reduces the risk of disease recurrence (by 10% at 10 years), no significant survival benefit has been demonstrated. Progress in this field is likely to be dependent on improved understanding of the biological differences between the various pathologies, and individualization of therapy according to molecular predictors of behaviour and response to treatment.

Radiotherapy

Most adult soft tissue sarcomas are only moderately radiosensitive. The most important role for radiotherapy is in the post-operative adjuvant setting, particularly for high-grade sarcomas treated by wide excision. Even when excision margins are clear, non-contiguous microscopic residual tumour may be present within the muscle compartment. Post-operative radiotherapy to the conserved limb may be delivered using a shrinking field technique, phase I 50 Gy/25 fractions, phase II 10–16 Gy. A strip of normal tissue along the length of the limb should be left unirradiated to reduce the risk of chronic lymphoedema. Lower doses of radiation are given following resection of retroperitoneal sarcomas, limited by normal tissue tolerance of the abdominal contents (e.g. 50 Gy/25 fractions). A number of investigators are examining the potential benefits of intra-operative radiotherapy after resection of sarcomas at a number of sites.

Novel therapies

Gastrointestinal (GI) stromal tumours are the commonest sarcomas in the GI tract and account for 5% of soft tissue sarcomas.

- Incidence 10–20 per million.
- 20–30% malignant.
- Most commonly arise in the stomach or small bowel.
- Rarely familial or associated with NF1 or Carney's triad.
- The majority have a gain of function mutation in the proto-oncogene *KIT*, which encodes the transmembrane receptor for stem cell factor.
- *KIT* expression can be detected by immunohistochemistry with CD117.
- Imatinib inhibits the KIT tyrosine kinase.
- Mainstay of treatment of these tumours is surgery.
- Inoperable recurrence or metastatic disease is unresponsive to conventional chemotherapy with median survival 10–20 months.
- Objective response rate with imatinib 400 mg daily ~50% with median survival time >36 months.
- Common mild/moderate toxicities: oedema, anaemia, nausea, lethargy, diarrhoea, skin rash, myelosuppression.

- Imatinib-resistant disease can respond to increased-dose imatinib (albeit with increased toxicity).
- Some evidence that even resistant disease benefits from continued therapy, with rapid acceleration of tumour growth after cessation of imatinib.
- Other targeted agents, e.g. sunitinib, have demonstrated activity in refractory disease.
- Individualization of therapy may be possible in the next few years according to the mutation of *c-KIT*.
- Trials of adjuvant therapy have been completed and mature results are awaited.
- Imatinib also active against unresectable dermatofibrosarcoma protruberans (DFSP).

Treatment outcome and prognostic factors for soft-tissue sarcomas

Treatment outcomes worse with:
- large tumours
- deep vs superficial tumours
- high-grade sarcoma
- intralesional excision
- visceral/retroperitoneal vs limb primary
- metastatic disease at presentation.

Overall the 5-year survival is around 70%, but 50% for stage III, and around 20% for stage IV. Patients who relapse with only pulmonary meta-stasis may be cured by metastatectomy.

Rhabdomyosarcoma

- Commonest soft tissue tumour in childhood and adolescence.
- >50% in children under 10 years.
- Rare in adults over 40 years.
- Male:female ratio 1.3:1.
- Arises from primitive mesenchymal cells with the capacity for rhabdomyoblastic development.
- Commonest sites of origin are:
  - head and neck
  - genitourinary tract
  - retroperitoneal
  - extremities.
- Disease is locally invasive (e.g. spreads from the orbit to the meninges and central nervous system).
- Disseminates to lymph nodes, lungs, bones, marrow, and brain.
- Aggressive malignancy requiring multimodality treatment.
- Outlook depends on the disease site and histological subtype.
- All cases should be managed by an experienced multidisciplinary sarcoma team within a cancer centre, ideally.

Diagnosis

- Presents with soft-tissue swelling or other local symptoms, e.g. displacement of the eye, vaginal bleeding, or dysuria.
- For histological diagnosis it is advisable to obtain fresh tissue for chromosomal studies.

Embryonal RMS

- About 60% of cases.
- Mainly in children under 15 years.
- Head and neck (including orbit), genitourinary tract, retroperitoneal.
- Spectrum of cells from primitive round cells to rhabdomyoblasts.
- Botryoid RMS is a subtype characterized by polypoid growth, like a 'bunch of grapes' usually found in hollow organs, e.g. vagina, bladder, and nasopharyngeal sinuses.

Alveolar RMS

- Poorly differentiated round or oval cells forming irregular spaces and separated by fibrous septae, giving the appearance of 'alveoli'.
- Sometimes this appearance is absent but the uniform appearance of the cells is distinct from that of the embryonal variety.
- Diagnosis may be confirmed by the presence of a t(2;13) (q37;q14) or variant t(1;13) (p36;q14) chromosomal translocation.
- Significantly worse prognosis than embryonal RMS.

Pleomorphic RMS

- Rare adult soft-tissue tumour.
- Behaves similarly to other adult soft-tissue sarcomas.
- May be curable if localized, with surgery and radiotherapy.
- Poor prognosis for locally advanced or metastatic disease.

Staging

- MRI or CT of the primary site.
- CT scan of the thorax.
- Isotope bone scan.
- Bone marrow aspirate and trephine.
- Stage is usually assigned using the International Society of Paediatric Oncology (SIOP)–International Union Against Cancer (UICC) TNM (tumour, nodes, metastases) staging system.

Prognostic factors

The prognosis in RMS depends on pathology, site, size, extent of spread, and response to chemotherapy (see Table 26.4). Overall 5-year survival has improved considerably from 25% in the 1960s to 70% currently, largely through the introduction of systemic chemotherapy.

Management

Treatment is tailored according to the prognosis, balancing the need for effective local and systemic treatment against the late morbidity particularly of radiotherapy and chemotherapy.

Chemotherapy

- Often given before definitive local surgery.
- Vincristine and actinomycin D (dactinomycin) only for good-prognosis disease.
- Other drugs added for worse prognosis disease (e.g. ifosfamide, doxorubicin).
- High-dose chemotherapy may have a role in metastatic disease.

Local treatment

- Surgery ideally with complete removal of all local disease and lymph node sampling. Extensive surgery involving significant morbidity is **not** essential in embryonal RMS as this tumour is radio- and chemosensitive.
- Surgery may not be feasible because of tumour extent or may lead to unacceptable mutilation/loss of function.
- Given concomitant with chemotherapy, doses of 40–50 Gy will achieve local disease control.

Table 26.4 Prognostic factors in rhabdomyosarcoma

Good	Poor
Orbit, paratesticular, vagina, extremities	Parameningeal, retroperitoneal
Localized to tissue of origin	Contiguous spread, nodal or metastatic disease
Complete resection feasible	Unresectable
Embryonal histology	Alveolar histology
Infant or child	Adult
Complete response to chemotherapy	Poor response to chemotherapy

- However, serious long-term sequelae are associated with the combined modality treatment in children:
  - late damage to sensitive organs, e.g. bladder, eye, brain, testis, ovary, thyroid
  - risk of second malignancy
  - impaired bone growth.
- Radiotherapy may be safely omitted in infants and children with localized favourable-prognosis disease, e.g. embryonal RMS of the orbit.
- Extremity tumours, alveolar histology, and parameningeal tumours require radiotherapy.

Further reading

Casali PG, Jost L, Sleijfer S, et al. (2008) Soft tissue sarcomas: ESMO clinical recommendations for diagnosis, treatment and follow-up. *Ann Oncol* **19(Suppl)**, 89–93.

Siegel HJ, Sessions W, Casillas MA, et al. (2007) Synovial sarcoma: clinicopathologic features, treatment and prognosis. *Orthopedics* **30**, 1020–5.

Cancer of unknown primary (CUP)

Confirming the diagnosis

- Carcinoma of unknown primary tumour can be defined as: '*histologically confirmed metastases in the absence of identifiable primary tumour despite a standardized diagnostic approach*'.
- Common oncological problem representing up to 10% of all referrals.
- Male>female.
- Median age at presentation is ~60 years.
- Clinical presentation is usually with symptoms arising from the site of metastasis.

The priority is to:

- exclude potentially curable malignancies, e.g. germ cells, lymphomas, thyroid cancer
- only perform investigations that will change management, e.g. colonoscopy in a patient without obstructive bowel symptoms but with metastatic adenocarcinoma of probable lower gastrointestinal (GI) origin may **not** influence treatment choice
- identify specific clinical syndromes that predict responsiveness to therapy. These account for 20% of patients with CUP, e.g. squamous cell carcinoma metastatic to cervical lymph nodes treated as advanced head and neck cancer.

Before accepting the diagnosis of cancer of unknown primary site it is important that all patient undergo:

- a thorough history, including detailed family history
- a full physical examination, including pelvic, breast, and rectal examination
- minimum additional investigations, which are likely to include:
  - full blood count (FBC)
  - serum biochemistry including liver function tests (LFTs)
  - chest X-ray (CXR)
  - ultrasound scan (USS)/computerized tomography (CT) of the abdomen
  - positron emission tomography (PET) – has an increasing role with some studies reporting it has identified likely primary tumour sites in up to 40% of cases
- further investigations, including tumour markers, will depend on the clinical scenario. Common tumour markers, e.g. CA125, CA15-3, carcinoembryonic antigen (CEA), CA19-9, have only a limited role in diagnosis and prognosis
- discussion at appropriate multidisciplinary team (MDT) meeting, including review of available histology.

Investigation of metastases to lymph nodes and peritoneum

Metastases to lymph nodes are more common than presentation with visceral/bony metastases.

Axillary lymph nodes in women

- Metastatic adenocarcinoma in axillary lymph nodes may indicate an occult breast cancer, even with a negative mammogram.
- Magnetic resonance imaging (MRI) of the breasts should be considered if the mammogram is normal.
- Oestrogen receptor (ER)/progesterone receptor (PR) staining should be performed on the biopsy sample, either fine needle aspiration (FNA), ultrasound-guided core biopsy, or open biopsy.
- In the absence of distant metastatic disease, management is as for stage II breast carcinoma and is likely to include loco-regional therapy with surgical excision and radiation, with or without chemotherapy.
- This group remains potentially curable.

Cervical lymph nodes

- Squamous or undifferentiated carcinoma in cervical lymph nodes should:
  - have open biopsy instead of FNA if there is a possibility of lymphoma
  - be referred for full ear, nose, and throat (ENT) examination under anaesthetic with direct laryngoscopy and nasopharyngoscopy and biopsy of the naso-, oro-, and hypopharynx
  - usually be treated as head and neck cancer with involved neck nodes – radical loco-regional radiotherapy can result in median survival of several years especially if the nodes are high in the neck.
- PET scanning may also have a role.
- Thyroid cancer can be excluded by staining for thyroglobulin.
- Supraclavicular lymph node metastases are usually associated with widespread malignancy and have a poor prognosis.

Inguinal lymph nodes

- Careful examination of most patients with squamous cell carcinoma in inguinal nodes will demonstrate a detectable primary site in the anorectal or genital region.
- DRE (digital rectal examination), proctoscopy, and examination of the penis or vulva/vagina/cervix should be performed.
- Small anal cancers remain potentially curable despite local lymph node involvement.
- Treatment often includes inguinal node dissection and combined modality treatment with chemo-radiotherapy (as for locally advanced cervical cancer in women).
- Primary skin cancer should also be considered.

Retroperitoneal or mediastinal lymph nodes in men

- Elevated serum human chorionic gonadotropin (HCG) and alpha-fetoprotein (AFP) may suggest a germ cell origin.
- Poorly differentiated adenocarcinoma with feature of extragonadal germ cell malignancy is treated as non-seminomatous extragonadal germ cell malignancy.
- Intent is curative.
- Intensive chemotherapy, e.g. with bleomycin, etoposide, and cisplatin, should be given and is often associated with an excellent response, even in the absence of histological confirmation of germ cell cancer or elevated serum tumour markers.

Peritoneal carcinomatosis in women

- Adenocarcinoma with diffuse peritoneal disease has a gynaecological origin in 55% of cases (the majority from ovaries) and is often treated as stage III ovarian carcinoma — a trial of platinum-based chemotherapy with palliative intent may be pragmatic and good responses can be achieved.
- Other possibilities include:
  - primary peritoneal disease (occurs more commonly in women with *BRCA1* mutations),
  - the GI tract (particularly if mucin secreting)
  - breast.
- Serum CA125 and pelvic ultrasound may be useful but are not specific.
- Laparoscopy has an investigative role in selected cases to inspect intra-abdominal (especially gynaecological) organs and to take adequate biopsies.
- Debulking surgery should be considered if disease is large volume.
- Malignant ascites in women, even without evidence of solid disease, is treated as advanced ovarian cancer, often with long-term survival.

Investigation of metastases to other sites

Lung
- Identified on CXR or CT thorax.
- Bronchoscopy – for central lesions. Brushings or ideally biopsy for visible tumours. Washings if tumour not visible. Lymph nodes may be accessible by transbronchial needle aspiration ± USS guidance.
- CT- or USS-guided percutaneous biopsy – for peripheral lesions.
- Sputum cytology – low yield. Reserve if bronchoscopy not appropriate.
- Immunohistochemistry – may help identify primary:
  - CK-7, lung/breast
  - CK-20, colorectal
  - TTF-1, lung (surfactant apoprotein)
  e.g. CK-7 **and** TTP-1 positive – phenotype 94% specific for lung.
- PET may be useful for staging particularly if a lung primary is suspected or if the primary is not identified on CT.
- Primaries commonly metastasizing to lung including head and neck squamous cell carcinoma, breast, kidney, and large bowel.
- Resection of solitary metastases occasionally produces long-term survivors, e.g. from colorectal/renal primaries.

Liver
- Present in 20–30% of patients with CUP.
- Usually identified on USS or CT scan.
- Completion of staging investigations is required (see 📖 Confirming the diagnosis, p.600) to determine extent of disease and any obvious primary.
- Biopsy under image guidance after correction of coagulation is usually needed if treatment is to be considered. This guides prognosis and allows selection of therapy (core biopsy under image guidance gives more pathological information than FNA).
- Liver resection, often with pre-operative chemotherapy, can sometimes be considered for solitary or limited hepatic metastases with a resectable colorectal primary in the absence of disease elsewhere – this group remains potentially curable and requires involvement of an appropriate tertiary centre, usually via the local MDT.
- Common primary sites include GI tract and breast.
- If the patient appears disproportionately well for the volume of liver disease, consider atypical diagnoses, e.g. neuroendocrine tumours such as carcinoid.
- Otherwise, a group of patients with a poor prognosis.

Bone

- Isotope bone scans:
  - caution must be exercised in the interpretation of isotope bone scans, and correlation with the plain radiographs should always be made
  - multiple 'hot spots' in the presence of a clear history of malignancy almost certainly represent metastatic disease
  - certain non-neoplastic disorders, e.g. Paget's disease, may also demonstrate multi-focal uptake
  - the differential diagnosis for a solitary 'hot spot' is broad
  - conversely, multiple myeloma and certain other aggressive tumours may present with a 'normal' bone scan
  - MRI may give more information
  - Discussion with the orthopaedic team is advised before biopsy of a bone tumour of unknown aetiology. This is to prevent a poorly planned biopsy from jeopardizing the potential for a subsequent curative procedure or limb-salvage surgery.
- If adenocarcinoma on biopsy primary sites include:
  - commonly lung, prostate and breast
  - less frequently kidney and thyroid.
  - measure prostate-specific antigen (PSA) in men with metastases predominantly affecting bone, particularly if lesions are osteoblastic. Biopsy tissue may also stain for PSA. Even if PSA is not elevated consider treating as advanced prostate carcinoma.
- A solitary bone metastasis occasionally warrants radical treatment such as high-dose radiotherapy or resection with endoprosthetic replacement, e.g. may permit long-term survival in the occasional patient with a solitary metastasis from renal cell carcinoma.

Brain

- Metastases are the commonest form of intracranial tumour.
- Prognosis is often dictated by the extent of extracranial disease.
- Common potential primary sites include lung, breast, and melanoma.
- Leptomeningeal disease: also most commonly due to breast, lung and melanoma as well as large-cell lymphomas and leukaemias. Up to 7% remain of unknown primary despite investigations.

Investigation of a pleural effusion

- Send fluid for cytology and biochemistry.
- Malignancy is more likely to be the cause if:
  - the patient is older
  - there are other risk factors, e.g. smoking, past history of asbestos exposure
  - the effusion is an exudate.
- If the fluid is a transudate other diagnoses which can be considered include:
  - congestive cardiac failure
  - constrictive pericaridits
  - hypoalbuminaemia
  - nephrotic syndrome, etc.
- The differential diagnosis of an undiagnosed exudative effusion includes:
  - infection, e.g. bacterial pneumonia, tuberculosis
  - pulmonary embolism
  - inflammatory disorders, e.g. sarcoidosis, pancreatitis
  - metabolic causes, e.g. hypothyroidism.
- Malignant causes include:
  - metastatic carcinoma, e.g. breast or lung primary
  - lymphoma
  - mesothelioma
  - leukaemia
  - chylothorax
  - Meigs' syndrome (ovarian fibroma, ascites, pleural effusion)
  - paraproteinaemia, e.g. multiple myeloma.
- CT chest – to assess for:
  - thoracic lymphadenopathy
  - pulmonary/pleural primary
  - metastatic disease.
- Percutaneous pleural biopsy ± image guidance – under local anaesthetic. This has a low sensitivity for malignant mesothelioma.
- Thoracoscopy – much more sensitive, particularly for malignant causes of effusions.
- Open pleural biopsy – occasionally necessary.
- Bronchoscopy – rarely helpful unless the patient has imaging to suggest a parenchymal lesion or symptoms suggestive of intrapulmonary pathology, e.g. haemoptysis.

Aetiology and pathology of CUP

- Undetected primary site most likely to unusual metastatic potential of the tumour. Occasionally there has been regression of the primary (well recognized in melanoma). Primary may remain undetected even after post-mortem examination (25%).
- Pattern of metastatic disease is often very different from cases where the primary site is known, e.g. lung cancer causes bone metastases ten times more often when the primary site is known than when the lung cancer is occult.
- Mean age at diagnosis is 60 years. Third commonest cancer presentation in those ≥70 years old. Rare if ≤40 years old.
- Median survival of 4 months in most series. However, some clinical scenarios are associated with much longer survival and it is these that are important to identify.
- Diagnosis encompasses tumours from many primary sites with varying biologies.

Favourable prognostic factors

- Female sex
- Fewer sites of metastatic disease especially lymph node/soft tissue rather than liver /bone
- Good performance status
- Normal serum lactate dehydrogenase (LDH), albumin and white cell count

Light microscopy

Five broad groups can be identified by light microscopy and this guides further investigation:

- adenocarcinoma (60–70%)
- poorly differentiated carcinoma (20–30%) – can be confused with seminoma, amelanotic melanoma, and epidermal carcinoma
- undifferentiated malignancy (<5%) – further staining required to exclude lymphoma
- squamous carcinoma (<5%)
- neuroendocrine carcinoma – uncommon:
  - high-grade, poorly differentiated, e.g. most patients with metastatic small-cell anaplastic carcinoma have a bronchial primary identified either via CT thorax or on bronchoscopy
  - Low-grade well-differentiated, e.g. atypical carcinoid – see 🕮 p.342.

Immunohistochemistry

- Essential where germ-cell cancer or lymphoma are possibilities.
- Initial panel of stains likely to use antibodies to:
  - CEA
  - PSA
  - cytokeratin
  - vimentin
  - common leucocyte antigen (CLA).

e.g. CLA stain can usually make the distinction between carcinoma and lymphoma (see Table 27.1).

- ER/PR staining should be requested if presentation is compatible with metastatic breast cancer. However, other primary sites may be ER/PR positive, e.g. ovarian or endometrial.
- May help decide between possible primary sites although unfortunately few stains are specific, e.g. neuroendocrine markers and chorionic gonadotrophin may be found on many tumours other than small-cell lung cancer and germ-cell cancer, respectively.

Electron microscopy

- Useful for distinguishing lymphoma from carcinoma.
- Can sometimes assist in identifying neuroendocrine tumours, melanomas, and poorly differentiated sarcomas.

Genetic analysis

- A promising technique but currently not in mainstream clinical use.
- Identification of specific genetic abnormalities is limited to a few tumours at present, e.g. Ewing's sarcoma, rhabdomyosarcoma, non-Hodgkin's lymphoma.

Table 27.1 Site-specific immunohistochemical stains

Stain	Tumour
Common leucocyte antigen (CLA)	Lymphoma
B- and T-cell gene rearrangement	Non-Hodgkin's lymphoma
Prostate-specific antigen (PSA)	Prostate
Thyroglobulin	Thyroid

Management of CUP

- The priority is to identify:
  - curable malignancies
  - clinical syndromes that respond well to specific therapies, e.g. some patients fall into the categories described earlier and this guides management, e.g. adenocarcinoma in axillary lymph nodes in women is usually treated as stage II breast carcinoma (see 📖 Axillary lymph nodes in women, p.602).
- After appropriate investigation, if the patient still has a diagnosis of CUP and does not fall into any of the subgroups described previously, then empiric treatment can be considered. See Figure 27.1.
- The heterogeneity of this patient population makes interpretation of trial data difficult.
- With treatment, median survival is generally <1 year.
- Involvement of palliative care services is usually appropriate for all patients.

Local therapy

- **Radiotherapy**: for symptomatic metastases should be considered, e.g. for painful bone metastases or for brain metastases.
- **Surgery**: only a single metastatic site of disease may be identified despite full staging investigations. In most instances, other metastases become clinically evident within a short time. However, if no further disease is identified then resection should be considered. This approach occasionally produces long disease-free intervals. This approach requires careful discussion with the patient and assessment at a multidisciplinary meeting.

Systemic treatment

- Select appropriate patients who may benefit from chemotherapy with palliative intent, dependent on:
  - tumour characteristics (chemo-responsiveness)
  - patient characteristics including organ function, performance status, and quality-of-life issues
  - discussion with the patient and often their family.
- There are relatively few randomized trials of chemotherapy in CUP.

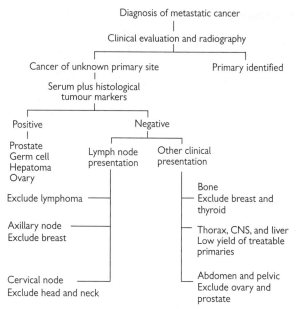

Fig. 27.1 Identification of treatable cancer of unknown primary site. Reproduced with permission from Cassidy J, Bissett D, Spence RAJ (1995) *Oxford Textbook of Oncology*, 1st edn. Oxford: Oxford University Press.

Further reading

Pavllidis N, Fizazi K (2005) Cancer of unknown primary (CUP). *Crit Rev Oncol Hematol* **54(3)**, 243–50.

Lazaridis G, Pentheroudakis G, Fountzilas G, Pavlidis N (2008) Liver metastases from cancer of unknown primary (CUPL): a retrospective analysis of presentation, management and prognosis in 49 patients and systematic review of the literature. *Cancer Treat Rev* **34**, 693–700.

Fizazi K (2008) Treatment of patients with specific subsets of carcinoma of inknown primary site. *Ann Oncol* **17(Suppl 10),** 177–80.

Paraneoplastic syndromes

Introduction

- These syndromes are caused by a cancer but are not due to direct local infiltration or metastatic spread.
- Occur in approximately 10% of cancer patients overall.
- Important to recognize because they may be the presenting feature of an undiagnosed cancer.

Cancers commonly associated with paraneoplastic syndromes (PS):

- lung: small cell (SCLC) and non-small cell (NSCLC)
- pancreatic
- lymphoma: non-Hodgkin's (NHL) and Hodgkin's lymphoma (HL)
- breast
- prostate
- ovary.

Although the mechanisms of PS are not fully understood, there appear to be two main causes:

- the inappropriate secretion of hormones and/or growth factors
- the production of anti-tumoural antibodies that cross-react with normal tissue antigens.

Endocrine paraneoplastic syndromes

Syndrome of inappropriate ADH (SIADH)

The most common endocrine PS is due to inappropriate secretion of antidiuretic hormone (arginine–vasopressin).

Cancer types
- SCLC (10% of patients), pancreatic, prostate, NHL, HL.

Presentation
- Often asymptomatic. CNS effects – fatigue, headaches; progressing to altered mental state, confusion, and seizures.

Diagnosis
- Exclude non-malignant causes, e.g. central nervous system (CNS) disease (infection, trauma, vascular), pulmonary disease (infections, cystic lesions, asthma), drug-induced (thiazides, cytotoxics, narcotics); clinically euvolaemic; laboratory studies.

Management
- Fluid restriction (0.5–1.0 l/day); democlocycline (150–300 mg, 8 hourly).

Laboratory criteria for diagnosis of SIADH
- Hyponatraemia Na+ <130 mmol/l
- Normal serum albumin and glucose
- Serum hypo-osmolarity <275 mmol/kg
- Urine osmolarity > serum osmolarity
- Urinary sodium >25 mmol/l
- Non-suppressed ADH

Cushing's syndrome

Inappropriate overproduction of adenocorticotrophic hormone (ACTH) precursors.

Cancer types
- SCLC, NSCLC, pancreatic, thymic, and carcinoid tumours

Presentation
- Rapid onset, marked weakness secondary to proximal myopathy, hyperpigmentation, metabolic disturbances (e.g. hyperglycaemia, hypokalaemic alkalosis)

Diagnosis
- Clinical features, especially hyperpigmentation, myopathy; hypo-kalaemia and metabolic alkalosis; high 24-h urinary cortisol, high plasma ACTH/precursors, no response to high-dose dexamethasone suppression or corticotrophin-releasing hormone stimulation

Management
- Specific anti-tumour treatment. Decrease cortisol secretion either surgically (bilateral adrenalectomy) or medically (metyrapone, octreotide, ketoconazole)

Hypercalcaemia

A common problem that in many cases is due to bony metastases. True paraneoplastic hypercalcaemia is due to tumour production of parathyroid hormone-related protein. This syndrome is called humoral hypercalcaemia of malignancy (HHM).

Cancer types
- NSCLC, head and neck, renal, other squamous cancers (rare in breast cancer where hypercalcaemia is usually due to bone metastases)

Presentation
- Rapid onset of nausea, polyuria, polydipsia, dehydration, cardiac arrhythmias

Diagnosis
- Serum Ca^{2+} >2.7 mmol/l, serum chloride low, hypercalcuria, high urinary phosphate, low/undetectable plasma parathyroid hormone

Management
- Saline hydration, IV pamidronate (60–120 mg)

Hypocalcaemia

Associated with tumours with lytic bone metastases (breast, prostate, and lung); can also occur with calcitonin-secreting medullary carcinomas of the thyroid. Usually asymptomatic. Rarely develop tetany and neuromuscular irritability. Treatment with calcium infusions.

Hypoglycaemia

Rarely caused by non-islet cell pancreatic tumours; often associated with mesenchymal tumours of the mediastinum and retroperitoneum and with hepatic cancers. Most likely cause is tumour production of the precursor to insulin-like growth factor II. Treatment with glucose infusions, tumour debulking.

Neurological paraneoplastic syndromes

- Common, occurring in up to 7% of cancer patients. Most common syndromes are:
  - peripheral neuropathy
  - proximal myopathy.
- Thought to be secondary to autoimmune mechanisms via production of anti-tumour antibodies.
- Treatment is based upon treatment of the cancer and decreasing antibody production by immune system suppression.
- Response to treatment is often poor (except for Lambert–Eaton myasthenic syndrome (LEMS)).

Peripheral neuropathy (PN)

Asymptomatic PN is common; symptomatic PN less so. Usually occurs after diagnosis of cancer has been made and caused by axonal degeneration or demyelination. Many types of PN, e.g. motor, sensory, autonomic, sensorimotor.

- **Cancer types**: SCLC, myeloma, HD, breast, GI cancers
- **Presentation**: depends upon type and site
- **Diagnosis**: exclude non-paraneoplastic causes; nerve conduction studies, nerve biopsy – look for inflammatory infiltrates; serum anti-Hu antibodies in some cases
- **Management**: corticosteroids; treat underlying cancer.

Encephalomyelopathies

Perivascular inflammation and selective neuronal degeneration at several levels of the nervous system. Can affect the limbic system, brainstem, and spinal cord.

- **Cancer types**: SCLC (75% of cases), breast, ovary, NHL
- **Presentation**: slow, subacute onset; progressive
- **Diagnosis**:
  - cerebrospinal fluid (CSF) – raised protein/immunoglobulin G (IgG) level, pleocytosis
  - serum – anti-Hu antibody
  - MRI
- **Management**: anti-tumour therapy.

Paraneoplastic cerebellar degeneration (PCD)

- **Cancer types**: breast, SCLC, ovary, Hodgkin's disease (HD)
- **Presentation**: rapid onset and progression; usually prior to cancer diagnosis; bilateral cerebellar signs; late diplopia and dementia
- **Diagnosis**:
  - CT – cerebellar atrophy (late)
  - serum autoantibodies – anti-Yo, -Tr, and -Hu
- **Management**: response to anti-tumour treatment, steroids, plasmapheresis.

Cancer-associated retinopathy (CAR)

- **Cancer types**: SCLC, breast, melanoma
- **Presentation**: visual defects, i.e. blurred vision, episodic visual loss, impaired colour vision; leads to progressive painless visual loss; usually precedes cancer diagnosis
- **Diagnosis**: loss of acuity; scotomata; abnormal electroretinogram; anti-retinal antibodies
- **Management:** corticosteroids.

Lambert–Eaton myasthenic syndrome (LEMS)

Disorder of the neuromuscular junction; reduced pre-synaptic calcium-dependent acetylcholine release. About 60% of patients with LEMS have underlying cancer.

- **Cancer types**: SCLC (60–70%), breast, thymus, GI tract cancers
- **Presentation**: proximal muscle weakness
- **Diagnosis**: electromyography (EMG) – normal conduction velocity with low-amplitude compound muscle action potentials that enhance to near normal following exercise
- **Management**: cancer treatment, corticosteroids, plasma exchange (high response rate).

Dermatomyositis/polymyositis

Inflammatory myopathies, often present prior to cancer diagnosis.

- **Cancer types**: NSCLC, SCLC, breast, ovary, GI tract cancers
- **Presentation**: proximal myopathy, skin changes, other systemic features; cardiopulmonary conditions, arthralgias, retinopathy
- **Diagnosis**:
  - serum – high creatine kinase (CK), LDH, aldolase
  - muscle biopsy – myositis
  - EMG – fibrillation, insertion irritability, short polyphasic motor units
- **Management**: search for and treat tumour; corticosteroids, azathioprine.

Haematological paraneoplastic syndromes

Red cell disorders

Erythrocytosis

Common, often secondary to increased erythropoietin production, e.g. renal cell carcinoma, hepatoma. Treat with venesection if required.

Haemolytic anaemia

- Autoimmune: secondary to lymphoproliferative disorders (treatment – corticosteroids)
- Micro-angiopathic: secondary to vascular tumours, acute pro-myelocytic leukaemia, or widespread metastatic adenocarcinoma. Treat the tumour; replace coagulation factors; IV heparin.

Red cell aplasia

Seen in thymoma, chronic lymphocytic leukaemia (CLL); rare in solid tumours.

White cell disorders

- Autoimmune neutropenia (rare)
- Granulocytosis: secondary to haemopoietic growth factor-secreting tumours (e.g. squamous cell cancers of lung, thyroid)
- Eosinophilia: in patients with HL.

Platelet disorders

- Thrombocytosis: $>450 \times 10^9/l$ is common and usually asymptomatic; in some cases may be secondary to interleukin-6 (IL-6) production
- Idiopathic thrombocytopenia: associated with leukaemias and lymphomas.

Coagulopathy

- Minor abnormalities of fibrin and fibrinogen degradation products are common.
- Overt disseminated intravascular coagulation is rare, and is associated with acute myelocytic leukaemia and adenocarcinomas.
- Diagnosed by triad of thrombocytopenia, abnormal prothrombin time, and hypofibrinoginaemia.
- Management is controversial.

Dermatological paraneoplastic syndromes

Pruritus
Common; characteristic of HL, leukaemias, CNS tumours, NHL.

Pigmentation
- **Acanthosis nigricans**: itchy brown hyperkeratotic plaques, mainly in flexures; may precede cancers by many years; associated with GI tract tumours, e.g. gastric adenocarcinoma.
- **Vitiligo**: patchy depigmentation, especially face, neck, and hands; associated with malignant melanoma; possibly due to anti-melanoma immune response.

Erythematous
- **Necrolytic migratory erythema**: islet cell tumour
- **Exfoliative dermatitis**: cutaneous T-cell lymphoma.

Bullous
- **Pemphigus**: characteristic bullous lesions on skin and mucous membranes; associated with lymphoma, Kaposi's sarcoma, thymic tumours
- **Dermatitis herpetiformis**: chronic, intensely itchy vesicles over elbows, knees, and lower back; precede tumour by many years; associated with lymphomas, e.g. NHL of the small intestine.

Other syndromes

Hypertrophic osteoarthropathy

Characterized by finger clubbing, periosteal new bone formation, and arthropathy.

- **Cancer types**: lung cancer, especially NSCLC
- **Presentation**: painful, swollen joints
- **Diagnosis**:
  - clinical – X-ray showing periosteal shadowing
  - bone scan – increased uptake
- **Management**: anti-tumour therapy, non-steroidal anti-inflammatory drugs (NSAIDS), corticosteroids, radiation.

Constitutional symptoms

Fever (pyrexia of unexplained origin (PUO))

Can be presenting feature of lymphoma, hepatoma, renal cell carcinoma; mediated by IL-1; treat with NSAIDS, corticosteroids; exclude other causes.

Cachexia

Very common, >10% loss of body weight is associated with poor prognosis; due to complex, multifactorial metabolic derangements; treat with enteral caloric supplements and appetite stimulants, e.g. corticosteroids, megesterol acetate.

Further reading

John WJ, Patchell RA, Foon KA (1994) Paraneoplastic syndromes. In: DeVita VT, Hellman S, Rosenberg SA, eds. *Cancer: principles and practice of oncology*, 5th edn. Philadelphia: Lippincott-Raven, pp. 2397–422.

MacCaulay VM, Smith IE (1995) Paraneoplastic syndromes. In: Peckham M, Pinedo H, Veronesi U, eds. *Oxford Textbook of Oncology*. Oxford: Oxford University Press, pp. 2228–53.

Multiple authors (1997) A series of articles on paraneoplastic syndromes in *Semin Oncol* **24**, 265–381.

AIDS-related malignancies

Introduction

Human immunodeficiency virus (HIV) represents the worst pandemic of the last quarter of a century.

- ~33 million people, including 2.5 million children, are currently living with HIV/AIDS.
- 2007 figures estimate that 2.7 million people worldwide were newly infected with the virus, including >130 000 living in Europe.
- Rate of new cases in some countries is stabilizing but in others, e.g. parts of Eastern Europe, the incidence continues to increase.
- Prevalence in sub-Saharan Africa is particularly great (5–25 % of the adult population, females > males). However, the pandemic has reached nearly all populations worldwide.
- <1% of HIV patients in the developing world have access to highly active antiretroviral therapy (HAART).

Malignant disease is observed in 25–40% of all HIV-infected patients at some stage in their illness and may be causative in almost one-third of HIV-related deaths. Currently four malignancies define the onset of AIDS:

- Kaposi's sarcoma (KS)
- intermediate and high-grade non-Hodgkin's lymphoma (NHL) of B-cell or unknown immunological phenotype
- primary CNS lymphoma (PCNSL) (in patients >60 years old positive HIV serology is required to define the onset of AIDS)
- invasive cervical cancer in HIV-positive females.

Other tumours have an increased incidence in HIV-positive individuals, e.g. anal cancer, Hodgkin's disease, but are not AIDS defining.

Management of the patient with an AIDS-related malignancy requires a multidisciplinary approach with consideration of:

- the cancer
- the underlying immune deficiency
- any co-existent complex psychological and social issues.

Effects of HAART

The evolution of highly active antiretroviral therapy (HAART) made it possible to achieve near-complete suppression of viral load and to maintain CD4 lymphocyte counts. Although the death rate from AIDS-related causes in developed countries is falling, an increasing number of deaths in HIV patients can be attributed to non-AIDS-related diseases. Observations have included:

- ↓ incidence of opportunistic infections
- ↑ proportion of HIV-related deaths attributable to cancer. Pre-HAART, this figure was 10%. Currently 25–30% of deaths in patients with HIV are due to malignancy. Possible explanations for this include a reduction in competing causes of deaths, an ageing population, the effects of chronic immunosuppression, and the increasing influence of other oncogenic viruses, e.g. Epstein–Barr (EBV), human papilloma (HPV), and hepatitis B (HBV) viruses
- ↓ incidence of KS
- no consistent change in the incidence of non-Hodgkin's lymphoma or non-AIDS-defining malignancies.

Kaposi's sarcoma

- The most common malignancy seen in patients with HIV infection.
- Incurable multifocal soft tissue sarcoma of vascular origin with a highly variable clinical course.
- Cutaneous involvement is characteristic and disease progression may be slow. However, it can behave aggressively, affecting visceral sites and causing significant morbidity and mortality.

Epidemiology and aetiology

Four clinical settings recognized:

- **classical form**: often indolent. Affects predominantly the extremities of older men from the Mediterranean, Middle East, or Eastern Europe
- **endemic African variant**: pre-dating HIV. Also male predominance. May be indolent or aggressive
- **iatrogenic**: seen in patients receiving immunosuppressive therapy, e.g. in organ transplant recipients typically 1–2 years after transplant. The tumour may regress when this treatment is reduced. Again, male predominance
- **epidemic AIDS-related form**: now the commonest form in the developing world:
  - in the West, principally a disease of men-who-have-sex-with-men (MSM)
  - associated with infection with human herpes virus (HHV-8). Infection precedes and is predictive of development of KS although its precise role in pathogenesis is not understood – increasing anti-HHV-8 antibody titres and absence of neutralizing antibodies have both been associated with a greater risk of disease. Transmission is likely to be both sexual and non-sexual. DNA from HHV-8 has been identified in KS lesions, semen, blood, and bronchial washings from affected patients
  - the incidence of KS is declining with the development of HAART. However, morbidity and mortality ascribed to KS has increased. Visceral KS accounts for the death of 1 in 4 HIV-positive MSM.

Presentation

May be precipitated/exacerbated by exogenous steroids.

Cutaneous

- Multiple non-painful red-purple lesions
- Flat → plaques → nodules with oedema. Up to several centimeters in diameter
- Typically affecting upper body, face, oral mucosa, genitalia, and legs.

Systemic

- Pulmonary: cough, breathlessness, chest pain, incidental finding on chest X-ray (CXR) (effusion, infiltration, lymphadenopathy), occasionally haemoptysis
- Gastrointestinal (GI) (40% at diagnosis): weight loss, pain, obstruction, diarrhoea, obstruction, bleeding
- Lymphoedema.

Investigations

- Skin biopsy
- CXR ± bronchoscopy if pulmonary KS suspected
- Faecal occult blood test (FOB) ± endoscopy if GI KS suspected
- CD4 count and viral load (necessary for accurate staging and appropriate treatment selection).

Pathology

- Key histological features of all forms of KS:
  - inflammatory infiltrate
  - angiogenesis
  - proliferation of spindle cells
  - A diagnostic feature is the intradermal proliferation of abnormal vascular structures lined with large, spindle-shaped endothelial cells.
  Also:
- micro-haemorrhages
- haemosiderin deposition.

Staging

The Aids Clinical Trials Group (ACTG) has developed a staging classification designed to assist with prognosis (see Table 29.1).

Table 29.1 ACTG guidelines

	Good prognosis – all of:	Poor prognosis – any of
Tumour	Skin only ± lymph nodes and/or minimal oral disease	Oedema/ulceration, extensive oral disease, visceral KS
Immunological	CD4 >200/µl	CD4 <200/ µl
Symptoms	Nil, Karnofsky >70	Opportunistic infection or thrush, B symptoms, Karnofsky <70, other HIV-related illness

Management

Treatment is palliative in intent with the primary goal being to stabilize tumour growth while maintaining quality of life.

Local therapy for local control and cosmesis

- Cryotherapy and laser, especially if lesions are ≤1 cm.
- Topical, e.g. with 9-cis retinoic acid (alitretinoin). This may produce local disease response after 4–8 weeks of treatment. The advantage is this is a patient-administered therapy with low toxicity – the main side-effect is local irritation.
- Intralesional chemotherapy, e.g. with vinblastine. Injection into the KS lesion can produce short-term regression in ~75% of cases. Mean duration of palliation is typically 3–4 months.
- Radiotherapy: a response rate equal to intralesional chemotherapy can be achieved with single fraction doses of 8 Gy. This can be repeated if

there is recurrence or insufficient regression. Palatal lesions can also be irradiated using iridium wire moulds.

Systemic therapy

If cutaneous disease is widespread, local treatment has failed, or there is extensive symptomatic oedema or visceral disease.

HAART

- ~60% of patients respond to immune restoration if treated with antiretroviral therapy alone. Lesions may fully or partially regress and there may be disappearance of baseline HHV-8 viraemia. Response rates may be greater if HAART is combined with appropriate chemotherapy.

Chemotherapy

- Consider if there is extensive disease or significant systemic symptoms unresponsive to HAART. Liposomal anthracyclines (e.g. pegylated liposomal doxorubicin, Caelyx®) are 1st-line choice.
- Response rates of 30–60% have been observed and may be greater if given in combination with HAART.
- Treatment is usually well tolerated, and cardiotoxicity with the new liposomal preparations is less than for conventional anthracyclines.
- Paclitaxel (Taxol®) can be considered as 2nd-line treatment in selected patients.

Biological therapies

- Immunotherapy:
  - interferon-α (IFN-α): most effective if disease is non-visceral and CD4 count is >200/μl. Response rates of 20–40% have been observed. Potential toxicity includes 'flu-like symptoms', marrow suppression, and depression
  - interleukin-12 (IL-12): disease response reported when used in small non-randomized trials either as single-agent treatment or in combination with standard chemotherapy.
- Anti-angiogenic agents: small clinical trials only so far, e.g. with thalidomide – response rates up to 40% reported.
- Imatinib (Glivec®): orally active tyrosine kinase inhibitor; again, only studied in small early-phase trials so far.

Supportive care

- Camouflage with cosmetics
- Psychosocial support
- Palliation of symptoms.

Systemic non-Hodgkin's lymphoma

Epidemiology and aetiology

- Second most common malignancy to affect those with AIDS. Almost half of patients will previously have had an AIDS-defining illness.
- Risk of a person with HIV developing lymphoma is 60–160 times greater than in the seronegative population.
- Incidence of systemic NHL increases with worsening immunosuppression. NHL also has a higher incidence in individuals who are immunocompromised for other reasons.
- Close association between the development of NHL in AIDS and infection with the EBV. EBV proteins can be demonstrated in ≥50% of lymphomas, particularly immunoblastic and large-cell lymphomas. It is thought that the proliferation of EBV-infected cells in the immune-deficient host may proceed unchecked.
- Oncogenic mutations have also been identified, e.g. in the *p53* tumour suppressor gene and *C-myc* gene.

Presentation

- Typically seen in advanced HIV infection (CD4 ≤ 100/µl).
- Frequently involves extranodal sites: ~80% have stage IV disease at presentation, e.g. involving the GI tract, bone marrow, central nervous system (CNS) including lymphomatous meningitis, liver, or recurrent effusions (primary effusion lymphoma is a variant of NHL).
- Constitutional 'B' symptoms are common.
- Differential diagnoses include tuberculosis and cytomegalovirus.

Pathology

- ~80% of AIDS-associated NHL is high grade.
- ≥90% are diffuse large B-cell (immunoblastic subtype) or Burkitt's-like lymphoma.
- Not all lymphomas in the immunocompromised patient are monoclonal. Some tumours may comprise polyclonal cell populations that demonstrate metastatic potential.

Investigations and staging

- Bloods including lactate dehydrogenase (LDH)
- CXR
- Computerized tomography (CT) head, abdomen, and pelvis
- Consider positron emission tomography (PET) – may assist in accurate staging
- Lymph node biopsy (ideally not fine needle aspiration (FNA)) and bone marrow biopsy
- Lumbar puncture and cerebrospinal fluid (CSF) examination even if asymptomatic.

Poor prognostic factors
- Prior AIDS-defining diagnosis or CD4 count <100/μl
- Karnofsky performance score <70
- Age >35 years
- Extranodal disease including bone marrow involvement
- ↑ LDH
- Immunoblastic subtype.

Management
- Optimal management should be co-ordinated in a centre with specialist expertise in AIDS-associated lymphomas.
- Concomitant HAART reduces the incidence of opportunistic infections and improves survival.
- Potentially curative local treatments can be considered for patients presenting with stage I or II NHL (see 📖 Chapter 25 on 'Haematological malignancies').
- Vast majority of patients with AIDS-associated NHL present with stage IV disease and require systemic therapy.
- Treatment for advanced disease is with combination chemotherapy, e.g. CHOP – cyclophosphamide, doxorubicin, vincristine, and prednisolone given on a 3-weekly schedule is a commonly used regime although many other combinations have been tried.
- Baseline immunodeficiency and reduced bone marrow reserve means more-intensive chemotherapy regimens tend to be poorly tolerated.
- Leptomeningeal involvement requires intrathecal chemotherapy, usually with methotrexate and cytarabine. Intrathecal prophylaxis remains controversial but can be considered in those at high risk of meningeal involvement (e.g. patients with Burkitt's lymphoma, paraspinal or paranasal disease, bone marrow infiltration or EBV detected in their CSF).
- Response rates to treatment and time to progression are less good in patients with AIDS than in seronegative patients treated for lymphomas of similar histology. However the routine use of HAART plus cobination chemotherapy has improved the outlook a little; 2–3-year survival is now 40–60%, with death usually due either to recurrent lymphoma or opportunistic infection. Those who achieve a complete response with chemotherapy have a survival benefit ranging from 6 to 20 months, with a small percentage of long-term survivors.
- Rituximab: a monoclonal antibody used in the standard treatment of NHL in the general (non-immunosupressed) population. However, its role in AIDS-associated NHL is controversial with no phase III data yet supporting its use and evidence to suggest it may decrease CD4 counts, increase viral load, and increase infectious complications.

Primary CNS lymphoma

Epidemiology and aetiology
- Affects at least 2–6% of HIV-positive individuals (autopsy series suggest the incidence may be greater).
- Accounts for 15% of NHLs in HIV-infected patients (as opposed to 1% of NHLs seen in the HIV-negative population).
- Usually a late manifestation of AIDS (CD4 ≤50/μl) and patients often have other serious opportunistic infections.
- Falling incidence in the developed world since the introduction of HAART.

Presenting symptoms
- Focal, e.g. hemiparesis, aphasia, focal seizures, deafness, cranial nerve palsies.
- Non-focal, e.g. confusion, lethargy, headaches.
- Constitutional, 'B' symptoms identified in ~80% of cases.

Pathology
- Diffuse B-cell lymphoma is the most common subtype.
- Histology is similar to that of AIDS-related NHL except that almost all cases are associated with EBV. This is very different to primary CNS lymphoma in seronegative patients, which is not associated with EBV.
- Disease limited to the CNS.

Investigations
- Magnetic resonance imaging (MRI) is the investigation of choice. Typical appearance is of a well-defined enhancing focal lesion, which may be indistinguishable from cerebral toxoplasmosis.
- CSF cytology ± amplification of EBV DNA in CSF sample.
- Toxoplasmosis serological testing.
- Single-photon emission computed tomography (SPECT) scanning, e.g. using thallium-201. Under investigation as a means of non-invasively differentiating between PCNSL and toxoplasmosis.
- Consider slit-lamp examination to assess for ocular involvement (reported in up to 15% of patients).
- Stereotactic brain biopsy is occasionally necessary, particularly if there has been no response to antitoxoplasma therapy.

Management

- Empirical treatment with antitoxoplasma therapy pending results of other investigations.
- Delay the use of steroids until after investigations have been completed, if at all possible. Exogenous corticosteroids may reduce tumour size and provide symptomatic benefit. They can also reduce radiological enhancement after contrast injection and diagnostic yield at biopsy.
- Treatment should be combined with appropriate HAART. There is evidence to show that an increase in CD4 count combined with tumour-specific therapy increases survival. It may also affect disease distribution, e.g. reduction in leptomeningeal involvement. Unfortunately multidrug resistance is common in the group of patients whose immunosuppression puts them at greatest risk of developing PCNSL.
- Standard 1st-line treatment for AIDS-associated PCNSL is whole-brain radiotherapy in combination with corticosteroids. Complete response rates as high as 50% have been reported.
- Intrathecal chemotherapy is occasionally used. There is little evidence to support the use of systemic chemotherapy.
- Entry into clinical trials should be offered wherever possible.
- Untreated, typical survival is 1–2 months. With treatment, median survival from diagnosis remains just 2–4 months. This is largely due to the context of severe immunocompromise in which PCNSL typically develops – death is usually due to opportunistic infections.
- A good performance status at diagnosis is associated with longer survival – palliation for up to 18 months may occasionally be possible.

Cervical cancer in HIV-positive females

- Moderate/severe cervical dysplasia is classed as an early symptomatic HIV condition in seropositive females.
- The prevalence of cervical intra-epithelial neoplasia (CIN) is up to 40% in HIV-infected women.
- All HIV-positive women should be encouraged to participate in screening programmes whereever possible. It is advisable to screen patients frequently, e.g. every 6–12 months.
- Effective antiretroviral therapy is usually associated with regression of CIN, particularly in women who are less immunocompromised when the lesion is diagnosed.
- Cervical cancer in seropositive females is an AIDS-defining diagnosis. Its increased prevalence may be because both HIV virus and the oncogenic human papillomavirus (HPV) are sexually transmissible. The incidence of all HPV-associated cancers is increased in AIDS. The incidence of cervical cancer is also inversely related to CD4 count.
- A potential major clinical issue in sub-Saharan Africa where there is no routine access to screening. However, at present (with limited availability of HAART), the most common cause of death in these regions is opportunistic infection.

Non-AIDS-defining malignancies

Hodgkin's disease

- Incidence of Hodgkin's disease (HD) in HIV-positive patients is 5–9 times greater than in the general population.
- The most common histological variant in patients with HIV is the mixed cellularity subtype (cf nodular sclerosis in non-HIV-infected patients with HD).
- Development of HD is associated with worsening immunosuppression, as with the AIDS-defining malignancies.
- More commonly observed in patients where transmission of HIV has been by intravenous drug use.
- Strong association with EBV infection.
- Often advanced at presentation with bone marrow involvement present in ~50% and widely disseminated extranodal disease in >75%.
- Combination chemotherapy should be combined with appropriate HAART. Complete remission following therapy is possible. However, median survival is only 12–18 months, with death due to relapse or opportunistic infection.

Anal cancer

- Anal cancer is independently associated with both HIV and HPV. MSM are a group at particular risk. The incidence of anal cancer in HIV-positive MSM is approximately twice that seen in seronegative MSM. There is often a preceding history of anal warts.
- Treatment of anal dysplasia in HIV-infected individuals is controversial. Low-grade lesions can be followed clinically by serial anoscopy and biopsy, while high-grade lesions, when immune function is preserved, can be treated by excision and laser ablation (if dysplasia is limited).
- Anal intra-epithelial neoplasia (AIN) developing at the epithelial transformation zone is the pre-invasive condition believed to progress to anal cancer (analogous to CIN in cervical cancer). However, the association between the risk of AIN and the CD4 count remains unclear. Effective antiretroviral treatment does not correlate with regression of AIN (unlike CIN).
- Anal cancer may be asymptomatic. Alternatively, presentation with tenesmus, bleeding, pruritus, or pain may occur.
- Treatment is with HAART and chemo-radiotherapy.

Other solid malignancies

Evidence suggests an ↑ incidence of other solid tumours in patients with concomitant HIV infection including:

- non-small-cell lung cancer
- skin cancers, particularly basal cell carcinoma
- testicular tumours
- squamous cell head and neck cancers.

It is unclear whether this reflects a genuine causative association with HIV infection or whether there may confounding factors, e.g. the greater incidence of smoking in the seropositive population.

The AIDS-defining malignancies are generally associated with advanced immunosuppression. It is now emerging that even patients with controlled HIV are at an increased risk of incurable solid malignancies.

Further reading

Aoki Y, Tosato G (2004) Neoplastic conditions in the context of HIV-1 infection. *Curr HIV Res* **56**, 343–9.

Berretta M, Cinelli R, Martellotta F, *et al.* (2003) Therapeutic approaches to AIDS-related malignancies. *Oncogene* **22**, 6646–59.

Biggar RJ, Chaturvedi AK, Goedert JJ, Engels EA (2007) AIDS-related cancer and severity of immunosuppression in persons with AIDS. *J Natl Cancer Inst* **99**, 962.

Department of Health (2008) *HIV Post-exposure Prophylaxis: guidance from the UK Chief Medical Offiicer Expert Advisory Group on AIDS*. London: Department of Health. Gruhlich AE, van Leeuwen MT, Falster MO, Vajdic CM (2007) Incidence of cancers in patients with HIV/AIDS compared with immunosuppressed transplant recipients: a meta-analysis. *Lancet* **370**, 59.

Quinn TC (2008) HIV Epidemiology and the effects of antiretroviral therapy on long-term consequences. *AIDS* **22(Suppl 3)**, S7–S12.

Childhood cancers presenting in adults

Introduction

Uncommonly, malignant tumours of pathology identical to childhood cancers occur in adults, usually aged 20–40 years, and these present a variety of particular challenges:

- often present with advanced disease
- pathological diagnosis may be difficult, and may require expert central review by a paediatric pathologist, and confirmatory cytogenetics
- scant evidence base to direct management in adults, no randomized trials, and few published historical series, often reflecting changes in management over several decades
- usually present through adult multidisciplinary teams who may lack experience and expertise in the treatment of these tumours, no designated national centres
- lack of research/novel therapy development because of their rarity and Cinderella status with the pharmaceutical industry.

In general, management will be broadly based on current practice in paediatric patients, but this must be modified to account for:

- frequently aggressive tumour pathology and natural history with relatively poor prognosis in adult patients compared with children
- age-related intolerance to intensive therapies
  - these patients may best be treated with granulocyte colony-stimulating factor (G-CSF) and/or broad-spectrum antibiotics as primary prophylaxis against febrile neutropenia during chemotherapy
  - cumulative myelosuppression and non-haematological toxicities (neuro- and cardiotoxicity) commonly limit the number of cycles of chemotherapy that can be safely delivered
- relative safety and breadth of experience with radiation therapy in adults compared with children at most tumour sites:
  - in particular fewer concerns with regard to late effects of treatment on growth, fertility, and risk of secondary malignancy.

This chapter will cover the solid tumours of childhood that can occur in adults; for haematological malignancies see 📖 Chapter 25.

Embryonal tumours

Medulloblastoma

- ~2% of adult central nervous system (CNS) tumours.
- Median age 30 years, very occasionally aged greater than 60 years.
- Usually present with disease in the lateral cerebellar hemisphere (vermis usual site in children).
- Differentiate from metastasis and glioma.
- Majority are treated by surgical resection followed by craniospinal radiotherapy:
  - 35 Gy to whole brain and spine
  - boost to 54 Gy to posterior fossa.
- Chemotherapy reserved for metastatic disease or recurrence.
- Late relapse in the posterior fossa is a common feature.
- 10-year survival ~50%:
  - prognosis worse with invasion of brainstem or 4th ventricle.

Radiation therapy should be planned and delivered by a team experienced in the delivery of craniospinal radiotherapy.

Retinoblastoma

- Very rare after the age of five years.
- Median age in adults 38 years (range 20–74 years).
- Present with loss of vision.
- Visible white tumour mass arising from the choroids.
- Differential diagnosis – lymphoma, amelanotic melanoma, metastatic carcinoma, benign retinocytoma, and inflammatory conditions.
- Should be managed in national specialist centres for ocular oncology (in the UK, Moorfield and Barts or Liverpool).
- Biopsy can be performed prior to definitive treatment.
- Enucleation is often the most appropriate treatment.

Neuroblastoma

- Arise in adrenal gland or elsewhere in the sympathetic nervous system.
- Differentiate from adrenal adenoma, adrenal metastasis, adenocarcinoma, and phaeochromocytoma.
- Surgical resection only for localized disease.
- Adjuvant chemotherapy and radiotherapy indicated for:
  - stage II–IV
  - high-risk pathology, i.e. undifferentiated tumours
  - amplification of the *MYCN* oncogene.
- Pathology and genetic analysis can be carried out on image-guided core biopsy.
- Recently agreed image-defined risk factors can be used in patients being considered for neoadjuvant therapy:
  - ipsilateral tumour extension within two body compartments (neck-chest, chest-abdomen, abdomen-pelvis)
  - neck tumours encasing major vessels, extending to skull base, or compressing trachea
  - cervico-thoracic junction tumours encasing brachial plexus or major vessels
  - thoracic tumours encasing major arteries, compressing major airway, or invading rib/spine

- abdominal or pelvic tumours infiltrating adjacent organs, major vessels, sciatic nerve
  - intra-spinal tumour.
- Metastatic disease has a poor prognosis with no MS (spread of disease confined to the skin, liver, bone marrow with relatively good prognosis) stage in patients greater than 18 months.
- Chemotherapy regimens include high-dose cyclophosphamide or ifosfamide, doxorubicin, cisplatin, and etoposide.
- External beam radiotherapy can be used with considerably greater freedom to improve local control than in young children:
  - therapy dose radiolabelled meta-iodobenzylguanidine (MIBG) may be useful in palliation of advanced disease
  - metastatic disease may also respond well to short courses of palliative radiotherapy by external beam.

The staging system for neuroblastoma is shown in Table 30.1.

Table 30.1 Neuroblastoma – international staging system (adults)

Stage	Description
1	Localized tumour with complete gross excision including any involved lymph nodes
2A	Localized tumour with incomplete gross excision, node negative
2B	Localized tumour with residual ipsilateral involved nodes
3	Unresectable unilateral tumour infiltrating across midline or with contralateral lymph node involvement
4	Disseminated disease (distant lymph nodes, bone, bone marrow, liver, skin, etc.)

Wilms' tumour

- Median age 26 years (range 16–73 years).
- Prognosis depends on stage and pathology.
- Pathological diagnosis of poor prognosis (Wilms' tumour with anaplasia) can be difficult to differentiate from sarcomatoid carcinoma:
  - need for central paediatric review of pathology.
- Worse prognosis stage for stage compared with children, particularly with unfavourable histology.
- Radiotherapy 40–50 Gy to the renal bed after incomplete resection.
- Adjuvant chemotherapy as per paediatric protocols with some provisos:
  - adults tolerate weekly vincristine poorly, rapidly developing peripheral and autonomic neuropathy
  - first-line therapy vincristine, actinomycin, doxorubicin, ± cyclophosphamide, carboplatin, etoposide.
- Reported overall 5-year survival >80%.
- Occasionally late lung secondaries have been reported over 20 years after the primary resection.

Soft-tissue sarcomas

Rhabdomyosarcoma

Sarcomas arising from muscle are relatively rare in adults, and the majority bear little resemblance to the embryonal rhabdomyosarcoma of childhood in terms of natural history and behaviour.

- Only comprises 2% of soft-tissue sarcomas >16 years.
- Median age 45 years, with bimodal distribution (one peak in the late teens, the other in the 60s).
- Majority are of pleomorphic pathology
  - then in order embryonal, followed by alveolar.
- Pathological diagnosis may be difficult and need central review
  - cytogenetics can be helpful (1:13 and 2:13 translocations in alveolar rhabdomyosarcoma).
- 1 in 3 present with metastatic disease, most often blood-borne to lung.
- 1 in 5 have lymph node spread, relatively unusual in sarcomas.
- Truncal and limb sites predominate, but can arise in head and neck/ genitourinary tract.
- Chemotherapy recommended for all patients if fit, e.g. doxorubicin-ifosfamide-based regimens.
- Response rate up to 80%, with complete responses in 30–40%.
- Best outcome with tumours <5 cm, good response to chemotherapy, and embryonal pathology (see Table 30.2).
- Localized tumours have a 30–50% local recurrence rate.
- Overall 5-year survival only 35%.
- Because this tumour is chemosensitive, surgery is used for biopsy and excision where practical without causing extensive morbidity. Repeat excision of limb and trunk tumours and debulking retroperitoneal tumours may provide some survival advantage.

Table 30.2 Rhabdomyosarcoma – pathology and behaviour

Pathological type	%	Site	Response to chemotherapy
Pleomorphic	36	Limb, trunk	Sensitive
Alveolar	23	Limb, trunk	Resistant
Embryonal	28	Head and neck, trunk	Highly sensitive
Other	13		

Further reading

Helman LJ, Malkin D (2008) Cancers of childhood. In: DeVita VT, Lawrence TS, senberg SA, eds. *Cancer – Principles and Practice of Oncology*. Philadelphia: Lippincott, Williams and Wilkins, pp. 2033–83.

Izawa JI, Al-Omar M, Winquist E, *et al.* (2008) Prognostic variables in adult Wilms tumour. *Can J Surg* **51**, 252–6.

Padovani L, Sunyach MP, Perol D, *et al.* (2007) Common strategy for adult and pediatric medulloblastoma: a multicenter series of 253 adults. *Int J Radiat Oncol Biol Phys* **68**, 433–40.

Parambil J, Aughenbaugh GL, Pereira JC (2005) Solitary pulmonary metastasis presenting 20 years after primary resection of Wilms tumour. *Mayo Clin Proc* **80**, 1514–16.

Simon JH, Paulino AC, Ritchie JM, Mayr NA, Buatti JM (2003) Presentation, prognostic factors and patterns of failure in adult rhabdomyosarcoma. *Sarcoma* **7**, 1–7.

Spinal cord compression and bone marrow suppression

Spinal cord compression

Spinal cord compression is a medical emergency. Treatment must begin within hours, not days, to maximize the chance of neurological recovery.

Presentation
- Bone involvement from cancer
- Common in these malignancies:
  - breast
  - prostate
  - lung
  - myeloma
  - lymphoma
- Less common in:
  - thyroid
  - kidney
  - bladder
  - bowel
  - melanoma
  - primary bone tumours
- May be the first presentation of malignancy – prostate, breast, myeloma
- Crush fracture and/or soft tissue tumour extension common
- Occasional direct extension from malignant retroperitoneal or mediastinal lymphadenopathy, e.g. lymphoma
- Occasional extradural tumour mass causing cord compression in absence of bone involvement
- Occasional intramedullary metastases or primary tumour
- 66% of cases occur in the thoracic cord.

Symptoms (see Table 31.1)
- Pain, typically radicular, exacerbated by coughing or straining and not relieved by bed rest, frequently precedes neurological symptoms or signs.
- Any patient with cancer who develops severe back pain with a root distribution should be considered at risk of spinal cord compression and urgently investigated.
- Patients with known bone metastases should be encouraged to self-refer without delay.
- Weakness of the legs (and arms if the lesion is cervical), sensory loss, retention, dribbling, or incontinence of urine or faeces, are late symptoms.

Table 31.1 Spinal cord compression syndromes

Complete compression

Sensory level just below level of lesion

Loss of all sensory modalities – may be variable at onset

Bilateral upper motor neurone weakness below lesion

Bladder and bowel dysfunction

Anterior compression

Partial loss of pain and temperature below lesion

Bilateral upper motor neurone weakness below lesion

Bladder and bowel dysfuncion

Posterior compression

Loss of vibration and position below lesion

Relative sparing of pain, temperature, and touch

Band of dysthaesia at level of lesion

Lateral compression (Brown–Séquard syndrome)

Contralateral loss of pain and temperature (touch relatively spared)

Ipsilateral loss of vibration and position

Ipsilateral upper motor neuron weakness

Cauda equina syndrome
- The spinal cord ends at the level of L1 or L2.
- Tumours below this level may produce cauda equina compression with sciatic pain (often bilateral), bladder dysfunction with retention and overflow incontinence, impotence, sacral (saddle) anaesthesia, loss of anal sphincter tone, and weakness and wasting of the gluteal muscles.
- The symptoms may be vague and the diagnosis difficult to make without imaging of the spine.

Examination
The following may be present:
- visible or palpable gibbus at the site of a wedged or collapsed vertebra
- pain and tenderness on palpation or percussion of the vertebra over the site of compression
- band of hyperaesthesia at the level of the lesion
- sensory and motor loss (with defects of power and sensation) at and below the level of the lesion
- the lesion may be partial or complete and the nature of the defect may depend on the portion of the cord compressed.

Investigations

- Plain X-rays may demonstrate destruction and/or collapse of a vertebra. Paravertebral masses may sometimes also be shown. In 15–20% of cases, plain films show no abnormality.
- Magnetic resonance imaging (MRI) scanning is the investigation of choice. It is particularly useful in cases of cauda equina syndrome.
- Where MRI is not available or contraindicated, myelography will show the anatomical location of a spinal cord lesion and whether a block is complete or not, but computerized tomography (CT) scanning will frequently yield sufficient information without delay. Simultaneous myelography improves the sensitivity of the investigation.

Management

- Speed is of the essence in the management of spinal cord compression.
- Fewer than 10% of patients with established paraplegia from metastatic disease walk again.
- Dexamethasone 16–20 mg should be given immediately. This can reduce peri-tumoural oedema.
- If immediate surgery is not contemplated, neurological status should be assessed at least daily so that deterioration may be detected early and surgical intervention considered.
- Best outcomes reported with surgical decompression/stabilization of spine, followed by radiotherapy.
- However, surgery is neither feasible nor appropriate in many, e.g. frailty, extensive bone destruction, extensive disease in other sites, etc.
- Surgery indicated particularly for:
  - acute-onset paraplegia
  - patients with good performance status
  - small-volume bone disease
  - fracture dislocation
  - radioresistant tumours
  - spinal cord compression progressing during radiotherapy or recurrence after radiotherapy
  - to provide tissue diagnosis where cord compression is the presenting symptom of malignancy.
- Radiation-induced oedema may exacerbate symptoms during radiotherapy – may require increase in the dose of steroids during radiotherapy.
- Chemotherapy rarely indicated in the treatment of spinal cord compression, e.g. chemosensitive primary tumour such as Ewing's.

Bone marrow suppression

- The major dose-limiting toxicity of cancer chemotherapy is bone marrow suppression.
- Normally between 1010 and 1012 cells are produced by the bone marrow every hour in a carefully controlled manner.
- Cytotoxic-induced bone marrow failure usually produces a pancytopenia.
- First problems relate to neutropenia, usually 7–10 days after the start of chemotherapy.
- Risk of sepsis relates to the severity and duration of neutropenia.
- If chemotherapy causes coincident mucosal damage, e.g. stomatitis or diarrhoea, this may provide a portal for bacteraemia.
- Day 10–14 may develop thrombocytopenia.
- Anaemia due to marrow suppression commonly occurs day 14–21.
- Bone marrow compromise may also result from wide-field radiotherapy.
- Certain specific cytotoxics cause preferential damage to stem cells leading to delayed and prolonged myelosuppression, e.g. 1-(2-chloroethyl)-3-cyclohexyl-1-nitrosourea (CCNU).
- Myelosuppression related to chemotherapy can be graded using defined criteria – a process useful in clinical trials and in judging risk in dose-intensive therapy (see Table 31.2).

Causes of bone marrow failure

- Depletion of anatomical and physiological elements, e.g. myelofibrosis, myelodysplasia
- Intrinsic stem cell/precursor cell failure, e.g. aplastic anaemia, paroxysmal nocturnal haemoglobinuria
- Iatrogenic, e.g. chemotherapy, irradiation
- Bone marrow infiltration, e.g. malignancy
- Peripheral consumption, e.g. hypersplenism
- Autoimmune diseases, e.g. systemic lupus erythematosus
- Vitamin deficiency, e.g. megaloblastic anaemia.

Pancytopenia in the cancer patient

- Neutropenia – life-threatening bacterial infections (see Table 31.3)
- Associated with:
  - poor nutrition
  - mucosal barrier defects
  - central venous lines
  - abnormal host colonization.
- Qualitative and quantitative defects
- Defects in chemotaxis, neutrophil degranulation.

Table 31.2 National Cancer Institute of Canada – Clinical Trials Group (NCIC–CTG) expanded common toxicity criteria

Toxicity grade	0	1	2	3	4
Hb g/dl	WNL	10.0–normal	8.0–9.9	6.5–7.9	<6.5
Platelets × 10^9/l	WNL	7.5–normal	50.0–74.9	25.0–49.9	<25.0
WCC × 10^9/l	≥4.0	3.0–3.9	2.0–2.9	1.0–1.9	<1.0
Granulocytes	≥2.0	1.5–1.9	1.0–1.4	0.5–0.9	<0.5
Lymphocytes	≥2.0	1.5–1.9	1.0–1.4	0.5–0.9	<0.5

Hb = haemoglobin; WCC = white cell count; WNL = within normal limits.

Table 31.3 Most common micro-organisms in neutropenic patients

Gram-negative bacilli	Gram-positive bacilli	Fungi
E. coli	Staphylococcus aureus	Candida spp.
Klebsiella spp	Staphylococcus epidermidis	Aspergillus spp.
Enterobacter spp	Streptococcus pneumoniae	Mucorales
Proteus spp	Viridans streptococci	
P. aeruginosa	Enterococci	
	Corynebacterium	

Management of fever in a neutropenic patient

- Fever is common in patients with cancer.
- Commonly caused by infection.
- Can also be related to underlying malignancy, blood product transfusion, and pyrogenic medications.
- Untreated sepsis in a neutropenic patient can be rapidly fatal.

Generally, antibiotics are administered empirically after careful physical examination and the following simple investigations:

- blood cultures (peripheral and central, if line in situ)
- sputum culture
- urine analysis and culture
- chest X-ray
- swabs from Hickman line exit site.

Treatment should then be instituted without delay, with empirical intravenous broad-spectrum antibiotic therapy, particularly if the patient is toxic or haemodynamically compromised. The widespread adoption of this approach has reduced the mortality of neutropenic sepsis to less than 10%.

- The selection of initial antibiotic regimen should be determined by a locally agreed protocol guided by the bacteriology department, according to the prevalence of antibiotic sensitivity/resistance.

- Fulminant sepsis requires intensive supportive therapy with close monitoring and correction of hypoxia, hypotension, fluid balance, acid–base balance, renal function, coagulopathy, etc.
- If the fever is unremitting at 48 h, or there is any clinical deterioration, an empirical change of antibiotics to a second-line antibiotic regime should be performed.
- If infection is associated with a central venous access line, removal of the line may be required if there is not a prompt response to appropriate antibiotics.
- Failure to resolve the fever within 5 days may suggest other opportunistic infections such as fungi or parasites such as *Pneumocystis carinii*. Careful consideration of these diagnoses, in close consultation with a microbiologist, is required, and may require more invasive investigation, e.g. bronchoscopy and bronchoalveolar lavage.
- Often, resolution of neutropenia is associated with resolution of refractory fever. This process can be accelerated by the prophylactic use of haemopoietic growth factors (e.g. granulocyte colony-stimulating factor (G-CSF)) started one day post chemotherapy. There is no evidence that administering G-CSF at the time of neutropenic sepsis improves the outcome.

Thrombocytopenia in the cancer patient

- Thrombocytopenia is commonplace in patients receiving cytotoxic chemotherapy.
- The trigger level to transfuse platelets is not always absolute.
- Spontaneous bleeding is unlikely if platelets are $>20 \times 10^9$/l, but the risk of traumatic bleeding is greater if $<40 \times 10^9$/l.
- Most clinicians would transfuse when platelets are $<10 \times 10^9$/l. However, if there is active bleeding or sepsis, platelet transfusion should be considered if platelets $<20 \times 10^9$/l.

Careful consideration of the patient's vascular status, clotting status, and disease-specific risks (e.g. gastric carcinoma) will determine the threshold for transfusion in an individual patient. Cross-matching is not required since patients generally receive random, pooled, donor platelets.

Some patients may become refractory after repeated transfusions and human leucocyte-associated antigen (HLA)-matched platelets should be used for these. Four units of fresh platelets, (doubled if platelets greater than 3 days old), should raise the count to >24–40×10^9/l in an adult. Although frequently part of the differential diagnosis of refractoriness, HLA allo-immunization is only one of many causes. Others include the presence of:

- anti-platelet antibodies
- disseminated intravascular coagulation
- concomitant drugs, e.g. septrin
- hypersplenism.

Red cell transfusion in cancer patients

- A low haemoglobin in a patient with cancer is also common and requires careful diagnostic evaluation.
- Elimination of obvious causes such as bleeding from a gastrointestinal malignancy is important before repeated red cell transfusions are given.
- A one-unit blood transfusion should raise the haemoglobin by approximately 1 g/dl.
- Transfusion may reduce the platelet count, so platelet transfusion may be required before or after blood transfusion.
- Red cell transfusion should be based on clinical criteria rather than absolute trigger values, but usually only given when Hb <10 g/dl.
- The use of erythropoietin to maintain haemoglobin values in patients with cancer is possible. Recent research suggests that some cancers may also be stimulated by erythropoietin, so it is used with more caution that previously.

Chapter 32

Superior vena cava obstruction and raised intracranial pressure

Superior vena cava obstruction (SVCO)

Aetiology

The superior vena cava (SVC) can be obstructed by:
- **external compression of the SVC**: accounts for >80% of cases of SVCO, e.g. from primary tumour (most commonly in the right paratracheal region) or from metastatic (particularly paratracheal) lymphadenoapthy
- **direct invasion of the SVC**: from the same causes
- **thrombus within the SVC**: e.g. due to central venous catheterization (Hickman or peripherally inserted central catheter (PICC) lines etc) or secondary to compression
- any combination of the above.

The most common underlying diagnosis is bronchogenic carcinoma. Small-cell lung carcinoma (SCLC) is a particularly frequent cause of SVCO (up to 20% of patients with SCLC) as this commonly develops within central rather than peripheral airways and often has extensive lymph node spread. However, any tumour involving the mediastinal nodes can cause SVCO, e.g. non-Hodgkin's lymphoma, thymoma, and mediastinal germ cell tumours.

Benign causes of SVCO are much less common but include sarcoidosis, post-radiotherapy fibrosis, and unusual infections, e.g. aspergillosis.

Clinical features

Symptoms
- Dyspnoea is the most commonly reported symptom. This is due to associated tracheal or bronchial obstruction/compression.
- Swelling of the neck, face, and arms, especially in the morning and often exacerbated by bending forwards or lying down.
- Cough.
- Headache.
- Visual disturbance.
- Acuteness of presentation is dependent upon the rate at which obstruction of the SVC occurs compared to recruitment of venous collaterals.

Signs
- Fixed engorgement of external and internal jugular veins
- Collateral veins over anterior and lateral chest wall (alternative pathways for the return of venous blood to the right atrium)
- Facial plethora
- Papilloedema (late feature).

Differential diagnoses
- **Heart failure:** jugular veins pulsating not fixed; other cardiac signs; dependent oedema
- **Cardiac tamponade:** characteristic symptoms/signs and chest X-ray (CXR) appearances
- **External jugular vein compression**: no facial oedema; no collaterals; usually supraclavicular fossa nodes.

Investigations

Up to 60% of patients with SVCO due to underlying cancer present without a known diagnosis of malignancy. Unless the patient has very severe and life-threatening symptoms (e.g. respiratory failure due to stridor), treatment should not start until a clear diagnosis (including pathology if possible) has been made.

- **CXR** typically shows a right paratracheal mass, mediastinal lymphadenopathy, or other indications of lung cancer, e.g. pleural effusion. Abnormal in >80% of cases.
- **Computerized tomography (CT) thorax**, ideally with contrast, to define the level and degree of venous blockage. Assists in identifying the cause of SVCO. Can help with staging of the cancer (especially if abdomen also imaged) and hence with appropriate further management. Percutaneous biopsy may confirm the diagnosis.
- **Venogram** needed if there is no obvious mass causing external compression, or if thrombolysis or stent insertion are planned.
- **Cytology** samples should be taken from any easily accessible tumour, e.g. stem cell factor (SCF) lymphadenopathy. Pleural fluid can also be sent for cytology. The priority is to obtain a histological diagnosis by the most minimally invasive method possible.
- **Bronchoscopy** essential if the clinical picture and CXR suggest lung cancer but no histopathology has been obtained.
- **Mediastinal biopsy** (mediastinoscopy, mediastinotomy, mini-thoracotomy, or CT-guided core biopsy) provides an alternative method of obtaining histology if other attempts have failed.

Management

Most patients present with symptoms of insidious onset and there is time to establish the diagnosis and extent of disease prior to commencing treatment. Prognosis is dependent on tumour histology and stage of disease at presentation, rather than the presence of SVCO *per se*.

If a patient is severely compromised consider the possibility that there is concomitant tracheal compression (see 📖 Chapter 33, 'Stridor'). In the acute situation:

- sit the patient up, establish intravenous access, and give them 100% O_2 if appropriate
- **dexamethasone 8 mg bd PO/IV**: to reduce any peritumoural oedema. This is common practice although evidence supporting it is lacking
- CXR and CT thorax remain essential
- **stenting**: an expanding metal stent can be manoeuvred into the SVC at the point of stricture. If an interventional cardiologist or radiologist can provide a rapid service this is the treatment of choice for patients with severe symptoms. Palliation is usually within 24–48 h. Endovascular stenting can also be used for recurrent SVCO in a previously irradiated field. Repeated stent insertion is possible
- **thrombolysis**: if a venogram confirms the presence of clot. Usually combined with stent insertion if possible, although morbidity is increased. Where thrombus has formed around a Hickman line, removal of the line alone will usually lead to resolution of SVCO

- **radiotherapy**: occasionally used in the absence of a histological diagnosis. However, it is important to stress this will **not** provide immediate symptomatic benefit. Anticipated life expectancy must be several weeks to see the full benefit. Radiotherapy may make subsequent histology difficult to obtain.

In practice it is rare for the clinical situation to be so acute as to prevent appropriate work-up. Therefore, treatment can be tailored according to the underlying diagnosis as in the following examples.

- **Small-cell lung cancer**: these are typically chemosensitive tumours. If the patient is fit enough, systemic chemotherapy is the appropriate first-line management producing palliation of symptoms within 1–2 weeks. Palliative radiotherapy is used in patients of poorer performance status or on relapse after previous chemotherapy.
- **Non-small cell lung cancer**: the presence of SVCO is usually associated with locally advanced (and hence incurable) disease. Surgery is unlikely to be appropriate. Occasionally, radical radiotherapy for central, localized cancers may be possible but generally radiotherapy is palliative in intent.
- **Non-Hodgkin's lymphoma**: usually chemotherapy.
- **Mediastinal germ cell tumour**: chemotherapy.

Raised intracranial pressure (ICP)

Clinical presentation

The rigid bony skull surrounding the brain is resistant to any increase in the volume of its contents, with any such change leading to a rise in intra-cranial pressure (ICP) and/or displacement of brain structures. The skull contents comprise:

- the brain and interstitial fluid (80%)
- intravascular blood (10%)
- cerebrospinal fluid (CSF) (10%).

An increase in volume of one component may be accommodated by reduction in another in order to maintain physiological ICP (10–20 cm H_2O). When malignancy involves the brain, these physiological regulatory mechanisms are commonly overcome, leading to raised ICP.

Clinical features

- Early stages: typically symptoms are of headache and nausea/vomiting.
- Often worse in the morning because of cerebral venous congestion associated with lying supine.
- Coughing or sneezing may aggravate the headache.
- As pressure increases, there may be cognitive impairment and drowsiness, heralding a more rapid neurological deterioration.
- Herniation of cerebral tissue through the tentorium may cause midbrain compression with coma associated with pupillary and oculomotor signs, and altered regulation of respiration and cardiovascular control, with bradycardia and hypertension.
- Fundoscopy will reveal papilloedema in 50%, and there may be associated neurological deficit.
- Specific signs may suggest the site of pathology, e.g. Parinaud's syndrome, with limitation of upward gaze associated with pineal tumours.
- Raised ICP may cause hyponatraemia through secretion of inappropriate antidiuretic hormone (SIADH).
- When increase in ICP is more gradual, presentation may be with memory loss, behavioural changes, and altered gait.
- Meningeal malignancy commonly causes cranial nerve palsies in addition to raised ICP.

Pathogenesis

The three commonest causes of increased ICP are:

- space-occupying lesion
- hydrocephalus (due to obstruction of CSF circulation)
- benign intracranial hypertension.

It should be remembered that patients with malignancy may be at risk of developing non-malignant raised ICP as a consequence of treatment, e.g. coagulopathy-associated intracranial haemorrhage or CNS infection in an immunocompromised individual.

Of the neoplastic lesions causing raised ICP:

- 50% are due to metastatic disease
- remainder are primary brain tumours, of which gliomas are the commonest.

Malignant disease in the central nervous system (CNS) can produce a rise in intracranial pressure through:
- mass effect
- vasogenic oedema: capillary leakage is associated with the abnormal tumour vasculature
- haemorrhage from the tumour (especially melanoma, choriocarcinoma, renal cancer)
- hydrocephalus:
  - obstruction of CSF flow, e.g. pineal tumour obstructing the aqueduct of Sylvius prevents drainage of CSF from the 3rd to the 4th ventricle
  - meningeal metastases may reduce the reabsorption of CSF with resulting communicating hydrocephalus.

Diagnosis
Contrast-enhanced computerized tomography (CT) or magnetic resonance imaging (MRI) scan.
- Unenhanced CT may show mass lesion(s) and associated haemorrhage (hyperdense).
- Surrounding oedema and/or hydrocephalus.
- CT with IV contrast demonstrates enhancement in the majority of CNS malignancies.
- MRI undoubtedly has superior sensitivity in the detection of CNS malignancy.
- Where CT shows a solitary tumour, MRI will reveal more than one lesion in at least 20%.
- On MRI, tumour appears iso- or hypodense on T_1-weighted images, hyperdense on T_2, and enhances with contrast.
- MRI gives superior definition of anatomical detail and may demonstrate meningeal spread of malignancy.

Management
- Early management:
  - reduce vasogenic oedema with high-dose dexamethasone (16 mg daily) with proton pump inhibitor (PPI) gastroprotection
  - in non-responding patients osmotic diuresis with IV mannitol (100 ml 20% solution over 1–2 h)
- Further management will depend on the diagnosis and may include:
  - neurosurgical intervention
  - systemic chemotherapy for chemosensitive disease, e.g. CNS lymphoma
  - cranial radiotherapy
  - symptom control only if poor prognosis.

In general, CNS tumours presenting with raised intracranial pressure require a tissue diagnosis, either by biopsy which may be stereotactic or by craniotomy and removal of the tumour. Ventricular shunting may be useful in patients with hydrocephalus due to lesions situated in areas difficult to access surgically. However, if at all possible, histological confirmation should be sought, as it has a major bearing on the therapeutic approach.

High-grade gliomas may have a substantial cystic component that in the setting of recurrent disease may be drained to provide rapid relief of elevated ICP.

Stridor

Aetiology

Malignant
- Intrinsic upper airway disease:
  - primary tumours of the upper airway (e.g. bulky intraluminal bronchogenic carcinomas non-small-cell lung cancer (NSCLC), small-cell lung cancer (SCLC)), larynx, (e.g. laryngeal carcinoma), hypopharynx, subglottis, trachea or local extension of a bronchial tumour invading the carina
  - metastatic endobronchial disease affecting the upper airway, e.g. bronchogenic, breast, melanoma, renal cell
  - occasionally carcinoid tumours
- Extrinsic compression:
  - mediastinal neoplasm (e.g. anaplastic thyroid cancer, germ cell tumour, thymic carcinoma, oeophageal cancer)
  - lymphadenopathy, e.g. from (typically non-Hodgkin's) lymphoma or metastatic carcinoma.

Benign
- Lymphadenopathy, e.g. sarcoidosis, tuberculosis
- Inhaled food/foreign body/mucus plug/blood clot
- Tracheal stenosis, e.g. post-tracheostomy, granulation tissue
- Bilateral vocal cord palsy, e.g. post-thyroid surgery
- Infective, e.g. epiglottitis.

Presentation

Usually insidious, e.g. slow compression by mediastinal tumour. Occasionally history is acute, e.g. rapid deterioration when sub-critical obstruction further compromised, e.g. by haemorrhage, infection or swelling.

Symptoms

- Shortness of breath, wheeze unresponsive to bronchodilators
- Cough ± sputum production ± haemoptysis
- Recurrent (incompletely resolving) pneumonias
- Difficulty swallowing or drooling
- Drowsiness, collapse.

Signs

- Stridor: a high-pitched noise generated by the turbulent flow of air through a partially obstructed airway. Timing of stridor may suggest the site of the obstruction
  - **inspiratory stridor**: with extra-thoracic, supraglottic or glottic obstruction
  - **biphasic stridor**: with glottic or subglottic obstruction
  - **expiratory stridor**: with intrathoracic tracheal obstruction
- Dyspnoea, tachycardia, cyanosis
- Features of underlying malignancy, e.g. goitre, clubbing, weight loss, Horners's syndrome, disseminated lymphadenopathy.

Management and investigation

- **Priority is to stabilize a distressed patient** – sit them up, check arterial blood gases (ABGs; to assess for ventilatory failure – involve intensive therapy unit (ITU) or ear, nose and throat (ENT) if exhausted or in respiratory failure i.e. arterial oxygen tension (P_aO_2) ≤10 kPa, arterial carbon dioxide tension (P_aCO_2) ≥6 kPa), give 100% O_2, establish intravenous access. Very occasionally, emergency tracheostomy may be required to preserve the airway before appropriate treatment is initiated.

Remember diagnosis/staging of underlying malignancy may not have been confirmed. **If the patient is stable** consider the following:

- **full blood count (FBC) –** exclude anaemia as an exacerbating factor
- **chest X-ray (CXR)** – may demonstrate mediastinal widening (lymphadenopathy), primary lung cancer, or other evidence of underlying malignancy, e.g. pleural effusion
- **computerized tomography (CT) scan of thorax** – may identify the site of obstruction and indicate the extent of disease (prognostic implications)
- **indirect laryngoscopy** – mobility of cords
- **bronchoscopy** – direct visualization confirms airway obstruction. Differentiates between intrinsic and extrinsic lesions. May allow histological confirmation of diagnosis
- **fibreoptic nasoendoscopy**
- **mediastinoscopy**.

Treatment of malignant airways obstruction in stable patients

- Dependent upon the underlying cause
- **Supplemental O$_2$:** assess need using pulse oximetry/ABGs
- **Patient comfort:** consider opiates for the sensation of breathlessness ± anxiolytics, typically benzodiazepines. Co-existent bronchospasm may respond to nebulized bronchodilators, e.g. salbutamol. Suction to remove pooled secretions if patients tolerates
- **High-dose steroids:** aiming to reduce peri-tumoural oedema and relieve obstruction, e.g. dexamethasone 8 mg bd PO/IV. Little evidence base for this approach and no immediate benefit
- **External beam radiotherapy:** used for most patients with NSCLC, usually with palliative intent. Appropriate in some other cancers, e.g. renal cell cancer. May be initiated in the absence of histology in urgent circumstances. Therapeutic effects are delayed. Anecdotal concern that radiotherapy may initially worsen peri-tumoural oedema and all such patients should receive steroids
- **Endobronchial brachytherapy** (single fraction) is also an option in recurrent obstruction, including following external beam radiotherapy
- **Chemotherapy:** appropriate primary treatment for airway obstruction due to chemosensitive tumours, e.g. small-cell carcinoma, lymphoma, germ cell tumours
- **Laser debulking:** helpful in bulky exophytic laryngeal tumours prior to definitive treatment or if the cancer is radio-resistant, e.g. metastatic melanoma. If sole therapy, then effects tend not to be long-lasting
- **Endoluminal stenting by bronchoscopy:** may produce useful palliation in cases of recurrent malignancy affecting the trachea or in obstruction due to extrinsic causes. Can be repeated if subsequently fails due to tumour overgrowth or stent migration
- **Surgical resection:** limited role as salvage therapy for recurrent laryngeal cancer and, more rarely, primary carcinoid tumour of the trachea or a solitary renal cell metastasis.

Further reading

Gasper WT, Jamshidi R, Theodore PR (2007) Palliation of thoracic malignancies. *Surg Oncol* **16(4)**, 259–65: includes sections on pleural and pericardial effusions and oesophageal obstruction.

Thromboembolic and cardiac emergencies

Thromboembolic disease and cancer

Scale of the problem

- Up to 90% of cancer patients exhibit activation of the coagulation pathways.
- 4–20% develop deep vein thrombosis and/or pulmonary embolus (venous thromboembolism or VTE).
- Risk has increased over the last 20 years, likely due to anti-cancer treatments e.g. hormone therapy, chemotherapy, and, more recently, targeted therapies against angiogenesis.
- Arterial thrombotic events are also increased (1–4%).
- May account for 9% of deaths in patients receiving chemotherapy.
- Prophylactic treatment should be effective for many at-risk patients.
- Patients who present with idiopathic thrombosis without a history of malignancy are at increased risk of occult cancer, and warrant chest X-ray, full physical examination including rectal and gynaecological assessment, faecal occult bloods (FOBs) and prostate-specific antigen (PSA) (only patients with positive clinical findings require further investigation e.g. computerized tomography (CT) scan).

Mechanisms of coagulopathy

The molecular basis is uncertain, proposed causes include:
- activation of coagulation by tissue factor in tumours
- factor X-activating cysteine protease
- mucinous glycoproteins
- *MET* oncogene activation.

Prevention of venous thromboembolism

Prophylaxis with low molecular weight heparin (e.g. dalteparin 3400–5000 U s/c daily) reduces the risk of VTE by 40–80% and is recommended for:
- patients undergoing major cancer surgery
- patients with cancer confined to bed, e.g. acute medical admissions
- ambulatory patients receiving chemotherapy deemed to be at high risk (see Table 34.1):
  - high-risk pathology
  - high-risk treatments
  - past history of deep vein thrombosis (DVT).

Contraindications to prophylactic anticoagulation include:
- active bleeding, e.g. primary tumour, central nervous system (CNS) metastasis, peptic ulcer
- thrombocytopenia or clotting dysfunction, e.g. hepatic metastases.

Randomized trials using an alternative approach – low-dose warfarin 1 mg daily – in patients receiving chemotherapy via central venous access, have shown this to be ineffective in reducing thrombotic events, although some have demonstrated reduction in line-related costs. Indeed experience has shown that it is necessary to frequently monitor the international normalized ratio (INR) when warfarin is given during chemotherapy, not least because of interactions between several cytotoxics and warfarin.

Table 34.1 Risk factors for VTE in patients with malignant disease

Patient-related factors:
- co-morbidity e.g. obesity, infection, chronic obstructive pulmonary disease (COPD), arteriopathy
- past history of VTE

Cancer-related factors:
- primary site gastrointestinal (GI) tract, brain, lung, gynaecological
- metastatic disease

Treatment-related factors
- recent surgery
- current hospitalization
- ongoing chemotherapy or hormone therapy
- anti-angiogenic therapy
- central venous catheter

Treatment of venous thromboembolism in cancer patients

Standard treatment of VTE with initial therapeutic dose low molecular weight heparin and warfarin is problematic in cancer patients because of:
- unpredictable response to warfarin, e.g. deranged hepatic metabolism in metastatic disease, drug interactions, e.g. capecitabine
- inconvenience of frequent monitoring of INR
- high rate of recurrent VTE on warfarin
- high rate of bleeding on warfarin
- for many patients the preferred option is long-term therapeutic dose low molecular weight heparin injections, and promising results with this approach suggest it may also have an added benefit of enhancing the anti-tumour effects of chemotherapy, e.g. in small-cell lung cancer (SCLC).

Thrombolytic treatment

Urokinase infusion indicated if:
- pulmonary embolus with severe right ventricular dysfunction
- massive iliofemoral thrombosis with the risk of limb gangrene

Vena cava filter

- Indicated for patients with VTE and contraindication to anticoagulant therapy
- Also patients with recurrent VTE despite adequate therapy with low molecular weight heparin.

Both thrombolysis and inferior vena cava (IVC) filter insertion require the assistance of interventional radiologists.

Heparin-induced thrombocytopenia (HIT)

Falling platelet counts during heparin therapy can be associated with severe thrombotic tendency, even resulting in massive thrombosis and limb gangrene. Management comprises:
- withdraw heparin
- consider switch to danaparoid rather than warfarin, particularly if the platelet count does not rise immediately.

Arterial thromboembolic disease

During the early randomized studies of adjuvant chemotherapy and hormone therapy for breast cancer in the 1970–80s, it was noted that 1.6% of pre-menopausal women developed arterial thromboses when treated with both chemotherapy and tamoxifen. Since then, other observations have included:

- sporadic cases of myocardial infarction and cerebrovascular accident (CVA) reported during chemotherapy for testicular cancer since 1980
- association with smoking, obesity, elevated cholesterol, diabetes
- more frequent cases of acute lower limb ischaemia as well as cardiac and cerebrovascular events following cisplatin-based chemotherapy for e.g. lung cancer and other smoking-related malignancies
- carboplatin appears less likely to cause vascular damage
- mechanism underlying acute ischaemia post chemotherapy still uncertain
- other cytotoxics e.g. 5-fluorouracil and capecitabine associated with coronary artery spasm rather than thrombosis.

There have been no formal trials of prophylactic therapy against arterial thromboembolism, but it would seem prudent to adopt the following:

- low-dose aspirin and a statin should be considered for smokers not already taking these who are receiving chemotherapy, in particular cisplatin
- unless there is strong evidence of inferior anti-cancer efficacy (e.g. testicular cancer), carboplatin should be considered instead of cisplatin for patients with existing vascular disease requiring platinum-based chemotherapy.

Disseminated intravascular coagulation and malignant disease

Definition
Disseminated intravascular coagulation (DIC) is an acquired disorder characterized by widespread activation of coagulation, resulting in:
- intravascular formation of fibrin
- thrombotic occlusion of small and mid-sized vessels
- multi-organ failure
- severe bleeding.

Aetiology in cancer patients
- Septicaemia usually in combination with neutropenia
- Direct effect of malignancy:
  - 5%, particularly prostate and GI cancers
  - 15% of patients with acute leukaemia (especially acute promyelocytic leukaemia).

Pathogenesis
- Thrombin generation is mediated by plasma tissue factor, released in response to infection or by tumour itself.
- Anticoagulation pathways are impaired, with low levels of antithrombin III.
- Fibrinolysis is suppressed by plasminogen activator inhibitor type 1.
- The combination of increased formation of fibrin and its inadequate removal results in disseminated intravascular thrombosis.

Clinical and laboratory features
- Bleeding tendency
- Thrombotic organ damage
- Renal failure
- Thrombocytopenia
- Prolonged clotting times
- Presence of fibrin degradation products in plasma
- Low plasma antithrombin III.

Management
- Mainstay of treatment is to tackle the underlying cause:
  - appropriate antibiotic therapy for sepsis
  - effective treatment for the underlying malignancy.
- Supportive measures appropriate to the individual presentation:
  - heparin anticoagulation
  - replace platelets and clotting factors (fresh frozen plasma if bleeding)
  - anti-fibrinolytic agents, e.g. tranexamic acid.

Unless the underlying pathology is sensitive to treatment, the prognosis is very poor indeed.

Cardiac disease and cancer

Patients with cancer frequently develop common cardiac problems such as infarction, failure, or arrhythmias. This can be unrelated to their malignancy, due to smoking, ageing, infection, etc. Alternatively, cardiac problems may arise through:

- direct tumour extension to the pericardium, heart or great vessels
- thromboembolic disease, e.g. pulmonary embolus
- tumour embolus, e.g. from hepatic metastasis to right side of heart
- metabolic effects of cancer, e.g. hypokalaemic alkalosis due to ectopic adrenocorticotrophic hormone (ACTH) production, release of adrenaline by phaeochromocytoma, or of 5-hydroxytryptamine ($5-HT_3$) by carcinoid tumour
- effects of treatment
  - post-operative arrhythmias
  - chemotherapy, e.g. anthracyclines, trastuzumab, sunitinib may all reduce left ventricular ejection fraction
  - radiotherapy, e.g. chest wall irradiation after surgery for breast cancer with late effects on coronary arteries and cardiac muscle.

Pericardial effusion

Thoracic malignancies such as lung cancer, mesothelioma, or metastatic disease can result in pericardial effusion.

- Presents with acute dyspnoea ± central chest pain.
- Rapid accumulation of fluid or pericardial stiffening due to tumour can result in tamponade, with worsening symptoms including orthopnoea, cough and syncope.
- Heart sounds muffled ± pericardial rub and apex beat not detectable.
- Low blood pressure and pulsus paradoxus.
- Low-voltage electrocardiogram (ECG).
- Typical chest X-ray (CXR) appearances – increased cardiothoracic ratio, enlarged globular heart.
- Confirm by echocardiography.
- Aspiration and cytological examination of the effusion may aid diagnosis.
- Symptomatic collections may require urgent assessment and intervention.
- Can be drained by needle (usually under radiological control) or by surgical procedure of 'pericardial window' formation.
- Treat underlying cancer.

Marantic endocarditis

Non-bacterial thrombotic endocarditis is characterized by:

- platelet-fibrin vegetations on the cardiac valves (especially mitral and aortic)
- 40% have emboli (digital arteries, spleen, kidney, brain, heart)
- may have associated DIC.

Treat with low molecular weight heparin and if possible effective systemic treatment for malignancy.

Tumours of the heart and great vessels

- Metastatic disease involving the heart is found in 1.5–21% of autopsies.
- Primary cardiac tumours are rare.
- Present with arrhythmias, heart failure, valvular dysfunction and murmurs, and arterial emboli.
- 75% benign, e.g. atrial myxoma.
- 25% malignant
  - rhabdomyosarcoma, leiomyosarcoma
  - poor prognosis with high risk of metastatic disease.
- Tumours of large arteries and veins also very rare, the latter presenting with extensive deep vein thrombosis.

Further reading

Lee AY (2007) The effects of low molecular weight heparins on venous thromboembolism and survival in patients with cancer. *Thromb Res* **120(Suppl 2)**, S121–7.

Lyman GH, Khorana AA, Falanga A, *et al.* (2007) American Society of Clinical Oncology guideline: recommendations for venous thromboembolism prophylaxis and treatment in patients with cancer. *J Clin Oncol* 25, 5490–505.

Mandala M, Falanga A, Roila F (2008) Management of venous thromboembolism in cancer patients: ESMO clinical recommendations. *Ann Oncol* **19(Suppl 2)**, ii126–7.

Obstruction

Intestinal obstruction

Aetiology

Predominantly associated with pelvic cancers and most commonly found in ovarian (6–42%), cervical (5%), and colonic cancers (10–30%). Cause is either intraluminal disease (more common in colonic cancer) or extramural compression. In ovarian and cervical cancer there are often multiple levels of obstruction. Obstruction in a patient with previous cancer may also be due to non-malignant causes (such as adhesions), and this diagnosis requires careful consideration.

Obstruction may be complete, subacute, or functional; it may be intermittent. Functional obstruction may be caused by a cancer-related or drug-related (vincristine) autonomic neuropathy, by direct involvement of the mesenteric plexus, or ileus (e.g. due to perforation). The most frequent cause of intestinal obstruction is the cancer itself, which may invade the lumen of the bowel, may extrinsically compress the bowel, or may disrupt the neurological supply to the bowel wall muscle. The common primary sites, causing gastric intestinal problems, are colorectal and ovarian cancers.

However, it is important to remember that less common, but reversible, causes include electrolyte disturbances, faecal impaction, post-operative adhesions, or herniae. The commonly implicated electrolyte disturbance is that of hypercalcaemia and hypokalaemia.

Presentation

- Symptoms: nausea, vomiting, colicky pain, constipation, increased bowel sounds
- Signs:
  - distension, dehydration, splash, bowel sounds variable
  - gastric outlet obstruction – large-volume projectile vomiting
  - large bowel obstruction; faeculent vomiting.

Investigations

Erect and supine plain abdominal views may confirm the diagnosis. Where the diagnosis is not clear, contrast barium studies may be indicated. If surgery is a possibility and there is doubt about the number of levels of obstruction or the site of the lesion, computerized tomography (CT) can be helpful. Appropriate resuscitation will be guided by clinical and biochemical assessment of dehydration and electrolyte disturbance. Occasionally, endoscopy of the upper or lower intestinal tract may allow visualization of the area of obstruction.

Management options

If active treatment is appropriate, surgery may need to be considered after careful multidisciplinary discussion. Intravenous fluids and nasogastric suction are usually instigated but **may** not be necessary if surgery is not an option. The patient may not wish surgery or, due to the extent of disease, surgery may not be appropriate. Laser therapy may be useful to debulk obstructing oesophageal, gastric, and rectal carcinomas. However, this approach requires repeated treatment. Plastic tubes or expandable metal stents can also be considered and are generally of use in oesophageal or oesophagogastric lesions. There is now increasing use of colonic stents inserted via colonoscopy.

Medical management

- Inoperable intestinal obstruction can be managed medically. This may permit the patient to be cared for at home. The patient can eat and drink small amounts. Treatment approaches vary depending on whether subacute obstruction or complete obstruction is present. The aim is to remove the debilitating feeling of nausea and to reduce the frequency of vomiting to a level acceptable to the patient.
- The symptoms to be palliated are nausea, vomiting, pain, and constipation. Oral medication is poorly absorbed in gastrointestinal obstruction and the subcutaneous or rectal route should be used.

Pain

For colic, an anti-spasmodic – Buscopan® (hyoscine butylbromide) 80–120 mg over 24 h via continuous subcutaneous infusion – is usually effective. Avoid pro-kinetic anti-emetics (metoclopramide), if colic is a problem. Pain from cancer or metastases usually requires parenteral analgesics (e.g. diamorphine given subcutaneously over 24 h via a syringe driver, or transdermal fentanyl).

Nausea and vomiting

- If partial obstruction without colic is present, metoclopramide, 80–120 mg over 24 h s/c, may stimulate effective bowel motility. This can be combined with high-dose dexamethasone, 16 mg/24 h, to reduce peri-tumour oedema and also serve as an anti-emetic. As vomiting is controlled, introduce oral laxatives as tolerated.
- If obstruction is complete or if colic is present, cyclizine, 100–150 mg/24 h s/c, is given with Buscopan® (hyoscine butylbromide). Haloperidol, 5–15 mg/24 h, is a suitable alternative. Haloperidol, cyclizine, and hyoscine are all miscible with diamorphine in a driver syringe.
- Levomeprazine is a highly specific 5-hydroxytryptamine (5-HT$_2$) antagonist and has inhibitory effects on other emetic pathway receptors. It is a useful alternative to the aforementioned anti-emetics and is also miscible with diamorphine. If vomiting persists then octreotide, 300–600 mg/24 h via continuous s/c infusion – a somatostatin analogue – can be used. This drug is anti-secretory and promotes reabsorption of electrolytes and, hence, water from the bowel.
- In difficult cases a nasogastric tube should be considered for short-term use. If all else fails to control the vomiting and it is distressing to the patient, then a venting gastrostomy must be considered, taking into account the patient's prognosis, current condition, and, above all, their own wishes. With a gastrostomy *in situ*, the patient can take oral liquids, which can be drawn off via the gastrostomy, as needed. In selected patients, endoscopic insertion of a percutaneous endoscopic gastrostomy (PEG) tube may be indicated. All patients with malignant bowel obstruction who fail to recover bowel function with conservative management should be considered for surgery if the clinical status of the patient permits and the patient wishes

further, more invasive, therapy. Even in those fit for surgery, 25% will die peri-operatively. The use of a colonic stent is helpful to avoid an open procedure. However laparoscopic creation of a stoma may lead to a more rapid recovery. This problem is best managed with a multidisciplinary team, involving surgeons, cancer specialists, and palliative care physicians along with discussions with the patient and his/her family. The risks and benefits must be discussed.

- If the obstruction is due to a very chemosensitive tumour, such as a lymphoma, small-cell, or testicular cancer, a trial of chemotherapy may be appropriate. However, this is potentially hazardous and requires close monitoring.
- The patient with oesophageal obstruction or duodenal obstruction may benefit from local radiotherapy or stent insertion. Often, the stent should be inserted first, followed by radiotherapy, as the benefit from the latter may not be seen for 6 weeks.

Surgical treatment

Surgical options include the following:
- obstruction in the oesophagus:
  - oesophagectomy (only in very selected patients)
  - stent insertion
  - laser treatment
- duodenal obstruction:
  - surgical bypass
  - stent insertion
  - ileal obstruction
  - resection of obstruction and re-anastomosis
  - division of adhesions
  - defunctioning ileostomy (via the laparoscope)
- colon – resection of obstruction and re-anastomosis
- defunctioning colostomy – stent.

Risks of bowel surgery in patients with advanced cancer include:
- multiple levels of bowel obstruction due to intraperitoneal tumour seeding
- poor anaesthetic risk due to generalized debility
- poor surgical healing due to malnutrition, chemotherapy, or tumour seeding
- high risk of thromboembolic events
- early mortality and morbidity.

The increasing use of laparoscopic procedures to deal with obstruction is useful with more rapid recovery, but must be done by specialized, experienced surgeons, as this is difficult, minimally invasive surgery.

Urinary tract obstruction

Aetiology

The following are the most common causes of urinary obstruction in patients with cancer:

- carcinoma of the prostate or bladder when the urethra or ureteric orifices become occluded
- carcinoma of the cervix or other carcinoma involving the pelvis obstructing the lower ureter
- para-aortic nodes or retroperitoneal tumour compressing the ureters
- transitional cell carcinoma of one or both ureters
- fibrosis following surgery, chemotherapy, or radiotherapy.

Symptoms

The gradual onset of unilateral ureteric obstruction is often asymptomatic, only diagnosed radiographically as hydronephrosis. Acute ureteric obstruction may cause painful spasm or dull aching in the flank, and the pain may radiate in the distribution of the L1 nerve root. Bilateral gradual obstruction becomes symptomatic as the serum urea rises above 25 mmol/l, ultimately leading to anuria and renal failure, with lethargy, drowsiness, confusion, nausea, and twitching.

Investigations

Selective use of abdominal ultrasound, intravenous urography (IVU) (contraindicated in uraemic patients), cystoscopy and retrograde ureteric studies, isotope renogram (assesses function of each kidney), and computerized tomography (CT) scan of the abdomen are helpful. CT of the abdomen with intravenous (IV) contrast as a single modality provides most information by defining any extra-ureteric pathology (although care must be taken with the use of IV contrast in renal impairment). CT is now replacing IVU as the imaging of choice. Cystoscopy is essential in those patients who are going to require active management.

Management options

Bladder outlet obstruction causes symptoms of acute urinary retention or chronic obstruction, with overflow incontinence relieved by urethral or suprapubic catheterization. Palliative transurethral resection of a prostate or bladder tumour may be necessary to provide symptomatic relief.
Ureteric decompression can be accomplished by:

- percutaneous nephrostomy with, or without, antegrade stenting
- cystoscopy and retrograde placement of an internal ureteric stent.

Ureteric stents need to be replaced every 6 months in patients with cancer, although modern stents may last longer.

Percutaneous nephrostomy is a temporary measure, appropriate in the following specific circumstances:

- undiagnosed malignant disease
- prostatic or cervical primary, with an available treatment modality with a reasonable chance of response
- in patients with malignancy in the pelvis, it may be impossible to cannulate the ureters and a nephrostomy may be essential.

Patients with advanced cancer can gain symptomatic benefit from nephrostomy/ureteric stent insertion. However, since a nephrostomy drain may remain *in situ* for several months, it is prone to dislodgement, infection, and leakage around the site. Double pigtail ureteric stents should be inserted in preference to a long-term nephrostomy (where possible).

Complications include transient bacteraemia, sepsis, haemorrhage, and obstructive encrustations. Care must be taken in these patients to ensure dehydration, fluid overload, and hyperkalaemia are corrected. The latter is a true emergency and ultimately it will lead to arrhythmias and cardiac arrest.

- In very selected patients there are indications for dialysis, such as increasing hyperkalaemia, fluid overload resistant to diuretics, and severe renal failure and acidosis. Other problems may include a significant bleeding tendency due to platelet dysfunction. Hypertension is occasionally a problem and requires fluid management and/or antihypertensives.
- Any manipulation of the obstructed urinary tract requires antibiotic cover as these patients are prone to septicaemia.
- Patients with urinary tract obstruction require multidisciplinary team management; prolonged survival, even with pelvic malignant disease, is still possible. In one series median survival was 26 weeks.
- There were four groups in this series:
  - group 1 – primary untreated malignancy.
  - group 2 – recurrent malignancy with further treatment options.
  - group 3 – recurrent malignancy with no further treatment options.
  - group 4 – benign disease as a consequence of previous treatment.
- Patients in groups 1 and 2 had similar survival: median survival 27 and 20 weeks, 5-year survival 20% and 10%, respectively.
- Patients in group 3 had a poor prognosis with median survival 6 weeks, with no patient surviving beyond 1 year.
- Patients in group 4 had the best outlook with 5-year survival of 64%.

If the patient has advanced pelvic maligancy for which there is no treatment, then quality of life and the patient's own wishes should determine whether to intervene (or not).

Obstructive jaundice

Aetiology

There are many causes of jaundice in the patient with malignant disease. Classically, the causes can be divided as follows:

- increased production of bilirubin, haemolytic anaemia
- decreased uptake of bilirubin:
  - Gilbert's syndrome
  - drugs
  - portacaval shunts
- decreased excretion of bilirubin:
  - hepatotoxic drugs
  - viral hepatitis
  - malignant infiltration of biliary tree or liver and extrahepatic biliary obstruction.

It is important in principle not to focus only on cancer causes in every patient with jaundice who has a history of cancer. Jaundice is not always due to the recurrence of the cancer or complications of same.

Patients must be carefully assessed, by a multidisciplinary team, to ensure that they are adequately investigated (where appropriate) so that non-cancerous causes of the obstructive jaundice can be dealt with appropriately.

History

- Abdominal pain.
- Duration of jaundice and whether the jaundice fluctuates.
- Fever.
- Itching.
- Dark stools and pale urine.
- In particular, it is important to assess whether or not the patient has signs of sepsis.
- A careful drug history is important as a number of drugs can cause hepatic toxicity, for example, cisplatin, oxaliplatin, can cause cholestasis. Similarly, some of the anti-metabolites, such as cytarabine, may cause self-limiting abnormalities of liver function, often with a cholestatic pattern. A similar pattern can arise with mercaptopurine and methotrexate:
  - some hormonal agents, such as tamoxifen, can occasionally cause abnormal liver function with a fatty liver
  - it is also important to take a detailed history of other drug therapies, such as paracetamol, antibiotics, and antifungal agents, all of which can cause liver abnormalities
  - total parenteral nutrition can cause fatty infiltration and intrahepatic cholestasis.

Examination

Signs of recurrence of the previous cancer: clinical jaundice, anaemia, signs of chronic liver disease, palpable liver, palpable gall bladder, the presence of ascites, and palpable spleen are all important findings.

Investigations

Depending upon the history and the examination, investigations should include the following:

- routine blood tests, including haemoglobin, white cell count
- liver function tests, including transaminases, gamma-glutamyl transpeptidase (GGT), bilirubin, alkline phosphatase
- autoantibody screen is important to investigate autoimmune disease (where appropriate); electrophoresis and other investigations for haemolysis in selected patients where indicated
- all patients who are undergoing active management and treatment require coagulation studies, because of deficiency of the vitamin K-dependent coagulation factors
- the most important screening radiological investigation is ultrasound, which can diagnose:
  - gallstones
  - demonstrate intra- or extrahepatic biliary dilatation
  - tumour masses in the region of the pancreas (better seen on computerized tomography (CT))
  - liver metastases
  - nodes around the porta hepatis, although the lower end of the common bile duct is not well visualized.

Other investigations include the following:

- magnetic resonance imaging (MRI) scanning gives excellent visualization of the biliary tree and is non-invasive
- CT scanning is excellent for liver and pancreatic lesions
- generally an endoscopic retrograde cholangiopancreatography (ERCP) (after discussion with the patient and family, and following discussion at a multidisciplinary team meeting) is the next step (provided the patient is going to require active management):
  - ERCP is an excellent diagnostic technique that can diagnose pancreatic, intrinsic biliary, extrinsic biliary, and hepatic lesions
  - brushings for cytology and biopsies can be taken.
  - ERCP is also an excellent therapeutic modality, which can be used to dilate strictures, place stents, extract gallstones from the common bile duct
  - occasionally, percutaneous transhepatic cholangiography is used in conjunction with ERCP to insert stents for difficult high hilar lesions, either intrinsic, such as cholangiocarcinoma (Klatskin's tumour), or extrinsic (nodes at porta hepatis). A good working relationship between the gastroenterologist and interventional radiologist is essential.

Points of caution

- Intrahepatic duct dilatation does not occur readily in extrinsic biliary obstruction, when there are multiple liver metastases compressing the ducts, when there is sclerosing cholangitis, and when there is liver cirrhosis.
- Any invasive endeavours around the bilary tree, including ERCP and biliary stenting, must be covered with antibiotics as there is a risk of sepsis. Coagulation must be checked and corrected as necessary.
- Serum amylase should be performed pre- and post-ERCP.

- Occasionally, liver biopsy is appropriate. This can be ultrasound guided, laparoscopic, or transjugular (in patients with coagulopathies).

Management

Management depends on the cause of the jaundice. It is crucial that these patients, who are highly complex, are managed in a multidisciplinary team setting. The patient's views and their family's wishes should be considered, especially when the jaundice is due to recurrence of a previous carcinoma.

Each cause of jaundice should be treated in its own right, depending on the patient's general condition and wishes. For example, a stone in the common bile duct can be removed at ERCP and the patient can undergo laparoscopic cholecystectomy at a later date, should that be appropriate. However, many patients with obstructive jaundice in the setting of cancer require palliation. Once drug causes have been excluded and if the patient does have an irresectable tumour problem causing the obstruction, often the best mode of palliation is endoscopic stenting. This tends to have a lower early morbidity and mortality than an open surgical bypass. With advances in laparoscopic surgery, laparoscopic biliary bypass is now technically feasible in selected patients, in experienced hands.

The main problem with stents is that they occlude with subsequent recurrence of jaundice and sepsis, although the more modern expandable metal stents have decreased bacterial colonization and are more resistant to tumour ingrowth.

Hepatorenal syndrome

- Classically this syndrome occurs in obstructive jaundice and it is essentially acute oliguric renal failure, occurring without intrinsic renal disease.
- There is intense renal cortical vasoconstriction with increased renal vascular resistance, decreased glomerular filtration rate, peripheral vasodilatation, and sodium and water retention.
- This diagnosis should be considered in patients with liver dysfunction, obstructive jaundice, rising serum creatinine in the absence of fluid losses, dehydration, renal disease, or nephrotoxic drugs, and in patients who are not septic.
- Investigations should exclude other causes of renal insufficiency: serum and urinary electrolytes, creatinine clearance, blood cultures, urinary tract ultrasound (to exclude urinary obstruction).
- Investigations usually reveal high serum creatinine, low creatinine clearance, low serum sodium, low urinary output, and low urinary sodium.
- Management is complex and should be in the setting of a multidisciplinary team involving renal physicians. Nephrotoxic drugs should be withdrawn. Sepsis should be corrected. Fluid and electrolyte imbalance should be corrected.
- Selected patients may warrant dialysis with correction of the obstructive jaundice. However, prognosis is often poor with only a 20% 3-month survival rate.
- Discussion with the patient and family, in a multidisciplinary team setting, with colleagues from the appropriate specialties, is essential for these ill patients with a poor prognosis.

Further reading

Agarwal AK, Mandal S, Singh S (2007) Biliary obstruction in gallbladder cancer is not sine qua non of inoperability. *Ann Surg Oncol* **14**, 2831–7.

Baron JH (2001) Expandable metal stents for the treatment of cancerous obstructions of the gastrointestinal tract. *N Engl J Med* **344**, 1681–17.

Dubovsky EV, Russell CD (1992) Advances in radionuclide evaluation of urinary tract obstruction. *Abdom Imaging* **23**, 17–26.

Garden OJ (2007) *Hepatobiliary and Pancreatic Surgery*. Edinburgh: Elsevier, Saunders, pp. 323–330.

Helyer LK, Lae CHL, Butler M, *et al.* (2007) Surgery as a bridge to palliative chemotherapy in patients with malignant bowel obstruction from colorectal cancer. *Ann Surg Oncol* **14**, 1264–71.

Hosono S, Ohtani H, Arimoto Y, *et al.* (2007) Endoscopic stenting versus gastroenterotomy for palliation of malignant gastroduodenal obstruction: A meta analysis. *J Gastroenterol* **42**, 283–90.

Lau MW, Temperley S, Mehta R, *et al.* (1995) Urinary tract obstruction and nephrostomy drainage in pelvic malignant disease. *Br J Urol* **76**, 565–9.

McIntyre JF, Eifel PJ, Levenback C (1995) Ureteral stricture as a late complication of radiotherapy for stage 1B carcinoma of uterine cervix. *Cancer* **75**, 836–43.

Rubin SC (2000) Management of intestinal obstruction in the patient with ovarian cancer. *Oncology* **14**, 1159–63.

Sohn TA, Lillemoe KD, Cameron JC, *et al.* (1999) Surgical palliation of unresectable periampullary adenocarcinoma in the 1990's. *J Am Coll Surg* **188**, 658–66.

Tilney HS, Lovegrove RE, Purkayastha S, *et al.* (2007) Comparison of colonic stenting and open surgery for malignant large bowel obstruction. *Surg Endosc* **21**, 225–33.

Watanapa P, Williamson RCN (1992) Surgical palliation for pancreatic cancer—developments during the past two decades. *Br J Surg* **79**, 8–20.

Yachia D (1997) Overview: role of stents in urology. *J Endourol* **11**, 379–82.

Biochemical crises

Malignant hypercalcaemia

Urgent intervention is required if free Ca^{2+} ≥3.0 mM.
- Hypercalcaemia complicates 10–20% of all cancers.
- Occurs in solid tumours and leukaemias.
- Especially associated with breast, myeloma, carcinoma of the lung (especially squamous cell), prostate cancer and lymphoma.
- Unusual as the presenting feature of malignancy.
- Leads to multi-system dysfunction.
- Effective treatment improves quality of life.

NB Free (ionic) Ca^{2+} is dependent on serum albumin and arterial pH.

$$\text{Free (ionic) } Ca^{2+} \text{ (mM)} = \text{measured } Ca^{2+} \text{ (mM)} + [(40 - \text{albumin}) \text{ (g/l)} \times 0.02]$$

Aetiology

- **Osteolysis**: local increased bone resorption induced by lytic bone metastases. Attributed to activation of osteoclasts via tumour cell cytokine production (particularly interleukins and tumour necrosis factor). Likely to be the dominant mechanism in certain malignancies, e.g. lymphoma, non-small cell lung cancer. Serum PO_4^{3-} is usually normal.
- **Humoral mediators**: systemic release of factors activating osteoclasts even in the absence of bony metastases e.g. parathyroid hormone-related peptide (PTHrP) seen particularly in squamous cell carcinoma of the lung. Often associated with ↓PO_4^{3-} due to inhibition of PO_4^{3-} reabsorption.
- **Dehydration**: exacerbates hypercalcaemia. Ca^{2+} is a potent diuretic causing salt and water loss. As diuresis continues, Ca^{2+} levels increase, causing further volume depletion etc.
- **Tumour-specific mechanisms**: e.g. myeloma – secretion of an osteoclast-activating factor ± deposition of Bence–Jones proteins → renal impairment → ↓Ca^{2+} excretion; e.g. some lymphomas (usually T-cell) – produce active metabolites of vitamin D → ↑ intestinal absorption of Ca^{2+}.

Often, more than one mechanism contributes, e.g. in breast cancer both osteolytic and humoral mechanisms may be important.

Presentation

- Acute or insidious or an incidental finding.
- **Neurological**: malaise, fatigue, drowsiness, weakness, depression, cognitive dysfunction, seizures, coma.
- **Gastrointestinal**: nausea, vomiting, anorexia, abdominal pain, constipation, including paralytic ileus, pancreatitis, peptic ulceration.
- **Renal**: polydipsia, polyuria, dehydration, signs of uraemia, renal colic (secondary to renal calculi).
- **Cardiac**: arrythmias, ↑blood pressure (BP) **or** ↓BP or postural hypotension.

Investigations

- Urea and electrolytes (U&Es), corrected serum Ca^{2+}, PO_4^{3-}, Mg^{2+}, liver function tests (LFTs), amylase.
- Full blood count (FBC) – a normal haemoglobin (Hb) will fall once the patient is rehydrated.
- Plasma PTH – this is appropriately undetectable in malignant hypercalcaemia. Remember non-malignant causes of hypercalcaemia are common and may co-exist with a diagnosis of cancer e.g. 1° or 3° hyperparathyroidism, hyperthyroidism.
- Electrocardiogram (ECG): may be abnormal including ↑PR interval, ↓QT, wide QRS.

Management

- Intervention likely to improve symptoms in all patients other than those entering the last few hours of life.
- **Rehydration is the priority**: to produce volume expansion, restore glomerular function and increase urinary Ca^{2+} excretion. Fluid deficit may be many litres. Aim for 3–6 l/24 h if cardiac function and urine output permit. Use 0.9% saline and reassess fluid status regularly.
- **Monitor U&Es**: renal impairment should improve with fluid resuscitation. K^+ and Mg^{2+} may fall with rehydration and require intravenous replacement (K^+ 20–40 mmol/l, Mg^{2+} up to 2 mmol/l of normal saline). Check Ca^{2+} and albumin daily.
- **Bisphosphonates**: consider if Ca^{2+} remains ≥3.0 mmol/l despite rehydration. Cause inhibition of osteoclast activity → ↓Ca^{2+}. Typical schedule: pamidronate 60–90 mg infused in a litre of normal saline over 2–24 h, provided renal function adequate following 24 h of rehydration. Then continue fluids. Onset of action from 48 h and usually normocalcaemic within 3–7 days, hence fluid resuscitation is the critical step in acute managment. Cannot repeat dose for 7 days. Optimal interval is ≥3 weeks (avoid repeating within a week). Side-effects: transient fever, hypocalcaemia. Zolendronic acid (4 mg IV over 15 min) is superseding pamidronate as the biphosphonate of choice in malignant hypercalcaemia due to its shorter infusion time and greater potency.
- **Loop diuretics** e.g. forosemide po/iv, ↓Ca^{2+} (↓ reabsorption in loop of Henle), maintains diuresis once patient rehydrated.
- **Steroids**: little role. May be helpful in haematological malignancies such as myeloma (e.g. prednisolone 30–60 mg od).
- **Avoid immobility**: lack of weight-bearing induces increased osteoclastic activity while reducing bone formation.
- **Dietary Ca^{2+} restriction**: not appropriate – gut Ca^{2+} absorption usually ↓ appropriately. Rare exception – some patients with lymphoma associated with ↑ vitamin D metabolites.
- **Salmon calcitonin**: → ↑ renal Ca^{2+} excretion and ↓ bone reabsorption. IM or s/c administration. Efficacy limited to initial 48 h of treatment (tachyphylaxis). Very uncommonly used.
- **Treat the underlying malignancy**: if appropriate. Hypercalcaemia is usually associated with advanced disease. Palliative systemic therapy or radiotherapy for symptomatic bony lesions may improve quality of life.

Hyponatraemia

Aetiology

With low plasma osmolality

With normal or increased plasma volume

- Excess antidiuretic hormone (ADH):
  - **ectopic tumour production of ADH** – most commonly associated with small-cell lung cancer (SCLC). Also described in many other cancers including carcinoid tumours, lymphomas, leukaemias, and pancreatic cancer
  - **syndrome of inappropriate ADH secretion (SIADH)** – reducing excretion of ingested H_2O ± re-setting of the osmostat (maintaining serum Na^+ at a stable, lower level). Multiple causes including: major surgery, pulmonary disease (e.g. concurrent pneumonia), and raised intracranial pressure. Apparent idiopathic SIADH is often associated with occult malignancy, particularly SCLC
  - **stimulation of ADH secretion** – can be caused by drugs used in the treatment of cancer, e.g. ifosfamide, vincristine, high-dose IV cyclophosphamide, opioids.
- **Metabolic causes including glucocorticoid insufficiency**, e.g. following rapid withdrawal of long-term exogenous steroid (may be accompanied by ↑K^+ ± metabolic acidosis) or hypothyroidism.
- **Excess intravenous fluid replacement** with hypotonic fluids or primary polydipsia.
- **Organ failure** including renal failure, congestive cardiac failure, hepatic cirrhosis with ascites.

With reduced plasma volume

- ↑ **renal Na^+ loss**, e.g. nephropathy following cisplatin chemotherapy, Addison's (mineralocorticois deficiency), renal tubular acidosis.
- ↑ **non-renal Na^+ loss**, e.g. diarrhea and vomiting, repeated ascitic drainage.

With normal or high plasma osmolality (pseudohyponatraemia)

For example, secondary to hyperglycaemia, very elevated serum paraproteins, or retention of hypertonic mannitol used in pre-hydration regimes for chemotherapy – this produces high plasma osmolality, drawing intracellular H_2O out into the circulating volume and hence producing apparent hyponatraemia. There is no hypo-osmolality, therefore no osmotic movement of water into the brain and hence no risk of cerebral oedema. Treatment directed at correcting the serum Na^+ is therefore not indicated.

Presentation

Often asymptomatic. Presence of symptoms dependent on:
- degree of hyponatraemia (↑ symptoms if Na <125 mmol/l)
- rapidity of onset
- age and sex of patient – pre-menopausal women most at risk.

If unwell, symptoms tend to be primarily neurological:
- nausea, malaise and weakness
- confusion, headache and drowsiness
- seizures, coma and respiratory arrest.

Examination and investigations

- Assess hydration status. May appear dehydrated ($\downarrow$ skin turgor, postural hypotension, tachycardic), or hypervolaemic (oedematous, ascites etc) depending on aetiology.
- Plasma and urinary Na^+.
- Plasma and urinary osmolality.
- LFTs, glucose, amylase, thyroid function.
- Cortisol ± short synacthen test if adrenal failure suspected.
- SIADH: low serum Na^+ and osmolality with inappropriately normal/ high urinary Na^+ and osmolality in a euvolaemic patient with normal adrenal, renal and thyroid function.

Management

With normal or increased plasma volume

- **Fluid restriction**: to approx 0.5–1 l/day (i.e. to below the level of urine output) is often sufficient, particularly in asymptomatic patients with serum Na^+ >125 mmol/l.
- **Optimize remaining electrolytes**.
- **Inhibition of the action of ADH on the renal tubule**, e.g. with demeclocycline (e.g. 250 mg po tds) to increase water excretion. Only consider in occasional patients with persistent significant hyponatraemia who cannot tolerate water restriction. Renal function needs to be monitored.
- **Infusion of hypertonic (3%) saline**: only to be considered if hyponatraemia is life threatening, and then only under senior or specialist supervision. Overly rapid correction must be avoided, particularly in chronic hyponatraemia. Not appropriate in most malignant causes of hyponatraemia as Na^+ handling is intact in SIADH. Administered Na^+ will simply be excreted unless the osmolality of the administered fluid exceeds urine osmolality.

With reduced plasma volume

- Intravenous infusion of normal (0.9%) saline with close monitoring of plasma volume.

Further reading

Verbalis JG, Goldsmith SR, Greenberg A, et al. (2007) Hyponatraemia treatment guidelines 2007: expert panel recommendations. Am J Med **120**, S1

Hyperkalaemia

Aetiology

- **Renal failure**: probably the most frequent cause.
- **Tumour lysis syndrome**: usually following initiation of therapy for large-volume treatment-sensitive disease (📖 p.706) or occasionally due to spontaneous tumour cell necrosis.
- **Concurrent septicaemia**.
- **Adrenal insufficiency**: usually secondary to glucocorticoid withdrawal or, rarely, adrenal destruction by a tumour.
- **Acute graft-versus-host disease**: following allogeneic bone marrow transplantation.
- **Drugs** e.g. diuretics such as spironolactone.

Presentation

- Often asymptomatic
- Occasionally muscle cramps/weakness
- Cardiac dysrhythmias and arrest
- Signs and symptoms of underlying cause.

Management

- **12-lead electrocardiogram (ECG) and continuous cardiac monitoring**: effects of $\uparrow K^+$ on cardiac conducting tissue include tented T-waves, broadening of the QRS complex, flattened P-waves and heart blocks.
- **Establish IV access and give 10 ml of 10% calcium gluconate iv**: this is cardio-protective. Can be repeated every 10 min until ECG normalizes (up to 50 ml may be required).
- **50 ml of 50% dextrose with 10 U Actrapid® insulin infused over 15–30 min** ($\uparrow$ movement of K^+ into cells).
- **5 mg nebulized salbutamol**.
- **Polystyrene sulphonate resin enema (Calcium Resonium®)**: increases gut K^+ losses.
- **If associated renal failure**: consider IV rehydration, need for central access and possibly IV sodium bicarbonate to correct acidosis (e.g. 50–100 ml 8.4% bicarbonate IV over 30 min via central line). This usually requires senior or specialist supervision.
- **Haemodialysis**: occasionally necessary.

Hyperglycaemia and hypoglycaemia

- **Corticosteroid administration**: corticosteroids are used in the treatment of some malignancies and as part of the routine anti-emetic prescription in highly and moderately emetogenic chemotherapy regimes. Will increase insulin requirements in patients with diabetes mellitus and may precipitate the need for hypoglycaemic medication in those with (often previously unidentified) impaired glucose tolerance.
- **Loss of appetite, nausea, and vomiting**: may complicate management of blood sugars in the diabetic patient.
- **Inappropriate insulin production**: from islet cell tumours and pancreatic APUDomas (amine precursor uptake and decarboxylation). Large metastatic tumours, particularly in the liver, rarely can produce insulin-like growth factors (IGF) which are released into the circulation, especially in response to treatment.

Acute renal failure

Certain causes of acute renal failure may be seen more commonly in the patient with malignant disease. Identification of treatable causes is the priority. Causes can be divided into the following categories although frequently renal impairment is multifactorial:

- **pre-renal**: hypovolaemia due to e.g. dehydration due to vomiting or hypercalcaemia, haemorrhage, concomitant sepsis causing impaired renal perfusion
- **renal**: renal parenchymal damage due to cytotoxic agents, e.g. platinum-based chemotherapy, and other nephrotoxic drugs, e.g. non-steroidal anti-inflammatory analgesia. Tumour lysis syndrome (calcium phosphate crystals) or myeloma (Bence–Jones proteins) causing deposition within the tubules. Glomerulonephritis secondary to underlying malignancy
- **post-renal**: e.g. obstruction secondary to a pelvic tumour, retroperitoneal fibrosis or pathological lymphadenopathy. Renal vein thrombosis.

Presentation

- Nausea/vomiting, anorexia, lethargy
- Oliguria/anuria
- Fluid overload: peripheral/ pulmonary oedema, ↑ jugular venous pressure (JVP) **or** volume depletion if pre-renal aetiology is dominant: ↓ skin turgor, postural hypotension, dry mucous membranes
- Confusion or seizures
- Symptoms related to specific electrolyte abnormalities observed due to renal tubular dysfunction, e.g. $\downarrow Ca^{2+}$, $\downarrow Mg^{2+}$, $\downarrow K^+$, $\downarrow Na^+ \rightarrow$ perioral/ limb dysaesthesiae, tetany/carpopedal spasm, muscle weakness, arrythmias etc. Patients receiving certain chemotherapy drugs, e.g. cisplatin, ifosfamide, are at particular risk of renal tubular dysfunction and require close monitoring of renal function and electrolyte levels.

Investigations

- U&Es, LFTs, Ca^{2+}, Mg^{2+}, PO_4^{3-}, bicarbonate, FBC
- Arterial blood gases (ABGs): establish degree of metabolic acidosis
- Chest X-ray (CXR): fluid overload, underlying diagnosis.
- Urinalysis: haematuria, proteinuria, crystals, casts, pus cells, Bence–Jones protein
- ECG: signs of $\uparrow K^+$ (see separate section)
- Investigations for underlying causes: may include septic screen, vasculitic screen, renal ultrasound scan (USS) Doppler imaging to assess blood flow, intravenous urography (IVU), renal biopsy. Computerized tomography (CT) abdo/pelvis may identify filling defects consistent with inferior vena cava (IVC) thrombus and establish extent of malignant disease.

Management

Appropriate management may include:

- **resuscitatation**: correction of life-threatening electrolyte derangement (see other sections in this chapter) and establishment of euvolaemia if possible
- **monitoring**: urine output (usually requiring catheterization). Cardiac monitor until electrolytes within the normal range. Consider central venous pressure (CVP) monitoring
- **treat the underlying causes if possible**: this should include treatment of suspected infection and review of all potentially nephrotoxic drugs:
  - **pre-renal**: aggressive fluid replacement to optimize renal perfusion and minimize ischaemic injury. Requires frequent assessment for volume overload and prompt involvement of the renal team if oliguria persists despite euvolaemia
  - **post-renal**: bladder catheterization (per urethra or supra-pubic) to relieve obstruction of the lower urinary tract. Retrograde ureteric stenting or percuatneous nephrostomy placement for drainage of the upper urinary tract. Diuresis may follow relief of obstruction
- **dialysis/haemofiltration**: indicated in refractory hyperkalaemia or fluid overload or symptomatic uraemia (e.g. encephalopathy). Early involvement of the renal team.

Management of these patients is likely to require discussion with senior colleagues. Information regarding primary cancer diagnosis and stage, realistic assessment of future treatment options, anticipated prognosis and quality of life are all likely to have a bearing on decisions made. If treatment options for the underlying malignancy are limited, aggressive intervention for their renal failure is likely to be inappropriate.

If uraemia is present at the end of life, then minimally invasive nursing and symptomatic management should be the focus of care:

- nausea (e.g. haloperidol, cyclizine)
- itching (e.g. topical emollients)
- myoclonic jerks (e.g. low-dose benzodiazepines).

Tumour lysis syndrome

Aetiology

- A syndrome of metabolic abnormalities and renal impairment due to massive lysis of rapidly proliferating tumour cells resulting in release of intracellular contents into the circulation.
- Suspect in patients with large-volume malignant disease developing acute renal failure in the presence of hyperuricaemia and/or hyperphosphataemia.
- Most commonly associated with bulky chemosensitive disease, e.g. poorly differentiated lymphomas, high blast-count leukaemias, metastatic germ cell tumours.
- Also described in many other cancers, e.g. breast, myeloma.
- Onset usually within hours or days of commencing chemotherapy.
- Can also occur:
  - after steroid monotherapy – e.g. in lymphoma or lymphoblastic leukaemia
  - following radiotherapy – for a similar range of cancers
  - spontaneously – in tumours with high cell turnover (typically without hyperphosphataemia).

Metabolic abnormalities

- **Hyperuricaemia**: release of nucleic acids metabolized to uric acid. Relative insolubility in water results in crystal deposition in renal tubules → acute uric acid nephropathy and oliguric acute renal failure.
- **Hyperphosphataemia**: secondary to release of intracellular phosphorus. Malignant cells have significantly higher concentrations of phosphorus than normal tissues. Can precipitate with calcium causing deposition of calcium phosphate e.g. in renal tubules (→ acute renal failure (ARF)), the skin (→ gangrene) and the heart (→ arrhythmias).
- **Hyperkalaemia**: exacerbated by deteriorating renal function. Can cause cardiac arrhythmias.
- **Hypocalcaemia/hypomagnesaemia**: secondary to $\uparrow PO_4^{3-}$ and precipitation of calcium phosphate. Symptoms include muscle weakness ± tetany. Contributes to cardiac dysrhythmias.
- **Acute renal failure**: due to urate crystal deposition and/or $\uparrow PO_4^{3-}$. May be exacerbated by underlying renal dysfunction due to e.g. tumour mass causing obstructive nephropathy, or malignant infiltration of the renal parenchyma.
- **Metabolic acidosis**.

Prophylaxis

- **PREVENTION IS THE PRIORITY**
- **Identify patients at risk**:
  - patient specific – baseline metabolic abnormaility, e.g. hyperuricaemia. Suboptimal renal function, e.g. dehydrated, obstructive nephropathy
  - tumour specific – large volume disease, rapid cell turnover, anticipated chemosensitivity
  - most commonly affected tumour types – high-grade lymphomas, leukaemias with high peripheral blast count, some germ cell tumours.

- **Optimize renal function before and during treatment**: relieve urinary tract obstruction if possible. Correct electrolyte abnormalities, e.g. hypercalcaemia. Ensure adequate fluid replacement. This usually involves intravenous hyperhydration to maintain high urine output (ideally 100 ml/h). The osmotic diuretic mannitol is sometimes used in pre-treatment hydration regimes. Loop diuretics (e.g. furosemide) can also help maintain appropriate diuresis during therapy.
- **If low risk (absence of pre-treatment hperuricaemia) – allopurinol**: xanthine analogue → competitive inhibition of xanthine oxidase → reduces metabolism of xanthine and hypoxanthine to uric acid e.g. 300 mg PO od. Pre-treatment for 48 h prior to chemotherapy results in a marked decrease in the incidence of post-treatment hyperuricaemia.
- **If high risk (pre-treatment hyperuricaemia) – rasburicase**: administration of recombinant urate oxidase causes ↑ degradation of uric acid to more water-soluble catabolites, e.g. 200 µg/kg od – duration of treatment dependent on serum uric acid level , usually 1 to 7 days. Contrainidcated in glucose-6-phosphate dehydrogenase (G6PD) deficiency.
- **Leucophoresis**: if peripheral blast count high.
- **Urinary alkalinization**: no good evidence.

The Cairo–Bishop definition of tumour lysis syndrome is ≥2 abnormal serum biochemistry results (see Table 36.1) occurring from 3 days prior to treatment until 7 days after commencing treatment.

Table 36.1 Cairo–Bishop definition of laboratory tumour lysis syndrome

Metabolite	Value	Compared to baseline
Uric acid	≥476 µmol/l	25% ↑
K^+	≥6 mmol/l	25% ↑
PO_4^{3-}	≥1.45 mmol/l (adults)	25% ↑
Ca^{2+}	≤1.75 mmol/l	25% ↓

Symptoms

- Reflect the underlying metabolic derangement
- Gastrointestinal (GI): anorexia, nausea, vomiting, diarrhoea
- Neurological: lethargy, paraesthesiase, confusion, seizures, hallucinations, coma
- Musculosleletal: muscle cramps or tetany
- Renal: flank pain, haematuria, oliguria/anuria, oedema
- Cardiac: heart failure, syncope, arrhythmias, sudden death.

Management

- Urgent correction of hyperkalaemia: see 🕮 p.702.
- Monitor fluid balance: urinary catheterization may be helpful. Careful assessment of circulating volume and intravenous rehydration if volume depleted.
- Urinalysis: may demonstrate uric acid crystals but may be normal due to oliguria from obstructed nephrons.
- Exclude post-renal causes of renal failure with USS, e.g. ureteric obstruction. Suspect this particularly if there is flank pain.
- Monitor electrolytes and urate: at least twice daily until stable. Patients receiving rasburicase require serum for uric acid to be transported on ice directly for analysis.
- Calcium supplementation not usually necessary unless there is neuromuscular irritability.
- Consider alkalinizing the urine: e.g. with acetazolamide or sodium bicarbonate. This reduces uric acid precipitation by converting uric acid to the more soluble urate salt. Evidence is controversial and hospital policies may vary. Likely to require senior or specialist supervision.
- Assess need for haemodialysis to remove excess circulating uric acid: consider referral if metabolic derangement persists despite appropriate care, ongoing metabolic acidosis, oliguria, or symptomatic uraemia despite rehydration and diuretics. Early dialysis is associated with a high chance of complete recovery of renal function.

Further reading

Cairo MS, Bishop M (2004) Tumour lysis syndrome: new therapeutic strategies and classification. *Br J Haematol* **127**, 3–11.

Coiffer B, Althman A, Pui C-H, Younes A, Cairo MS (2008) Guidelines for the management of pediatric and adult tumor lysis syndrome: an evidence-based review. *J Clin Oncol* **26**, 2767–8.

Complications of long-term central venous lines and chemotherapy extravasation

Complications of long-term central venous lines

Cancer patients commonly require intravenous therapy over a period of many months. This may be in the form of regular infusions in hospital or as a continuous portable infusion at home. Vascular access may be difficult in this group of patients due to either their primary diagnosis or complications of their treatment, e.g. lymphoedema, previous radiotherapy, etc.

An alternative to frequent (and often painful) peripheral cannulation is insertion of a long-term venous catheter terminating in the proximal superior vena cava (SVC). This is most commonly a tunnelled catheter (e.g. Hickman, Groshong) passing via the subclavian vein and exiting the skin at the chest wall, with a Dacron 'cuff' to secure it just inside the exit site. Alternatives include a totally implantable device, also tunnelled beneath the chest skin but with a subcutaneous infusion reservoir accessed by needle puncture (e.g. Port-a-cath) or a peripherally inserted central catheter (PICC) exiting in the antecubital fossa.

Infection of central venous lines

Local

- Presenting with purulent discharge from the exit site, local pain, and erythema ± tenderness overlying the subcutaneous tunnel tract.
  Beware – immunocompromised patients may demonstrate few signs of local infection until bone marrow recovery.
- Optimal management is with removal of the line. However, antibiotic therapy without removal of the line is a reasonable approach if the line is still needed for therapy and provided the patient is monitored for any signs of systemic infection.
- Flucloxacillin 500 mg qds PO for at least a week (unless penicillin-allergic) pending results from swabs/cultures is an appropriate starting regime in a well patient although local guidelines should be consulted.

Systemic

- Presenting with signs and symptoms of systemic sepsis often including pyrexia, rigors, and hypotension. Signs of local catheter infection may also be present. Rarely, there may be distant complications such as metastatic abscesses or endocarditis.
- Confirmation of the diagnosis is by isolation of the same micro-organism from blood cultures taken from the catheter and from peripheral samples, without identification of an alternative source.
- Resuscitation and empiric antibiotic treatment must commence immediately. Again, local protocols should be consulted. However, an example of an appropriate regime pending sensitivities would be vancomycin in combination with an aminoglycoside, e.g. gentamicin, with dosing dependent on renal function and serum levels.
- Line removal is optimal – the tip should be sent for culture. However, in an uncomplicated bacteraemia with a still-functioning line, antibiotic therapy alone may be reasonable. Antibiotics should be administered down the line and the patient should be monitored closely. Seek advice

from microbiology once sensitivities are known regarding changing therapy and ideal duration of treatment.
- Line removal becomes imperative in certain situations including failure to improve within 48 h, suspicion of infection with fungi or Gram-negative bacilli, especially *Pseudomonas aeruginosa*, septic thrombophlebitis, metastatic abscesses, and endocarditis.

Thrombosis of central venous lines

Thrombus related to long-term venous catheterization of patients with cancer is relatively common, e.g. studies suggest a 3–30% incidence of catheter-induced axillo-subclavian vein thrombosis. This is a population already prone to thrombosis in which a thrombogenic focus has been introduced.

Presentation
- Commonly asymptomatic: high index of suspicion needed
- Local symptoms, e.g. unilateral hand/arm oedema, shoulder pain, prominent collateral veins visible on chest wall
- Distant embolization.

Investigation
- Usually by duplex ultrasound examination
- Occasionally with a venogram. However, this requires adequate peripheral access, the absence of which is often the reason the catheter was inserted in the first place.

Management
- **Line removal**: if at all possible, i.e. removal of the thrombogenic stimulus. Commonly this is a decision that potentially complicates treatment of the underlying cancer and therefore needs to be addressed on an individual basis.
- **Anticoagulation** with low-molecular weight heparin or warfarin. The duration of anticoagulant therapy is dependent on past medical history, ongoing presence of the venous catheter, other risk factors, etc.
- **Catheter-directed thrombolysis**: there is no current evidence that this is superior to conservative management. However, it can be considered in selected patients, particularly those with a good prognosis from their cancer who have significant acute thrombus-related symptoms.

Prophylaxis
Warfarin 1 mg od without routine international normalized ratio (INR) monitoring is a commonly used prophylactic regime in cancer patients with long-term venous catheters. There is randomized prospective double-blind data to support this as a method for reducing the incidence of catheter-related thrombus in patients receiving chemotherapy. It is generally well tolerated with a low complication rate. However, it should be remembered that, even at this low dose, warfarin may prolong the INR to potentially dangerous levels – for instance, with concomitant broad-spectrum antibiotic therapy or with certain chemotherapy regimes, e.g. containing 5-fluorouracil (5-FU).

Thrombus of the catheter lumen

Inability to withdraw blood from or infuse into a venous catheter is common. CXR will help exclude kinking or line migration. Instillation of a fibrinolytic agent into the line, e.g. urokinase or equivalent, may clear intraluminal thrombus.

Chemotherapy extravasation

Many chemotherapy drugs are rather poorly soluble in aqueous media and are vesicant (literally causing a drying effect – tissue necrosis) to tissues. Great care must be taken to ensure that drugs are given into a free-flowing vascular access. This can be done by ensuring that intravenous fluids (usually normal saline) run in without restriction, resistance, or local pain. This is particularly important to check if patients have lines that have been *in situ* for many days. If any doubt exists about patency, the venous catheter should not be used. A new venous access should be obtained and checked for patency. Despite these precautions extravasation of drugs will still occur in rare cases. Some drugs are less likely to cause tissue problems (e.g. 5-FU) than others. Some agents can cause extensive tissue damage that requires debridement and even subsequent tissue grafting. Particular care should be exercised with anthracyclines and vinca alkaloids. Local protocols exist in cancer centres for management of extravasation.

For all IV drugs:
* stop infusion if pain at injection site
* frequently test patency of IV device by allowing blood flow back and free flow of IV solution such as saline if delivering IV bolus drugs
* avoid unattended infusions of known highly vesicant drugs such as Adriamycin® or vincristine
* if extravasation suspected immediately stop infusion
* massage tissue to extrude any obvious fluid from the IV site.

Controversy exists as to the use of ice packs, needle aspiration of tissues, and/or use of hyaluronidase to cause diffusion of substances away from injection site. Follow local policies if available.

Early involvement of plastic surgery is advisable in all patients who have significant tissue injury.

Further reading

Zingg W, Cartier-Fassler V, Walder B (2008) Central venous catheter-associated infections. *Best Practice & Research Clinical Anaesthesiology* **22**(3), 407–421.

Acedo Sanchez JD, Battle JF, Feijoo JB (2007) Catheter-related thrombosis: a critical review. *Supportive Cancer Therapy* **4**(3), 145–51.

Part 6

The way forward

Novel therapeutic strategies

New drug discovery

The process of drug discovery is driven by three main factors:
- conventional therapies have reached a plateau of effectiveness and therapeutic index
- opportunities for novel molecular targets opened up by our new understanding of the molecular biology of cancer
- the range of new technologies that are available allow for rapid-throughput testing of many thousands of potential drug compounds.

Contemporary approaches to drug discovery

The increasing trend is for a given drug discovery project to be aimed at a particular molecular target (e.g. a specific oncogene product), the hope being that pharmacological intervention might deliver a particular desired biological or phenotypic effect (e.g. inhibition of proliferation, cell cycle progression, motility, invasion, angiogenesis, and metastasis; or the induction of apoptosis or differentiation) rather than a more general cytotoxic or cytostatic effect.

This new molecular target-orientated approach is now dominant in the pharmaceutical and biotechnology companies. Contemporary mechanism-based drug discovery can be divided into the following phases (see Fig. 38.1).

Target identification and validation

The objective is to identify genes and their associated proteins that are directly responsible for cancer causation and progression. Having identified a gene that is either mutated or shows deregulated expression, a variety of experiments can be carried out to validate the target – that is, to provide evidence that it is indeed involved in the disease process in humans and to increase the level of confidence that pharmacological manipulations of the target would lead to an anti-tumour effect.

Lead identification

The objective of this phase is to identify a chemical structure that has some activity against the molecular target. This may be done by screening chemically diverse compounds in automated, high-throughput assays or by rational design based on a known substrate or ligand. Much of this part can now be done *in silica* by exploration of public access databases.

Lead optimization

The aim is to improve and refine the desired properties of the lead (e.g. solubility, potency, and selectivity) and eliminate undesirable features. This is done by making chemical derivatives or analogues of the lead compound.

In vivo testing

The final stage of testing will involve seeking evidence of regression or growth arrest/delay in a human tumour xenograft. Depending on the biological effect sought, more complex tests such as orthoptic or metastatic models may be useful. Transgenic mouse models can be valuable, as can surrogate non-tumour endpoints.

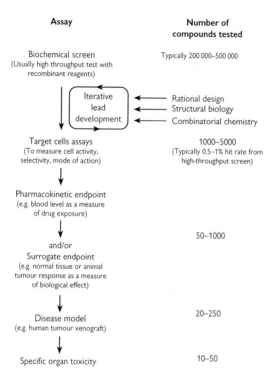

Assay	Number of compounds tested

Biochemical screen
(Usually high throughput test with
recombinant reagents)

Typically 200 000–500 000

Iterative
lead
development

← Rational design
← Structural biology
← Combinatorial chemistry

Target cells assays
(To measure cell activity,
selectivity, mode of action)

1000–5000
(Typically 0.5–1% hit rate from
high-throughput screen)

Pharmacokinetic endpoint
(e.g. blood level as a measure
of drug exposure)

and/or

Surrogate endpoint
(e.g. normal tissue or animal
tumour response as a measure
of biological effect)

50–1000

Disease model
(e.g. human tumour xenograft)

20–250

Specific organ toxicity

10–50

Fig. 38.1 Structure of a contemporary mechanism-based drug discovery test cascade.

Usually, activity will be sought in at least a small panel of tumours, including human xenografts. Ideally, these would be characterized for the molecular target and pathway involved, together with any other relevant features.

There is increasing use of so-called transgenic models which are considered to be more representative of the human disease than older xenograft models.

Preclinical drug development

Following selection of a potential clinical candidate, a number of preclinical development activities must be carried out:

- formulation: choice of formulation is influenced by solubility, stability, and dosage requirements
- preclinical pharmacology: more detailed pharmacokinetic/absorption, distribution, metabolism, excretion (ADME) studies will be carried out
- preclinical toxicology to define qualitative and quantitative organ toxicities.

Conclusion

Despite major advances in methodology, the drug discovery and development process is still likely to take around 7 years from new target to regulatory approval. With the trend away from empirical screening for anti-cancer activity to new mechanism-based approaches targeted to specific molecular abnormalities responsible for cancer, we are now screening a range of exciting new agents emerging for clinical evaluation.

The explosion of molecular knowledge about cancer pathophysiology is now beginning to yield new agents that strike at specific target pathways that are expressed within the cancer.

Clinical trials (refer to 📖 Chapter 11)

The primary aim of the phase I trials is to establish the safety and tolerability of the compound being tested and to define an optimum dose and schedule for further (phase II) studies. Other, secondary objectives may be to investigate the pharmacokinetics of the drug in humans and study the efficacy of the drug in the patients.

Phase I

Phase I studies are generally dose-escalation trials, where the initial dose level is calculated from the preclinical toxicology studies. This starting dose aims to be low enough to ensure the safety of the patients, but high enough to minimize the number of patients treated at ineffective (too low) doses.

The endpoint of the phase I trial is normally toxicity (maximal tolerated dose) (MTD) and dose-limiting toxicity (DLT) will be defined in the protocol, except for non-cytotoxic agents, when the endpoint may be the optimum activity of the drug as defined by its mechanism of action, unless unacceptable toxicity is observed first. For example, this may be inhibition of an enzyme or reduction of plasma levels of a hormone.

On completion of the phase I trial, the basic toxicity profile of the agent in question should be known and an appropriate dose for further trials identified.

It is still unusual in oncology for phase I studies to be done in normal volunteers – but in certain circumstances with drugs in which we can monitor a biological effect this does now occur.

Phases II and III

Unless the drug has proved to be unacceptably toxic, it will then be subject to phase II and, if successful, phase III testing. The aim of phase II trials is to assess the efficacy of the drug. Each phase II trial will be undertaken in patients with one particular tumour type and they will all be treated with the same dose and schedule. While toxicity will continue to be monitored, the patients' disease will also be assessed for response.

There is a trend to perform randomized phase II trials in oncology of intermediate size between the traditional 30–40 patient phase II and the much bigger full scale phase III randomized controlled trial (RCT). Usually this is done to give an earlier indication of whether the novel agent actually does hit the target that was intended, or to allow for introduction of patient selection criteria that could enrch the trial population in order to maximize that chance that the drug will have demonstrable anti-cancer activity.

The aim of phase III trials is to compare the new agent with existing best treatment for the disease in question.

Novel radiotherapeutic approaches

Radiotherapy is an effective anti-cancer treatment modality. Increasing the dose delivered to the tumour while sparing the surrounding normal tissue will commonly improve local tumour control. Novel radiotherapeutic approaches aim to:
- increase the dose delivered to the tumour
- more accurately localize that radiotherapy onto the cancer
- increase the biological effectiveness of radiation by use of radiosensitization agents
- use different forms of radiation that have improved biological effects
- use alternative schedules of radiation to increase the differential between tumour kill and normal tissue damage.

Targeted radiotherapy

The biological properties of the tumour itself provide the basis for selective irradiation. In principle, this strategy should be capable of eradicating tumour cells anywhere in the body, but it is currently at an early stage of development for many sites.
- Iodine (well-differentiated thyroid carcinomas)
- Monoclonal antibodies to cancer cell surface antigens (B-cell lymphoma)
- Catecholamine precursor analogue meta-iodobenzylguanidine (MIBG) (neuroblastoma)
- Somatostatin (neuroendocrine tumours).

Improvements in external-beam radiotherapy delivery

Improvements in focusing the external radiotherapy beam on the tumour and avoiding normal tissue should allow a safe increase in the dose of radiotherapy delivered. The principle IS similar to stereotactic surgery – in fact the so-called gamma-knife has been developed with a focus on use in central nervous system (CNS) tumours to avoid radiotherapy to nearby vital structures.

Conformal therapy

This technique uses three-dimensional image reconstruction and treatment planning to conform a high dose of radiotherapy to the target volume (often irregularly shaped) but maintain a low dose to the non-target tissues of the patients. Early clinical results suggest that normal tissue side-effects can be reduced and dose escalation is possible, e.g. in the treatment of localized prostate cancer.

Intensity-modulated radiation therapy (IMRT)

Here the intensity of the radiotherapy beam is varied across the treatment field to ensure that a uniform dose can be achieved in a regular- or irregular-shaped target. Essentially, this may add to conformal therapy by further reducing the dose to sensitive structures.

Intra-operative radiotherapy

Radiotherapy can be delivered to a tumour volume under direct visual localization during an open operation within a designated radiotherapy suite. A large single dose is delivered at the one procedure. The potential advantage of a targeted boost (given in addition to external-beam fractionated therapy) is balanced by the theoretical limitations of the biological effects of the single large dose.

Improvements in radiotherapy fractionation

In general, tumours and critical normal tissues (those that limit the dose that may safely be delivered in a course of radiotherapy) are associated with different fractionation sensitivities.

Studies have demonstrated fast rates of growth in certain tumours such that clonogens have potential doubling times of less than 5 days. This implies that the time taken to deliver a radical course of conventionally fractionated radiotherapy should not be extended. Indeed, clinical trials have demonstrated benefits with treatment acceleration, where a radical course of treatment may be completed in 2 weeks (with thrice-daily fractions), rather than the more usual 4–6 weeks.

Radiosensitization

If tumour cells can be made more sensitive to the delivered radiotherapy, improvements in local control can be gained only if radiosensitization is selective for the tumour.

Hypoxic cell sensitizers

Hypoxic tumour cells are resistant to radiation. The delivery of hypoxic cell sensitizers should theoretically improve tumour cell kill. Recently, trials with, for example, tirapazamine, have demonstrated benefit, but these agents are still under evaluation.

Synchronous chemotherapy

Chemotherapy delivered with radiotherapy may provide benefit over and above the addition of more cell kill. This may be due to the inhibition of DNA repair by the agent or some other mechanism of tumour radiosensitization. More clinical studies are required to define the optimal combination of chemotherapy and radiotherapy and to ensure that this is a selective improvement for the tumour and does not just produce additive toxicity. However, the approach is widely used in some cancers, e.g. rectal cancer which is locally advanced.

Targeted radiotherapy

Targeted radiotherapy means the selective irradiation of tumour cells by radionuclides that are conjugated to tumour-seeking molecules (targeting agents).

Targeting agents

Tumour targeting depends on the existence of biological differences between normal and tumour cells. Several categories of targeting agent have been used, or are under development (see Table 38.1).

- Monoclonal antibodies:
  - limited discriminatory ability
  - poor penetration of tumour mass
  - murine antibodies provoke host response
  - used in cancer of ovary, colon, brain with modest response
  - best response in B-cell lymphoma
- MIBG:
  - taken up by catecholamine-synthesizing cells of sympathetic nervous system
  - taken up by neuroblastoma, phaeochromocytoma
  - diagnostic and therapeutic
- Future:
  - melanoma
  - glioma, squamous cell carcinoma: overexpressed cell receptor epidermal growth factor (EGF)

Radionuclides for therapy

Radionuclides that have potential for targeted therapy are the α, β, and Auger particle emitters (see Table 38.2). Though particle-emitting radionuclides usually produce some γ-ray photons as well, the photons make little contribution to the therapeutic effect.

The physical half-life of a targeting radionuclide must be long enough to allow radiochemical conjugation and the homing of the conjugate to its target tumour cells. In practice, clinical experience with targeted radiotherapy is largely confined to β-emitters, particularly ^{131}I and, to a lesser extent, ^{90}Y. The advantages of ^{131}I are its availability, ease of conjugation, and clinical familiarity.

α-emitters have high radiobiological effectiveness and short-range emissions but are difficult to obtain and have inconveniently short half-lives. Experience with α-emitters is so far confined to the laboratory, but encouraging clinical potential has been demonstrated.

Auger electron emitters have been little used for targeted therapy because the short range of the Auger electron requires a DNA-targeting agent.

Table 38.1 Targeting agents for targeted radiotherapy

Biological differential	Targeting agent	Target tumour
Epitope	Antibodies	Various
Noradrenaline transporter	MIBG	Neuroblastoma
Melanin synthetic pathway	Methylene blue	Melanoma
EGF receptor overexpression	EGF	Squamous carcinoma, glioma
Proliferative differential	IudR	Brain tumours
Oestrogen nuclear receptor	Oestrogen	Breast cancer
Genomic aberration	Oligonucleotide	?

Table 38.2 Radionuclides for targeted radiotherapy

Radionuclide	Half-life	Emitted particles	Particle range
^{90}Y	2.7 days	β	5 mm
^{131}I	8 days	β	0.8 mm
^{67}Cu	2.5 days	β	0.6 mm
^{199}Au	3.1 days	β	0.3 mm
^{211}At	7 h	α	0.05 mm
^{212}Bi	1 h	α	0.05 mm
^{125}I	60 days	Auger electrons	1 µm
^{123}I	15 h	Auger electrons	1 µm

Combined modalities

Targeted radiotherapy using β-emitters inevitably results in a whole-body radiation dose because of limited targeting specificities (cross-targeting to normal tissues) and because of radionuclide in the general circulation.

These concepts are now being applied in the targeted radiotherapy of neuroblastoma using ^{131}I-MIBG in combination with total body irradiation (TBI) or high-dose chemotherapy. Combined modality treatment of B-cell lymphoma using radiolabelled antibodies, TBI, or systemic chemotherapy and haemopoietic rescue may be an appropriate next step.

Gene therapy and immunotherapy for cancer

Introduction

- New anti-cancer strategies are needed as most cancers ultimately become resistant to conventional treatment modalities.
- Increasing insight into the control and growth of human cells and their deregulation in cancer have coincided with advances in recombinant DNA technology.

Gene therapy is the transfer and expression of genetic material into a cell, tissue, or organ for a therapeutic purpose.

- Strategies may include introduction of genes which:
  - correct a somatic error
  - alter expression levels of relevant genes
  - affect cell differentiation or survival.
- Successful gene therapy will require:
  - a method of delivering that gene into the correct cell
  - a mechanism of controlling expression of that gene
- The vast majority of clinical trials have been at phase I or II level only.
- In the UK clinical gene therapy trials are closely regulated by the Gene Therapy Advisory Committee (GTAC).
- UK: There are currently no gene therapy treatments approved for main-stream clinical use.
- Worldwide: the first gene therapy product to be approved for use is Gendicine® (see 🕮 Somatic correction of gene defect, p.736)
- Early clinical trials are typically undertaken in those with advanced disease but it seems likely that any future role for gene therapy will be greatest in those patients with low volume or resected disease (i.e. the adjuvant setting).
- Ongoing development of new techniques means that there is over-lap between techniques used in gene therapy and in specific immuno-therapy, with novel approaches drawing on both methods (immunogenetic strategies).

Immunotherapy aims to use immune mechanisms to influence the course of a disease. This may either be by enhancing natural host immune responses or by the use of exogenous biological agents. Immunotherapy may be:
- non-specific (see 🕮 Chapter 10, 'Biological and targeted therapies'), or
- specific – targeting a tumour-related antigen.

- The concept of a vaccine against cancer first arose when the infectious aetiology of certain malignancies was identified. Examples include:
  - human papilloma virus in cervical cancer
  - hepatitis B virus in hepatocellular cancer
  - Epstein–Barr virus in Burkitt's lymphoma and nasopharyngeal cancer.
- It was then proposed that cancers with no recognizable infectious aetiology may be targeted with cancer vaccines designed against tumour-specific antigens.

- The potential advantage of this strategy is that local delivery of a gene-vector inoculation may generate a tumour-specific response that would be amplified and disseminated – targeting tumour cells at distant sites.
- The majority of current gene therapy trials involve immunogenetic techniques.
- Much effort goes into the design and implementation of cancer gene therapies and immunogenetic strategies. However our incomplete understanding of the biological system means we have a limited ability to predict true targets *in vivo*.

Strategies for cancer gene therapy

- Somatic correction of gene defect:
  - expression of tumour suppressor gene
  - anti-sense oligonucleotide to mutant oncogene
- Genetic pro-drug activation
- Genetic immunomodulation:
  - non-specific immunotherapy (📖 Chapter 10, 'Biological and targeted therapies')
  - specific immunotherapy

Somatic correction of gene defect

Expression of tumour suppressor gene

- Tumour suppressor genes are genes whose function is lost in carcinogenesis. Both allele copies must be inactivated before the tumour suppressor function is completely lost, with potential initiation or progression of a cancer.
- Replacement with normal non-mutated copies of tumour suppressor genes using viral vectors has resulted in suppression and/or reversal of the malignant phenotype in *in vivo* tumour models.
- **An example is the *p53* tumour suppressor gene:**
  - many trials of cancer gene therapy have concentrated on *p53*
  - Gencidine® is a recombinant adenovirus expressing *p53* and is approved for use in China for the treatment of head and neck cancers
  - phase I and II trials in which patients with non-small cell lung cancer (NSCLC) with mutations in *p53* have undergone intratumoural injection of a retroviral vector containing wild-type *p53* have produced no consistent clinical benefit.
- There is some suggestion that combining successful restoration of genes such as wild-type *p53* and sequential administration of chemotherapy (such as cisplatin) may be synergistic in reducing the malignant expression in these cell lines.

Correction of mutant oncogenes

- Proto-oncogenes are genes whose function becomes enhanced in carcinogenesis. The gene product is typically a protein with an essential role in controlling cellular proliferation, e.g. growth factors or transcription factors. A hereditary or acquired mutation in only one copy of the oncogene disrupts normal regulation of cellular replication.
- Anti-sense DNA oligonucleotides are short, synthetic nucleotide sequences that are complementary to specific DNA or RNA sequences and are specifically engineered to target individual oncogenes. The aim is to inhibit transcription into mRNA or translation of the mRNA message into protein. This limits gene expression and hence limits expression of the gene product.
- **An example is the tumour suppressor gene *bcl-2*:**
  - an apoptotic inhibitor upregulated in certain types of cancer and specifically over-expressed through chromosomal translocation in some non-Hodgkin's lymphomas
  - identified as playing a role in the development of tumour drug resistance
  - G3139 (oblimersen or Genasense®) is an anti-sense oligonucleotide targeting the initiation codon region the *bcl-2* mRNA, and is undergoing clinical trials in many malignancies including advanced prostate cancer, melanoma, lymphoma, and leukaemia.

Genetic pro-drug activation (GPAT)

- The fundamental problem with current chemotherapy is its lack of selectivity and hence its associated toxicity. Targeting of therapy can potentially be increased by gene transfer techniques. The aim is to maximize cell kill while minimizing toxicity.
- This method is variously known as:
  - genetic pro-drug activation therapy (GPAT)
  - gene-directed enzyme pro-drug system (GDEPT)
  - virus-directed enzyme pro-drug therapy (VDEPT), if gene transfer is via a viral vector
  - suicide gene therapy.
- Targeting could be achieved by the sequence of events shown in Fig. 39.1.

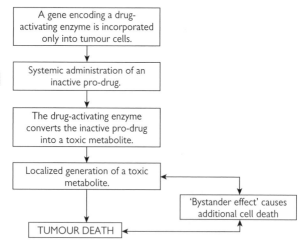

Fig. 39.1 Potential mechanisms of tumour targeting using a pro-drug system in combination with gene therapy. Gene therapy techniques could enhance the specificity of anti-cancer agents by preferentially targeting malignant cells.

- Potential advantage of GPAT:
  - may permit success even in the absence of highly efficient gene transfer due to the 'bystander effect' whereby non-transduced cells in a mixed population die in the presence of a given pro-drug due to passive diffusion, active transport, or recruitment of a local immune response.

- Current limitations of GPAT include:
  - limited gene transfer efficiency at the tumour site by the vectors currently available
  - current requirement for direct intratumoural gene injection so that efficacy may be restricted to solitary tumours rather than disseminated disease.
- Early-phase trials are under way to investigate whether the theory of GPAT will translate into treatments with any real clinical benefit.
- An example of a prototype genetic pro-drug activation system is the bacterial enzyme nitroreductase:
  - the nitroreductase gene could be introduced into tumours by direct injection
  - the enzyme nitroreductase converts the pro-drug CB1954 (which can be safely administered intravenously or intraperitoneally) to a highly toxic alkylating agent nitrobenzamidine that cross-links DNA
  - systemic administration of CB1954 may could result in conversion to the cytotoxic nitrobenzamidine only where the activating gene had been incorporated
  - therapeutic efficacy has not yet been demonstrated, although trials are under way in patients with a range of cancers, including hepatocellular carcinoma and liver metastases from colorectal cancer.

Genetic immunomodulation

Non-specific immunotherapy

- Aims to increase immune responsiveness in general rather than directing a reaction against a particular antigen.
- The patient is immunized with materials that elicit an immune reaction capable of eliminating/delaying tumour growth.
- Examples of non-specific ummunotherapy include the use of the bacillus Calmette–Guérin (BCG) and cytokines e.g. interferon-α, interleukin-2 (see 📖 Chapter 10, 'Biological and targeted therapies').

Specific immunotherapy

Many techniques are being developed with the aim of generating an immune response to a specific tumour-associated antigen:
- Whole-cell tumour preparations
- peptide vaccinations
- DNA vaccines.

Methods are also being developed to improve the efficiency of antigen presentation to the immune system-associated antigen:
- dendritic cell vaccination.

Cancer vaccinations remain the focus of ongoing clinical trials.

- An ideal target antigen should have the following properties:
  - expressed solely in the tumour or only at very low levels elsewhere in the body
  - present in primary and metastatic disease
  - available to recognition by the immune system either by expression on the cell surface or by being processed by major histocompatibility complex (MHC) proteins.

Methods of generating tumour-specific immune reactions

Whole tumour cell preparations
- Individual preparation of vaccination for each patient using samples from their own tumour, usually administered with an adjuvant agent, e.g. BCG.
- Advantage: avoids the need to identify specific tumour-associated antigens.
- Disadvantages: high-intensity preparation so scope for widespread clinical application may be limited.
- Examples of the application of whole tumour cell include small-scale trials in patients with renal cell carcinoma and following resection of colorectal tumours – encouraging results with trends towards longer disease-free survival.

Peptide vaccinations
- If an appropriate antigen can be isolated and identified then specific peptides derived from that antigen could be developed into epitopes for immunotherapy. Subsequent exposure to the antigen should increase the possibility of tumour recognition by immune surveillance and hence rejection.

- So far, clinical trials have examined intradermal or subcutaneous administration, usually in combination with an immunological adjuvant such as BCG.
- Disadvantages: the need to identify specific tumour-associated antigens and to introduce the synthetic epitope in such a way as to stimulate an immune response.
- An example of a tumour-specific peptide antigen under investigation is Mucin-1: a large glycoprotein expressed on gastrointestinal (GI) mucosa and overexpressed in several cancers, including pancreatic and colorectal. Currently little evidence of clinical efficacy.

DNA vaccines

- Genes known to be over-expressed in malignancy can be targeted. The aim is to produce a recombinant DNA vaccine in which a vector is used to introduce DNA encoding tumour-associated proteins. Presentation of the antigen protein induces humoral and cell-mediated immune responses.
- Disadvantage: limited by the paucity of truly tumour-specific antigens. Most target antigens are tumour-**associated** rather than tumour-**specific** and are normal cellular genes that are inappropriately expressed in malignant cells.
- Examples of targets for DNA vaccination strategies include:
  - *p53*: a mutated tumour suppressor gene present in >50% of all human cancers.
  - **carcinoembryonic antigen (CEA)**: a cell surface glycoprotein overexpressed by the majority of colorectal cancer cells and also at low levels in normal colon and biliary epithelium. The gene encoding CEA has been incorporated into various vectors for use as a vaccine. Although many phase I and II trials confirm that the vaccine is well tolerated, there has not yet been clear evidence of clinical benefit.
  - **MAGE-1**: an embryonic gene product associated with breast cancer and malignant melanoma.
  - **Her-2/neu receptor**: an epidermal growth factor receptor with intracellular tyrosine kinase activity, over-expressed in several solid tumours including breast, stomach, and pancreatic cancer.

Method of optimizing antigen presentation
Dendritic cell vaccination

- Although appropriate antigen selection is vital, success is dependent on optimal presentation of those antigens to the immune system. The need to ensure efficient antigen presentation has led to antigen administration in association with dendritic cells (DCs).
- Dendritic cells have the following properties which make them appropriate for manipulation:
  - they are potent antigen-processing and antigen-presenting cells critical to the development of primary MHC-restricted T-cell immunity to infectious agents, in autoimmune diseases and anti-tumour immunity
  - they express high levels of MHC and co-stimulatory molecules

- they can be expanded *in vitro* from peripheral blood precursors and marrow, using cytokines. Cultured DCs are able to take up exogenous antigen (as tumour protein, peptide or RNA) or may be transduced with genes encoding tumour antigen using physical or viral methods of gene transfer.
- The hope is that co-administration of antigen with DCs will maximize subsequent T-cell response and hence host immune-recognition of the tumour-associated peptide.
- Disadvantage: DCs remain very labour-intensive to generate.
- Only small-scale early-phase trials have so far been conducted.

Gene delivery

Successful gene therapy requires a delivery system that is capable of efficient gene transfer without causing any associated pathological effects. Current delivery systems are discussed under the headings that follow.

Direct physical delivery of gene therapy

- Examples of physical means include:
  - injection of naked DNA into skeletal muscle by simple needle and syringe
  - DNA transfer by liposomes
  - DNA coated on the surface of gold pellets that are air-propelled into the epidermis (the 'gene gun').
- Advantages: convenience and safety.
- Disadvantages: low efficiency of gene transfer and the technique results in transient gene expression only.

Use of biological vectors for delivery of gene therapy

- Examples of biological vectors include:
  - bacterial vectors
  - viral vectors (see Table 39.1).
- Advantages: it is the most efficient, stable method and permits the integration of DNA into large numbers of target cells.
- Disadvantages: the safety issues, that it is technically more complex, and the potential generation of neutralizing immune responses and systemic toxicities.

Administration of gene therapy

- Is typically by local injection.
- Systemic administration is generally precluded by the high prevalence of cross-reacting antibodies and the high immunogenicity of the vectors.

Efficiency of transfer of therapeutic DNA varies and this will influence the choice of vector

For example:
- for gene replacement, high-efficiency viral vectors are desirable
- for short-term gene expression to prime an immune response or sensitize cells to radiotherapy, liposomal delivery may be adequate.

Delivery of gene therapy

This may be:
- *ex vivo* (outside the patient): transfer of a therapeutic gene into isolated cancer or non-cancer cells that are then re-implanted into the patient
- *in vivo*: delivery of genes to target cancer cells by exploiting transcriptional differences of specific genes between cancer and normal cells. This technique is less efficient for gene transfer.

Table 39.1 Viral vectors for gene therapy

	Retrovirus	Adenovirus	Adeno-associated virus	Lentivirus	Herpes virus
Advantages					
	Small genome	High viral titres	Small genome	Small genome	High viral titres
	Carries 10 kb insert	Carries 8–30 kb insert	Carries 4–5 kb insert	Can infect non-dividing target cells	Carries up to 15 kb insert
	Stable colinear integration				
	Efficient gene transfer	Highly efficient gene transfer	Efficient gene transfer		Highly efficient gene transfer
			Can infect non-dividing cells		Can infect non-dividing cells
			Naturally replication-incompetent		Neural tropism
Disadvantages					
	Immunogenicity	Immunogenicity	Immunogenicity	Immunogenicity	Immunogenicity
	Requires actively dividing cells	Transient expression	Not well studied	Large genome	Large genome
	Small DNA sequences only carried	Small DNA sequences only carried	Small DNA sequences only carried		Lytic virus
	Poor transduction efficiency in human tumours				
	Low titre, transient expression				
	Random integration				
	Insertional mutagenesis				

Further reading

Bassett EA, Wang W, Rastinejad F, El-Deiry WS (2008) Structural and functional basis for therapeutic modulation of p53 signaling. Clin Cancer Res **14**, 6376–86.

Dougan M, Dranoff G (2009) Immune therapy for cancer. *Annu Rev Immunol* **27**, 83–117.

Guinn BA, Mulherkar R (2008) International progress in cancer gene therapy. *Cancer Gene Ther* **15**, 765–75.

Yip KW, Reed JC (2008) Bcl-2 familf proteins and cancer. *Oncogene* **27**, 6398–406.

Auman JT, McLeod HL (2008) Applications of genomic tools to colorectal cancer therapeutics. *Curr Opin Mol Ther* **10**, 546–54.

Biomarkers and cancer

Biomarkers and cancer

Definition
A measurement which provides insight into the biological process underlying the cancer, and/or gives clinically useful information about an individual malignancy, additional to established clinical parameters such as performance status. This can be:
- diagnostic – marker specific for the cancer
- prognostic – marker correlates with extent of disease/natural history
- predictive – marker correlates with responsiveness/resistance to therapy
- response assessment – marker correlates with treatment efficacy or development of refractory disease.

Established biomarkers
A number of biomarkers are well established in oncological practice:
- serum alpha-fetoprotein (AFP), human chrionic gonadotrophin (HCG), and lactate dehydrogenase (LDH) are validated prognostic markers for germ-cell malignancies of the testis, and are key to monitoring patients during treatment and on surveillance
- tumour oestrogen receptor (ER), progesterone receptor (PR), and human epidermal growth factor receptor 2 (HER2), assessed by immunocytochemistry or fluorescence *in situ* hybridization (FISH), provide valuable predictors both of response to targeted therapy and prognosis in breast cancers.

Other commonly used tumour markers include:
- serum CA125 in ovarian cancer
- serum carcinoembryonic antigen (CEA) in colorectal cancer (but also elevated in e.g. non-small-cell lung cancer (NSCLC) and breast cancer)
- serum thyroglobulin in follicular and papillary thyroid cancer
- serum calcitonin in medullary carcinoma of the thyroid
- urinary 5-hydroxyindoleacid acid (5-HIAA) in carcinoid tumours.

Development of novel biomarkers
Progress in the understanding of the molecular biology of cancer has been paralleled by the development of laboratory technology in the fields of genomics and proteomics. Tissue micro-array technology was first described in 1987, and over the last 10 years has been refined so that currently it is possible to quantify the expression of several thousand genes in a single experiment, with only a few days delay between biopsy and automated analysis.

Similarly with advances in proteomics, it is estimated that plasma contains greater than 10 000 different proteins, with concentrations varying by 10 orders of magnitude. In order to study cancer-specific proteins, techniques have been developed to remove the abundant proteins (albumin, immunoglobulin, fibrinogen, etc) to allow separation and detection of tumour-related proteins, with quantification of not only individual proteins but their phosphorylation status, which can correlate with activity.

The past decade has also heralded in a new era in the understanding of gene regulation in diseases such as cancer. We now appreciate that normal human cells express thousands of non-coding RNAs and that cancer cells misexpress these RNAs. Many of the non-coding RNAs, epitomized by the miRNA, have regulatory functions in normal cells. The aberrant expression of miRNA promotes tumorigenesis, metastasis, and other features of cancer.

The presence of circulating tumour cells (CTCs) in the blood of patients with advanced cancer was noted more than 20 years ago. However it is only in the last few years, again through improved biotechnology, that fast and accurate assays of these have become available. CTCs are particularly abundant in advanced prostate cancer and breast cancer, where:
- number of cells predict duration of survival in metastatic disease
- fall in CTC correlates with response and response duration after chemotherapy
- change in CTC may be a useful surrogate endpoint for systemic treatment efficacy, superior to current assessment, e.g. axial imaging
- there is potential value of receptor studies on CTCs to predict subsequent responsiveness to therapies.

Signal transduction

Understanding of the cell signalling pathways that control cellular behaviour has provided many potential biomarkers for malignant disease. Most of these pathways can be triggered by extracellular factors binding to receptors, either on the cell surface or within the cell. The processes they control include:
- activation of genes
- changes in metabolism
- cellular proliferation
- cellular death
- cellular migration.

Gene activation can lead to a cascade of effects through production of:
- proteins with enzyme activity
- transcription factors which activate one or more genes downstream in the pathway (see Fig. 40.1).

With the advent of targeted therapies directed at growth factor receptors or their tyrosine kinases, it is becoming increasingly important to identify which components of the signal transduction pathways predominate in individual cancers. For example, most gastrointestinal (GI) stromal tumours are driven by mutation in *c-kit* which leads to constitutive activation of the KIT tyrosine kinase, the target for the tyrosine kinase inhibitor (TKI) imatinib. Clearly when the pathway is disrupted by alteration downstream from the growth factor receptor, agents targeted against the receptor or its specific tyrosine kinase are unlikely to have significant anti-tumour effects. For example, tumours driven by *kRAS* mutations do not respond to antibody therapy directed against membrane-bound growth factor receptors or to corresponding receptor TKIs.

Angiogenesis

Tumour growth and spread requires the development of new blood vessels by:
- sprouting
- recruitment of bone marrow cells
- co-option of normal vessels
- intussusception.

Commonly, malignant tumours have areas of highly vascularized tissue facilitating proliferation and growth, but other areas of low perfusion and hypoxia arise where tumour growth has outstripped angiogenesis, and these may contain tumour stem cells, relatively protected from chemotherapy and radiotherapy.

A variety of anti-cancer strategies target angiogenesis:
- antibody against vascular endothelial growth factor (VEGF), bevacizumab, inhibits sprouting
- VEGF receptor (VEGFR) TKIs have similar effects
- other agents, e.g. trastuzumab, lead to increase in thrombospondin 1, a natural inhibitor of angiogenesis.

Currently the best method of assessing their efficacy is imaging of tumour vascular permeability, e.g. using dynamic magnetic resonance imaging (MRI).

Biomarkers of antiangiogenesis agents under investigation include:
- serum VEGF
- soluble VEGFR
- hypoxia-inducible factors (HIFs)
- basic fibroblast growth factor (bFGF).

Pharmacological biomarkers

Deactivating enzymes

Measurement of drug-specific metabolic enzyme activities can be predictive of toxicity or efficacy for a number of anti-cancer drugs or:
- thiopurine methyltransferase – low levels predict toxicity unless 6-mercaptopurine doses are reduced in treatment of acute lymphoblastic leukaemia
- dihydropyridine dehydrogenase – deficiency leads to increased toxicity with 5-fluorouracil (5-FU) and capecitabine
- uridine diphosphate glucuronyltransferase – low levels predict toxicity from irinotecan.

DNA repair enzymes

DNA repair phenotype can influence:
- normal tissue susceptibility to malignant transformation, e.g. after environmental exposure to radiation or chemical carcinogens
- tumour genetic instability, leading to the loss of normal cellular controls, and acquired resistance to therapies
- toxicity with standard doses of cytotoxics or radiotherapy due to failure of normal DNA repair in healthy tissues
- tumour response/resistance to treatment with radiotherapy/chemotherapy.

Pharmacokinetics/pharmacodynamics

Increasingly, attempts are being made to move away from the use of anti-cancer drugs at their maximum tolerable dose, to the optimization of dosage of established and new agents according to their pharmacological and biological activity in individuals:

• therapeutic drug monitoring – knowledge and measurement of a target plasma level of the drug or its metabolites to allow dose adjustment
• direct measurement of biomarker of drug efficacy, e.g. protein phosphorylation
• use of surrogate endpoints i.e. biological measures which, although independent of tumour cell kill, correlate with this.

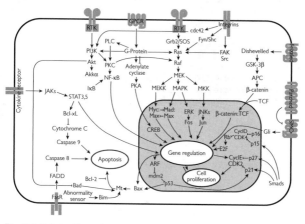

Fig. 40.1 Cell signalling pathways.

Imaging biomarkers

Traditionally, the assessment of treatment efficacy in oncology requires comparison of imaging-based measurements, to define complete response/partial response/stable disease/progressive disease:

- World Health Organization (WHO), original standard, using product of bidimensional measurements of tumour masses on CT or MRI
- Response Evaluation Criteria in Solid Tumors (RECIST), adopted in 2000, using uni-dimensional measurements
- 3D volumetric tumour assessments are currently being investigated.

Many targeted therapies exert anti-cancer effects which are cytostatic rather than cytotoxic, so that early responses are difficult to appreciate according to, e.g. RECIST criteria. Instead of conventional CT/MRI to assess novel therapies, specific imaging biomarkers are being developed and validated to demonstrate biological activity of the various classes of targeted therapy:

- dynamic contrast-enhanced CT and MRI – contrast agent allows the assessment of anti-angiogenic effects on tumour perfusion
- positron emission tomography (PET) can quantitatively measure tumour perfusion (^{15}O-labelled H_2O)
- measure tumour cell proliferation – ^{18}F-fluorothymidine
- PET imaging of molecular pathway receptors, e.g. VEGFR-2.

Clinical applications of biomarkers

With the widespread use of adjuvant therapy for modest benefit in e.g. breast and colorectal cancer, and the advent of costly targeted therapies which are active in only a minority of the cancer types for which they are licensed, there is increasing pressure to pursue the establishment of clinically relevant biomarkers for each cancer site, in order to rationalize individual treatments according to:

- predicted natural history of the cancer
- predominant drivers to malignant phenotype
- predicted responsiveness to available therapies.

Breast cancer

Tumour stage, ER, PR, and HER2 status remain key to the selection of adjuvant therapy, but there remains much uncertainty with regard to which individuals gain most/least from adjuvant chemotherapy, in particular among women with node-negative breast cancer. Recently, microarray technology has produced a 70-gene signature which has prognostic value in node-negative breast cancer, and trials are under way to prospectively evaluate its ability to improve selection of adjuvant therapy in such patients.

Similarly, with regard to adjuvant endocrine therapy, work is progressing to try to identify which patients may benefit from aromatase inhibitors instead of tamoxifen, whether some patients may be best treated by sequential hormonal therapy, and potential for other targeted therapies such as growth factor receptor TKIs either after failure of anti-oestrogens or in combination.

Other biomarkers under investigation include:

- the tumour suppressor PTEN is activated by binding of trastuzumab to ErbB2, and conversely mutation of *PTEN* confers resistance to trastuzumab
- expression of the truncated growth factor receptor p95HER2 also leads to trastuzumab resistance
- importance of stromal gene expression in prognosis.

Lung cancer

Although EGFR immunohistochemistry is positive in 85% of NSCLC, there is no correlation between its expression and response to e.g. cetuximab or EGFR TKIs. While FISH for gene copy number may be more informative, there is now good evidence that specific EGFR gene mutations (e.g. exon 19 deletion) predict response to TKIs; indeed these tumours respond better to targeted therapy than to docetaxel chemotherapy alone or paclitaxel plus carboplatin. Other observations include:

- k-RAS and *BRAF* mutations are highly specific predictors of primary resistance to EGFR tyrosine kinase inhibitors and monoclonal antibody against EGFR in NSCLC
- resistant EGFR mutant tumours may respond to irreversible TKIs which block other receptors e.g. erbB2 and 4
- acquired resistance to EGFR TKIs may be due to MET amplification and MET inhibitors are under development

- similarly for insulin-like growth factor-1 receptor (IGF1R) and its inhibitors
- cisplatin DNA damage is repaired by nucleotide excision repair, and high-level expression of one of the enzymes in this process, ERCC1 (excision repair cross-complementing rodent repair deficiency, complementation group 1), predicts poor response to adjuvant chemotherapy and to platinum-based chemotherapy for advanced disease.

Colorectal cancer

Currently only CEA is in common use as a biomarker. However, understanding of the three pathways to colorectal cancer, chromosomal instability, microsatellite instability, and gene silencing by hypermethylation (e.g. of DNA mismatch repair enzymes), is now complemented by research including:

- screening for early disease/local recurrence by detection of molecular markers of premalignant and malignant lesions in faeces
- microsatellite instability conveys better prognosis but paradoxically is a predictor of lack of benefit of 5-FU adjuvant therapy
- k-RAS mutations (45%) predict poor prognosis, but also failure of therapy targeted against EGFR, e.g. cetuximab; no apparent correlation with EGFR expression, but other potential biomarkers include BRAF and PTEN
- proteomic search for serum marker to replace CEA for follow-up/early diagnosis of relapse
- genomic markers to predict patients who do not require adjuvant therapy or close follow-up.

Renal cell cancer

Given the importance of angiogenesis in this disease, the current focus of biomarker research in this tumour type includes:

- serum VEGF – high level conveys poor prognosis irrespective of treatment; during sunitinib therapy, serum VEGF elevates (produced by non-malignant stroma), but falls on withdrawal (drug is normally taken daily for four weeks, then two weeks' rest), large fluctuations predict good response
- soluble VEGF receptor levels show an inverse pattern of fluctuation during treatment
- hypertension (frequent side-effect of anti-angiogenesis therapy) correlates with positive clinical outcome with e.g. sunitinib
- cellular hypoxia-inducible factors (HIFs)
- basic fibroblast growth factor bFGF
- VHL mutation and the von Hippel–Landau (VHL) protein – no proven correlation with therapeutic outcome.

CNS tumours

- Epigenetic silencing of the DNA repair gene methylguanine–DNA methyltransferase (MGMT) by promoter methylation is associated with temozolomide chemosensitivity in glioblastoma.
- 1p/19q deletions predict better survival and chemosensitivity in oligodendroglioma.

Controversies and limitations

While these developments provide great hope for the individualization of cancer therapies, they also present significant problems:

- realistically must have short turnaround time to allow integration of biomarker into the therapeutic decision-making process of the multidisciplinary team
- integration into conventional drug development and clinical trial design is challenging, and inevitably reduces rates of recruitment to trials where entry is limited to biomarker-positive patients
- combination therapy trials – how best to deliver conventional chemotherapy with targeted agents, sequentially or concomitant
- heterogeneity of tumour and limited availability of biopsy material, e.g. NSCLC commonly diagnosed on cytology rather than biopsy
- feasibility of genomic techniques with fine needle aspiration (FNA) versus core biopsy material
- heterogeneity between primary and metastasis, either re-biopsy or look at circulating tumour cells, e.g. FISH for genotype
- biotechnology quality control, centralized versus local laboratories
- setting limits for therapy, e.g. what is the smallest probability of survival benefit to justify adjuvant therapy
- acceptability of these to patients versus health economists.

Further reading

Hanahan D, Weinberg RA (2000) Hallmarks of cancer. *Cell* **100**, 57–70.

O'Connor JP, Jackson A, Asselin MC, *et al.* (2008) Quantitative imaging biomarkers in the clinical development of targeted therapeutics: current and future perspectives. *Lancet Oncol* **9**, 766–76.

Soreide K, Nedrebo BS, Knapp JC, *et al.* (2009) Evolving molecular classification by genomic and proteomic biomarkers in colorectal cancer: Potential implications for the surgical oncologist. *Surg Oncol* **18**, 31–50.

Appendices

Appendices

NCIC common toxicity criteria (CTC) grading system (March 1998, revised)

Common toxicity criteria (CTC)

Adverse event	Grade				
	0	1	2	3	4
ALLERGY/IMMUNOLOGY					
Allergic reaction/ hypersensitivity (including drug fever)	None	Transient rash, drug fever <38°C (<100.4°F)	Urticaria, drug fever ≥38°C (≥100.4°F), and/or asymptomatic bronchospasm	Symptomatic bronchospasm, requiring parenteral medication(s), with or without urticaria; allergy-related oedema/angioedema	—
Note: isolated urticaria, in the absence of other manifestations of an allergic or hypersensitivity reaction, is graded in the DERMATOLOGY/SKIN category					
Allergic rhinitis (including sneezing, nasal stuffiness, postnasal drip)	None	Mild, not requiring treatment	Moderate, requiring treatment	—	—
Autoimmune reaction	None	Serological or other evidence of autoimmune reaction but patient is asymptomatic (e.g. vitiligo), all organ function is normal, and no treatment is required	Evidence of autoimmune reaction involving a non-essential organ or function (e.g. hypothyroidism), requiring treatment other than immunosuppressive drugs	Reversible autoimmune reaction involving function of a major organ or other adverse event (e.g. transient colitis or anaemia), requiring short-term immunosuppressive treatment	Autoimmune reaction causing major grade 4 organ dysfunction; progressive and irreversible reaction; long-term administration of high-dose immuno-suppressive therapy required

Also consider hypothyroidism, colitis, haemoglobin, haemolysis

	None	—	—	Present	—
Serum sickness	None	—	—	Present	—

Urticaria is graded in the DERMATOLOGY/SKIN category if it occurs as an isolated symptom. If it occurs with other manifestations of allergic or hypersensitivity reaction, grade as Allergic reaction/hypersensitivity above

	None	Mild, not requiring treatment	Symptomatic, requiring medication	Requiring steroids	Ischaemic changes or requiring amputation
Vasculitis	None	Mild, not requiring treatment	Symptomatic, requiring medication	Requiring steroids	Ischaemic changes or requiring amputation
Allergy/immunology – Other (specify___)	None	Mild	Moderate	Severe	Life-threatening or disabling

AUDITORY/HEARING

Conductive hearing loss is graded as Middle ear/hearing in the AUDITORY/HEARING category

Earache is graded in the PAIN category

	Normal	External otitis with erythema or dry desquamation	External otitis with moist desquamation	External otitis with discharge, mastoiditis	Necrosis of the canal soft tissue or bone
External auditory canal	Normal	External otitis with erythema or dry desquamation	External otitis with moist desquamation	External otitis with discharge, mastoiditis	Necrosis of the canal soft tissue or bone

Note: changes associated with radiation to external ear (pinnae) are graded under Radiation dermatitis in the DERMATOLOGY/SKIN category

Adverse event	Grade				
	0	1	2	3	4
Inner ear/hearing	Normal	Hearing loss on audiometry only	Tinnitus or hearing loss, not requiring hearing aid or treatment	Tinnitus or hearing loss, correctable with hearing aid or treatment	Severe unilateral or bilateral hearing loss (deafness), not correctable
Middle ear/hearing	Normal	Serous otitis without subjective decrease in hearing	Serous otitis or infection requiring medical intervention; subjective decrease in hearing; rupture of tympanic membrane with discharge	Otitis with discharge, mastoiditis, or conductive hearing loss	Necrosis of the canal soft tissue or bone
Auditory/ hearing – Other specify,___	Normal	Mild	Moderate	Severe	Life-threatening or disabling
BLOOD/BONE MARROW					
Bone marrow cellularity	Normal for age	Mildly hypocellular or ≤25% reduction from normal cellularity for age	Moderately hypocellular or >25–≤50% reduction from normal cellularity for age or >2 but <4 weeks to recovery of normal bone marrow cellularity	Severely hypocellular or >50–≤75% reduction in cellularity for age or 4–6 weeks to recovery of normal bone marrow cellularity	Aplasia or >6 weeks to recovery of normal bone marrow cellularity

Normal ranges:

Children (≤18 years)	90% cellularity average			
Younger adults (19–59 years)	60–70% cellularity average			
Older adults (≥60 years)	50% cellularity average			

Note: grade bone marrow cellularity only for changes related to treatment not disease

CD4 count	Within normal limits (WNL)	<lower limit of normal (LLN)–500/mm³	200–<500/mm³	50–<200/mm³	<50/mm³
Haptoglobin	Normal	Decreased	—	Absent	—
Haemoglobin (Hb)	WNL	<LLN–10.0 g/dl <LLN–100 g/l <LLN–6.2 mmol/l	8.0–<10.0 g/dl 80–<100 g/l 4.9–<6.2 mmol/l	6.5–<8.0 g/dl 65–<80 g/l 4.0–<4.9 mmol/l	<6.5 g/dl <65g/l <4.0 mmol/l
For leukaemia studies or bone marrow infiltrative/myelophthisic processes, if specified in the protocol	WNL	10–<25% decrease from pre-treatment	25–<50% decrease from pre-treatment	50–<75% decrease from pre-treatment	≥75% decrease from pre-treatment

Adverse event	Grade 0	1	2	3	4
Haemolysis (e.g. immune haemolytic anaemia, drug-related haemolysis, other)	None	Only laboratory evidence of haemolysis [e.g. direct antiglobulin test (direct antiglobulin test (DAT), Coombs') schistocytes]	Evidence of red cell destruction and ≥2 g decrease in haemoglobin, no transfusion	Requiring transfusion and/or medical intervention (e.g. steroids)	Catastrophic consequences of haemolysis (e.g. renal failure, hypotension, bronchospasm, emergency splenectomy)
Also consider haptoglobin, haemoglobin					
Leucocytes (total white cell count, WCC)	WNL	<LLN–3.0 × 10^9/l <LLN–3000/mm³	≥2.0–<3.0 × 10^9/l ≥2000–<3000/mm³	≥1.0–<2.0 × 10^9/l ≥1000–<2000/mm³	<1.0 × 10^9/l <1000/mm³
For BMT studies, if specified in the protocol	WNL	≥2.0–<3.0 × 10^9/l ≥2000–<3000/mm³	≥1.0–<2.0 × 10^9/l ≥1000–<2000/mm³	≥0.5–<1.0 × 10^9/l ≥500–<1000/mm³	<0.5 × 10^9/l <500/mm³
For paediatric BMT studies (using age, race, and sex normal values), if specified in the protocol		≥75–<100% LLN	≥50–<75% LLN	≥25–50% LLN	<25% LLN
Lymphopenia	WNL	<LLN–1.0 × 10^9/l <LLN–1000/mm³	≥0.5–<1.0 × 10^9/l ≥500–<1000/mm³	<0.5 × 10^9/l <500/mm³	—

For paediatric BMT studies (using age, race, and sex normal values), if specified in the protocol	WNL	≥75–<100% LLN	≥50–<75% LLN	≥25–<50% LLN	<25% LLN
Neutrophils/granulocytes (ANC/AGC)	WNL	≥1.5–<2.0×10⁹/l ≥1500–<2000/mm³	≥1.0–<1.5×10⁹/l ≥1000–<1500/mm³	≥0.5–<1.0×10⁹/l ≥500–<1000/mm³	<0.5×10⁹/l <500/mm³
For BMT studies, if specified in the protocol	WNL	≥1.0–<1.5×10⁹/l ≥1000–<1500/mm³	≥0.5–<1.0×10⁹/l ≥500–<1000/mm³	≥0.1–<0.5×10⁹/l ≥100–<500/mm³	<0.1×10⁹/l <100/mm³
For leukaemia studies or bone marrow infiltrative/myelophthisic process, if specified in the protocol	WNL	10–<25% decrease from baseline	25–<50% decrease from baseline	50–<75% decrease from baseline	≥75% decrease from baseline
Platelets	WNL	<LLN–75.0×10⁹/l <LLN–75 000/mm³	≥50.0–<75.0×10⁹/l ≥50 000–<75 000/mm³	≥10.0–<50.0×10⁹/l ≥10 000–<50 000/mm³	<10.0×10⁹/l <10 000/mm³
For BMT studies, if specified in the protocol	WNL	≥50.0–<75.0×10⁹/l ≥50 000–<75 000/mm³	≥20.0–<50.0×10⁹/l ≥20 000–<50 000/mm³	≥10.0–<20.0×10⁹/l ≥10 000–<20 000/mm³	<10.0×10⁹/l <10 000/mm³
For leukaemia studies or bone marrow infiltrative/myelophthisic process, if specified in the protocol	WNL	10–<25% decrease from baseline	25–<50% decrease from baseline	50–<75% decrease from baseline	≥75% decrease from baseline

Adverse event	Grade				
	0	1	2	3	4
Transfusion: platelets	None	—	—	Yes	Platelet transfusions and other measures required to improve platelet increment; platelet transfusion refractoriness associated with life-threatening bleeding (e.g. HLA or cross-matched platelet transfusions)
For BMT studies, if specified in the protocol	None	1 platelet transfusion in 24 hours	2 platelet transfusions in 24 hours	≥3 platelet transfusions in 24 hours	Platelet transfusions and other measures required to improve platelet increment; platelet transfusion refractoriness associated with life-threatening bleeding. (e.g. HLA or cross-matched platelet transfusions)
Also consider platelets					
Transfusion: packed red blood cells (pRBCs)	None	—	—	Yes	—
For BMT studies, if specified in the protocol.	None	≤2 u pRBC in 24 h elective or planned	3 u pRBC in 24 h elective or planned	≥4 u pRBC in 24 h	Haemorrhage or haemolysis associated with life-threatening anaemia; medical intervention required to improve haemoglobin

For paediatric BMT studies, if specified in the protocol	None	≤15 ml/kg in 24 h elective or planned	>15–≤ 30 ml/kg in 24 h elective or planned	>30 ml/kg in 24 h	*Haemorrhage or haemolysis associated with life-threatening anaemia; medical intervention required to improve haemoglobin*

Also consider haemoglobin

Blood/bone marrow – Other (specify,____)	None	Mild	Moderate	Severe	Life-threatening or disabling

CARDIOVASCULAR (ARRHYTHMIA)

Conduction abnormality/ atrioventricular heart block	None	Asymptomatic, not requiring treatment (e.g. Mobitz type I second-degree atrioventricular (AV) block, Wenckebach)	Symptomatic, but not requiring treatment	Symptomatic and requiring treatment (e.g. Mobitz type II second-degree AV block, third-degree AV block)	Life-threatening (e.g. arrhythmia associated with congestive heart failure (CHF), hypotension, syncope, shock)
Nodal/junctional arrhythmia/ dysrhythmia	None	Asymptomatic, not requiring treatment	Symptomatic, but not requiring treatment	Symptomatic and requiring treatment	Life-threatening (e.g. arrhythmia associated with CHF, hypotension, syncope, shock)
Palpitations	None	Present	—	—	

Note: grade palpitations only in the absence of a documented arrhythmia

Adverse event	Grade			
	0	1	2	3	4
Prolonged QTc interval (QTc >0.48 s)	None	Asymptomatic, not requiring treatment	Symptomatic, but not requiring treatment	Symptomatic and requiring treatment	Life-threatening (e.g. arrhythmia associated with CHF, hypotension, syncope, shock)
Sinus bradycardia	None	Asymptomatic, not requiring treatment	Symptomatic, but not requiring treatment	Symptomatic and requiring treatment	Life-threatening (e.g. arrhythmia associated with CHF, hypotension, syncope, shock)
Sinus tachycardia	None	Asymptomatic, not requiring treatment	Symptomatic, but not requiring treatment	Symptomatic and requiring treatment of underlying cause	—
Supraventricular arrhythmias (supraventricular tachycardia (SVT)/atrial fibrillation/flutter)	None	Asymptomatic, not requiring treatment	Symptomatic, but not requiring treatment	Symptomatic and requiring treatment	Life-threatening (e.g. arrhythmia associated with CHF, hypotension, syncope, shock)
Syncope (fainting) is graded in the NEUROLOGY category					
Vasovagal episode	None	—	Present without loss of consciousness	Present with loss of consciousness	—
Ventricular arrhythmia (premature ventricular contractions (PVCs)/ bigeminy/ trigeminy/ ventricular tachycardia)	None	Asymptomatic, not requiring treatment	Symptomatic but not requiring treatment	Symptomatic, and requiring treatment	Life-threatening (e.g. arrhythmia associated with CHF, hypotension, syncope, shock)

Cardiovascular/arrhythmia – Other (specify____)	None	Asymptomatic, not requiring treatment	Symptomatic, but not requiring treatment	Symptomatic, and requiring treatment of underlying cause	Life-threatening (e.g. arrhythmia associated with CHF, hypotension, syncope, shock)

CARDIOVASCULAR (GENERAL)

Acute vascular leak syndrome	Absent	—	Symptomatic, but not requiring fluid support	Respiratory compromise or requiring fluids	Life-threatening; requiring pressor support and/or ventilatory support
Cardiac ischaemia/infarction	None	Non-specific T-wave flattening or changes	Asymptomatic, ST- and T-wave changes suggesting ischaemia	Angina without evidence of infarction	Acute myocardial infarction
Cardiac left ventricular function	Normal	Asymptomatic decline of resting ejection fraction of ≥10% but <20% of baseline value; shortening fraction ≥24% but <30%	Asymptomatic but resting ejection fraction below LLN for laboratory or decline of resting ejection fraction ≥20% of baseline value; <24% shortening fraction	CHF responsive to treatment	Severe or refractory CHF or requiring intubation

CNS cerebrovascular ischaemia is graded in the NEUROLOGY category

Cardiac troponin I (cTnI)	Normal	—	—	Levels consistent with unstable angina as defined by the manufacturer	Levels consistent with myocardial infarction as defined by the manufacturer
Cardiac troponin T (cTnT)	Normal	≥0.03–<0.05 ng/ml	≥0.05–<0.1 ng/ml	≥0.1–<0.2 ng/ml	≥0.2 ng/ml
Oedema	None	Asymptomatic, not requiring therapy	Symptomatic, requiring therapy	Symptomatic oedema limiting function and unresponsive to therapy or requiring drug discontinuation	Anasarca (severe generalized oedema)

Adverse event	Grade				
	0	**1**	**2**	**3**	**4**
Hypertension	None	Asymptomatic, transient increase by >20 mmHg (diastolic) or to >150/100* if previously WNL; not requiring treatment	Recurrent or persistent or symptomatic increase by >20 mmHg (diastolic) or to >150/100* if previously WNL; not requiring treatment	Requiring therapy or more intensive therapy than previously	Hypertensive crisis

Note: for paediatric patients, use age- and sex-appropriate normal values >95th percentile upper limit of normal (ULN)

Adverse event	Grade				
Hypotension	None	Changes, but not requiring therapy (including transient orthostatic hypotension)	Requiring brief fluid replacement or other therapy but not hospitalization; no physiological consequences	Requiring therapy and sustained medical attention, but resolves without persisting physiological consequences	↑Shock (associated with acidaemia and impairing vital organ function due to tissue hypoperfusion)

Also consider syncope (fainting)

Notes: angina or myocardial infarction (MI) is graded as Cardiac-ischaemia/infarction in the CARDIOVASCULAR (GENERAL) category

For paediatric patients, systolic blood pressure (BP) 65 mmHg or less in infants up to 1 year old and 70 mmHg or less in children older than 1 year of age, use two successive or three measurements in 24 h

Adverse event	Grade				
Myocarditis	None	—	—	CHF responsive to treatment	Severe or refractory CHF
Operative injury of vein/artery	None	Primary suture repair for injury, but not requiring transfusion	Primary suture repair for injury, requiring transfusion	Vascular occlusion requiring surgery or bypass for injury	Myocardial infarction; resection of organ (e.g. bowel, limb)

	None	Grade 1	Grade 2	Grade 3	Grade 4
Pericardial effusion/pericarditis	None	Asymptomatic effusion, not requiring treatment	Pericarditis (rub, ECG changes, and/or chest pain)	With physiological consequences	Tamponade (drainage or pericardial window required)
Peripheral arterial ischemia	None	—	Brief episode of ischaemia managed non-surgically and without permanent deficit	Requiring surgical intervention	Life-threatening or with permanent functional deficit (e.g. amputation)
Phlebitis (superficial)	None	—	Present	—	—

Notes: injection site reaction is graded in the DERMATOLOGY/SKIN category
Thrombosis/embolism is graded in the CARDIOVASCULAR (GENERAL) category

Syncope (fainting) is graded in the NEUROLOGY category

	None	Grade 1	Grade 2	Grade 3	Grade 4
Thrombosis/embolism	None	—	Deep vein thrombosis, not requiring anticoagulant	Deep vein thrombosis, requiring anticoagulant therapy	Embolic event including pulmonary embolism

Vein/artery operative injury is graded as operative injury of vein/artery in the CARDIOVASCULAR (GENERAL) category

	None	Grade 1	Grade 2	Grade 3	Grade 4
Visceral arterial ischaemia (non-myocardial)	None	—	Brief episode of ischaemia managed non-surgically and without permanent deficit	Requiring surgical intervention	Life-threatening or with permanent functional deficit (e.g. resection of ileum)
Cardiovascular/General – Other (specify,___)	None	Mild	Moderate	Severe	Life-threatening or disabling

COAGULATION

Note: see the HAEMORRHAGE category for grading the severity of bleeding events

Adverse event	Grade				
	0	1	2	3	4
DIC (disseminated intravascular coagulation)	Absent	—	—	Laboratory findings present with <u>no</u> bleeding	Laboratory findings <u>and</u> bleeding
Also consider platelets					
Note: must have increased fibrin split products or D-dimer in order to grade as DIC					
Fibrinogen	WNL	≥0.75–<1.0 × LLN	≥0.5–<0.75 × LLN	≥0.25–<0.5 × LLN	<0.25 × LLN
For leukaemia studies or bone marrow infiltrative/ myelophthisic process, if specified in the protocol	WNL	<20% decrease from pre-treatment value or LLN	≥20–<40% decrease from pre-treatment value or LLN	≥40–<70% decrease from pre-treatment value or LLN	<50 mg
Partial thromboplastin time (PTT)	WNL	>ULN–≤1.5 × ULN	>1.5–≤2 × ULN	>2 × ULN	—
Phlebitis is graded in the CARDIOVASCULAR (GENERAL) category					
Prothrombin time (PT)	WNL	>ULN–≤1.5 × ULN	>1.5–≤2 × ULN	>2 × ULN	—
Thrombosis/embolism is graded in the CARDIOVASCULAR (GENERAL) category					

Thrombotic microangiopathy (e.g. thrombotic thrombocytopenic purpura/TTP or haemolytic uraemic syndrome/HUS)	Absent	—	Evidence of RBC destruction (schistocytosis) without clinical consequences	Laboratory findings present without clinical consequences	Laboratory findings and clinical consequences, (e.g. central nervous system (CNS) haemorrhage/bleeding or thrombosis/embolism or renal failure) requiring therapeutic intervention
For BMT studies, if specified in the protocol.	—		Evidence of RBC destruction with elevated creatinine (≤3 × ULN)	Evidence of RBC destruction with creatinine (>3 × ULN) not requiring dialysis	Evidence of RBC destruction with renal failure requiring dialysis and/or encephalopathy

Also consider haemoglobin, platelets, creatinine
Note: must have microangiopathic changes on blood smear (e.g. schistocytes, helmet cells, red cell fragments)

Coagulation – Other (Specify,___)	None	Mild	Moderate	Severe	Life-threatening or disabling

CONSTITUTIONAL SYMPTOMS

Fatigue (lethargy, malaise, asthenia)	None	Increased fatigue over baseline, but not altering normal activities	Moderate (e.g. decrease in performance status by 1 ECOG level or 20% Karnofsky or Lansky) or causing difficulty performing some activities	severe (e.g. decrease in performance status by ≥2 ECOG levels or 40% Karnofsky or Lansky) or loss of ability to perform some activities	Bedridden or disabling

Note: see Performance status scales in 📖 Appendix 3

Adverse event	Grade				
	0	1	2	3	4
Fever (in the absence of neutropenia, where neutropenia is defined as AGC<1.0 ×10³/l)	None	38.0–39.0°C (100.4–102.2°F)	39.1–40.0°C (102.3–104.0°F)	>40.0°C (>104.0°F) for <24 h	>40.0°C (>104.0°F) for >24 h
Also consider allergic reaction/hypersensitivity Note: the temperature measurements listed above are oral or tympanic					
Hot flashes/flushes are graded in the ENDOCRINE category					
Rigors, chills	None	Mild, requiring symptomatic treatment (e.g. blanket) or non-narcotic medication	Severe and/or prolonged, requiring narcotic medication	Not responsive to narcotic medication	—
Sweating (diaphoresis)	Normal	Mild and occasional	Frequent or drenching	—	—
Weight gain	<5%	5–<10%	10–<20%	≥20%	
Also consider ascites, oedema pleural effusion (non-malignant)					
Weight gain associated with veno-occlusive disease (VOD) for BMT studies, if specified in the protocol	<2%	≥2<5%	≥5–<10%	≥10% or as ascites	≥10% or fluid retention resulting in pulmonary failure
Also consider ascites, oedema pleural effusion (non-malignant)					
Weight loss	<5%	5–<10%	10–<20%	≥20%	—
Also consider vomiting, dehydration, diarrhoea					

	None	Mild	Moderate	Severe	Life-threatening or disabling
Constitutional Symptoms – Other (specify, ____)					
DERMATOLOGY/SKIN					
Alopecia	Normal	Mild hair loss	Pronounced hair loss	—	—
Bruising (in absence of grade 3 or 4 thrombocytopenia)	None	Localized or in dependent area	Generalized	—	—
Note: bruising resulting from grade 3 or 4 thrombocytopenia is graded as petechiae/purpura and haemorrhage/bleeding with grade 3 or 4 HAEMORRHAGE category, not in the DERMATOLOGY/SKIN category					
Dry skin	Normal	Controlled with emollients	Not controlled with emollients	—	—
Erythema multiforme (e.g. Stevens-Johnson syndrome, toxic epidermal necrolysis)	Absent	—	Scattered, but not generalized eruption	Severe or requiring IV fluids (e.g. generalized rash or painful stomatitis)	Life-threatening (e.g. exfoliative or ulcerating dermatitis or requiring enteral or parenteral nutritional support)
Flushing	Absent	Present	—	—	—
Hand–foot skin reaction	None	Skin changes or dermatitis without pain (e.g. erythema, peeling)	Skin changes with pain, not interfering with function	Skin changes with pain, interfering with function	—
Injection site reaction	None	Pain or itching or erythema	Pain or swelling, with inflammation or phlebitis	Ulceration or necrosis that is severe or pro-longed, or requiring surgery	—

Adverse event	Grade				
	0	1	2	3	4
Nail changes	Normal	Discoloration or ridging (koilonychia) or pitting	Partial or complete loss of nail(s) or pain in nailbeds	—	—
Petechiae is graded in the HAEMORRHAGE category					
Photosensitivity	None	Painless erythema	Painful erythema	Erythema with desquamation	—
Pigmentation changes (e.g. vitiligo)	None	Localized pigmentation changes	Generalized pigmentation changes	—	—
Pruritus	None	Mild or localized, relieved spontaneously or by local measures	Intense or widespread, relieved spontaneously or by systemic measures	Intense or widespread and poorly controlled despite treatment	—
Purpura is graded in the HAEMORRHAGE category					
Radiation dermatitis	None	Faint erythema or dry desquamation	Moderate to brisk erythema or a patchy moist desquamation, mostly confined to skin folds and creases; moderate oedema	Confluent moist desquamation ≥1.5 cm diameter and not confined to skin folds; pitting oedema	Skin necrosis or ulceration of full thickness dermis; may include bleeding not induced by minor trauma or abrasion
Note: pain associated with radiation dermatitis is graded separately in the PAIN category as Pain due to radiation					
Radiation recall reaction (reaction following chemotherapy in the absence of additional radiation therapy that occurs in a previous radiation port)	None	Faint erythema or dry desquamation	Moderate to brisk erythema or a patchy moist desquamation, mostly confined to skin folds and creases; moderate oedema	Confluent moist desquamation ≥1.5 cm diameter and not Confined to skin folds; pitting oedema	Skin necrosis or ulceration of full thickness dermis; may include bleeding not induced by minor trauma or abrasion

	None/0	1	2	3	4
Rash/desquamation	None	Macular or papular eruption or erythema without associated symptoms	Macular or papular eruption or erythema with pruritus or other associated symptoms covering <50% of body surface or localized desquamation or other lesions covering <50% of body surface area	Symptomatic generalized erythroderma or macular, papular, or vesicular eruption or desquamation covering ≥50% of body surface area	Generalized exfoliative dermatitis or ulcerative dermatitis

Also consider allergic reaction/hypersensitivity

Note: Stevens–Johnson syndrome is graded separately as Erythema multiforme in the DERMATOLOGY/SKIN category

	None/0	1	2	3	4
Rash/dermatitis associated with high-dose chemotherapy or BMT studies.	None	Faint erythema or dry desquamation	Moderate to brisk erythema or a patchy moist desquamation, mostly confined to skin folds and creases; moderate oedema	Confluent moist desquamation ≥1.5 cm diameter and not confined to skin folds; pitting oedema	Skin necrosis or ulceration of full-thickness dermis; may include spontaneous bleeding not induced by minor trauma or abrasion

	None/0	1	2	3	4
Rash/desquamation associated with graft versus host disease (GVHD) for BMT studies, if specified in the protocol.	None	Macular or papular eruption or erythema covering <25% of body surface area without associated symptoms	Macular or papular eruption or erythema with pruritus or other associated symptoms covering ≥25–<50% of body surface or localized desquamation or other lesions covering ≥25–<50% of body surface area	Symptomatic generalized erythroderma or symptomatic macular, papular, or vesicular eruption, with bullous formation, or desquamation covering >50% of body surface area	Generalized exfoliative dermatitis or ulcerative dermatitis or bullous formation

Also consider allergic reaction/hypersensitivity

Note: Stevens–Johnson syndrome is graded separately as Erythema multiforme in the DERMATOLOGY/SKIN category

Adverse event	Grade 0	1	2	3	4
Urticaria (hives, welts, wheals)	None	Requiring no medication	Requiring PO or topical treatment or IV medication or steroids for <24 h	Requiring IV medication or steroids for ≥24 h	—
Wound – infectious	None	Cellulitis	Superficial infection	Infection requiring IV antibiotics	Necrotizing fasciitis
Wound – non-infectious	None	Incisional separation	Incisional hernia	Fascial disruption without evisceration	Fascial disruption with evisceration
Dermatology/skin – Other (specify,_____)	None	Mild	Moderate	Severe	Life-threatening or disabling
ENDOCRINE					
Cushingoid appearance (e.g. moon face, buffalo hump, centripetal obesity, cutaneous striae)	Absent	—	Present	—	—
Also consider hyperglycaemia, hypokalaemia					
Feminization of male	Absent	—	—	Present	—
Gynaecomastia	None	Mild	Pronounced or painful	Pronounced or painful and requiring surgery	—
Hot flashes/flushes	None	Mild or no more than 1 per day	Moderate and greater than 1 per day	—	—

Hypothyroidism	Absent	Asymptomatic, TSH elevated, no therapy given	Symptomatic or thyroid replacement treatment given for manifestations of hypothyroidism	Patient hospitalized	Myxoedema coma
Masculinization of female	Absent	—	—	Present	—
SIADH (syndrome of inappropriate antidiuretic hormone)	Absent	—	—	Present	—
Endocrine – Other (specify, ___)	None	Mild	Moderate	Severe	Life-threatening or disabling

GASTROINTESTINAL

Amylase is graded in the METABOLIC/LABORATORY category

Anorexia	None	Loss of appetite	Oral intake significantly decreased	Requiring IV fluids	Requiring feeding tube or parenteral nutrition
Ascites (non-malignant)	None	Asymptomatic	Symptomatic, requiring diuretics	Symptomatic, requiring therapeutic paracentesis	Life-threatening physiological consequences
Colitis	None	—	Abdominal pain with mucus and/or blood in stool	Abdominal pain, fever, change in bowel habits with ileus or peritoneal signs, and radiographic or biopsy documentation	Perforation or requiring surgery or toxic megacolon

Also consider haemorrhage/bleeding with grade 3 or 4 thrombocytopenia, haemorrhage/bleeding without grade 3 or 4 thrombocytopenia, melaena/gastrointestinal (GI) bleeding, rectal bleeding/haematochezia, hypotension

Constipation	None	Requiring stool softener or dietary modification	Requiring laxatives	Obstipation requiring manual evacuation or enema	Obstruction or toxic megacolon

	Grade			
Adverse event	**0**	**1**	**2**	**3**	**4**
Dehydration	None	Dry mucous membranes and/or diminished skin turgor	Requiring IV fluid replacement (brief)	Requiring IV fluid replacement (sustained)	Physiological consequences requiring intensive care; haemodynamic collapse
Also consider diarrhoea, vomiting, stomatitis/pharyngitis (oral/pharyngeal mucositis), hypotension					
Diarrhoea patients without colostomy:	None	Increase of <4 stools/day over pre-treatment	Increase of 4–6 stools/day, or nocturnal stools	Increase of ≥7 stools/day or incontinence; or need for parenteral support for dehydration	Physiological consequences requiring intensive care; or haemodynamic collapse
Patients with a colostomy:	None	Mild increase in loose, watery colostomy output compared with pre-treatment	Moderate increase in loose, watery colostomy output compared with pre-treatment, but not interfering with normal activity	Severe increase in loose, watery colostomy output compared with pre-treatment, interfering with normal activity	Physiologic consequences, requiring intensive care; or haemodynamic collapse
Diarrhea associated with graft versus host disease (GVHD) for BMT studies, if specified in the protocol	None	>500–≤1000 ml of diarrhoea/day	>1000–≤1500 ml of diarrhoea/day	>1500 ml of diarrhoea/day	Severe abdominal pain with or without ileus
For paediatric BMT studies, if specified in the protocol.		*>5–≤ 10 ml/kg of diarrhoea/day*	*>10–≤15 ml/kg of diarrhoea/ day*	*>15 ml/kg of diarrhoea/day*	—
Also consider haemorrhage/bleeding with grade 3 or 4 thrombocytopenia, haemorrhage/bleeding without grade 3 or 4 thrombocytopenia, pain, dehydration, hypotension					
Duodenal ulcer (requires radiographic or endoscopic documentation)	None	—	Requiring medical management or non-surgical treatment	Uncontrolled by outpatient medical management; requiring hospitalization	Perforation or bleeding, requiring emergency surgery

Adverse event	None	Mild	Moderate	Severe	
Duodenal ulcer (requires radiographic or endoscopic documentation)	None	—	Requiring medical management or non-surgical treatment	Uncontrolled by outpatient medical management; requiring hospitalization	Perforation or bleeding, requiring emergency surgery
Dyspepsia/heartburn	None	Mild	Moderate	Severe	—
Dysphagia, esophagitis, odynophagia (painful swallowing)	None	Mild dysphagia, but can eat regular diet	Dysphagia, requiring predominantly pureed, soft, or liquid diet	Dysphagia, requiring IV hydration	Complete obstruction (cannot swallow saliva) Requiring enteral or parenteral nutritional support, or perforation

Note: if the adverse event is radiation-related, grade *either* under dysphagia—oesophageal related to radiation or dysphagia—pharyngeal related to radiation

Adverse event	None	Mild	Moderate	Severe	
Dysphagia—*oesophageal* related to radiation	None	Mild dysphagia, but can eat regular diet	Dysphagia, requiring predominantly pureed, soft, or liquid diet	Dysphagia, requiring feeding tube, IV hydration, or hyperalimentation	Complete obstruction (cannot swallow saliva); ulceration with bleeding not induced by minor trauma or abrasion or perforation

Also consider pain due to radiation, mucositis due to radiation as Fistula—oesophageal

Note: fistula is graded separately as Fistula—oesophageal

Adverse event	None	Mild	Moderate	Severe	
Dysphagia—*pharyngeal* related to radiation	None	Mild dysphagia, but can eat regular diet	Dysphagia, requiring predominantly pureed, soft, or liquid diet	Dysphagia, requiring feeding tube, IV hydration, or hyperalimentation	Complete obstruction (cannot swallow saliva); ulceration with bleeding not induced by minor trauma or abrasion or perforation

Also consider pain due to radiation, mucositis due to radiation as fistula – pharyngeal

Note: fistula is graded separately as fistula – pharyngeal

Adverse event	Grade			
	0	1	2	3	4
Fistula—oesophageal	None	—	—	Present	Requiring surgery
Fistula—intestinal	None	—	—	Present	Requiring surgery
Fistula—pharyngeal	None	—	—	Present	Requiring surgery
Fistula—rectal/anal	None	—	—	Present	Requiring surgery
Flatulence	None	Mild	Moderate	—	—
Gastric ulcer (requires radiographic or endoscopic documentation)	None	—	Requiring medical management or non surgical treatment	Bleeding without perforation, uncontrolled by outpatient medical management; requiring hospitalization or surgery	Perforation or bleeding, requiring emergency surgery
Also consider haemorrhage/bleeding with grade 3 or 4 thrombocytopenia, haemorrhage/bleeding without grade 3 or 4 thrombocytopenia					
Gastritis	None	—	Requiring medical management or non-surgical treatment	Uncontrolled by out-patient medical management; requiring emergency hospitalization or surgery	Life-threatening bleeding, requiring emergency surgery
Also consider haemorrhage/bleeding with grade 3 or 4 thrombocytopenia, haemorrhage/bleeding without grade 3 or 4 thrombocytopenia					
Haematemesis is graded in the HAEMORRHAGE category					
Haematochezia is graded in the HAEMORRHAGE category as Rectal bleeding/haematochezia					
Ileus (or neuroconstipation)	None	—	Intermittent, not requiring intervention	Requiring non-surgical intervention	Requiring surgery
Mouth dryness	Normal	Mild	Moderate	—	—

Mucositis

Notes: mucositis not due to radiation is graded in the GASTROINTESTINAL category for specific sites: colitis, oesophagitis, gastritis, stomatitis/pharyngitis (oral/pharyngeal mucositis), and typhlitis; or the RENAL/GENITOURINARY category for vaginitis
Radiation-related mucositis is graded as mucositis due to radiation

Mucositis due to radiation	None	Erythema of the mucosa	Patchy pseudomembranous reaction (patches generally ≤1.5 cm in diameter and non contiguous)	Confluent pseudomembranous reaction (patches contiguous generally >1.5 cm in diameter)	Necrosis or deep ulceration; may include bleeding not induced by minor trauma or abrasion

Also consider pain due to radiation
Notes: grade radiation mucositis of the larynx here
dysphagia related to radiation is also graded as either Dysphagia – oesophageal related to radiation or Dysphagia – pharyngeal related to radiation, depending on the site of treatment

Nausea	None	Able to eat	Oral intake significantly decreased	No significant intake, requiring IV fluids	—
Pancreatitis	None	—	—	Abdominal pain with pancreatic enzyme elevation	Complicated by shock (acute circulatory failure)

Also consider hypotension
Note: amylase is graded in the METABOLIC/LABORATORY category

Pharyngitis is graded in the GASTROINTESTINAL category as stomatitis/pharyngitis (oral/pharyngeal mucositis)

Adverse event	Grade				
	0	1	2	3	4
Proctitis	None	Increased stool frequency, occasional blood-streaked stools or rectal discomfort (including haemorrhoids) not requiring medication	Increased stool frequency, bleeding, mucus discharge, or rectal discomfort requiring medication; anal fissure necessitating pads	Increased stool frequency/ diarrhoea requiring parenteral support; rectal bleeding requiring transfusion; or persistent mucus discharge,	Perforation, bleeding, or necrosis or other life-threatening complication requiring surgical intervention (e.g. colostomy)

Also consider haemorrhage/bleeding with grade 3 or 4 thrombocytopenia, haemorrhage/bleeding without grade 3 or 4 thrombocytopenia, pain due to radiation

Notes: fistula is graded separately as Fistula—rectal/anal

proctitis occurring more than 90 days after the start of radiation therapy is graded in the RTOG/EORTC Late Radiation Morbidity Scoring Scheme (see later in this appendix.)

Adverse event	Grade				
	0	1	2	3	4
Salivary gland changes	None	Slightly thickened saliva; may have slightly altered taste (e.g. metallic); additional fluids may be required	Thick, ropy, sticky saliva; markedly altered taste; alteration in diet required	—	Acute salivary gland necrosis
Sense of smell	Normal	Slightly altered	Markedly altered	—	—
Stomatitis/ pharyngitis (oral/ pharyngeal mucositis)	None	Painless ulcers, erythema, or mild soreness in the absence of lesions	Painful erythema, oedema, or ulcers, but can eat or swallow	Painful erythema, oedema, or ulcers requiring IV hydration	Severe ulceration or requires parenteral or enteral nutritional support or prophylactic intubation

	None				
For BMT studies, if specified in the protocol.	None	Painless ulcers, erythema, or mild soreness in the absence of lesions	Painful erythema, oedema, or ulcers but can swallow	Painful erythema, oedema, or ulcers preventing swallowing or requiring hydration or parenteral (or enteral) nutritional support	Severe ulceration requiring prophylactic intubation or resulting in documented aspiration pneumonia
Note: radiation-related mucositis is graded as mucositis due to radiation					
Taste disturbance (dysgeusia)	Normal	Slightly altered	Markedly altered	—	—
Typhlitis (inflammation of the caecum)	None	—	—	≥6 episodes in 24 h over pre-treatment; or need for IV fluids	Perforation, bleeding, or necrosis or other life-threatening complication requiring surgical intervention (e.g. colostomy)
Also consider haemorrhage/bleeding with grade 3 or 4 thrombocytopenia, haemorrhage/bleeding without grade 3 or 4 thrombocytopenia, hypotension, febrile neutropenia					
Vomiting	None	Over pre-treatment	2–5 episodes in 24 h over pre-treatment	≥6 episodes in 24 h over pre-treatment; or need for IV fluids	Requiring parenteral nutrition; or physiological consequences requiring intensive care; haemodynamic collapse
Also consider dehydration					
Weight gain is graded in the CONSTITUTIONAL SYMPTOMS category					
Weight loss is graded in the CONSTITUTIONAL SYMPTOMS category					
Gastrointestinal—Other (specify, _____)	None	Mild	Moderate	Severe	Life-threatening or disabling

Adverse event	Grade			
	0	1	2	3	4

HAEMORRHAGE

Notes: transfusion in this section refers to pRBC infusion

For *any* bleeding with grade 3 or 4 platelets (<50 000), *always* grade hemorrhage/bleeding with grade 3 or 4 thrombocytopenia. Also consider platelets, transfusion: pRBCs, and transfusion: platelets in addition to grading severity by grading the site or type of bleeding

If the site or type of haemorrhage/bleeding is listed, also use the grading that incorporates the site of bleeding: CNS haemorrhage/bleeding, haematuria, haematemesis, haemoptysis, haemorrhage/bleeding with surgery, melaena/lower GI bleeding, petechiae/purpura (haemorrhage/bleeding into skin), rectal bleeding/haematochezia, vaginal bleeding

If the platelet count is ≥50 000/mm³ and the site or type of bleeding is listed, grade the specific site. If the site or type is not listed and the platelet count is ≥50 000/mm³, grade haemorrhage/bleeding without grade 3 or 4 thrombocytopenia and specify the site or type in the OTHER category

Adverse event	0	1	2	3	4
Haemorrhage/bleeding with grade 3 or 4 thrombocytopenia	None	Mild without transfusion		Requiring transfusion	Catastrophic bleeding, requiring major non-elective intervention

Also consider platelets, hemoglobin, transfusion: platelets, transfusion: pRBCs, site or type of bleeding. If the site is not listed, grade as haemorrhage —Other (specify site,_____)

Note: this adverse event must be graded for any bleeding with grade 3 or 4 thrombocytopenia

Adverse event	0	1	2	3	4
Haemorrhage/bleeding without grade 3 or 4 thrombocytopenia	None	Mild without transfusion		Requiring transfusion	Catastrophic bleeding, requiring major non-elective intervention

Also consider platelets, haemoglobin, transfusion: platelets. transfusion: pRBCs, haemorrhage – Other (specify site,_____)

Note: bleeding in the absence of grade 3 or 4 thrombocytopenia is graded here only if the specific site or type of bleeding is not listed elsewhere in the HAEMORRHAGE category. Also grade as Other in the HAEMORRHAGE category

					Haemorrhagic stroke or haemorrhagic vascular event (CVA) with neurological signs and symptoms
				Bleeding noted on computerized tomography (CT) or other scan with no clinical consequences	
CNS haemorrhage/ bleeding	None	—			Haemorrhagic stroke or haemorrhagic vascular event (CVA) with neurological signs and symptoms
Epistaxis	None	Mild without transfusion	—	Requiring transfusion	Catastrophic bleeding, requiring major non-elective intervention
Haematemesis	None	Mild without transfusion	—	Requiring transfusion	Catastrophic bleeding, requiring major non-elective intervention
Haematuria (in the absence of vaginal bleeding)	None	Microscopic only	Intermittent gross bleeding, no clots	Persistent gross bleeding or clots; may require catheterization or instrumentation, or transfusion	Open surgery or necrosis or deep bladder ulceration
Haemoptysis	None	Mild without transfusion	—	Requiring transfusion	Catastrophic bleeding, requiring major non-elective intervention
Haemorrhage/ bleeding associated with surgery	None	Mild without transfusion	—	Requiring transfusion	Catastrophic bleeding, requiring major non-elective intervention
Note: expected blood loss at the time of surgery is not graded as an adverse event					
Melaena/GI bleeding	None	Mild without transfusion	—	Requiring transfusion	Catastrophic bleeding, requiring major non-elective intervention

Adverse event	Grade				
	0	1	2	3	4
Petechiae/purpura (haemorrhage/bleeding into skin or mucosa)	None	Rare petechiae of skin	Petechiae or purpura in dependent areas of skin	Generalized petechiae or purpura of skin or petechiae of any mucosal site	—
Rectal bleeding/haematochezia	None	Mild without transfusion or medication	Persistent, requiring medication (e.g. steroid suppositories) and/or break from radiation treatment	Requiring transfusion	Catastrophic bleeding, requiring major non-elective intervention
Vaginal bleeding	None	Spotting, requiring <2 pads per day	Requiring ≥2 pads per day, but not requiring transfusion	Requiring transfusion	Catastrophic bleeding, requiring major non-elective intervention
Haemorrhage – Other (specify site,___)	None	Mild without transfusion		Requiring transfusion	Catastrophic bleeding, requiring major non-elective intervention
HEPATIC					
Alkaline phosphatase	WNL	>ULN–2.5 × ULN	>2.5–5.0 × ULN	>5.0–20.0 × ULN	>20.0 × ULN
Bilirubin	WNL	>ULN–1.5 × ULN	>1.5–3.0 × ULN	>3.0–10.0 × ULN	>10.0 × ULN
Bilirubin associated with graft versus host disease (GVHD) for BMT studies, if specified in the protocol.	normal	≥2–<3 mg/100 ml	≥3–<6 mg/100 ml	≥6–<15 mg/100 ml	≥15 mg/100 ml

GGT (γ-glutamyl transpeptidase)	WNL	>ULN–2.5 × ULN	>2.5–5.0 × ULN	>5.0–20.0 × ULN	>20.0 × ULN
Hepatic enlargement	Absent	—	—	Present	—
Note: grade haepatic enlargement only for treatment-related adverse event including veno-occlusive disease					
Hypoalbuminemia	WNL	<LLN–3 g/dl	≥2–<3 g/dl	<2 g/dl	—
Liver dysfunction/failure (clinical)	Normal	—	—	Asterixis	Encephalopathy or coma
Portal vein flow	Normal	—	Decreased portal vein flow	Reversal/retrograde portal vein flow	—
SGOT (AST) (serum glutamic oxaloacetic transaminase)	WNL	>ULN–2.5 × ULN	>2.5–5.0 × ULN	>5.0–20.0 × ULN	>20.0 × ULN
SGPT (ALT) (serum glutamic pyruvic transaminase)	WNL	>ULN–2.5 × ULN	>2.5–5.0 × ULN	>5.0–20.0 × ULN	>20.0 × ULN
Hepatic – Other (specify_____)	None	Mild	Moderate	Severe	Life-threatening or disabling

INFECTION/FEBRILE NEUTROPENIA

Catheter-related infection	None	Mild, no active treatment	Moderate, localized infection, requiring local or oral treatment	Severe, systemic infection, requiring iv antibiotic or antifungal treatment or hospitalization	Life-threatening sepsis (e.g. septic shock)

Adverse event	Grade			
	0	1	2	3	4
Febrile neutropenia (fever of unknown origin without clinically or micro-biologically docu-mented infection)	None	—	—	Present	Life-threatening sepsis (e.g. septic shock)
(ANC<1.0 × 10⁹/l, fever ≥38.5°C)					
Also consider neutrophils					
Note: hypothermia instead of fever may be associated with neutropenia and is graded here					
Infection (documen-ted clinically or microbiologically) with grade 3 or 4 neutropenia	None	—	—	Present	Life-threatening sepsis (e.g. septic shock)
(ANC<1.0 × 10⁹/l)					
Also consider neutrophils					
Notes: hypothermia instead of fever may be associated with neutropenia and is graded here					
In the absence of documented infection grade 3 or 4 neutropenia with fever is graded as febrile neutropenia					
Infection with unknown ANC	None	—	—	Present	Life-threatening sepsis (e.g. septic shock)
Note: this adverse event criterion is used in the rare case when ANC is unknown					

Infection without neutropenia	None	Mild, no active treatment	Moderate, localized infection, requiring local or oral treatment	Severe, systematic infection, requiring IV antibiotic or antifungal treatment, or hospitalization	Life-threatening sepsis (e.g. septic shock)

Also consider neutrophils

Wound infections is graded in the DERMATOLOGY/SKIN category

Infection/febrile neutropenia – Other (specify___)	None	Mild	Moderate	Severe	Life-threatening or disabling

LYMPHATICS

Lymphatics	Normal	Mild lymphoedema	Moderate lymphoedema requiring compression; lymphocyst	Severe lymphoedema limiting function; lymphocyst requiring surgery	Severe lymphoedema limiting function with ulceration
Lymphatics – Other (specify___)	None	Mild	Moderate	Severe	Life-threatening or disabling

METABOLIC/LABORATORY

Acidosis (metabolic or respiratory)	Normal	PH <normal, but ≥7.3	—	pH <7.3	pH <7.3 with life-threatening physiological consequences
Alkalosis (metabolic or respiratory)	Normal	PH >normal, but ≤7.5	—	PH >7.5	PH >7.5 with life-threatening physiological consequences

Adverse event	Grade				
	0	1	2	3	4
Amylase	WNL	>ULN–1.5 × ULN	>1.5–2.0×ULN	>2.0–5.0 × ULN	>5.0 × ULN
Bicarbonate	WNL	<LLN–16 mEq/dl	11–15 mEq/dl	8–10 mEq/dl	<8 mEq/dl
CPK (creatine phosphokinase)	WNL	>ULN–2.5 × ULN	>2.5–5 × ULN	>5–10 × ULN	>10 × ULN
Hypercalcaemia	WNL	>ULN–11.5 mg/dl >ULN–2.9 mmol/l	>11.5–12.5 mg/dl >2.9–3.1 mmol/l	>12.5–13.5 mg/dl >3.1–3.4 mmol/l	>13.5 mg/dl >3.4 mmol/l
Hypercholesterolaemia	WNL	>ULN–300 mg/dl >ULN–7.75 mmol/l	>300–400 mg/dl >7.75–10.34 mmol/l	>400–500 mg/dl >10.34–12.92 mmol/l	>500 mg/dl >12.92 mmol/l
Hyperglycaemia	WNL	>ULN–160 mg/dl >ULN–8.9 mmol/l	>160–250 mg/dl >8.9–13.9 mmol/l	>250–500 mg/dl >13.9–27.8 mmol/l	>500 mg/dl >27.8 mmol/l or acidosis
Hyperkalaemia	WNL	>ULN–5.5 mmol/l	>5.5–6.0 mmol/l	>6.0–7.0 mmol/l	>7.0 mmol/l
Hypermagnesaemia	WNL	>ULN–3.0 mg/dl >ULN–1.23 mmol/l	—	>3.0–8.0 mg/dl >1.23–3.30 mmol/l	>8.0 mg/dl >3.30 mmol/l
Hypernatraemia	WNL	>ULN–150 mmol/l	>150–155 mmol/l	>155–160 mmol/l	>160 mmol/l
Hypertriglyceridaemia	WNL	>ULN–2.5 × ULN	>2.5–5.0 × ULN	>5.0–10 × ULN	>10 × ULN
Hyperuricaemia	WNL	>ULN–<10 mg/dl ≤0.59 mmol/l without physiological consequences	—	>ULN–<10 mg/dl ≤0.59 mmol/l with physiological consequences	>10 mg/dl >0.59 mmol/l
Also consider tumour lysis syndrome, renal failure, creatinine, hyperkalaemia					
Hypocalcaemia	WNL	<LLN–8.0 mg/dl <LLN–2.0 mmol/l	7.0–8.0 mg/dl 1.75–<2.0 mmol/l	6.0–<7.0 mg/dl 1.5–<1.75 mmol/l	<6.0 mg/dl <1.5 mmol/l

	None / WNL	Mild	Moderate	Severe	Life-threatening
Hypoglycaemia	WNL	<LLN–55 mg/dl <LLN–3.0 mmol/l	40–55 mg/dl 2.2–<3.0 mmol/l	30–<40 mg/dl 1.7–<2.2 mmol/l	<30 mg/dl <1.7 mmol/l
Hypokalaemia	WNL	<LLN–3.0 mmol/l		2.5–<3.0 mmol/l	<2.5 mmol/l
Hypomagnesemia	WNL	<LLN–1.2 mg/dl <LLN–0.5 mmol/l	0.9–<1.2 mg/dl 0.4–<0.5 mmol/l	0.7–<0.9 mg/dl 0.3–<0.4 mmol/l	<0.7 mg/dl <0.3 mmol/l
Hyponatraemia	WNL	<LLN–130 mmol/l	—	120–<130 mmol/l	<120 mmol/l
Hypophosphatemia	WNL	<LLN–2.5 mg/dl <LLN–0.8 mmol/l	≥2.0–2.5 mg/dl ≥0.6–<0.8 mmol/l	≥1.0–<2.0 mg/dl ≥0.3–<0.6 mmol/l	<1.0 mg/dl <0.3 mmol/l

Hypothyroidism is graded in the ENDOCRINE category

	None / WNL	Mild	Moderate	Severe	Life-threatening
Lipase	WNL	>ULN–1.5 × ULN	>1.5–2.0 × ULN	>2.0–5.0 × ULN	>5.0 × ULN
Metabolic/ laboratory – Other (specify,____)	None	Mild	Moderate	Severe	Life-threatening or disabling

MUSCULOSKELETAL

Arthralgia is graded in the PAIN category

	None	Mild	Moderate	Severe	Disabling
Arthritis	None	Mild pain with inflammation, erythemal or joint swelling but not interfering with function	Moderate pain with inflammation, erythema, or joint swelling interfering with function, but not interfering with activities of daily living	Severe pain with inflammation, erythema, or joint swelling and interfering with activities of daily living	Disabling

WNL, within normal limits; ULN, upper limits of normal; LLN, lower limits of normal

Adverse event	Grade				
	0	1	2	3	4
Muscle weakness normal (not due to neuropathy)	Normal	Asymptomatic with weakness on physical exam	Symptomatic and interfering with function, but not interfering with activities of daily living	Symptomatic and interfering with activities of daily living	Bedridden or disabling

Myalgia (tenderness or pain in muscles) is graded in the PAIN category

Adverse event	0	1	2	3	4
Myositis (inflammation/ damage of muscle)	None	Mild pain, not interfering with function	Pain interfering with function, but not interfering with activities of daily living	Pain interfering with function and interfering with activities of daily living	Bedridden or disabling

Also consider CPK

Note: myositis implies muscle damage (i.e. elevated CPK)

Adverse event	0	1	2	3	4
Osteonecrosis none (avascular necrosis)	None	Asymptomatic and detected by imaging only	Symptomatic and interfering with function, but not interfering with activities of daily living	Symptomatic and interfering with activities of daily living	Symptomatic; or disabling
Musculoskeletal– Other none (specify, _____)	None	Mild	Moderate	Severe	Life-threatening or disabling

NEUROLOGY

Aphasia, receptive and/or expressive, is graded under speech impairment in the NEUROLOGY category

Arachnoiditis/meningismus/radiculitis	Absent	Mild pain not interfering with function	Moderate pain interfering with function, but not interfering with activities of daily living	Severe pain interfering with activities of daily living	Unable to function or perform activities of daily living; bedridden; paraplegia
Also consider headache, vomiting, fever					
Ataxia (incoordination) normal	Normal	Asymptomatic but abnormal on physical exam, and not interfering with function	Mild symptoms interfering with function, but not interfering with activities of daily living	Moderate symptoms interfering with activities of daily living	Bedridden or disabling
CNS cerebrovascular none ischaemia	None	—	—	Transient ischaemic event or attack (TIA)	Permanent event (e.g., cerebral vascular accident)
CNS haemorrhage/bleeding is graded in haemorrhage category					
Cognitive disturbance/ none learning problems	*None*	*Cognitive disability; not interfering with work/school performance; preservation of intelligence*	*Cognitive disability; interfering with work/school performance; decline of 1 SD (standard deviation) or loss of developmental milestones*	*Cognitive disability; resulting in significant impairment of work/ school performance; cognitive decline >2 SD*	*Inability to work/frank mental retardation*

Adverse event	Grade				
	0	1	2	3	4
Confusion	Normal	Confusion or disorientation or attention deficit of brief duration; resolves spontaneously with no sequelae	Confusion or disorientation or attention deficit interfering with function, but not interfering with activities of daily living	Confusion or disorientation interfering with function, but not interfering with activities of daily living	Confusion or delirium interfering with activities of daily living	Harmful to others or self; requiring hospitalization
Cranial neuropathy is graded in the NEUROLOGY category as Neuropathy–cranial					
Delusions	Normal	—	—	Present	Toxic psychosis
Depressed level of consciousness	Normal	Somnolence or sedation not interfering with function	Somnolence or sedation interfering with function, but not interfering with activities of daily living	Obtundation or stupor; difficult to arouse; interfering with activities of daily living	Coma
Note: syncope (fainting) is graded in the NEUROLOGY category					
Dizziness/ lightheadedness	None	Not interfering with function	Interfering with function, but not interfering with activities of daily living	Interfering with activities of daily living	Bedridden or disabling
Dysphasia, receptive and/or expressive, is graded under Speech impairment in the NEUROLOGY category					
Extrapyramidal/ involuntary movement/ restlessness	None	Mild involuntary movements not interfering with function	Moderate involuntary movements interfering with function, but not interfering with activities of daily living	Severe involuntary movements or torticollis interfering with activities of daily living	Bedridden or disabling
Hallucinations	Normal	—	—	Present	Toxic psychosis
Headache is graded in the PAIN category					

Insomnia	Normal	Occasional difficulty sleeping not interfering with function	Difficulty sleeping interfering with function, but not interfering with activities of daily living	Frequent difficulty sleeping, interfering with activities of daily living	—

Note: this adverse event is graded when insomnia is related to treatment. If pain or other symptoms interfere with sleep do not grade as insomnia

Irritability (children <3 years of age)	Normal	Mild; easily consolable	Moderate; requiring increased attention	Severe; inconsolable	—
Leucoencephalopathy associated radiological findings	None	Mild increase in SAS (subarachnoid space); and/or mild ventriculomegaly; and/or small (± multiple) focal T2 hyperintensities. Involving periventricular white matter or <1/3 of susceptible areas of cerebrum	Moderate increase in SAS; and/or moderate ventriculomegaly; and/or focal T2 hyperintensities or diffuse white matter hyperintensities or diffuse low attenuation (CT); focal white matter necrosis (cystic)	Severe increase in SAS; severe ventriculomegaly; near total white matter T_2 hyperintensities or diffuse low attenuation (CT); diffuse white matter necrosis (magnetic resonance imaging, MRI)
Memory loss	Normal	Memory loss not interfering with function	Memory loss interfering with function, but not interfering with activities of daily living	Memory loss interfering with activities of daily living	Amnesia
Mood alteration—anxiety, agitation	Normal	Mild mood alteration not interfering with function	Moderate mood alteration interfering with function, but not interfering with activities of daily living	Severe mood alteration interfering with activities of daily living	Suicidal ideation or danger to self

Adverse event	Grade				
	0	1	2	3	4
Mood alteration—depression	Normal	Mild mood alteration not interfering with function	Moderate mood alteration interfering with function, but not interfering with activities of daily living	Severe mood alteration interfering with activities of daily living	Suicidal ideation or danger to self
Mood alteration—euphoria	Normal	Mild mood alteration not interfering with function	Moderate mood alteration interfering with function, but not interfering with activities of daily living	Severe mood alteration interfering with activities of daily living	Danger to self
Neuropathic pain is graded in the PAIN category					
Neuropathy—cranial	Absent	—	Present, not interfering with activities of daily living	Present, interfering with activities of daily living	Life-threatening, disabling
Neuropathy—motor	Normal	Subjective weakness but no objective findings	Mild objective weakness interfering with function, but not interfering with activities of daily living	Objective weakness interfering with activities of daily living	Paralysis
Neuropathy—sensory	Normal	Loss of deep tendon reflexes or paraesthesia (including tingling) but not interfering with function	Objective sensory loss or paraesthesia (including tingling), interfering with function, but not interfering with activities of daily living	Sensory loss or paresthesia interfering with activities of daily living	Permanent sensory loss that interferes with function
Nystagmus	Absent	Present	—	—	
Also consider Vision—double vision					Toxic psychosis

	Normal	Change, but not disruptive to patient or family	Disruptive to patient or family	Disruptive to patient and family; requiring mental health intervention	Harmful to others or self; requiring hospitalization
Personality/ behavioural	Normal	Change, but not disruptive to patient or family	Disruptive to patient or family	Disruptive to patient and family; requiring mental health intervention	Harmful to others or self; requiring hospitalization
Pyramidal tract dysfunction (e.g. tone, hyperreflexia, positive Babinski, fine motor coordination)	Normal	Asymptomatic with abnormality on physical examination	Symptomatic or interfering with function but not interfering with activities of daily living	Interfering with activities of daily living	Bedridden or disabling; paralysis
Seizure(s)	None	—	Seizure(s) self-limited and consciousness is preserved	Seizure(s) in which consciousness is altered	Seizures of any type that are prolonged, repetitive, or difficult to control (e.g. status epilepticus, intractable epilepsy)
Speech impairment (e.g. dysphasia or aphasia)	Normal	—	Awareness of receptive or expressive dysphasia, not impairing ability to communicate	Receptive or expressive dysphasia, impairing ability to communicate	Inability to communicate
Syncope (fainting)	Absent	—	—	Present	—
Also consider CARDIOVASCULAR (ARRHYTHMIA), Vasovagal episode, CNS cerebrovascular ischaemia					
Tremor	None	Mild and brief or intermittent but not interfering with function	Moderate tremor interfering with function, but not interfering with activities of daily living	Severe tremor interfering with activities of daily living	—

Adverse event	Grade				
	0	1	2	3	4
Vertigo	None	Not interfering with function	Interfering with function, but not interfering with activities of daily living	Interfering with activities of daily living	Bedridden or disabling
Neurology – Other (specify, ___)	None	Mild	Moderate	Severe	Life-threatening or disabling
OCULAR/VISUAL					
Cataract	None	Asymptomatic	Symptomatic, partial visual loss	Symptomatic, visual loss requiring treatment or interfering with function	—
Conjunctivitis	None	Abnormal ophthalmological changes, but asymptomatic or symptomatic without visual impairment (i.e. pain and irritation)	Symptomatic and interfering with function, but not interfering with activities of daily living	Symptomatic and interfering with activities of daily living	—
Dry eye	Normal	Mild, not requiring treatment	Moderate or requiring artificial tears	—	—
Glaucoma	None	Increase in intraocular pressure but no visual loss	Increase in intraocular pressure with retinal changes	Visual impairment	Unilateral or bilateral loss of vision (blindness)
Keratitis (corneal inflammation/corneal ulceration)	None	Abnormal ophthalmological changes but asymptomatic or symptomatic without visual impairment (i.e. pain and irritation)	Symptomatic and interfering with function, but not interfering with activities of daily living	Symptomatic and interfering with activities of daily living	Unilateral or bilaterall loss of vision (blindness)

Tearing (watery eyes)	None	Mild: not interfering with function	Moderate: interfering with function, but not interfering with activities of daily living	Interfering with activities of daily living	—
Vision—blurred vision	Normal	—	Symptomatic and interfering with function, but not interfering with activities of daily living	Symptomatic and interfering with activities of daily living	—
Vision—double vision (diplopia)	Normal	—	Symptomatic and interfering with function, but not interfering with activities of daily living	Symptomatic and interfering with activities of daily living	—
Vision—flashing lights/floaters	Normal	Mild, not interfering with function	Symptomatic and interfering with function, but not interfering with activities of daily living	Symptomatic and interfering with activities of daily living	—
Vision—night blindness (nyctalopia)	Normal	Abnormal electro-retinography but asymptomatic	Symptomatic and interfering with function, but not interfering with activities of daily living	Symptomatic and interfering with activities of daily living	—
Vision—photophobia	Normal	—	Symptomatic and interfering with function, but not interfering with activities of daily living	Symptomatic and interfering with activities of daily living	—

Adverse event	Grade				
	0	1	2	3	4
Ocular/Visual – Other (specify, ___)	Normal	Mild	Moderate	Severe	Unilateral or bilateral loss of vision
PAIN					
Abdominal pain or cramping	None	Mild pain not interfering with function	Moderate pain: pain or analgesics interfering with function, but not interfering with activities of daily living	Severe pain: pain or analgesics severely interfering with activities of daily living	Disabling
Arthralgia (joint pain)	None	Mild pain not interfering with function	Moderate pain: pain or analgesics interfering with function, but not interfering with activities of daily living	Severe pain: pain or analgesics severely interfering with activities of daily living	Disabling
Arthritis (joint pain with clinical signs of inflammation) is graded in the MUSCULOSKELETAL category					
Bone pain	None	Mild pain not interfering with function	Moderate pain: pain or analgesics interfering with function, but not interfering with activities of daily living	Severe pain: pain or analgesics severely interfering with activities of daily living	Disabling

	None	Mild pain not interfering with function	Moderate pain: pain or analgesics interfering with function, but not interfering with activities of daily living	Severe pain: pain or analgesics severely interfering with activities of daily living	Disabling
Chest pain (non-cardiac and non-pleuritic)	None	Mild pain not interfering with function	Moderate pain: pain or analgesics interfering with function, but not interfering with activities of daily living	Severe pain: pain or analgesics severely interfering with activities of daily living	Disabling
Dysmenorrhoea	None	Mild pain not interfering with function	Moderate pain: pain or analgesics interfering with function, but not interfering with activities of daily living	Severe pain: pain or analgesics severely interfering with activities of daily living	Disabling
Dyspareunia	None	Mild pain not interfering with function	Moderate pain interfering with sexual activity	Severe pain preventing sexual activity	—
Dysuria is graded in the RENAL/GENITOURINARY category					
Earache (otalgia)	None	Mild pain not interfering with function	Moderate pain: pain or analgesics interfering with function, but not interfering with activities of daily living	Severe pain: pain or analgesics severely interfering with activities of daily living	Disabling
Headache	None	Mild pain not interfering with function	Moderate pain: pain or analgesics interfering with function, but not interfering with activities of daily living	Severe pain: pain or analgesics severely interfering with activities of daily living	Disabling

Adverse event	Grade				
	0	1	2	3	4
Hepatic pain	None	Mild pain not interfering with function	Moderate pain; pain or analgesics interfering with function, but not interfering with activities of daily living	Severe pain; pain or analgesics severely interfering with activities of daily living	Disabling
Myalgia (muscle pain)	None	Mild pain not interfering with function	Moderate pain; pain or analgesics interfering with function, but not interfering with activities of daily living	Severe pain; pain or analgesics severely interfering with activities of daily living	Disabling
Neuropathic pain (e.g. jaw pain, neurological pain, phantom limb pain, post-infectious neuralgia, or painful neuropathies)	None	Mild pain not interfering with function	Moderate pain; pain or analgesics interfering with function, but not interfering with activities of daily living	Severe pain; pain or analgesics severely interfering with activities of daily living	Disabling
Pain due to radiation	None	Mild pain not interfering with function	Moderate pain; pain or analgesics interfering with function, but not interfering with activities of daily living	Severe pain; pain or analgesics severely interfering with activities of daily living	Disabling
Pelvic pain	None	Mild pain not interfering with function	Moderate pain; pain or analgesics interfering with function, but not interfering with activities of daily living	Severe pain; pain or analgesics severely interfering with activities of daily living	Disabling

Pleuritic pain	None	Mild pain not interfering with function	Moderate pain; pain or analgesics interfering with function, but not interfering with activities of daily living	Severe pain; pain or analgesics severely interfering with activities of daily living	Disabling
Rectal or perirectal pain (proctalgia)	None	Mild pain not interfering with function	Moderate pain; pain or analgesics interfering with function, but not interfering with activities of daily living	Severe pain; pain or analgesics severely interfering with activities of daily living	Disabling
Tumour pain (onset or exacerbation of tumor pain due to treatment)	None	Mild pain not interfering with function	Moderate pain; pain or analgesics interfering with function, but not interfering with activities of daily living	Severe pain; pain or analgesics severely interfering with activities of daily living	Disabling
Tumour flare is graded in the SYNDROME category					
Pain – Other (specify,_____)	None	Mild	Moderate	Severe	Disabling
PULMONARY					
Adult respiratory distress syndrome (ARDS)	Absent	—	—	—	Present
Apnoea	None	—	—	Present	Requiring intubation

Adverse event	Grade				
	0	1	2	3	4
Carbon monoxide diffusion capacity (DL_{CO})	≥90% of pre-treatment or normal value	≥75–<90% of pre-treatment or normal value	≥50–<75% of pre-treatment or normal value	≥25–<50% of pre-treatment or normal value	<25% of pre-treatment or normal value
Cough	Absent	Mild, relieved by non-prescription medication	Requiring narcotic antitussive	Severe cough or coughing spasms, poorly controlled or unresponsive to treatment	—
Dyspnoea (shortness of breath)	Normal	—	Dyspnoea on exertion	Dyspnoea at normal level of activity	Dyspnoea at rest or requiring ventilator support
Forced expiratory volume in 1 s (FEV_1)	≥90% of pre-treatment or normal value	≥75–<90% of pre-treatment or normal value	≥50–<75% of pre-treatment or normal value	≥25–<50% of pre-treatment or normal value	<25% of pre-treatment or normal value
Hiccoughs (hiccups, singultus)	None	Mild, not requiring treatment	Moderate, requiring treatment	Severe, prolonged, and refractory to treatment	—
Hypoxia	Normal	—	Decreased O_2 saturation with exercise	Decreased O_2 saturation at rest, requiring supplemental oxygen	Decreased O_2 saturation, requiring pressure support (CPAP) or assisted ventilation
Pleural effusion (non-malignant)	None	Asymptomatic and not requiring treatment	Symptomatic, requiring diuretics	Symptomatic, requiring O_2 or therapeutic thoracentesis	Life-threatening (e.g requiring intubation)

Pleuritic pain is graded in the PAIN category

	None/Normal	Mild	Moderate	Severe	Life-threatening
Pneumonitis/pulmonary infiltrates	None	Radiographic changes but asymptomatic or symptoms not requiring steroids	Radiographic changes and requiring steroids or diuretics	Radiographic changes and requiring oxygen	Radiographic changes and requiring assisted ventilation
Pneumothorax	None	No intervention required	Chest tube required	Sclerosis or surgery required	Life-threatening
Pulmonary embolism is graded as Thrombosis/embolism in the CARDIOVASCULAR (GENERAL) category					
Pulmonary fibrosis	None	Radiographic changes, but asymptomatic or symptoms not requiring steroids	Requiring steroids or diuretics	Requiring oxygen	Requiring assisted ventilation
Note: radiation-related pulmonary fibrosis is graded in the RTOG/EORTC late radiation morbidity scoring scheme—lung (see later section of this appendix)					
Voice changes/stridor/larynx (e.g. hoarseness, loss of voice, laryngitis)	Normal	Mild or intermittent hoarseness	Persistent hoarseness, but able to vocalize; may have mild to moderate edema	Whispered speech, not able to vocalize; may have marked oedema	Marked dyspnoea/stridor requiring tracheostomy or intubation
Notes: cough from radiation is graded as cough in the PULMONARY category; radiation-related haemoptysis from larynx/pharynx is graded as grade 4 mucositis due to radiation in the GASTROINTESTINAL category; radiation-related haemoptysis from the thoracic cavity is graded as grade 4 Haemoptysis in the HAEMORRHAGE category					
Pulmonary – Other (specify, _____)	None	Mild	Moderate	Severe	Life-threatening or disabling

RENAL/GENITOURINARY

Adverse event	Grade			
	0	1	2	3	4
Bladder spasms	Absent	Mild symptoms, not requiring intervention	Symptoms requiring antispasmodic	Severe symptoms requiring narcotic	—
Creatinine	WNL	>ULN–1.5	ULN >1.5–3.0 × ULN	>3.0–6.0 × ULN	>6.0 × ULN
Note: adjust to age-appropriate levels for paediatric patients					
Dysuria (painful urination)	None	Mild symptoms requiring no intervention	Symptoms relieved with therapy	Symptoms not relieved despite therapy	—
Fistula or GU fistula (e.g. vaginal, vesicovaginal)	None	—	—	Requiring intervention	Requiring surgery
Haemoglobinuria	—	Present	—	—	—
Haematuria (in the absence of vaginal bleeding) is graded in the HAEMORRHAGE category					
Incontinence	None	With coughing, sneezing, etc.	Spontaneous, some control	No control (in the absence of fistula)	—
Operative injury to bladder and/or ureter	None	—	Injury of bladder with primary repair	Sepsis, fistula, or obstruction requiring secondary surgery; loss of one kidney; injury requiring anastomosis or re-implantation	Septic obstruction of both kidneys or vesicovaginal fistula requiring diversion

Proteinuria	Normal or <0.15 g/24 h	1+ or 0.15–1.0 g/24 h	2+ to 3+ or 1.0–3.5 g/24 h	4+ or >3.5 g/24 h	Nephrotic syndrome

Note: if there is an inconsistency between absolute value and dip stick reading, use the absolute value for grading

Renal failure	None	—	—	Requiring dialysis, but reversible	Requiring dialysis and irreversible
Ureteral obstruction	None	Unilateral, not requiring surgery	—	Bilateral, not requiring surgery	Stent, nephrostomy tube, or surgery
Urinary electrolyte wasting (e.g., Fanconi's syndrome, renal tubular acidosis)	None	Asymptomatic, not requiring treatment	Mild, reversible, and manageable with oral replacement	Reversible but requiring IV replacement	Irreversible, requiring continued replacement

Also consider Acidosis, Bicarbonate, Hypocalcaemia, Hypophosphataemia

Urinary frequency/urgency	Normal	Increase in frequency or nocturia up to 2 × normal	Increase >2 × normal but <hourly	Hourly or more with urgency, or requiring catheter	—
Urinary retention	Normal	Hesitancy or dribbling, but no significant residual urine; retention occurring during the immediate post-operative period	Hesitancy requiring medication or occasional in/out catheterization (<4× per week), or operative bladder atony requiring indwelling catheter beyond immediate post-operative period but for <6 weeks	Requiring frequent in/out catheterization (≥4× per week) or urological intervention (e.g. transurethral resection o0f the prostate (TURP), suprapubic tube, urethrotomy)	Bladder rupture

Adverse event	Grade				
	0	1	2	3	4
Urine colour change (not related to other dietary or physiological cause, e.g. bilirubin, concentrated urine, haematuria)	Normal	Asymptomatic, change in urine color	—	—	—
Vaginal bleeding is graded in the HAEMORRHAGE category					
Vaginitis (not due to infection)	None	Mild, not requiring treatment	Moderate, relieved with treatment	Severe, not relieved with treatment, or ulceration not requiring surgery	Ulceration requiring surgery
Renal/genitourinary – Other (specify,____)	None	Mild	Moderate	Severe	Life-threatening or disabling

SECONDARY MALIGNANCY

Adverse event	Grade				
	0	1	2	3	4
Secondary malignancy – Other (specify type,____) excludes metastasis from initial primary	None	—	—	—	Present

SEXUAL/REPRODUCTIVE FUNCTION

Dyspareunia is graded in the PAIN category

Dysmenorrhoea is graded in the PAIN category

	Normal/None	Mild	Moderate	Severe	Disabling
Erectile impotence	Normal	Mild (erections impaired but satisfactory)	Moderate (erections impaired, unsatisfactory for intercourse)	No erections	—
Female sterility	Normal	—	—	Sterile	—

Feminization of male is graded in the ENDOCRINE category

	Normal/None	Mild	Moderate	Severe	Disabling
Irregular menses (change from baseline)	Normal	Occasionally irregular or lengthened interval, but continuing menstrual cycles	Very irregular, but continuing menstrual cycles	Persistent amenorrhoea	—
Libido	Normal	Decrease in interest	Severe loss of interest	—	—
Male infertility	—	—	Oligospermia (low sperm count)	Azoospermia (no sperm)	—

Masculinization of female is graded in the ENDOCRINE category

	Normal/None	Mild	Moderate	Severe	Disabling
Vaginal dryness	Normal	Mild	Requiring treatment and/or interfering with sexual function, dyspareunia	—	—
Sexual/reproductive function – Other (specify,_____)	None	Mild	Moderate	Severe	Disabling

	Grade			
Adverse event	**0**	**1**	**2**	**3**	**4**

SYNDROMES (not included in previous categories)

Acute vascular leak syndrome is graded in the CARDIOVASCULAR (GENERAL) category

ARDS (adult respiratory distress syndrome) is graded in the PULMONARY category

Autoimmune reactions are graded in the ALLERGY/IMMUNOLOGY category

DIC (disseminated intravascular coagulation) is graded in the COAGULATION category

Fanconi's syndrome is graded as Urinary electrolyte wasting in the RENAL/GENITOURINARY category

Renal tubular acidosis is graded as Urinary electrolyte wasting in the RENAL/GENITOURINARY category

Stevens–Johnson syndrome (erythema multiforme) is graded in the DERMATOLOGY/SKIN category

SIADH (syndrome of inappropriate antidiuretic hormone) is graded in the ENDOCRINE category

Thrombotic microangiopathy (e.g. thrombotic thrombocytopenic purpura/TTP or haemolytic uraemic syndrome/HUS) is graded in the COAGULATION category

	None				Disabling
Tumour flare	None	Mild pain not interfering with function	Moderate pain; pain or analgesics interfering with function, but not interfering with activities of daily living	Severe pain; pain or analgesics interfering with function and interfering with activities of daily living	Disabling

Also consider Hypercalcaemia

Note: Tumour flare is characterized by a constellation of symptoms and signs in direct relation to initiation of therapy (e.g. anti-oestrogens/androgens or additional hormones). The symptoms/signs include tumour pain, inflammation of visible tumour, hypercalcaemia, diffuse bone pain, and other electrolyte disturbances

Tumour lysis syndrome	Absent	—	—	Present	—

Also consider Hyperkalaemia, Creatinine

Urinary electrolyte wasting (e.g. Fanconi's syndrome, renal tubular acidosis) is graded in the RENAL/GENITOURINARY category

	None	Mild	Moderate	Severe	Life-threatening or disabling
Syndromes –Other (specify,_____)	None	Mild	Moderate	Severe	Life-threatening or disabling

Adverse event module

To be implemented at the request of the study sponsor or principal investigator in the protocol or by protocol amendment when more detailed information is considered pertinent.

Adverse event:	Date of treatment:	Course number:
Date of onset:		Grade at onset:
Date of first change in grade:		Grade:
Date of next change in grade:		Grade:
Date of next change in grade:		Grade:
Date of next change in grade:		Grade:
Date of next change in grade:		Grade:
Date of next change in grade:		Grade:
Did adverse event resolve? If so, date of resolution of adverse event:	Yes_____ No_____	
Date of last observation (if prior to recovery):		
Reason(s) observations stopped (if prior to recovery):		
Was patient retreated?	Yes_____ No_____	
If yes, was treatment delayed for recovery? Date of next treatment?	Yes_____ No_____	
Dose reduced for next treatment?	Yes_____ No_____	
Additional comments:		

If module is being activated for new adverse event nor currently in CTC, please provide definitions for adverse event grading:

Grade 0 =

Grade 1 =

Grade 2 =

Grade 3 =

Grade 4 =

Infection module

To be implemented at the request of the study sponsor or principal investigator in the protocol or by protocol amendment when more detailed information is considered pertinent.

1. Use the common toxicity criteria definitions to grade the severity of the infection
2. Specify type of infection from the following (CHOOSE ONE):
   BACTERIAL   FUNGAL   PROTOZOAL   VIRAL   UNKNOWN

3. Specify site of infection from the following (CHOOSE ALL THAT APPLY):

   BLOOD CULTURE POSITIVE

   BONE INFECTION

   CATHETER (intravenous)

   CATHETER (intravenous), tunnel infection

   CENTRAL NERVOUS SYSTEM INFECTION

   EAR INFECTION

   EYE INFECTION

   GASTROINTESTINAL INFECTION

   ORAL INFECTION

   PNEUMONIA

   SKIN INFECTION

   UPPER RESPIRATORY INFECTION

   URINARY TRACT INFECTION

   VAGINAL INFECTION

   INFECTION, not otherwise specified (Specify site: _____)

4. Specify organism, if known: _____.
5. Prophylactic antibiotic, antifungal, or antiviral therapy administration
   Yes _____   No _____

   If prophylaxis was given prior to infection, please specify below:

   Antibiotic prophylaxis _____

   Antifungal prophylaxis _____

   Antiviral prophylaxis _____

   Other prophylaxis _____

Performance status scales/scores

PERFORMANCE STATUS CRITERIA

Karnofsky and Lansky performance scores are intended to be multiples of 10

ECOG (Zubrod)		Karnofsky		Lansky*	
Score	Description	Score	Description	Score	Description
0	Fully active, able to carry on all pre-disease performance without restriction	100	Normal, no complaints, no evidence of disease	100	Fully active, normal
		90	Able to carry on normal activity; minor signs or symptoms of disease	90	Minor restrictions in physically strenuous activity
1	Restricted in physically strenuous activity but ambulatory and able to carry out work of a light or sedentary nature, e.g. light housework, office work	80	Normal activity with effort; some signs or symptoms of disease	80	Active, but tires more quickly
		70	Cares for self, unable to carry on normal activity or do active work	70	Both greater restriction of and less time spent in play activity

2	Ambulatory and capable of all self-care but unable to carry out any work activities. Up and about more than 50% of waking hours	60	Requires occasional assistance, but is able to care for most of his/her needs	60	Up and around, but minimal active play; keeps busy with quieter activities
		50	Requires considerable assistance and frequent medical care	50	Gets dressed, but lies around much of the day; no active play; able to participate in all quiet play and activities
3	Capable of only limited self-care, confined to bed or chair more than 50% of waking hours	40	Disabled, requires special care and assistance	40	Mostly in bed; participates in quiet activities
		30	Severely disabled, hospitalization indicated. Death not imminent	30	In bed; needs assistance even for quiet play
4	Completely disabled. Cannot carry on any self-care. Totally confined to bed or chair	20	Very sick, hospitalization indicated. Death not imminent	20	Often sleeping; play entirely limited to very passive activities
		10	Moribund, fatal processes progressing rapidly	10	No play; does not get out of bed

*The conversion of the Lansky to Eastern Cooperative Oncology Group (ECOG) scales is intended for National Cancer Institute (NCI) reporting purposes only.

RTOG: Radiation Therapy Oncology Group.

RTOG/EORTC late radiation morbidity scoring scheme

Use for adverse event occurring more than 90 days after radiation therapy

Adverse event	Grade				
	0	1	2	3	4
Bladder – late RT morbidity scoring	No change from baseline	Slight epithelial atrophy/ minor telangiectasia (microscopic haematuria)	Moderate frequency/ generalized telangiectasia/ intermittent macroscopic haematuria	Severe frequency and dysuria/severe generalized telangiectasia (often with petechiae); frequent haematuria; reduction in bladder capacity (<150 ml)	Necrosis/contracted bladder (capacity <100 ml/ severe haemorrhagic cystitis
Bone – late RT morbidity scoring	No change from baseline	Asymptomatic; no growth retardation; reduced bone density	Moderate pain or tenderness; growth retardation; irregular bone sclerosis	Severe pain or tenderness; complete arrest of bone growth; dense bone sclerosis	Necrosis/spontaneous fracture
Brain – late RT morbidity scoring	No change from baseline	Mild headache; slight lethargy	Moderate headache; great lethargy	Severe headaches; severe CNS dysfunction (partial loss of power or dyskinesia)	Seizures or paralysis; coma
Oesophagus – late RT morbidity scoring	No change from baseline	Mild fibrosis; slight difficulty in swallowing solids; no pain on swallowing	Unable to take solid food normally; swallowing semi-solid food; dilation may be indicated	Severe fibrosis; able to swallow only liquids; may have pain on swallowing; dilation required	Necrosis/perforation; fistula

Eye – late RT morbidity scoring	No change from baseline	Asymptomatic cataract; minor corneal ulceration or keratitis	Symptomatic cataract; moderate corneal ulceration; minor retinopathy or glaucoma	Severe keratitis; severe retinopathy or detachment; severe glaucoma	Panophthalmitis; blindness
Heart – late RT morbidity scoring	No change from baseline	Asymptomatic or mild symptoms; transient T wave inversion and ST changes; sinus tachycardia >110 (at rest)	Moderate angina on effort; mild pericarditis; normal heart size; persistent abnormal T wave and ST changes; low QRS	Severe angina; pericardial effusion; constrictive pericarditis; moderate heart failure; cardiac enlargement; ECG abnormalities	Tamponade/severe heart failure/severe constrictive pericarditis
Joint – late RT morbidity scoring	No change from baseline	Mild joint stiffness; slight limitation of movement	Moderate stiffness; intermittent or moderate joint pain; moderate limitation of movement	Severe joint stiffness; pain with severe limitation of movement	Necrosis/complete fixation
	No change from baseline	Transient albuminuria; no hypertension; mild impairment of renal function; urea 25–35 mg%; creatinine 1.5–2.0 mg%; creatinine clearance >75%	Persistent moderate albuminuria (2+); mild hypertension; no related anaemia; moderate impairment of renal function; urea >36–60 mg%; creatinine clearance >50–74%	Severe albuminuria; severe hypertension; persistent anaemia (<10 g%); severe renal failure; urea >60 mg%; creatinine >4 mg%; creatinine clearance <50%	Malignant hypertension; uraemic coma/urea >100%
Larynx – late RT morbidity scoring	No change from baseline	Hoarseness; slight arytenoid oedema	Moderate arytenoid oedema; chondritis	Severe oedema; severe chondritis	Necrosis

Adverse event	Grade				
	0	1	2	3	4
Liver – late RT morbidity scoring	No change from baseline	Mild lassitude; nausea; dyspepsia; slightly abnormal liver function	Moderate symptoms; some abnormal liver function tests; serum albumin normal	Disabling hepatic insufficiency; liver function tests grossly abnormal; low albumin; oedema or ascites	Necrosis/hepatic coma or encephalopathy
Lung – late RT morbidity scoring	No change from baseline	Asymptomatic or mild symptoms (dry cough); slight radiographic appearances	Moderate symptomatic fibrosis or pneumonitis (severe cough); low grade fever; patchy radiographic appearances	Severe symptomatic fibrosis or pneumonitis; dense radiographic changes	Severe respiratory insufficiency/continuous O₂/assisted ventilation
Mucous membrane – late RT morbidity scoring	No change from baseline	Slight atrophy and dryness	Moderate atrophy and telangiectasia; little mucus	Marked atrophy with complete dryness; severe telangiectasia	Ulceration
Salivary glands – late RT morbidity scoring	No change from baseline	Slight dryness of mouth; good response on stimulation	Moderate dryness of mouth; poor response on stimulation	Complete dryness of mouth; no response on stimulation	Fibrosis
Skin – late RT morbidity scoring	No change from baseline	Slight atrophy; pigmentation change; some hair loss	Patchy atrophy; moderate telangiectasia; total hair loss	Marked atrophy; gross telangiectasia	Ulceration

Small/large intestine – late RT morbidity scoring	No change from baseline	Mild diarrhoea; mild cramping; bowel movement >5× daily; slight rectal discharge or bleeding	Moderate diarrhoea and colic; bowel movement >5× daily; excessive rectal mucus or intermittent bleeding	Obstruction or bleeding, requiring surgery	Necrosis/perforation fistula
Spinal cord – late RT morbidity scoring	No change from baseline	Mild Lhermitte's syndrome	Severe Lhermitte's syndrome	Objective neurological findings at or below cord level treatment	Mono-, para-, quadriplegia
Subcutaneous tissue – late RT morbidity scoring	No change from baseline	Slight induration (fibrosis) and loss of subcutaneous fat	Moderate fibrosis but asymptomatic; slight field contracture; <10% linear reduction	Severe induration and loss of subcutaneous tissue; field contracture >10% linear measurement	Necrosis
Radiation – Other (specify, _____)	None	Mild	Moderate	Severe	Life-threatening or disabling

Bone marrow transplantation (BMT): specific adverse events

Summary of BMT – specific adverse events that may be used **if specified by the protocol**. These differ from the standard CTC and may be more relevant to the transplant setting. They are listed here for the convenience of investigators writing transplant protocols. They are also included in the CTC document

Adverse event	Grade				
	0	1	2	3	4
Bilirubin associated with graft versus host disease for BMT studies	Normal	≥2–<3 mg/100 ml	≥3–<6 mg/100 ml	≥6–<15 mg/100 ml	≥15 mg/100 ml
Diarrhoea associated with graft versus host disease (GVHD) for BMT studies	None	>500–≤1000 ml of diarrhoea/day	>1000–≤1500 ml of diarrhoea/day	>1500 ml of diarrhoea/day	Severe abdominal pain with or without ileus
Diarrhoea for paediatric BMT studies		*>5–≤10 ml/kg of diarrhoea/day*	*>10–≤15 ml/kg of diarrhoea/day*	*>15 ml/kg of diarrhoea/day*	—
Hepatic enlargement	Absent	—	—	Present	—
Leucocytes (total white cell count (WCC) for BMT studies	Within normal limits (WNL)	≥2.0–<3.0 × 10⁹/l ≥2000–<3000/mm³	≥1.0–<2.0 × 10⁹/l ≥1000–<2000/mm³	≥0.5–<1.0 × 10⁹/l ≥500–<1000/mm³	<0.5 × 10⁹/l <500/mm³
Leucocytes (total WBC) for paediatric BMT studies (using age, race, and sex normal values)	≥75–<100% lower limit of normal (LLN)	≥50–<75% LLN	≥25–50% LLN	<25% LLN	

Lymphopenia for paediatric BMT studies (using age, race, and sex normal values)	mm³	≥75-<100% LLN	≥50-<75%LLN	≥25-<50% LLN	<25% LLN
Neutrophils/granulocytes (absolute neutrophil count (ANC)/absolute granulocyte count (AGC) for BMT studies	WNL	≥1.0-<1.5 × 10⁹/l ≥1000-<1500/mm³	≥0.5-<1.0 × 10⁹/l ≥500-<1000/mm³	≥0.1-<0.5 × 10⁹/l ≥100-<500/mm³	<0.1 × 10⁹/l <100/mm³
Platelets for BMT studies	WNL	≥50.0-<75.0 × 10⁹/l ≥50 000-<75 000/mm³	≥20.0-<50.0 × 10⁹/l ≥20 000-<50 000/mm³	≥10.0-<20.0 × 10⁹/l ≥10 000-<20 000/mm³	<10.0 × 10⁹/l <10 000/mm³
Rash/dermatitis associated with high-dose chemotherapy or BMT studies	None	Faint erythema or dry desquamation	Moderate to brisk erythema or a patchy moist desquamation, mostly confined to skin folds and creases; moderate oedema	Confluent moist desquamation, ≥1.5 cm diameter, not confined to skin folds; pitting oedema	Skin necrosis or ulceration of full-thickness dermis; may include spontaneous bleeding not induced by minor trauma or abrasion
Rash/desquamation associated with graft versus host disease (GVHD) for BMT studies	None	Macular or papular eruption or erythema covering <25% of body surface area without associated symptoms	Macular or papular eruption or erythema with pruritus or other associated symptoms covering ≥25-<50% of body surface or localized desquamation or other lesions covering ≥25-<50% of body surface area	Symptomatic generalized erythroderma or symptomatic macular, papular or vesicular eruption, with bullous formation, or desquamation covering ≥50% of body surface area	Generalized exfoliative dermatitis or ulcerative dermatitis or bullous formation

Adverse event	Grade				
	0	1	2	3	4
Stomatitis/pharyngitis (oral/pharyngeal mucositis) for BMT studies	None	Painless ulcers, erythema, or mild soreness in the absence of lesions	Painful erythema, oedema, or ulcers but can swallow	Painful erythema, oedema, or ulcers preventing swallowing or requiring hydration or parenteral (or enteral) nutritional support	Severe ulceration requiring prophylactic intubation or resulting in documented aspiration pneumonia
Transfusion: platelets for BMT studies	None	1 platelet transfusion in 24 h	2 platelet transfusions in 24 h	≥3 platelet transfusions In 24 h	Platelet transfusions and other measures required to improve platelet increment; platelet transfusion refractoriness associated with life-threatening bleeding, (e.g. human leucocyte antigen (HLA) or cross-matched Platelet (transfusions)
Transfusion: packed red blood cells (pRBCs) for BMT studies	None	≤2 u pRBC in 24h elective or planned	3 u pRBC in 24 h elective or planned	≥ 4 u pRBC in 24 h	Haemorrhage or haemolysis associated with life-threatening anaemia; medical intervention required to improve haemoglobin

Transfusion: pRBCs for paediatric BMT studies	None	≤15 ml/kg in 24 h elective or planned	>15–≤30 ml/kg in 24 h elective or planned	>30 ml/kg in 24 h	Haemorrhage or haemolysis associated with life-threatening anaemia; medical intervention required to improve haemoglobin
Thrombotic microangiopathy (e.g. thrombotic thrombocytopenic purpura/TTP or haemolytic-uraemic syndrome/HUS) for BMT studies	—	Evidence of RBC destruction (schistocytosis) without clinical consequences	Evidence of RBC destruction with elevated creatinine (≤3 × upper limit of normal (ULN))	Evidence of RBC destruction with creatinine (>3 × ULN) not requiring dialysis	Evidence of RBC destruction with renal failure requiring dialysis and/or encephalopathy
Weight gain associated with veno-occlusive disease (VOD) for BMT studies	<2%	≥2–<5%	≥5–<10%	≥10% or as ascites	≥10% or fluid retention resulting in pulmonary failure

Bone marrow transplantation: complex/multicomponent events

Adverse event	Grade			
	0	1	2	3	4

Note: the grading of complex/multicomponent events in bone marrow transplant will be defined in the protocol. The grading scale must use the CTC criteria for grading the specific component events (adverse events)

Adverse event	0	1	2	3	4
Failure to engraft	Absent	Mild	Moderate	Severe	Life-threatening

Also consider Haemoglobin, Neutrophils/granulocytes (ANC/AGC), Neutrophils/granulocytes (ANC/AGC) for BMT studies, if specified in the protocol, Platelets, Platelets for BMT studies, if specified in the protocol

Graft versus host disease	Absent	Mild	Moderate	Severe	Life-threatening

Also consider Fatigue, Rash/desquamation, Rash/desquamation associated with graft versus host disease (GVHD) for BMT studies, if specified in the protocol, Diarrhoea for patients without colostomy, Diarrhoea for patients with colostomy, Diarrhoea associated with GVHD for BMT studies, if specified in the protocol, Diarrhoea for pediatric BMT studies, if specified in the protocol, Bilirubin, Bilirubin associated with GVHD for BMT studies, if specified in the protocol

Stem cell infusion complications	Absent	Mild	Moderate	Severe	Life-threatening

Also consider Allergic reaction/hypersensitivity, Conduction abnormality/Atrioventricular heart block, Nodal/Junctional arrhythmia/dysrhythmia, Prolonged QTc interval (QTc >0.48 s), Sinus bradycardia, Sinus tachycardia, Supraventricular arrhythmias (SVT/atrial fibrillation/flutter), Vasovagal episode, Ventricular arrhythmia (premature ventricular contractions (PVCs)/bigemin/trigemin/ventricular tachycardia), Cardiovascular/Arrhythmia – Other (specify,_____), Hypertension, Hypotension, Fever (in the absence of neutropenia, where neutropenia is defined as AGC <1.0 × 10^9/l), Rigors/chills, Sweating (diaphoresis), Rash/desquamation, Rash/desquamation associated with GVHD for BMT studies, if specified in the protocol, Urticaria (hives, welts, wheals), Diarrhoea for patients without colostomy, Diarrhoea for patients with colostomy, Diarrhoea associated with GVHD for BMT studies, if specified in the protocol, Diarrhoea for pediatric BMT studies, if specified in the protocol, Nausea, Vomiting, Haemorrhage/bleeding with grade 3 or 4 thrombocytopenia, Haemorrhage/bleeding without grade 3 or 4 thrombocytopenia, Haemoptysis, Alkaline phosphatase, Bilirubin, Bilirubin associated with GVHD for BMT studies, if specified in the protocol, gamma-glutamyl transferase (GGT), serum glutamic oxaloacetic transaminase (SGOT) (aspartate aminotransferase, AST), serum glutamic pyruvic transaminase (SGPT) (alanine aminotransferase, ALT), Infection (documented clinically or microbiologically) with grade 3 or 4 neutropenia (ANC <1.0 × 10^9/l), infection without neutropenia, Hyperkalaemia, Hypernatraemia, Hypokalaemia, Depressed level of consciousness, Seizures, Abdominal pain, Headache, Creatinine, haemoglobinuria

	Absent	Mild	Moderate	Severe	Life-threatening
Veno-occlusive disease (VOD)					

Also consider Weight gain associated with VOD for BMT studies, if specified in the protocol, Bilirubin, Bilirubin associated with GVHD for BMT studies, if specified in the protocol, Depressed level of consciousness, Hepatic pain, Renal failure, Hepatic enlargement

Nomogram for determination of body surface area

Nomogram for determination of body surface from height and mass

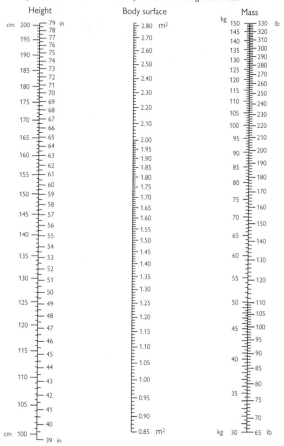

Fig. A2.1 Nomogram for determination of body surface area. Reproduced with permission from Lentner C, ed. *Geigy Scientific Tables*, 8th edn. Basel: Ciba Geigy Ltd, 1981. BNF body surface area calculator can be accessed on http://www.bnf.org/bnf/extra/current/450018.htm

Performance status

Many decisions in the management of patients with malignancy depend on the patients' general well-being. Various scoring systems exist which attempt to quantify this. The two most commonly used are the Karnofsky and the Eastern Cooperative Oncology Group (ECOG) systems.

Karnofsky score

The Karnofsky scoring system is detailed in 📖 Appendix 1, p.812.

Further reading

http://hospicepatients.org/karnofsky.html

Doyle D, Hanks G, Cherny NI, Calman K, eds (2005) Oxford Textbook of Palliative Medicine, 3rd edn. Oxford: Oxford University Press

Karnofsky DA, Burchenal JH (1949) The clinical evaluation of chemotherapeutic agents in cancer In: MacLeod CM, ed. *Evaluation of Chemotherapeutic Agents.* New York: Columbia University Press, p. 196.

ECOG score

0	Fully active. Able to carry on all pre-disease performance without restriction
1	Restricted in physically strenuous activity but ambulatory and able to carry out work of a light or sedentary nature
2	Ambulatory and capable of all self-care but unable to carry out any work activities. Up and about for >50% of waking hours
3	Capable of only limited self-care. Confined to bed or chair for >50% of waking hours
4	Completely disabled. Cannot carry out any self-care. Totally confined to bed or chair
5	Death

Further reading

Onken MM, Creech RH, Tormey DC, *et al.* (1982) Toxicity and response criteria of the Eastern Cooperative Oncology Group. *American Journal of Clinical Oncology* **5**, 649–55.

We credit the Eastern Cooperative Oncology Group, Robert Comis MD, Group Chair.

Support agencies' addresses and websites

- www.adjuvantonline.com – **Adjuvant! Online**: an American website aiming to provide a decision making tool for doctors to assist in weighing up the relative risks and benefits of adjuvant treatment depending on certain patient and tumour variables. Currently has protocols for breast, colon and lung cancers
- www.asco.org – **American Society of Clinical Oncology**
- www.cancerbackup.org.uk – **Cancerbackup**: up-to-date cancer information (including information about treatments), practical advice and support for cancer patients, their families and carers. Cancerbackup has now merged with Macmillan Support and is an approved NHS information partner. Also provides links to useful site-specific websites
- www.cancerresearchuk.org – **Cancer Research UK**
- www.cancerhelp.org.uk – patient information website: part of **Cancer Research UK**
- www.dh.gov.uk/en/Healthcare/NationalServiceFrameworks/Cancer/index.htm – **Department of Health National Health Service Framework for Cancer**
- www.eortc.be – EORTC, the **European Organisation for the Research and Treatment of Cancer**
- www.maggiescentres.org.uk – **Maggie's Cancer Caring Centres**: patient help with information, benefits and travel advice for those affected by cancer, and psychological support. Centres are in limited locations at present but more are planned and online support groups are available
- www.mariecurie.org.uk – **Marie Curie Cancer Care**: charitable organization providing free nursing care to cancer patients and those with terminal illnesses in their own homes
- www.cancer.gov – **National Cancer Institute**: comprehensive cancer information
- http://ctep.cancer.gov/protocolDevelopment/electronic_applications/ctc.htm – **National Cancer Institute (NCI) CTC toxicity scale** version 4.0 (updated May 2009)
- http://ncrndev.org.uk – the **National Cancer Research Network** aims to provide the NHS with an infrastructure to support high-quality cancer clinical studies
- www.ncpc.org.uk – **National Council for Palliative Care**
- www.nice.org.uk – **National Institute for Health and Clinical Excellence**: national guidance on services, interventions and management
- www.rcr.ac.uk – **The Royal College of Radiologists** home-page
- www.teenagecancertrust.org – **Teenage Cancer Trust UK**
- www.statistics.gov.uk/cci/nugget.asp?id=915 – **UK National Cancer Statistics**
- www.winstonswish.org.uk – **Winston's Wish**: leading childhood bereavement charity offering practical support and guidance to families, professionals and anyone concerned about a grieving child.

Index